The Musculoskeletal System in Health and Disease

HARPER & ROW, PUBLISHERS

HAGERSTOWN

Cambridge		*London*
New York		*Mexico City*
Philadelphia		*São Paulo*
San Francisco		*Sydney*

1817

The Musculoskeletal System in Health and Disease

Cornelius Rosse, M.D.
Professor, Department of Biological Structure
University of Washington

D. Kay Clawson, M.D.
Dean, College of Medicine
Professor, (Orthopedic) Surgery
University of Kentucky

with 10 Additional Contributors

Cover illustration reproduced by gracious permission of Her Majesty Queen Elizabeth II

Copyright © 1980, by Harper & Row, Publishers

ISBN 0-06-142287-8

Library of Congress Card Number 79-22437

Printed in the United States of America

1   3   5   6   4   2

Library of Congress Cataloging in Publication Data

Main entry under title:

The Musculoskeletal system in health and disease.

Includes index.
1. Musculoskeletal system–Diseases.
2. Musculoskeletal system.   I. Rosse, Cornelius.
II. Clawson, David Kay
RC925.M86   616.7   79-22437
ISBN 0-06-142287-8

Contents

Contributors

Sterling K. Clarren, M.D.
Director, Congenital Defects, Craniofacial Clinic; Children's Orthopedic Hospital and Medical Center; University of Washington; Seattle, Washington

D. Kay Clawson, M.D.
Dean, College of Medicine; Professor, Surgery (Orthopedic); College of Medicine; University of Kentucky, Lexington, Kentucky

Barbara J. de Lateur, M.D.
Professor, Department of Rehabilitation Medicine; University of Washington; Seattle, Washington

Abner Golden, M.D.
Professor and Chairman, Department of Pathology; College of Medicine; University of Kentucky; Lexington, Kentucky

Albert M. Gordon, Ph.D.
Professor, Department of Physiology; University of Washington; Seattle, Washington

George H. Kraft, M.D.
Professor, Department of Rehabilitation Medicine; University of Washington; Seattle, Washington

Russell Ross, Ph.D.
Professor, Department of Pathology; University of Washington; Seattle, Washington

Cornelius Rosse, M.D.
Professor, Department of Biological Structure; University of Washington; Seattle, Washington

Jane G. Schaller, M.D.
Professor, Department of Pediatrics; University of Washington; Seattle, Washington

Peter A. Simkin, M.D.
Associate Professor, Department of Medicine; University of Washington; Seattle, Washington

Walter C. Stolov, M.D.
Professor, Department of Rehabilitation Medicine; University of Washington; Seattle, Washington

Rosalind H. Troupin, M.D.
Associate Professor, Department of Radiology; University of Pennsylvania; Philadelphia, Pennsylvania

Preface

The predecessor of this volume, *Introduction to the Musculoskeletal System*, published 10 years ago, was the product of changing trends in medical education during the 1960s, and it was the first textbook which integrated all aspects of an organ system for the beginning student in the health professions. The integrated approach was met with enthusiasm both by students and teachers. However, in an attempt to remain concise and to concentrate on a core of basic information, the book fell short of being self-sufficient. Learning and courses based on it had to be supplemented substantially from other sources. The need for a more comprehensive presentation of the organ system became evident as the years went by and the growing pains of curricular changes abated. We hope that presenting the musculoskeletal system in greater depth will not obscure our original aims and will make learning more enjoyable and satisfying.

Several recent books deal with one or another aspect of the musculoskeletal system. We believe that interrelation of the various disciplines has profound benefits for the student who is being introduced to musculoskeletal health care, and at the same time, it generates an enhanced appreciation of problems for those who have been engaged for some time in health care delivery.

Introduction to the Musculoskeletal System was based on input provided by numerous members of the faculty at the University of Washington, and some of its chapters have been included in the present volume without much change. However, the majority of chapters are completely rewritten or are entirely new, lending a much wider scope to the book than its predecessor aspired to. Greater emphasis has been given to physiology, pathology, functional gross anatomy, and to the clinical evaluation of various regions of the musculoskeletal system. The book is primarily intended for medical students. It is especially designed for courses in which basic scientists and clinicians can collaborate extensively. Such courses fit as well into the early part of the curriculum, as they do later during the clerkships. A beginning student will gain appreciation for the necessity and applicability of the basic sciences in clinical medicine, while to a more advanced student the usefulness of the basic sciences will appear in a different light because he or she can apply and practice their principles on the wards and clinics. The book should, moreover, be a useful aid for individual learning, independent of courses.

Anatomy forms the basis of understanding function in the musculoskeletal system, and it is essential for understanding and eliciting physical signs. Functional anatomy accounts for the greatest bulk in these pages, and we have attempted to present it so that it should be of interest not only to the beginning student but also to those who have progressed from traditional anatomy courses to the clinical scene. We have not shied away from introducing some recent and yet controversial concepts in functional anatomy of the various regions. No doubt some of these will meet with criticism, which we invite, and others will be replaced by new ideas. Much remains to be learned about basic musculoskeletal functions at the molecular, tissue, and gross structural levels of organization. It is our intent to encourage students in such an endeavor. We hope that the book in its present format will appeal to residents in orthopedics, rehabilitation medicine, and other areas of musculoskeletal health care delivery, and will induce them to rethink the basic concepts for evaluating the musculoskeletal system clinically. Physiotherapists have found *Introduction to the Musculoskeletal System* well suited to their aims in education. Although the present text is more comprehensive, we hope that it retains its usefulness for their curricula.

The first eight chapters of the book discuss the functional units of the musculoskeletal system and deal also with the basic concepts of their clinical evaluation. Introductory chapters on the pathology and radiologic evaluation of the musculoskeletal system serve to put into perspective clinical examples used in Chapters 9–19, which describe the anatomic regions of the system. The subsequent chapters discuss the more important disease processes which affect the musculo-skeletal system, and the final chapter presents a comprehensive screening examination for the evaluation of musculoskeletal health. This manner of presentation inevitably leads to some repetitions, which are intentional. Repetition will seem redundant only to those readers who are specialists in one or other aspect of musculoskeletal health care. They are necessary for realizing our intention, which is to stimulate and facilitate learning. We hope that having accomplished that, we will have contributed toward improving the standard of medical care in the area of musculoskeletal disease.

CORNELIUS ROSSE
Seattle, Washington

D. KAY CLAWSON
Lexington, Kentucky

Acknowledgments

We wish to reiterate our indebtedness to many members of the faculty at the University of Washington on whose collaboration the predecessor of the present volume, *Introduction to the Musculoskeletal System*, was based. Without their contribution toward establishing an organ system oriented course, the present book would probably not have been written.

In addition to writing a chapter on radiologic evaluation of the musculoskeletal system, Dr. Rosalind H. Troupin, until recently Associate Professor of Radiology at the University of Washington, provided, with few exceptions, all the radiographs on which many of the chapters rely. The number and quality of the x-rays throughout the book speak for how much the entire book owes to her generosity and dedication. The majority of the illustrations prepared by Ms. Jessie Phillips for *Introduction to the Musculoskeletal System* have been retained. Grace von Drasek Ascher drew most of the new illustrations and it is a particular pleasure to acknowledge her talent and beautiful work. We are also grateful to Charlotte Kaiser and Robert Herndon for numerous illustrations. It is a pleasure to put on record our thanks to two of our medical students: Anthony C. Venbrux worked with dedication on several drawings and Dahveed W. Rubin sculpted the ingenious models of scoliosis. Roy Hayashi provided much valued skill in the preparation of the majority of photographs, and for this we are indebted to him. Our thanks are due to Doris Ringer who typed the manuscript, provided many valued editorial comments, and put her heart into the book beyond the call of duty.

Our publisher, Harper & Row has been patient, helpful, and supportive in this enterprise beyond our expectations.

C. R.
D. K. C.

The Musculoskeletal System in Health and Disease

1
The Musculoskeletal System

CORNELIUS ROSSE,   D. KAY CLAWSON

The musculoskeletal system is the mechanical effector system of the body which is in continuous interaction with its environment. The most important function of this system is to bring about movement of the body in its parts or as a whole, and as such to serve the purpose of locomotion. In addition, the musculoskeletal system provides support and protection for the entire body and for its other organ systems. These functional requirements are in essence reflected in the unique properties of the tissues which constitute this system. This is manifest by the various degrees of rigidity and resilience found in bone, cartilage, ligament, and tendon, and in the contractility of muscle.

Function in the musculoskeletal system, however, is entirely dependent upon the manner in which these tissues are welded into functional units and set into action by the nervous system. **The functional unit of the musculoskeletal system is the joint with its associated structures.** In this unit, bones acting as levers are held together by specialized connective tissues and are set into motion in relation to one another through muscle action initiated and controlled by nerves. Normal function within the unit is dependent on the integrity of each of these components and, above all, on their orderly and harmonious interaction. Conversely, injury or disease of any of the components results in the functional impairment of the entire unit. This principle of interdependence will be emphasized throughout this book in dealing with the individual regions of the musculoskeletal system. Such interdependence applies not only to the tissues, but also to individual joints and regions within the system. The functional effectiveness of the entire musculoskeletal system is important because the tasks of everyday life require integration of activity within the system. For instance, a torn ligament in the knee not only impairs the function of that joint, but puts the entire lower limb out of action. **Adaptations have to take place in the whole musculoskeletal system of the injured patient in order to compensate more or less effectively for the resulting disability.** Thus, the whole individual is affected, not only physically, but also psychologically and socioeconomically. This aspect of musculoskeletal health and disease relating to the individual as a whole cannot be given sufficient emphasis in this book. The student must learn to relate functional assessment of individual regions within the musculoskeletal system to the entire system and to the entire patient. This can be acquired only with experience.

The overall unity of the musculoskeletal system is illustrated not only by the functional interdependence of its parts, but also by the diseases which affect the system as a whole, exemplified by rheumatoid arthritis and degenerative joint disease. Such diseases may have effects on other organ systems as well. Conversely, there are diseases which primarily affect other organ systems but have secondary effects on the musculoskeletal system. For instance, diseases of the hematologic system such as hemophilia, gastrointestinal disorders such as ulcerative colitis, diseases of the skin such as psoriasis, and metabolic disturbances such as gout all may have joint manifestations and may even present initially with joint symptoms. These examples are intended to illustrate that in diagnosing and treating musculoskeletal diseases, the physician needs to look beyond this system and examine, investigate, and treat the whole patient.

It is virtually impossible to practice in any field of medicine and not meet musculoskeletal disease. Some of these diseases are so common that they are regarded as part of the normal aging process and affect all persons beyond a certain age, while others are medical curiosities. More medical manpower is expended in treating musculoskeletal problems than in treating disorders of any other single system. The magnitude of the problem created by the prevalence of musculoskeletal disease can be better appreciated when one considers the increasing numbers of congenitally defective children who are now kept alive; the ravages of trauma sustained at home, in industry, on the highways, and in continuing wars; and the effects of arthritis and the degenerative conditions that affect all in our aging population. Statistics from national health surveys show that arthritis is the nation's number one crippler and costs the United States economy several billion dollars a year.[1] In the United States in 1962, an estimated 40.5 million persons had radiologic changes indicative of degenerative joint disease, and an additional 3.6 million suffered from rheumatoid arthritis. Musculoskeletal conditions account for 41 percent of disorders leading to rehabilitation problems.[2] Federal statistics on the diagnosis of children served by the crippled children's program show that the musculoskeletal system is the most frequently involved organ system. According to recent surveys, around 63 million persons per year are injured, requiring medical attention or restriction of their usual activities.[3] The latest figure for the injury rate is 336 per 1000 population per year, each with an average of 6.3 days of restricted activity.[4] In a 1975 survey of ambulatory care, it was noted that 5.8 percent of all office visits were for disease of the musculoskeletal system. For people 65 years or older this figure was 9.3 percent. Of the morbidity-related problems, those affecting the limbs and the back are the most frequently seen in ambulatory care and account for 9 percent of all visits.[5]

It is obvious that not only special medical services, but also specially trained medical practitioners, are necessary to deal with a problem of this magnitude. This book is not primarily written for these specialists. Its aim is to lay the foundation for the appreciation and thorough understanding of **how the musculoskeletal system functions normally and how and why normal function is disturbed by trauma and disease.** Its aim is also to provide those basic tools of physical examination for the assessment of musculoskeletal function which every medical practitioner should know, regardless of his specialty. Such knowledge will enable him to establish a diagnosis of disturbed function and direct the patient to other medical personnel who can provide the needed attention.

REFERENCES

1. **Age Patterns in Medical Care, Illness and Disability,** United States, July 1963–June 1965. Washington DC, National Center for Health Statistics, Vital and Health Statistics, 1966, Series 10, No. 32
2. **Lehmann JF:** Patient care needs as a basis for development of objectives of physical medicine and rehabilitation teaching in undergraduate medical schools, J Chronic Dis, *21*:3, 1968.
3. **Persons Injured and Disability Days,** United States, 1971–1972. Washington DC, National Center for Health Statistics, Vital and Health Statistics, 1976, Series 10, No. 105
4. **Acute Conditions. Incidence and Associated Disability,** United States, July 1975–June 1976. Washington DC, National Center for Health Statistics, Vital and Health Statistics, 1978, Series 10, No. 120
5. **The National Ambulatory Medical Care Survey,** 1975 Summary. Washington DC, National Center for Health Statistics, Vital and Health Statistics, Series 13, No. 33

2
Tissues of the Musculoskeletal System

CORNELIUS ROSSE, RUSSELL ROSS

The musculoskeletal system is composed essentially of skeletal muscle tissue and of various types of specialized connective tissue, such as bone, cartilage, tendons, and ligaments. In each of these tissues, the cells and the extracellular matrix reflect in their structure functional adaptations that furnish one or more of the qualities required of the musculoskeletal tissues for supporting and moving the body. Loose connective tissue lacking such structural adaptation is widely dispersed among the specialized musculoskeletal elements. Nerves and blood and lymph vessels run in the loose connective tissue that surrounds and interlaces muscles, bones, and joints. Fluids, nutrients, and metabolites are exchanged between the specialized tissues and the circulation through loose connective tissue.

Nerves and blood vessels are essential for the maintenance and normal function of musculoskeletal tissues and are closely integrated with them anatomically and functionally. The musculoskeletal tissues depend on their nerve and blood supply for defense against trauma, infections, and other harmful agents. Following injury, healing and repair of musculoskeletal tissues depends on adequate blood supply and on cells that emigrate from the circulation or are resident in the surrounding loose connective tissue.

This chapter is concerned primarily with the structure and function of connective tissue proper, cartilage, and bone. Chapter 3 discusses the structure of skeletal muscle, together with neuromuscular physiology. Chapter 6 deals with the responses of musculoskeletal tissues to injury.

THE CONNECTIVE TISSUES

Connective tissue consists of cells dispersed in extracellular matrix produced by the cells. Connec-

tive tissue cells are derived from embryonic mesenchyme and throughout life will retain morphologic similarity in the various types of connective tissues. These apparently similar cells have differentiated at some point of embryonic development and are able to produce different types of extracellular matrices in different locations of the body. The special properties of the various types of connective tissue are determined by the composition of the extracellular matrix. Consequently, the classification of connective tissues is based on the differences in this matrix.

Extracellular matrix is composed of **fibers** and amorphous **ground substance.** Only two basic types of fibers are admixed in various proportions in all connective tissues: **collagen fibers** and **elastic fibers.** On the other hand, the composition and consistency of ground substance varies considerably between the different connective tissue types. These tissue types include 1) *ordinary* or *proper* connective tissues (e.g., loose connective tissue, tendon, ligament, fascia) and 2) *special* connective tissues, namely, cartilage and bone.

In connective tissue proper, the ground substance has the physical properties of a thin gel, while in cartilage it forms a firm gel of distinct chemical composition. The ground substance specific for bone tissue becomes impregnated by inorganic bone salts that lend rigidity to this tissue.

The density and type of the connective tissue fibers determine whether the particular tissue is of primary mechanical importance in musculoskeletal function or whether it forms loose packing material through which nutrients and cells can pass. **Loose connective tissue** consists of an open meshwork of fibers and cells, the interstices of which are filled by ground substance and can be greatly distended by abnormal amounts of tissue fluid (edema). Loose connective tissue is the pro-

3

totype of all the more specialized connective tissues and most closely resembles embryonic mesenchyme. Tendons and ligaments represent **dense connective tissue** in which collagen fibers are closely packed in a regular pattern. An ordered fiber network is also present in articular cartilage and bone. However, these fibers are masked by the staining properties of cartilage and bone matrix, and special methods are needed for their demonstration. Dense connective tissue also constitutes deep fascia and intermuscular septa, and the arrangement of fibers is quite regular.

Densely arranged elastic fibers make up the bulk of the extracellular matrix in **elastic tissue.** Elastic tissue is found in certain ligaments associated with the spine (ligamenta flava) and in the walls of certain arteries.

CELLS OF THE CONNECTIVE TISSUES

Principal Cell Types

The principal cells of connective tissue produce the matrices characteristic of connective tissue proper, cartilage and bone. The three cell types are known as **fibroblasts, chondroblasts** (or **chondrocytes**), and **osteoblasts** (or **osteocytes**), respectively. These cells are closely related and are distinguishable principally by the unique extracellular matrix each cell secretes. Unlike the terms chondrocyte and osteocyte, fibrocyte is rarely applied to mature cells of proper connective tissue. The blast forms of cartilage and bone cells differ from their more mature equivalents only in that they are capable of proliferation, while chondrocytes and osteocytes enclosed in semisolid or completely rigid matrix no longer divide.

Fibroblasts, chondrocytes, and osteocytes display different shapes, but this is largely determined by the environment in which each cell is located. Pertinent environmental factors are the amount, rigidity, and orientation of extracellular fibers; the molecular orientation within the ground substance (this is beyond the resolution of the light and electron microscope); and the mechanical forces that produce lines of stress in the tissue. It must be remembered, however, that deposition of the extracellular matrix in an ordered fashion is the function of the cells and, therefore, the cells are largely responsible for creating their environment.

Fibroblasts are found dispersed along bundles of collagen or elastic fibers; in loose connective tissue they are stellate, but in tendon and ligament the cells are compressed into elongated spindles by the parallel fiber bundles. **Chondrocytes** remain round or oval in the more or less regular cavities called lacunae they occupy in cartilage matrix, while **osteocytes** extend delicate processes from their cell body into canaliculi that interconnect with neighboring lacunae of bone.

All three cell types are involved in protein synthesis, which is reflected in their morphology (Fig. 2–1; compare with Figs. 2–10 and 2–11). In the nucleus, euchromatin predominates and the nucleoli are prominent. The cytoplasm contains extensive rough-surfaced endoplasmic reticulum and a well developed Golgi complex. Both organelles are characteristic of cells engaged in the synthesis and intracellular transport of secretory proteins, such as the proteins of connective tissue. The abundance of ribosomes along the cisternae of the endoplasmic reticulum explains the basophilic staining of the cytoplasm which is evident in the light microscope, especially in areas of active matrix deposition (e.g., wound healing, new bone formation).

Each of the cell types produces a matrix containing differing amounts of proteins, such as collagen, elastic fiber proteins, and glycosaminoglycans. The proteins secreted by fibroblasts in the different connective tissues are also different. For example, the fibroblasts of most tendons produce larger amounts of collagen and relatively little elastin. In contrast, fibroblasts from elastic ligaments such as the ligamentum flavum produce much elastin and relatively less collagen. Even with the electron microscope, it is not possible to discern morphologic differences between the two cells. Furthermore, it is now known that collagen secreted by fibroblasts of tendon and ligament or by osteocytes differs in its amino acid composition from collagen secreted by chondrocytes.

It is important to have an appreciation and an understanding of the various connective tissues at the fine structure and molecular level because it is becoming apparent that only at this level of resolution can many diseases of these tissues be understood.

Incidental Cells

The matrix of bone and cartilage contains only osteocytes and chondrocytes, respectively. This is quite different from loose connective tissue, where, in addition to fibroblasts, a variety of other cells are encountered. These incidental cells are not directly concerned with matrix formation but are important in defense, repair, and regeneration.

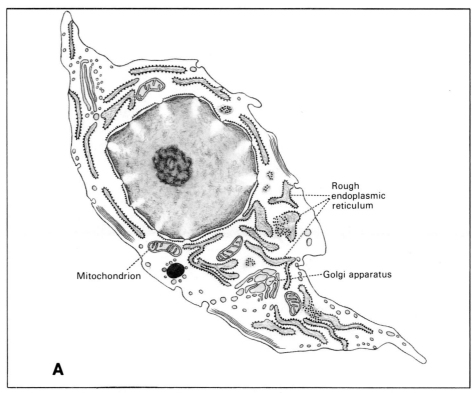

A

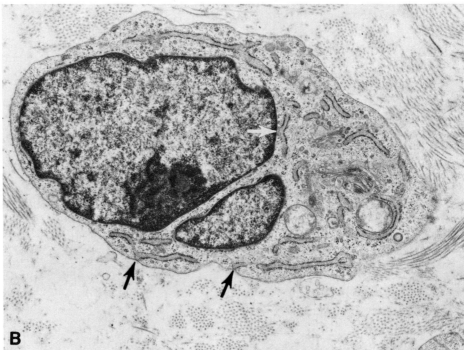

B

FIG. 2–1. **A.** An idealized schematic representation of a fibroblast identifying the characteristic organelles. **B.** An electron micrograph of a fibroblast in human dermis. The plane of section is tangential to a slight indentation in the nucleus. The rough endoplasmic reticulum appears to be continuous with the nuclear envelope **(white arrow)** and some of its cisternae are apparently in fusion with the cell membrane **(black arrows)** suggesting a secretory process. Note collagen fibrils and ground substance in the extracellular matrix. (**B** Courtesy of Dr. Karen A. Holbrook) (× 18,800)

Such cells are brought into association with bone and cartilage via the loose connective tissue present in the cavities of bone (haversian canals, medullary cavity) or via the periosteum and perichondrium. Incidental cells include mesenchymal cells, fat cells, synovial cells, mononuclear phagocytes, lymphocytes, neutrophil and eosinophil granulocytes, and mast cells.

Mesenchymal cells are thought to be primitive connective tissue cells that retain into adult life the potential of differentiating into fibroblasts, osteoblasts, and chondroblasts. They are difficult to distinguish morphologically from fibroblasts and may be identical with them.

Fat cells are specialized for the synthesis and storage of fat. The volume of the fat droplets enclosed by the cell may be many times greater than the volume of its own nucleus and cytoplasm. Fat cells are most likely derived from mesenchymal cells or fibroblasts and their incidence is variable in different parts of the body. They are abundant in superficial fascia, where they account for the bulk of the tissue. The variety of loose connective tissue laden with fat cells is known as **adipose tissue.** In the musculoskeletal system, adipose tissue serves special mechanical functions in two places: over the soles of the feet and palms of the hands, where it acts as padding against pressure, and in synovial joints, where compressable fat pads assist in the even spreading of synovial fluid during movement of the joint.

Synovial cells develop along certain planes of habitual movement, where friction is generated within loose connective tissue. Such cells are derived from either mesenchymal cells or fibroblasts and are specialized for secreting synovial fluid, which serves as a lubricant. Synovial cells characteristically line synovial joints and will be discussed in that context more fully, but they may develop anywhere. The cells align themselves to form a pocket or bag that is moistened by their secretion. Such a connective tissue structure is known as a **bursa.**

Mononuclear phagocytes are common in loose connective tissue. They are formed in the bone marrow, enter the circulation as monocytes, and migrate through the capillary wall into loose connective tissue. When the cell becomes phagocytic, it is known as a **macrophage.** Some macrophages apparently reside in connective tissue for some time and such cells used to be distinguished by the name *fixed* macrophages. This notion was based on the interpretation of fixed histologic specimens,

and modern experiments have proved it to be meaningless. Macrophages are indiscriminate scavengers and they dispose of dead cells, degraded components of the matrix, and foreign organic and inorganic materials. They are known to release a number of enzymes concerned in tissue breakdown and they participate in the immune response by processing and storing antigens. In addition, they have been shown to be capable of secreting a mitogen that may play a role in the proliferation of connective tissue.

Lymphocytes are immunocompetent cells. They gain access to antigens located in connective tissue by emigrating from capillaries. Lymphocytes are formed initially in the thymus or bone marrow and circulate through the connective tissues by leaving blood capillaries and entering lymphatic capillaries, which pervade loose connective tissue. Following their sensitization they may kill foreign cells, tissues (grafts), or organisms in the connective tissue, or they may differentiate into **plasma cells** responsible for the secretion of antibodies. Plasma cells are abundant in lymph nodes and the spleen, but they may also accumulate in connective tissue.

Polymorphonuclear neutrophils, eosinophils, and **mast cells** play an important role in inflammatory reactions. Neutrophils and eosinophils are derived from the blood, but mast cells are believed to be of connective tissue origin. Neutrophils display marked antibacterial activity and contribute to abscess and pus formation.

EXTRACELLULAR MATRIX

Hardness may be obtained in a tissue by the transformation of its cells into rigid units as in keratinization. Such a process, however, renders the cells metabolically inactive. The production of extracellular materials, on the other hand, makes possible the synthesis of substances of all degrees of hardness, plasticity, and elasticity and, at the same time, metabolically active cells can be retained in the tissue. These cells will be able to provide for growth and remodeling. In the musculoskeletal system, mechanical requirements have been met by the versatility of connective tissue cells in secreting extracellular materials that possess varied mechanical properties. Apart from the inorganic bone salts, all the structurally important extracellular substances are glycoproteins, and interference with protein synthesis, posttranslational modification, or assembly of the subunits of these specialized molecules results in functional impairment of the musculoskeletal system.

The two main fiber types of extracellular matrix, collagen fibers and elastic fibers, each have a unique amino acid composition. Each type of fiber displays a highly characteristic arrangement of macromolecular subunits which accounts for its distinct behavior in response to mechanical stress. Much less is known about the molecular configuration of the various types of glycoproteins in the amorphous ground substance.

Collagen Fibers

Collagen is the principal protein constituent of extracellular matrix in all connective tissues except in elastic tissue. It is the main fibrous protein in the body and it is widely distributed. Apart from fibroblasts, osteoblasts, and chondroblasts, collagen is also synthesized by smooth muscle cells, reticular cells, corneal and vascular endothelium, epithelial cells, and many other differentiated cells. Collagen functions to contribute integrity and strength to all tissues, and in many instances, it provides the morphologic model for developing tissues and organs.

Collagen fibers are white and flexible, exemplified by tendons which consist almost exclusively of large bundles of collagen fibers. Collagen fibers have a high tensile strength and are nonextensible. In connective tissue, they are aggregated into rather coarse bundles (Fig. 2–2A), but in other tissues they form a delicate network of fibers, known as a reticulum, which supports the cells. (Basement membrane, though nonfibrillar, subserves the same function.) The fine fibers called **reticular fibers** have a different amino acid composition from the coarser collagen fibers of connective tissue, such as those in the dermis.

Structure of Collagen Fibers. Each collagen fiber consists of numerous **collagen fibrils** of 200–1000 A in diameter, resolved only by the electron microscope (Fig. 2–2B). The electron microscope reveals a periodic banding pattern along collagen fibrils. The major bands are separated by distances of approximately 700 A (Fig. 2–2C). This periodicity can be demonstrated also by x-ray diffraction. The visible banding pattern is the result of the highly ordered aggregation of collagen molecules. The mechanical properties of collagen fibers are determined by intermolecular cross linking. When

collagen fibers break under stress, they probably do so because collagen molecules separate from one another.

Biosynthesis of Collagen. The biosynthetic pathway of collagen is complex, but it illustrates the types of mechanisms that are involved in the assembly of proteins (Fig. 2–3). Polypeptide chains consisting of about 1600 amino acids (known as pro–α chains) are synthesized on ribosomes of the rough endoplasmic reticulum in connective tissue cells. These chains are of two types ($\alpha1$ and $\alpha2$) and both are rich in the amino acids glycine, proline, and hydroxyproline, but are lacking tryptophan. This unusual amino acid composition favors the formation of a long asymmetric molecule which consists of three α chains arranged in a triple helix. Depending on the type of collagen, the constituent chains are characteristically different.

Three polypeptide chains become aligned and united in a triple helix by interchain hydrogen bonds to form a **procollagen** molecule. This macromolecule is larger than the final form of collagen due to the presence of extensive nonhelical amino acid sequences at both the amino and carboxy termini of the molecule. The procollagen molecule is secreted through the Golgi complex by the cell. At the site of secretion the connective tissue cell also releases proteolytic enzymes (procollagen peptidases) which cleave off the nonhelical terminal segments from the procollagen molecule. The remaining helical protein is collagen.

It is thought that the nonhelical terminal segments prevent the procollagen molecules from aggregating into larger units before they have been secreted from the cell. Once the cleavage of the two ends has been achieved, the collagen molecules can aggregate into collagen fibrils. The alignment of the polarized, asymmetric collagen molecules takes place in register, resulting in the visible banding pattern characteristic of the collagen fibril (Fig. 2–2C). Intermolecular cross links are established by specific enzymes acting on specific amino acids located in the polypeptide chains of two adjacent collagen molecules. Both the cells and the extracellular environment play a role in this fibril formation.

Types of Collagen. The type of collagen present in different tissues is determined by the cell that synthesizes the molecule. For instance, type I collagen (two $\alpha1[I]$ + one $\alpha2$ chains) is prevalent in tendon, ligament, loose connective tissue, bone and skin,

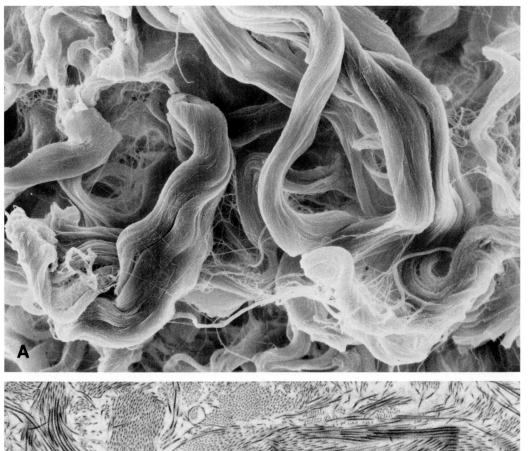

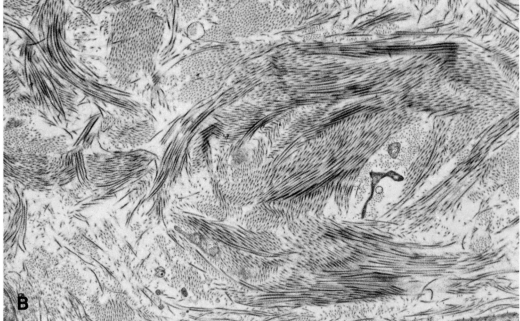

(continued)

FIG. 2–2. Collagen fibers seen at different magnification with the electron microscope. **A.** Bundles of collagen fibers of the dermis revealed by scanning electron microscopy. (× 1350) **B.** At higher magnification the transmission electron microscope resolves these large bundles into collagen fibrils which exhibit characteristic banding patterns. **C.** This banding pattern of the fibrils is shown to better advantage after the specimen has been "shadowed" with chromium. The repeat period of the cross striations within the fibrils is about 700 Å. (**A** and **B** Courtesy of Dr. Karen A. Holbrook; **C** courtesy of Dr. Jerome Gross) (× 60,000)

but type II collagen (three α1[II] chains) is largely confined to cartilage. Type III collagen (three α1[III] chains) is present principally in the wall of large blood vessels. Other types of collagen have also been described which occur alone or admixed with types I, II, and III. Basement membrane collagen has been identified as type IV and has yet a different amino acid composition.

It is possible to demonstrate these closely related but distinct proteins by biochemical analysis of the tissue and by antibodies which have been experimentally raised against each type (Fig. 2–4). It has been shown that in developing chick cartilage some individual connective tissue cells synthesize type I collagen whereas other cells synthesize only type II collagen (Fig. 2–5). When one type of connective tissue (e.g., cartilage) is transformed into another type (e.g., bone), the collagen characteristic of the new tissue is evidently synthesized by a different population of cells than in the precursor tissue, although some cells have been shown to be able to synthesize at least two types of collagen.

In certain types of disorders of connective tissue, the production of a particular type of collagen may be impaired, resulting in a clinical and pathologic picture which can only be explained if the tissue distribution of the particular collagen is understood. Other defects of collagen fiber formation may be attributed to the lack of certain enzymes necessary for converting procollagen into collagen or for establishing the specific cross linking between the polypeptide chains.

Defects in Collagen Fiber Production. Because collagen is so ubiquitously associated with all types of tissues, the clinical and pathologic picture that results from defective collagen fiber production may present in a great variety of ways. Musculoskeletal tissues are usually affected. Such patients may show abnormalities in bone formation, hypermobility of joints due to weakness of the ligaments, and destruction of component tissues of joints (Fig. 2–6).

The defects in collagen fiber production are not yet fully understood, nor is it entirely clear how important and common such defects may be in the various clinically recognized diseases of connective tissue. The types of defects fall into three categories: 1) defective polypeptide chain synthesis, 2) defects in molecular cross linking due to enzyme abnormalities, and 3) defects in aggregation. The causative agents may be gene defects, deficiency of vitamins and other substances, and certain types of drugs which may inhibit enzymes or compete with amino acids necessary for collagen synthesis.

(continued)

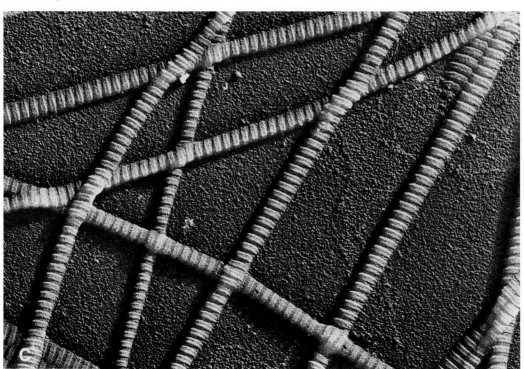

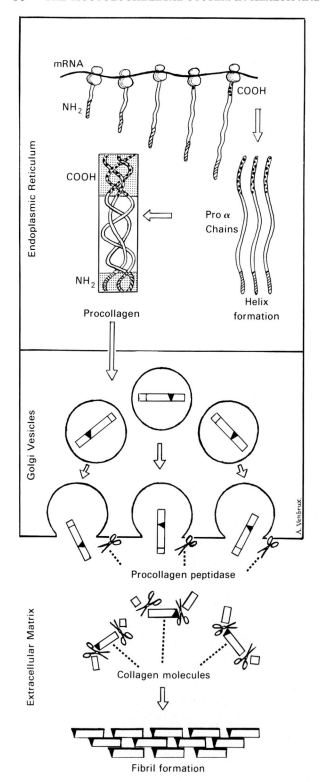

Examples of such defects are a severe autosomal recessive form of osteogenesis imperfecta. In this condition, type I collagen is not produced normally because of a defect in polypeptide chain synthesis. In scurvy, collagen fibril production is defective because vitamin C, which is necessary for the hydroxylation of proline and lysine, is not available. As a result hydroxyproline and hydroxylysine are not formed and the molecule is unstable. When the enzyme procollagen peptidase is lacking, procollagen molecules cannot be converted into collagen and fibril formation is altered. One or more enzymes necessary for establishing intermolecular cross links in collagen may be lacking. The appearance of some abnormal types of collagen fibers is shown in Figure 2–7. Diseases in which collagenous tissue destruction is a major manifestation (e.g., rheumatoid arthritis, degenerative joint disease) probably share in common the fact that collagenases are released at an abnormally high rate and at unusual sites.

Breakdown of Collagen. It has been found recently that different cells can secrete enzymes which specifically degrade collagen fibrils and the collagen molecule. These enzymes have been termed **collagenases.** Mammalian collagenase cleaves the collagen molecule into three–quarter and one–quarter length segments. As a result, the molecule which normally is resistant to other proteolytic enzymes denatures and can now be broken down.

The types of cells that have been found to produce collagenase include macrophages, neutro-

FIG. 2–3. Schematic representation of collagen synthesis. The information for assembling the amino acids is carried by messenger RNA (mRNA). Three polypeptide chains are synthesized by ribosomes of the endoplasmic reticulum. When both the carboxy (COOH) and amino (NH₂) termini are complete, the chains are released into the cisternae of the reticulum. Three such chains become helically associated and form a procollagen molecule. This molecule is transferred to Golgi vesicles and becomes secreted from the cell surface. It is possible that some secretion may also occur directly from the cisternae of the endoplasmic reticulum as suggested by some profiles in Fig. 2–1 **(black arrows).** Assembly into a fibril is preceded by enzymatic splitting of both ends of the procollagen molecule after it is released from the cell.

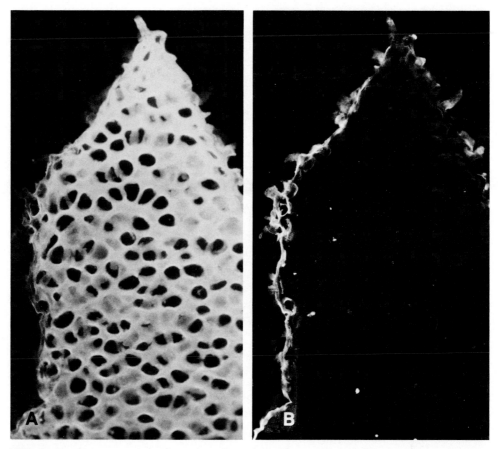

FIG. 2–4. Demonstration of type I and type II collagen in a spicule of cartilage which is beginning to ossify in the tibia of a 13-day-old chick embryo. The same spicule shows staining in **A** with an antiserum raised in the rabbit against type II collagen of the chick and in **B** with a similar antiserum raised against type I collagen. Type II collagen is present throughout the cartilage matrix (chondrocytes have fallen out of their lacunae during the staining process). Type I collagen has only been formed at this stage around the periphery of the cartilage spicule where bone matrix is being laid down by endochondral ossification. Binding of the two different antisera to the same specimen is demonstrated in the fluorescent microscope under ultraviolet light by the use of double staining with fluoresceinated and rhodaminated antisera which can be excited at different wave lengths using appropriate filters. (von der Mark K, von der Mark H: J Bone Joint Surg 59(B)(4):458, 1977) (× 190)

phils, and even fibroblasts. It appears that fibroblasts play an important role in collagen turnover and tissue remodeling not only through synthesizing collagen but also through breaking it down with specific collagenolytic enzymes. The collagenolytic activity of macrophages and neutrophils clearly plays an important role in the pathogenesis of inflammatory diseases of connective tissue.

Elastic Fibers

Elastic fibers derive their name from the elastic properties they demonstrate when they are stretched. When released, they return to their original length. Unlike collagen fibers, they have low tensile strength and when they break each fragment retracts. Elastic fibers play an important role in maintaining the shape of distensible and

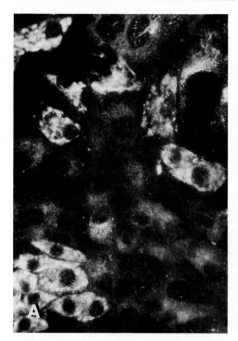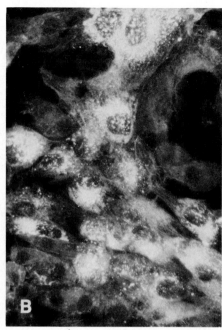

FIG. 2–5. Chick sternal chondrocytes have been cultured for 2 weeks and have been doubly stained with antisera raised against type I and type II collagen using the same procedure as described in Figure 2–4. The same microscopic field is shown in **A** and **B**. In **A** the cytoplasm of cells that synthesize type II collagen is fluorescent and appears bright, while in **B** cells engaged in type I collagen synthesis are fluorescent. The majority of cells synthesize only one or the other type of collagen; very few cells show fluorescence with both antibodies simultaneously. (von der Mark K, Gauss V, von der Mark H, Müller P: Nature 267:531, 1977) (× 360)

stretchable organs (lungs, blood vessels, certain ligaments) and are universal components of the extracellular matrix in all types of connective tissue including tendons and ligaments. They are particularly numerous in elastic tissue.

Unlike collagen fibers, elastic fibers demonstrate no periodicity when viewed in the electron microscope (Fig. 2–8). They consist of two different morphologic components: microfibrils, visible only with the electron microscope, and elastin, the dominant protein of each elastic fiber. **Elastin** is an unusual protein in that it behaves like a protein rubber. It is amorphous in appearance in the electron microscope and contains very few polar amino acids, but is rich in neutral amino acids such as valine, alanine, and glycine.

The **microfibrils** of the elastic fiber surround the core of amorphous elastin and are embedded in it. They differ in their amino acid composition from elastin, since they are particularly rich in polar amino acids and contain a large amount of cystine.

It was learned from the study of the morphogenesis of embryonic elastic tissue that the two components of the elastic fiber appear in two successive stages. The microfibrils are the first component to be synthesized. During the first stage of elastic tissue morphogenesis, bundles of microfibrils are found adjacent to the surface of fibroblasts in developing ligamentum nuchae. These microfibrils conform to the shape and direction of the developing presumptive elastic fiber. In the second stage of morphogenesis, small amounts of amorphous elastin are secreted by the same cells, and are cross-linked between and around the existing microfibrils. With increasing maturity of the elastic fiber, increasing amounts of elastin are added. Ninety percent of the fully formed elastic fiber consists of elastin and only 10 percent of microfibrils (Fig. 2–8).

It appears that the form and direction of elastic fibers may be determined by the cell through the laying down of microfibrils. Because of their opposite charge, microfibrils attract the secreted elastin. The elastin is then rendered insoluble by cross-linking enzymes secreted by the cell, similar to those that cross-link collagen. Elastin itself could not adopt a clear fibrillar form; otherwise it could not behave as an elastomer. The behavior of elastin as an elastomer is due to specific association and cross-linking of elastin molecules with one another, which permits them to become aligned when stretched and to recoil when released, thus furnishing elastomeric properties to the fiber.

Elastic fiber proteins are synthesized by smooth muscle cells in arteries, by fibroblasts in tendons, ligaments, and loose connective tissue, and by chondroblasts in cartilage.

Ground Substance

The amorphous ground substance in which the cells and fibers of connective tissue are embedded is difficult to demonstrate histologically. Ground substance contains variable amounts of water, soluble extracellular proteins, sugars, and calcium salts but its most important constituents are **proteoglycans.** Proteoglycans are formed by proteins joined to **glycosaminoglycans** (polysaccharides that contain amino sugars, especially hexosamine). The differences in relative amounts of glycosaminoglycans found in bone, cartilage, and other connective tissues appear to be responsible in part for the different physical properties demonstrated by each of these tissues. The most important glycosaminoglycans are 1) chondroitin sulfate, 2) keratan sulfate, 3) hyaluronic acid, and 4) dermatan sulfate. Chondroitin sulfate, keratan sulfate, and hyaluronic acid are common constituents of cartilage and bone, while dermatan sulfate is found in the dermis and blood vessels.

Proteoglycans rich in hyaluronic acid have high viscosity in aqueous solutions and play an important role in determining the viscosity of ground substance. Hyaluronic acid is also an important constituent of synovial fluid. Acting as a lubricant it reduces friction not only in joints but probably also between connective tissue fibers.

Since the large proteoglycan molecules are entangled with fibrous elements of the matrix they are important in maintaining the integrity of the tissue and its components. An example of this is presented by the myotendinal junction. Collagen fibers of tendon are separated by a definite interval from the sarcolemma (cell wall) of the muscle fiber (Fig. 2-9). Ruthenium red, a reagent with special affinity for glycosaminoglycans, demonstrates that collagen fibers are secured to the sarcolemma by a substance which stains with ruthenium red.

TENDON, LIGAMENT AND FASCIA

Tendons and ligaments are similar structures. Both represent a form of dense connective tissue

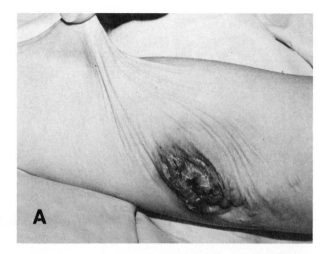
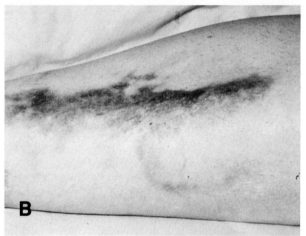
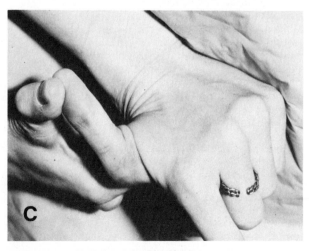

FIG. 2-6. Photograph of a 26-year-old woman suffering from type I Ehlers–Danlos syndrome, a disease in which collagen fiber production is defective. She has fragile skin which is thin and markedly hyperextensible (**A**); she bruises easily and her scars are often hyperpigmented and appear thin and atrophic (**B**). Her joints are extremely lax (**C**). (Courtesy of Dr. P. H. Byers)

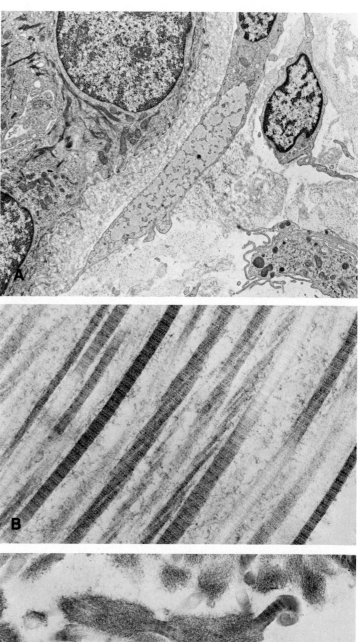

FIG. 2–7. Abnormal collagen production. **A.** A long, narrow fibroblast from the dermis of a patient suffering from a type IV Ehlers-Danlos syndrome. The cisternae of the endoplasmic reticulum are grossly dilated suggesting defective collagen release into the extracellular matrix. **B.** Abnormal configuration of collagen fibrils in the dermis of a cat due to deficiency of procollagen peptidase. The same disorder occurs also in man. Because the nonhelical termini of the procollagen molecule are not split off, fibril assembly is defective. The central fibril is apparently normal but those on either side are thicker, spiraled, and frayed. **C.** A collagen fibril from the dermis of a patient suffering from a disorder that affects primarily bones and joints as well as a number of other tissues (spondyloepiphyseal dysplasia). Along the fibril there are abnormally associated portions in which the filaments of the fibril are visible. These irregularities as well as the terminal whorls are highly abnormal. (**A** and **B** courtesy of Dr. Karen A. Holbrook; **C,** Byers PH, Holbrook KA, Hall JG et al: Human Genetics 40:157, 1978)

FIG. 2–8. The morphology of elastic fibers. **A.** Electron micrograph of human dermis. The central bundle consists of typical collagen fibrils and on either side are elastic fibers. (× 14,000) **B.** A large elastic fiber at higher magnification surrounded by collagen fibrils. Microfibrils (mf) surround the amorphous elastin component (a) of the fiber. (**A** courtesy of Dr. Karen Holbrook) (× 40,000)

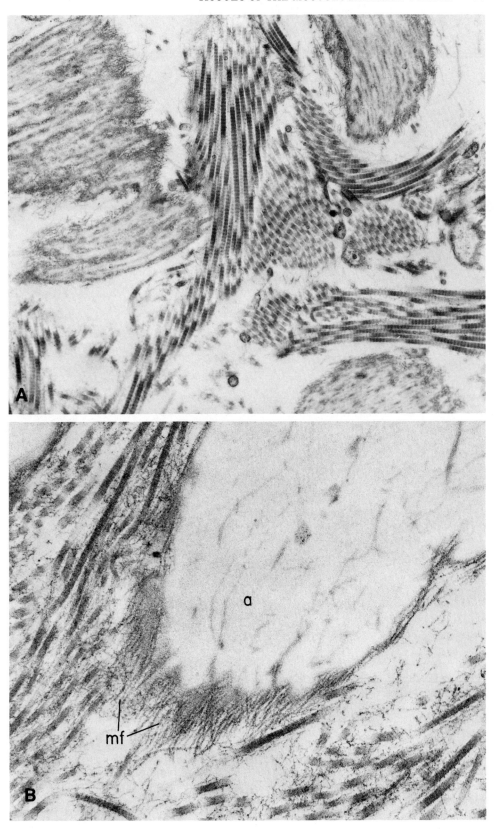

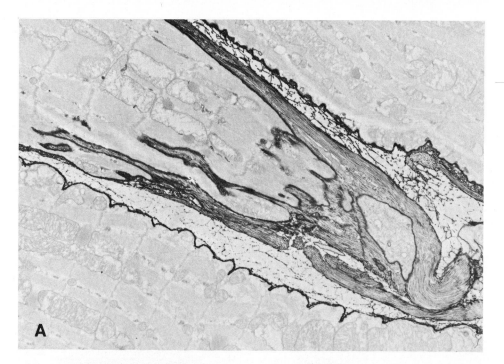

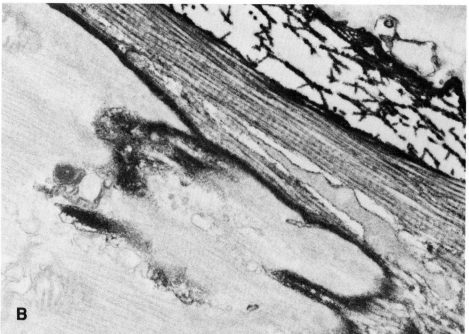

FIG. 2–9. Myotendinal junction in the diaphragm of the mouse. The specimen has been treated with ruthenium red but is otherwise unstained. Despite the absence of staining, muscle tissue and collagen are clearly identifiable. In **A** the distal end of the central muscle fiber can be seen interdigitating with its tendon. In **B,** which represents an enlarged area of **A,** the banding pattern of collagen fibrils in the tendon is evident. Certain components of the ground substance have a high affinity for ruthenium red which is highly electron dense. This electron dense material is present as a precipitate between the muscle fibers on the surface of the sarcolemma and is particularly prominent at the interface between the muscle cell and the tendon. Presumably, the material stained with ruthenium red is responsible for affixing collagen fibers to the muscle cell. (Courtesy of Dr. John H. Luft) (**A,** × 9,250; **B,** × 29,000)

that is flexible and yet offers great resistance to a pulling force. **Tendons** attach muscle to bone and **ligaments** attach bone to bone. Layers or sheets of connective tissue visible to the naked eye, which envelop various organs and their parts and separate them from one another, are known as **fascia.** The dense connective tissue membrane which invests the limbs and the neck like a stocking is known as **deep fascia.** The same type of tissue surrounds individual muscles forming their epimysium and is known also as deep fascia. The layer of adipose tissue between the deep fascia and the skin is the **superficial fascia.** Deep fascia extends in the form of septa in between muscle groups of the limbs. Some of these intermuscular septa are quite substantial and separate the limb musculature into compartments.

Tendons and ligaments consist primarily of thick bundles of collagen fibers packed closely and parallel with one another. Few elastic fibers and little loose connective tissue intervene. Fibroblasts are sparse and are arranged in long parallel rows along the fibers. Because of this longitudinal arrangement of all elements, it is difficult to suture torn tendons and ligaments. The primary difference in the structure of a tendon and a ligament is that fiber bundles are less regularly arranged in the ligament with some crossing over in different planes. Ligaments contain more loose connective tissue than tendon.

Sheetlike muscles tend to have sheetlike tendons. These are known as **aponeuroses.** Histologically, aponeuroses are similar to tendons.

The arrangement of fibers in deep fascia forms a more or less regular, widely open lattice pattern. Although elastic fibers are more numerous than in tendon, deep fascia provides a firm support for muscles. It has been shown that the power of muscle contraction is diminished when its deep fascia is stripped. Because of the limited compliance of deep fascia, pressure rises in the muscle compartment during muscle contraction. The intermittent increase in pressure aids venous return from pendant limbs. Excessive pressure in a compartment due to swelling or hematoma compresses the veins, leading to edema, and eventually will endanger the arterial blood supply of the musculature. The muscle cells will die unless the deep fascia is incised and the pressure released.

Tendons and ligaments have a low vascularity and their capacity for regeneration is limited. A torn tendon or ligament heals by scar tissue formation. The stresses acting on the scar tissue may align some of its fibers with those of the tendon or ligament.

CARTILAGE

Cartilage acts as a material which retains the shape of organs (ear, nose, trachea, intervertebral disk). It is able to resist compression and bending forces to a considerable extent. It is located on the articular surfaces of practically all joints where its resiliency protects the bone from direct compression and permits smooth movement of skeletal pieces against each other.

During prenatal and postnatal development, including adolescence, cartilage provides a site of bone formation and by its own growth determines the height of the individual.

Cartilage has a relatively low rate of metabolism. Under experimental conditions it arises from loose connective tissue when oxygen tension is low, while bone arises from the same tissue when oxygen is supplied plentifully.

The cartilage cells called **chondrocytes** are enclosed by the matrix which they form (Fig. 2–10). The small cavities, so-called **lacunae,** which surround the cells in conventional light microscopic preparations are artifacts of poor fixation. The nourishment of chondrocytes and metabolic exchange take place by diffusion across the matrix. Cartilage is usually described as an avascular tissue. However, this is true only for articular cartilage. The cartilage templates of many bones, as well as the cartilaginous epiphyses of long bones, are penetrated by **cartilage canals** which contain arterioles, capillaries, and venules embedded in loose connective tissue.

Cartilage is enclosed by a dense fibrous connective tissue everywhere except where it is exposed to synovial fluid in joints. This connective tissue envelope is rich in blood vessels and nerves and is called the **perichondrium.** Blood vessels and connective tissue of the cartilage canals are derived from the perichondrium. Nerves, however, have not been demonstrated in the canals.

There are three types of cartilage: hyaline, fibrous, and elastic. **Hyaline cartilage** constitutes the models of the developing bones, growth plate cartilage, and articular cartilage. The tracheal rings and bronchial and laryngeal cartilages are also hyaline. The name is derived from the semitransparent, glassy nature of hyaline cartilage. In its apparently homogeneous matrix is concealed a dense system of collagen fibers which is highly ordered in articular cartilage and will be discussed in Chapter 5.

Fibrocartilage is, in a sense, a mixture of hyaline cartilage and ligament. Histologically, it consists of islands of hyaline cartilage in a dense mass of

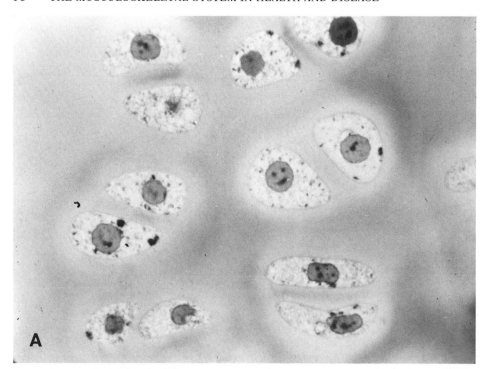

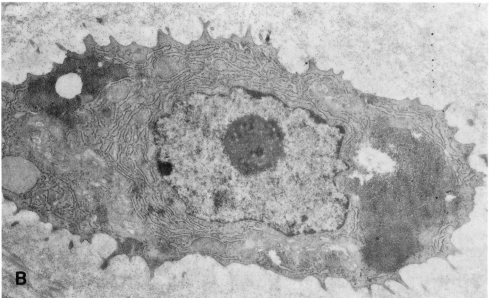

FIG. 2-10. Hyaline cartilage. **A.** The chondrocytes are embedded in amorphous matrix which exhibits different staining properties in the vicinity of the cells and in acellular regions. The fibrous components of the matrix are not visible in such light microscopic preparations. Most of the chondrocytes occur in pairs suggesting that they became entrapped soon after mitosis. (Courtesy of Dr. John H. Luft) (× 700) **B.** In this electron micrograph of a chondrocyte from hyaline cartilage, the similarity to a fibroblast is quite evident (Fig. 2–1). Note the euchromatic nucleus, prominent nucleolus, extensive rough surfaced endoplasmic reticulum, and Golgi apparatus. The cell contains two large and several smaller accumulations of glycogen granules. Note also the amorphous matrix. (Silberman M: J Anat [London]:Jan, 1978) (× 8000)

collagen fibers not surrounded by, and therefore not obscured by, cartilaginous ground substance. Functionally, it combines the tensile strength of ligament with the resistance of compression and shearing forces of cartilages. It occurs in intervertebral and other intraarticular disks.

Elastic cartilage contains elastic fibers in addition to other components. It is found in the pinna of the ear and in the epiglottis.

Calcification normally occurs in hyaline cartilage in advance of endochondral bone formation. It also occurs as a normal age change. The laryngeal cartilages may begin to calcify as early as 20 years of age, but calcification in articular cartilage normally does not occur even in advanced age.

BONE

Bones of the skeleton are discrete organs which have anatomically defined parts and consist of several tissues. The gross anatomy of bones is discussed together with the skeleton in Chapter 7. The subject matter of this section is the principal tissue of bones, namely **bone tissue** and the tissues directly concerned with its *de novo* formation and growth. Bone is formed either in embryonic mesenchyme or in hyaline cartilage, and its growth depends on the proliferation of cartilage and on matrix deposition by the periosteum.

Bone is a mineralized connective tissue whose cells, the **osteocytes,** are enclosed in lacunae of the rigid matrix, maintain contact with one another by cytoplasmic processes, and in their morphology are similar to fibroblasts (Fig. 2–11). Osteoblasts and osteocytes secrete all the organic components of bone matrix, 90 percent of the protein of which is collagen. This collagen is identical to that found in tendon, ligament, fascia, and loose connective tissue, but it is distinct from the collagen of cartilage (see Fig. 2–4). On the other hand, bone matrix shares with hyaline cartilage the notable property of being calcifiable. It is important to recognize, however, that bone differs qualitatively from calcified cartilage, and the difference lies chiefly in the architecture of the two tissues and in their content of proteoglycans. While cartilage is essentially of homogeneous construction and relatively avascular, bone is highly porous and highly vascular.

Unlike chondroblasts and fibroblasts, osteoblasts are polarized cells in that they secrete matrix initially only from the cell surface facing the bone. Subsequently, the matrix is refashioned into thin **lamellae,** the architectural arrangement of which meets precisely the mechanical stresses to which a particular bone is subjected. Such adaptability is wanting in calcified cartilage. Thus bone is a living tissue—hard, supportive, and protective, yet also plastic, resilient, changeable, and reparable. It also serves as an important store of quickly usable calcium and other electrolytes.

Ossification

All bones develop in preexisting connective tissue templates. With the exception of the shaft of the clavicle and a number of bones of the skull, all bones of the human skeleton are preformed in hyaline cartilage and the first nidus of ossification appears in these cartilaginous templates at a time which is predetermined and is characteristic for each bone. Thus, the vast majority of bones are formed by a process known as **endochondral ossification.** In the remaining few, the connective tissue template of the bone is not cartilage but embryonic mesenchyme, and hence the process of their development is known as **mesenchymal ossification** (or **intramembranous ossification** since the majority of these bones are the squamous or *membrane* bones of the vault of the skull).

It should be emphasized before discussing these processes in detail that the cellular and extracellular events of bone tissue formation are essentially identical in mesenchymal and endochondral ossification. In both instances the source of osteogenic cells capable of secreting bone matrix is embryonic, perivascular, loose connective tissue or mesenchyme. Although cartilage proliferation is necessary for the growth of bones preformed in cartilage, once growth is accomplished the cartilage becomes calcified, serving merely as an inert scaffolding upon which immigrant, mesenchymal osteogenic cells deposit bone matrix. Cartilage is *never* transformed into bone; it is eliminated and replaced by newly formed bone.

Despite the basic similarity in mesenchymal and endochondral ossification, it is useful to consider the two processes separately, not only for the sake of clarity but because different genetically determined mechanisms seem to regulate them. For instance, in cleidocranial dysostosis the congenital defect in bone formation affects mesenchymal ossification, in achondroplasia endochondral bone is defective, while in osteogenesis imperfecta both are abnormal.

Mesenchymal (Intramembranous) Bone Formation. The mesenchyme representing the primordium of membrane bones and of the clavicle becomes well vascularized before ossification begins.

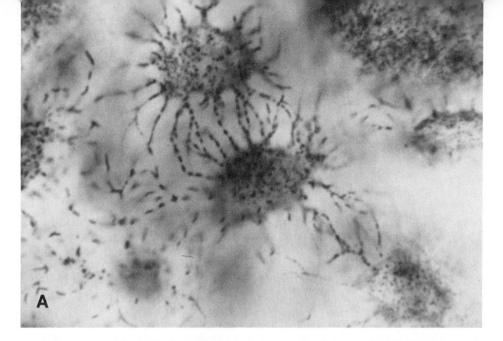

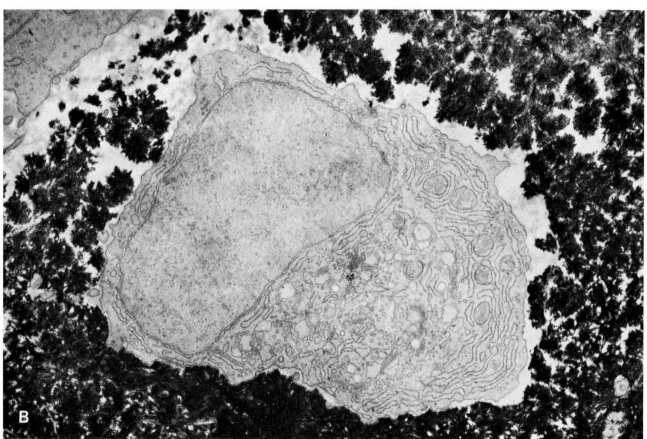

FIG. 2–11. **A.** Osteocytes in the newly ossified parietal bone of the fetal mouse skull. The thin calcified matrix is transparent to the light microscope and osteocytes can be seen maintaining contact with one another through processes that occupy canaliculi. (Courtesy of Dr. H. Kashiwa) (× 700) **B.** Electron micrograph of an osteoblast. Electron dense hydroxyapatite crystals in the matrix almost completely surround the cell. The matrix in the immediate vicinity of the cell is uncalcified and in the light microscope would appear as a lacuna. Note the extensive rough endoplasmic reticulum and the Golgi apparatus. Compare with Figures 2–1 and 2–10. (× 6000)

The perivascular mesenchymal cells proliferate, enlarge, develop prominent nucleoli, numerous ribosomes, rough surfaced endoplasmic reticulum, and begin the active synthesis of a new type of matrix. This **osteoid matrix** is identifiable by its staining properties that differentiate it from the surrounding mesenchyme. Such a focus is known as an **ossification center** and the differentiated cells may now be regarded as **osteoblasts.** They align themselves almost like an epithelium along the strands of the osteoid matrix, maintaining contact with each other through cytoplasmic processes. The production of collagen and proteoglycans continues, and soon thin, needlelike crystals of hydroxyapatite make their appearance in the osteoid matrix. The crystals develop from calcium phosphate, and they are deposited under the influence of osteoblasts both in relation to the collagen fibrils and proteoglycans. The mineralized bone trabeculae form an interlacing network (primary spongiosa). As calcification progresses many of the osteoblasts become surrounded by hydroxyapatite crystals within the calcifying matrix. Once entrapped, these cells lose their capacity for proliferation and are designated as **osteocytes.** Osteocytes occupy small lacunae in the bone and retain cell contact with their fellows through minute **canaliculi.** Bone tissue is thus established. The spaces remaining in this primitive bony labyrinth are filled with vascular mesenchyme which develops into hemopoietic bone marrow.

Since interstitial growth in the rigid matrix is not possible, growth of this tissue proceeds by progressive incorporation and transformation of surrounding mesenchyme. This type of newly formed bone is often called **woven bone** because of the coarse, interlacing network of collagen fibers within its matrix. Later, the collagen fibers are deposited in regular parallel bundles determined by the vascular channels and the lines of stress. In this process, the trabeculae are also remodeled establishing the definitive architecture of **spongy** or **cancellous bone.** The vascular, rather dense, connective tissue membrane surrounding the bone retains osteogenic cells throughout life and it is known as the **periosteum.** A more delicate layer of cells, the **endosteum,** lines the spaces of the bony labyrinth and contributes to bone deposition but its chief role in the remodeling process of bone is resorption.

Endochondral Bone Formation. Bone is formed within and upon the hyaline cartilage models which foreshadow the shape of definitive bones.

These bars or masses of cartilage have developed earlier from mesenchyme and are surrounded by a fibrovascular membrane, the **perichondrium.** The sequence of events of ossification is shown schematically in Figure 2–12. The first signs of imminent ossification in the cartilage template, for instance of a femur, are heralded by the enlargement and subsequent degeneration of chondrocytes in the center of the shaft. The lacunae of dying chondrocytes also enlarge, and the vacuolated cartilage matrix soon begins to calcify. Osteoid matrix is first deposited circumferentially upon the surface of the shaft, creating a *collar* around the calcifying cartilage matrix. The osteogenic cells are derived from the perichondrium—now properly called the periosteum—and the osteoblasts enact the entire scenario of mesenchymal bone formation, complete with mineralization of the deposited osteoid.

This thin, subperiosteal, bony collar is hardly formed when it is broken through by blood vessels surrounded by periosteal mesenchyme containing osteogenic cells. The vascular sprouts penetrate into the degenerating cartilage and ramify within its spaces. The immigrant osteogenic cells align themselves along the surfaces of the calcified partitions in the cartilage matrix and begin the laying down of osteoid (Fig. 2–13). Thus a so-called **primary ossification center** is formed.

The areas of central and subperiosteal bone formation soon became confluent and extend toward the two ends of the bone. The calcified cartilage matrix entrapped within the bony trabeculae will be completely eliminated as the trabeculae are eroded (Fig. 2–13C) and the mesenchyme-filled spaces become confluent, creating the **medullary cativy.** The mesenchyme differentiates into endosteum and hemopoietic bone marrow which later in life is transformed into fatty marrow.

The unossified terminal cartilage grows by proliferation of chondroblasts and interstitial synthesis of new cartilage matrix, apace with radial growth of the bone through subperiosteal bone matrix formation. In the majority of bones sooner or later new ossification centers appear within the terminal cartilage at one or both ends (Figs. 2–12 and 2–14A). These are the **secondary ossification centers.** In most long bones such centers are multiple but they eventually fuse into a single mass of bone. The ossification process recapitulates that described for the primary center, albeit without subperichondral bone collar formation. The bones remain cartilaginous at their articular ends and the vascular osteogenic mesenchyme breaks

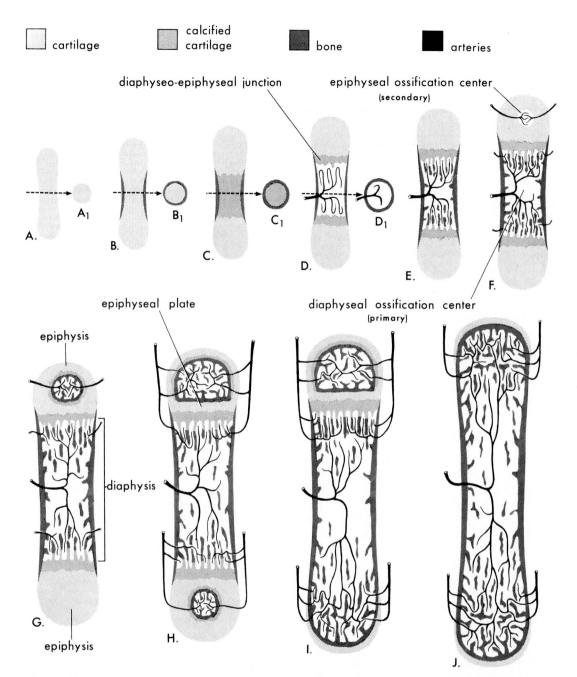

FIG. 2–12. Schematic representation of endochondral ossification and the development of a typical long bone. **A** to **J** are longitudinal sections and **A₁** to **D₁** are cross sections at the levels indicated. **A.** Cartilage model of the bone. **B.** Subperiosteal collar of bone appears. (Hypertrophy of cartilage is not illustrated.) **C.** Cartilage begins to calcify. **D.** Vascular osteogenic mesenchyme enters the calcified cartilage and the primary ossification center is established. **E.** Calcification of cartilage advances toward the ends of the bone primordium, followed by ossification. The medullary cavity is established. **F.** Blood vessels and osteogenic mesenchyme enter the upper epiphysis. **G.** The epiphyseal or secondary ossification center is established, with epiphyseal plate interposed between it and the diaphyseal (primary) ossification center. **H.** A secondary ossification center develops in the lower epiphyseal cartilage. **I.** The lower epiphyseal plate is ossified but growth proceeds at the upper epiphyseal plate. **J.** The upper epiphyseal plate ossifies. (Moore KL: The Developing Human, 2nd ed. Philadelphia, WB Saunders, 1977. Based on Bloom W, Fawcett DW: A Textbook of Histology, 10th ed. Philadelphia, WB Saunders, 1975)

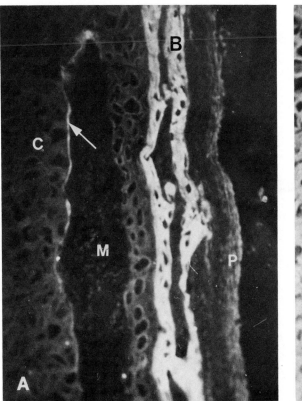

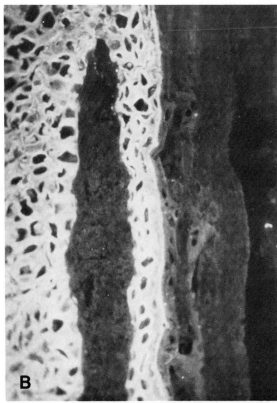

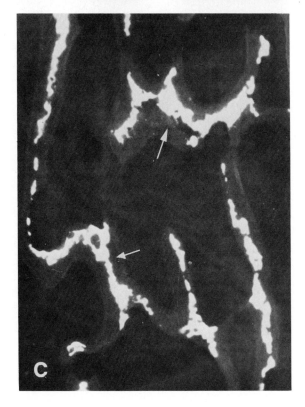

FIG. 2-13. Ossification of the chick's tibia. **A** and **B** represent the same microscopic field from a section of a 19-day-old embryo. The specimen has been stained for type I and type II collagen, respectively (see description in Fig. 2–4) to illustrate the distribution of cartilage and osteoid matrix. (B = bone; C = calcified hypertrophic cartilage; M = mesenchyme and primitive bone marrow; P = periosteum) In **A** bone matrix is fluorescent and is present immediately subjacent to the periosteum. Osteoid matrix has been deposited also as a thin layer on the calcified cartilage by osteogenic cells of the mesenchyme. In **B** cartilage matrix is fluorescent. Section **C** is from a 3-week-old chick stained for type II collagen (cartilage matrix). The brightly stained trabeculae of the calcified cartilage matrix are being resorbed as osteoid matrix **(arrows)** is being deposited upon their surfaces from the mesenchyme-filled spaces. (Courtesy of Dr. K. von der Mark) (× 200)

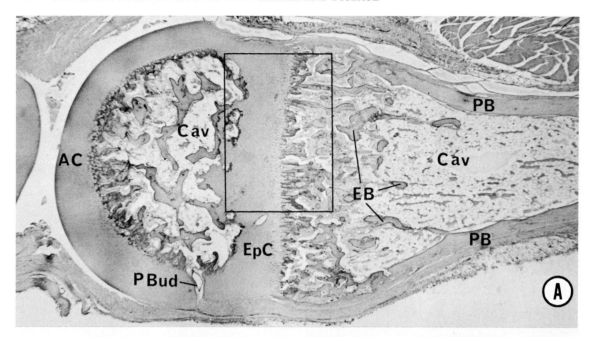

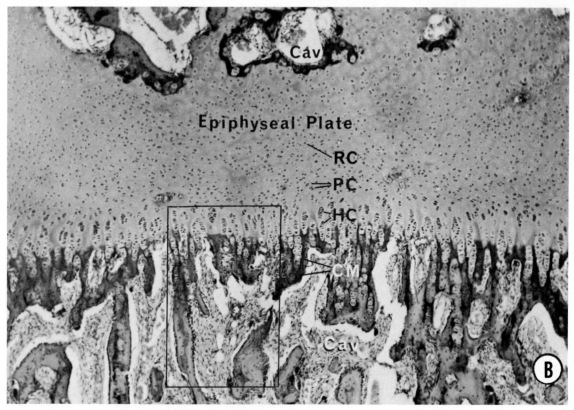

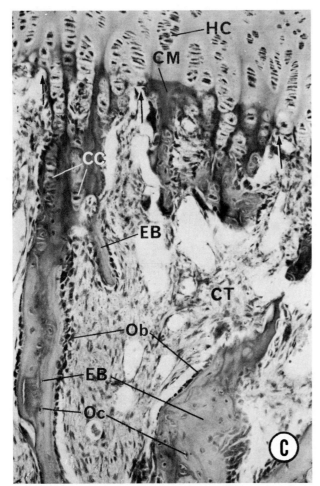

◀ FIG. 2–14. Photomicrographs of endochondral ossification and bone growth in a long bone of monkey at increasing magnifications. **(A)** The epiphyseal growth plate (EpC) separates the epiphysis, covered by articular cartilage (AC), from the diaphysis, surrounded by periosteal bone (PB). The endochondrally formed bone (EB) contains vascular connective tissue and differentiated marrow cells in its cavities (Cav) in both the epiphysis and the metaphysis. **(B)** In the epiphyseal plate, layers of proliferating (PC) and hypertrophied (HC) chondrocytes are found only on the side of the metaphysis. Toward the epiphysis the chondrocytes are resting (RC). **(C)** Arrows indicate areas of resorption of calcified cartilage matrix (CM). Cartilage cells (CC), osteoblasts (Ob), and osteocytes (Oc) are also labeled. (Reith EJ, Ross MH: Atlas of Descriptive Histology. New York, Harper and Row, 1977) (**A,** × 16; **B,** × 40; **C,** × 160)

through this cartilage and invades the calcified matrix of the secondary ossification center (Fig. 2–14A).

The shaft of the bone developing from the primary ossification center may now be defined as the **diaphysis,** and the secondary ossification centers, which by their growth come to occupy most of the articular ends of the bones, form the **epiphyses.**

Bone Growth

It is characteristic of bone growth that new tissue is added to existing surfaces, interstitial expansion being precluded by the rigid, mineralized matrix. This process is relatively simple in mesenchymal ossification exemplified by the growth of membrane bones and the radial growth of bones ossified in cartilage. Longitudinal growth of endochondral bones takes place by the addition of new bone at their ends, and this depends on the proliferation of cartilage.

A layer of modified cartilage persists between the diaphysis and epiphysis for a period of time. This cartilage is the **epiphyseal plate** or **growth plate** (Fig. 2–14). Although the epiphyseal plate grows with the bone in a transverse direction as the diaphyseal diameter enlarges, its *raison d'être* is to determine the *longitudinal* growth of bones and ultimately the height of the individual.

Chondrocytes of the epiphyseal plate are aligned in longitudinal rows or palisades (Fig. 2–14C), but the functional organization of the growth plate is transverse. This is important to appreciate because vertical splitting of a growth plate involved in a fracture will not distort growth significantly but transverse or shearing trauma can arrest growth and lead to permanent deformity (see Chap. 28).

The **zone of growth** is adjacent to the epiphysis and is characterized by interstitial growth of the cartilage and proliferation of chondroblasts. Their division in the long axis of the bone generates the palisades of chondrocytes and is responsible for longitudinal growth. The **zone of ossification** is adjacent to the diaphysis. Here the enlarged lacunae have been vacated by dead chondrocytes and the calcified cartilage matrix is being invaded by vascular osteogenic mesenchyme from the medullary cavity. Between these two zones is the **zone of transformation** characterized by chondrocyte hypertrophy, degeneration, and endochondral calcification. Thus, bone is formed by the same process as in the primary and secondary ossification centers. The newly formed bone is remodeled and the medullary cavity extends into this zone of remodeling. The advancing front of ossification is a particularly vascular area of the bone, and it corresponds to the region of a bone known as the **metaphysis.**

Growth hormone plays a part in controlling the growth rate of epiphyseal cartilage. Pituitary malfunction leads to gross skeletal abnormalities such as dwarfism, gigantism, and acromegaly. Other hormones, including estrogen, testicular and adrenal androgens, and thyroxin also influence skeletal growth directly or indirectly. The longitudinal growth of bones is halted by fusion of the epiphysis with the diaphysis, an event also under hormonal control. The time of epiphyseal fusion is characteristic of individual bones and is achieved by ossification of the epiphyseal plate. The line of fusion remains recognizable in many bones as a dense line throughout the life of the individual (see Fig. 7–4).

Circumferential or radial growth is accomplished by subperiosteal bone formation. This process is precisely coordinated with longitudinal growth and bone resorption. During their growth bones attain their characteristic shape and their medullary cavity enlarges. The mechanisms of

FIG. 2–15. A section of decalcified human lamellar bone stained with hematoxylin and eosin. The marrow cavity is seen on either side of this bony trabecula. In **A** the section is viewed in normal illumination and some of the lacunae and canaliculi are clearly discernible. In **B** the lamellar structure of the trabecula is more dramatically demonstrated by viewing the same section in polarized light. As the inorganic bone salts have been removed, the lamellae consist of collagen fibers embedded in osteoid ground substance. (Hancox NM: Biology of Bone. Cambridge, Cambridge University Press, 1972)

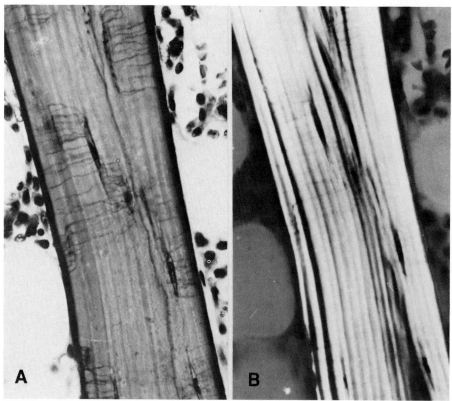

bone remodeling and the establishment of definitive bone structure are the concern of the following section.

Bone Resorption and Deposition

Bone resorption begins as soon as bone is first formed, whether by mesenchymal or endochondral ossification. Bone formation and resorption will go on hand-in-hand throughout the life of the individual, for decades after bone growth has ceased. These two dynamic processes determine the adaptable structure of mature lamellar bone and, to a large extent, also the homeostasis of calcium and phosphate ions in blood and extracellular fluid. The latter will be the concern of Chapter 21 while this section deals with how the definitive structure of bone is established.

Deposition of Lamellar Bone. The woven bone first deposited in ossification centers, under the periosteum, or in a healing fracture always becomes replaced by **lamellar bone.** Lamellar bone consists of 5–7μm thick sheets or plates of bone tissue in which collagen fibers and hydroxyapatite crystals associated with the fibers are arranged in regular, parallel arrays that run within the plane of the lamella (Fig. 2–15).

The formation of lamellar bone is always preceded by endosteal resorption of existing bone. The most active osteolytic agents are specialized, multinucleate phagocytic cells, known as **osteoclasts.** These cells were believed to have common mesenchymal ancestors with osteoblasts, but recent evidence suggests that they may be derived from macrophages.

In cancellous bone, while resorption proceeds on one surface of a trabecula, a new lamella is being deposited on the other surface by osteogenic activity of the endosteum. Several parallel lamellae make up each trabecula and these lamellae are not penetrated by blood vessels. The nourishment of osteocytes entrapped in the lamellae depends on diffusion from the vascular bone marrow. Mechanical stress acting on the bone plays a major role in determining the orientation of the newly deposited lamellae (Fig. 2–16). This is probably mediated in part by a *piezoelectric effect.* In crystalline sub-

FIG. 2–16. The upper end of the femur showing the definite arrangement of bony lamellae in cancellous bone. The specimen shown in **A** has been prepared by John Hunter, an 18th century anatomist and surgeon. It has been decalcified and cut in the coronal plane. Only the fixed osteoid matrix remains. **B** is an x-ray of a femur which exhibits a lamellar architecture. Therefore inorganic bone salts are responsible for generating this image. The deposition of the mineral phase of bone conforms to the orientation of the organic matrix which is secreted by the cells.(**A** Courtesy of Huntarian Museum, Royal College of Surgeons, London; **B** courtesy of Dr. Rosalind H. Troupin)

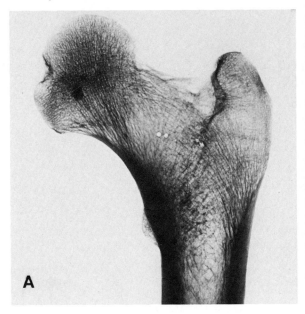

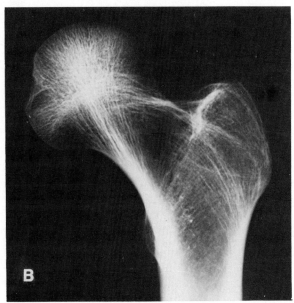

stances small electric currents are generated when they are deformed. It is possible that such currents polarize osteolytic and osteogenic cells in such a way that bone is reorganized to resist the force tending to deform it.

The woven bone of the subperiosteal collar over the diaphysis is resorbed by endosteum as the bone grows and the medullary cavity expands. New bone is deposited by the periosteum in a lamellar form. Several such circumferential lamellae remain immediately underneath the periosteum (Fig. 2–17). To these lamellae is anchored the periosteum and also by stronger fibers (Sharpey's fibers), tendons, and ligaments. However, deeper lamellae become replaced by smaller units as diaphyseal bone becomes thicker and is pervaded by blood vessels. Most of the blood vessels are de-

rived from the periosteum, and they traverse the lamellae in so-called **Volkmann's canals.** New concentric lamellae are deposited around the terminal, capillary branches of these vessels forming cylindrical, paper-scroll-like units. The majority of these units are oriented in the long axis of the bone and are known as **osteons** or **haversian systems.** So-called **interstitial lamellae** which are the unabsorbed portions of circumferential lamellae or of previous osteons remain identifiable as the relics of the preexisting bone.

Each osteon consists of a central **haversian canal** (containing an arteriole or capillary) and 4–20 concentric lamellae (Fig. 2–18). Canaliculi connect osteocytes within a lamella and also between adjacent lamellae. The structure of the lamellae is identical to that of the trabeculae in cancellous bone

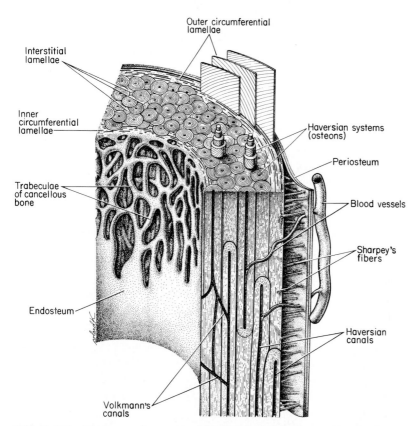

FIG. 2–17. Diagram of a sector of the shaft of a long bone illustrating the disposition of the lamellae in the osteons or haversian systems, the interstitial lamellae, and the outer and inner circumferential lamellae. (Bloom W, Fawcett DW: A Textbook of Histology, 10th ed. Philadelphia, WB Saunders, 1975)

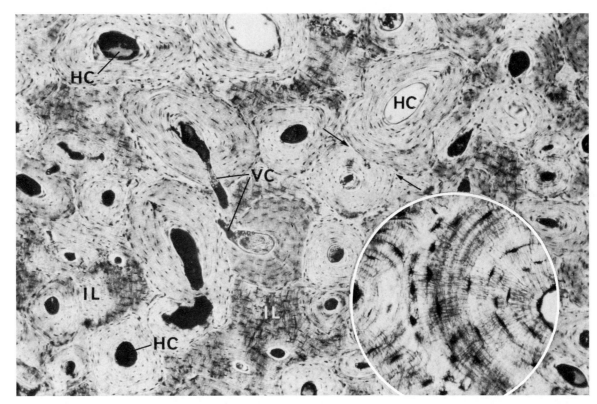

FIG. 2–18. Photomicrograph of a ground section of compact bone. The section was treated with India ink. Volkmann's canals (VC) transmit blood vessels to haversian canals (HC), and both as well as the lacunae of osteocytes appear black. The osteocytes situated in concentric lamellae are interconnected by minute canaliculi (inset). Arrows point to an osteon which is being resorbed. Interstitial systems or interstitial lamellae (IL) are evident between the haversian systems. (Reith EJ, Ross MH: Atlas of Descriptive Histology, 3rd ed. Harper & Row, 1977)

but the *arrangement* of the lamellae is profoundly different. In distinction from cancellous or spongy bone, bone constructed of osteons is known as **compact bone,** and it is found characteristically on the surface of all bones, being the thickest in the shaft of long bones where spongy bone is trivial or nonexistent.

Resorption and deposition of osteons takes place from the haversian canal, both potentially osteolytic and osteogenic cells being present in the pericapillary connective tissue. The canal enlarges during resorption, while newly deposited lamellae constrict it. A sharp line, the cement line, indicates the frontier to which resorption progressed before reverting to bone deposition. Most recently formed lamellae are the most central and, being less mineralized, are less radioopaque and tracer elements incorporated into bone (radioisotopes, alizarin red, tetracyclenes) are first detectable in them (Fig. 2–19). These are important parameters in the evaluation of bone biopsies (see Chap. 21).

TURNOVER AND REGENERATION IN CONNECTIVE TISSUES

In all tissues a continuous input and output process takes place on the molecular, cellular, and tissue level. This process is called turnover. In a stable equilibrium, the input is quantitatively equal to the output. Turnover occurs in all levels of biologic organization.

Cellular turnover in the various forms of connective tissue is slow. Fibroblasts, osteocytes, and

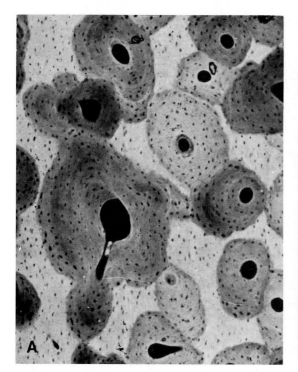 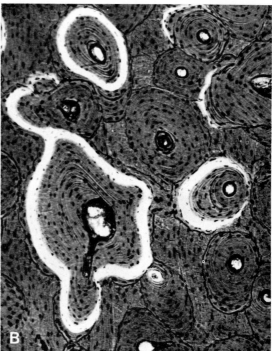

FIG. 2-19. Sections of bone from the midshaft of the human fibula. **A** In this historadiogram differing shades of gray in the scales from nearly white to nearly black reflect the differing concentrations of calcium. In the haversian canals there has been no absorption of the x-rays and the film is therefore black. The most recently deposited haversian systems are incompletely calcified and appear dark gray, whereas older ones containing high concentrations of calcium are lighter. The old interstitial lamellae being fully calcified are most highly absorbent and therefore appear white. **B** The 14-year-old girl from whom this specimen was taken had been given a daily dose of the antibiotic Achromycin for 15 consecutive days at one period of her illness. Amputation of the leg was carried out about 230 days later. Achromycin is incorporated into the matrix of bone being deposited at the time of its administration and imparts a fluorescence to the newly formed bone. In the section shown here, transilluminated with ultraviolet light in a fluorescent microscope, the white areas represent areas of bone laid down during the 15-day Achromycin treatment. The nonfluorescent central portion of the same haversian systems represents bone deposited after cessation of the treatment. (Bloom W, Fawcett DW: A Textbook of Histology, 10th ed. Philadelphia, WB Saunders, 1975)

chondrocytes normally do not proliferate in the fully grown individual. However, in wound healing or fracture repair, dividing connective tissue cells can be observed. Because of this proliferative potential, the regenerative capacity of loose connective tissue and bone is excellent. On the other hand, regeneration is limited in cartilage, tendon, and ligaments. In these tissues scar formation is achieved by the associated loose connective tissue and any regeneration is due to the reorganization and transformation of this tissue.

Despite the proliferative inactivity of connective tissue cells, the active and continuous synthesis of extracellular proteins provides for uninterrupted molecular turnover in the matrix of ordinary connective tissue, cartilage, and bone. Such turnover is readily documented with pulse and chase studies using radioactive amino acids (Fig. 2–20). Degradation of connective tissue proteins by specific enzymes maintains the tissue in equilibrium with the synthetic process. The same cell may be involved in the regulation of both phenomena.

Due to the unique amino acid composition of collagen and other connective tissue proteins, analysis of degradation products in the blood and urine can give an assessment of the turnover of

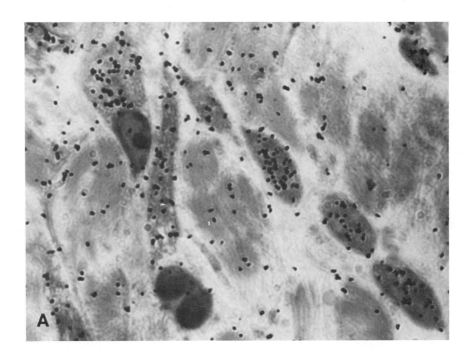

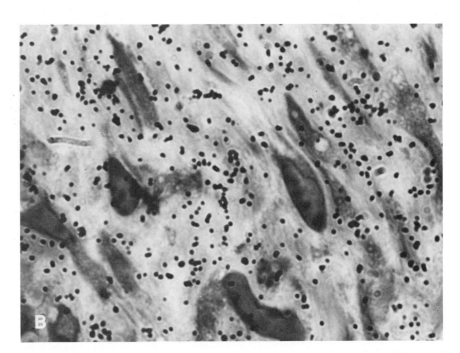

FIG. 2–20. Radioautographs prepared from sections of a 10-day-old wound in the skin of a guinea pig. The animal was injected with ³H-proline, an amino acid incorporated into collagen. Section **A** was obtained 30 min after the injection and the radioautographic grains are concentrated over the cytoplasm of fibroblasts, an evidence of the uptake of ³H-proline. Section **B** was obtained 4 hours after the injection, by which time the labeled material has been secreted into the matrix as collagen. The cells are now unlabeled.

these proteins. For instance, blood and urinary levels of hydroxyproline and hydroxylysine can be used to determine the turnover of collagen in various disease states. Under physiologic conditions and following injury the mechanisms of turnover provide the means for remodeling the connective tissues in response to environmental factors.

An appreciation of tissue turnover is essential to the understanding of both the pathogenesis and the treatment of musculoskeletal abnormalities, particularly the response to injury. The normal balance in turnover may be disturbed in certain disease states. Excessive amount of scar formation by the connective tissue of various organs may seriously interfere with their function. This is the case, for instance, in cirrhosis of the liver and in damaged cardiac and skeletal muscle. Regeneration of liver and muscle cells is limited by the excessive amount of fibrous tissue formed. It is essential to gain an understanding of the mechanisms that regulate tissue turnover in order to be able to control such pathologic phenomena.

The turnover of bone is of particular importance and this is discussed further in Chapter 21. Bone turnover, including organic and inorganic components is 2–3 percent of the skeletal mass per year in adults, but after the fifth decade bone resorption exceeds deposition, and bone loss may proceed at 5–10 percent per decade.

The exchange of ions between bone salts and the tissue fluid and circulation is an important factor upon which homeostasis of various electrolytes relies. Only 1 percent of total body calcium is not in bone and bone also contains, for instance, half of the body sodium. Exchange of ions between the tissue fluid and bone matrix is assured over an enormous surface area, some 100 acres, represented by the crystals of bone salts that are exposed in haversian canals and on bony trabeculae. The factors which control homeostasis of calcium and phosphate ions and regulate the turnover of these substances in bone, are discussed in Chapter 21.

SUGGESTED READING

Bell GH: Living bone as an engineering material. Adv Sci 26:1, 1969–1970
Discusses the types of forces bone is subjected to and the factors which give bone mechanical strength.

Bloom W, Fawcett DW: A Textbook of Histology, 10th ed. Philadelphia, WB Saunders, 1975
The chapter on connective tissue, cartilage and bone give well-written, well-illustrated accounts of these tissues with bibliography.

Bornstein P, Byers, PH: Disorders of collagen metabolism. In Bondy P, Rosenberg L (eds): Metabolic Control and Disease, 8th ed. Philadelphia, WB Saunders 1979
An up-to-date treatise correlating various steps in collagen synthesis with a number of diseases in which connective tissue abnormalities can be identified.

Hancox NM: Biology of Bone. Cambridge, Cambridge University Press, 1972
A very readable small book.

O'Rahilly R, Gardner E: The embryology of bone and bones. In Ackerman LV, Spuit HJ, and Abell MR (eds): Bones and Joints. Baltimore, Williams & Wilkins, p 1, 1976
Beautifully illustrated brief account based on human embryos of the Carnegie collection.

Prockopp DJ, Guzman NA: Collagen diseases and the biosynthesis of collagen. Hosp Pract 12:61, 1977
A concise exposition of the major steps in collagen synthesis, correlated with some known collagen defects and their clinical manifestations.

Ramachandran GN, Reddi AH (eds): Biochemistry of Collagen. New York Plenum Press, 1976
An up-to-date, multi-author, comprehensive treatise, dealing with the organization and chemistry of connective tissue.

Ross R, Bornstein P: Elastic fibers in the body. Sci Am 224:44, 1971

Sandberg LB, Gray WR, Frangblau C (eds): Elastin and Elastic Tissue. New York, Plenum Press, 1977
An excellent collection of papers covering all aspects of what is known about elastic tissue.

von der Mark KH, von der Mark H, Gay S: Study of differential collagen synthesis during development of the chick embryo by immunofluorescence. Dev Biol 53:153, 1976
One of the more recent studies dealing with the synthesis of collagens of different types during osteogenesis.

3
Skeletal Muscle

ALBERT M. GORDON, CORNELIUS ROSSE

Almost half of the body weight of man is constituted of skeletal muscle tissue. The fundamental property of this tissue is contractility and its primary function is to generate force and thereby produce and prevent movement of the body and of its parts. This large tissue mass is divided into several hundred discrete muscles each of which may be considered a true organ with a specific function. The function of individual muscles is to control the movement of specific parts of the skeleton.

Muscles attach to bones via tendons and cross one or more joints. When contraction shortens the muscle, movement is produced at the joint, but when contraction occurs without a change in muscle length, the joint will be stabilized and movement by other forces will be resisted. In either event, stored chemical energy is converted by the muscle into mechanical energy.

Skeletal muscles are under the direct control of the voluntary nervous system. Activation of muscle contraction is achieved by impulses that arise in the central nervous system, proceed along axons, and are transmitted to the muscle at specialized neuromuscular junctions. Afferent impulses are generated within muscles and tendons by changes in length, tension, and speed of movement, and these impulses are fed back to the central nervous system. Through the reflex arcs thus established the voluntary movements are monitored, and at the same time other muscles are activated reflexly which cancel out or prevent unwanted movements. This chapter deals with the structure and physiology of muscle as a tissue. The control of muscle contraction is the subject of Chapter 4.

THE STRUCTURE AND FORM OF MUSCLES

The contractility and structure of skeletal muscle cells or muscle fibers is similar in all muscles. The infinitely graded variety of actions muscles are capable of exerting in terms of power, range, and precision of movement largely depends on the three-dimensional arrangement of muscle fibers and fiber bundles. The pattern is defined by connective tissue septa that interlace muscles and delineate their macroscopic and microscopic subunits.

Anatomic Subunits of Muscles

Connective Tissue of Muscles. All muscles are ensheathed by a continuous layer of deep fascia, or **epimysium,** which defines the muscles anatomically and facilitates their sliding on surrounding structures. Connective tissue septa extend inward from the muscle's fascia and this **perimysium** subdivides the muscle into macroscopically visible fiber bundles or **fasciculi.** In their finest extensions the septa surround all individual muscle fibers, the cellular units of skeletal muscle, and constitute the **endomysium** (Fig. 3–1).

This extensive connective tissue stroma subserves three important functions.

1. It largely determines the extent of stretching and deformability in a relaxed muscle, lending it elasticity and a certain degree of stiffness.
2. It constitutes the pathways for nerves, blood vessels, and lymphatics.
3. It transmits the forces generated by the muscle to bones and functions as a spring or the *series elastic element.*

Nerve and Blood Supply. Nerves and blood vessels enter muscles at one or two well defined points (neurovascular hila) by piercing the muscle's fascia and then arborizing in the connective tissue septa. The capillaries embedded in endomysium surround individual muscle fibers, and the terminal branching of axons takes place also in this tissue. The nerve that enters the muscle contains both sensory and motor fibers (see Fig. 4–2). The motor fibers are the axons of numerous anterior

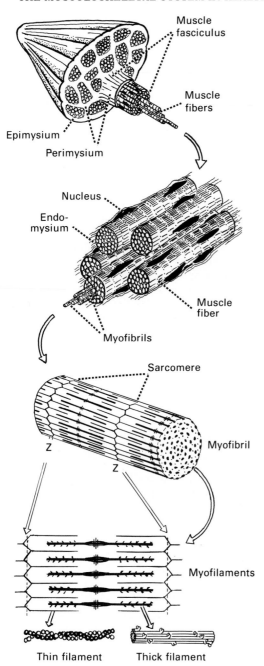

FIG. 3-1. Diagrammatic representation of the organization of skeletal muscle from the gross anatomic to the submicroscopic level. Subunits of a whole muscle are shown with the associated connective tissue elements. (Redrawn from Warwick R, Williams PL (eds): Gray's Anatomy, 35th ed. Philadelphia, WB Saunders Co, 1973)

horn cells (motor neurons) and are gathered from one or as many as four spinal cord segments (Chaps. 10 and 12).

The Motor Unit. Each muscle fiber is innervated by one of the terminal branches of an axon. The collection of muscle fibers supplied by the terminal branches of one axon derived from a motor neuron is called a **motor unit.** The motor unit is the unit of contraction in skeletal muscle, and when the motor neuron fires, all its fibers contract synchronously. Several motor units are included in a muscle fasciculus and these units are activated in turn during normal muscle action.

The size of the motor unit is determined by the number of muscle fibers innervated by a single motor neuron. Motor unit size is large (several hundred fibers per nerve cell) in the large lower limb muscles, and small (under 10) in muscles concerned with fine movements such as the muscles of the eye. Powerful muscles have a coarse texture due to large muscle fasciculi, whereas in muscles concerned with precise movements, the fasciculi are fine.

Muscle-Tendon Relationship. The anchoring of the muscle is accomplished via its connective tissue stroma which condenses into a tendon at the muscle's site of origin and insertion. With few exceptions, such as the muscles of the tongue, facial expression, or certain voluntary sphincters, the origin and insertion of most muscles are on bone. At the myotendinal junction (see Fig. 2–9), force is transmitted from the muscle fibers to the endomysium, to the tendon, and then to the periosteum and bone. Collagen fibers of the tendon can be traced directly into the bone matrix as Sharpey's fibers.

Some muscle fibers are as long as the muscle (more than a foot long in the sartorius for instance), while others terminate in the muscle's connective tissue stroma. Tendon is always present at muscle attachments even though macroscopically this attachment appears to be entirely fleshy. On the other hand, in muscles which exert their action at a distance the tendon may be longer than the muscle itself.

Arrangement of Muscle Fasciculi

The overall size and shape of a muscle and the arrangement of its fasciculi are adapted to the

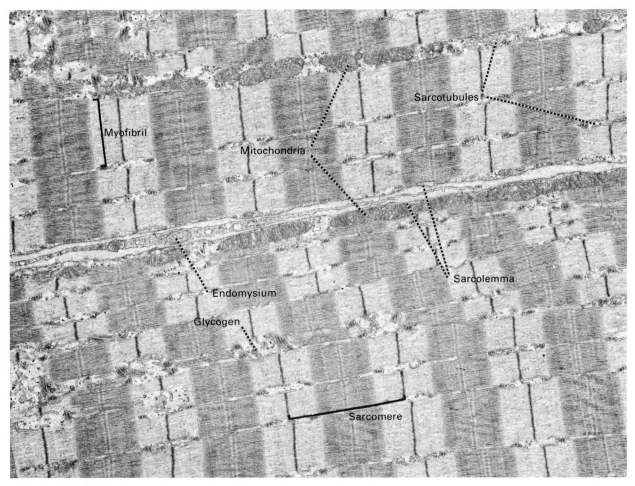

FIG. 3-2. Electron micrograph of a longitudinal section of two adjacent muscle fibers from guinea pig vastus muscle. A fibroblast in the endomysium is interposed between the two muscle fibers. The basement membrane is discernible on the outer surface of the sarcolemma as a glycoprotein coating slightly more electron dense than the connective tissue matrix between the fibers. The myofibrils are stacked in less than perfect register. Their banding pattern and their filamentous structure is evident at this magnification but is more clearly illustrated in Figure 3–3. Large mitochondria are aligned longitudinally beneath the sarcolemma and they are seen also among the myofibrils, lying in both transverse and longitudinal directions. This section does not include any muscle cell nuclei which lie subjacent to the sarcolemma in the same plane as the mitochondria. Note also profiles of sarcotubules and glycogen granules in between the myofibrils. The extent of a sarcomere is indicated. (Courtesy of B. R. Eisenberg, A. M. Kuda and Journal of Ultrastructural Research) ($\times$ 12,000)

range of movement and strength required at the joint it serves. The range of effective movement is dependent on the length of muscle fibers. Since muscle fibers can shorten to approximately half their length, long muscles produce a greater range of movement than short ones. This direct relationship holds true only if the fasciculi are more or less parallel to the muscle's line of pull as in strap muscles (rectus abdominis) or in fusiform muscles (biceps brachii). When the fasciculi are oblique to the line of pull, represented usually by the tendon of insertion, only a proportion of the force generated is effective in producing movement. However, this arrangement lends itself to increasing the number of muscle fibers without unduly increasing the muscle's diameter.

Oblique muscle fiber arrangements include forms that resemble a triangle, a half or complete feather form (*unipennate* and *bipennate*, respectively), and composite or *multipennate* forms where several tendons receive the obliquely set fasciculi. The loss of efficiency in force transmission to the tendon is outweighed in practice by the large number of short fibers such muscles are composed of. Powerful movements of limited range are executed, as a rule, by muscles composed of obliquely set fibers. Some muscles are twisted or spiralized. Their contraction untwists them, usually resulting in rotation of the bone they move.

The actual range and type of movement produced by a muscle is modified by factors independent of the muscle's architecture. These factors include 1) the shape of articular surfaces at the joint served by the muscle, 2) leverage, and 3) the action of stabilizing, synergistic and antagonistic muscles. These factors are discussed in Chapters 4 and 5, while our present objective is to explain the mechanism of contraction which is the basic property of the muscle fiber.

THE MUSCLE FIBER

The Muscle Cell

The muscle fiber is a multinucleated cell highly specialized for contraction. Muscle fibers are long, cylindrical cells ranging in diameter from 10–100μm. Each may contain several hundred nuclei.

Around 80 percent of the fiber volume is constituted by contractile protein fibrils, the **myofibrils,** longitudinally arranged in the fiber. The myofibrils possess a highly regular banding pattern revealed by the electron microscope (Fig. 3–2). Be-

cause the myofibrils are stacked in register, the entire muscle fiber acquires a transversely striated appearance (Figs. 3–1 and 3–2). The transverse striations are visible in the optical microscope whether the fiber is examined in the fixed or living state.

Mitochondria are sandwiched between the myofibrils or are displaced together with all the nuclei to the peripheral part of the cytoplasm (known as the **sarcoplasm**) and lie subjacent to the **sarcolemma** which is the limiting membrane (i.e., plasmalemma) of the muscle cell. Outside the sarcolemma is an external coating of glycoproteins or basement membrane and a fine network of reticular fibers, an integral part of the endomysium.

In addition to the sarcolemma, two membrane-bound tubular systems play an important role in the initiation of contraction. The first consists of the **sarcotubules** and constitutes the **sarcoplasmic reticulum,** which surrounds the myofibrils and is similar to the endoplasmic reticulum of other cells but has relatively few ribosomes associated with it. The second is characterized by tubular invaginations of the sarcolemma, which tunnel through the muscle fiber in transverse direction and are known as **transverse tubules** or **T-tubules.** Both membrane systems will be discussed further, and they are illustrated in Figure 3–3.

The sarcoplasm contains scattered ribosomes necessary for protein synthesis, clusters of glycogen granules (a source of energy in muscle), Golgi bodies, lysosomes, and lipid granules. Besides the principal proteins of the myofilaments, the sarcoplasm contains some myoglobin as well as other

---

FIG. 3–3. Electron micrograph of guinea pig soleus muscle. In **A** the muscle is cut longitudinally while **B** through **D** are transverse sections across the appropriate bands of the sarcomere. The I band contains only thin filaments. Tortuous mitochondria and sarcotubules interlace between the myofibrils in this band **(B).** In the lateral portions of the A band, the arrays of thick and thin filaments are telescoped into one another **(A),** and a transverse section cut slightly obliquely at this level **(C)** reveals the two types of myofilaments more clearly. In the upper part of **C** the hexagonal arrangement of the thin filaments around the thick ones can be made out; whereas below, the section has passed into the H zone where only thick filaments are present. The complex dense structure of the Z line is illustrated in **D.** Numerous sarcotubules course through the Z disk between bundles of thin filaments. The M line is discernible in the center of the H zone in the longitudinal section **(A).** Compare with Figure 3–1. (Courtesy of B. Eisenberg, A. M. Kuda, J. B. Peter; J. Cell Biol. [**A**] and 30th Annual Proceedings of Electron-Microscopy Society of America [**B. C. D.**])

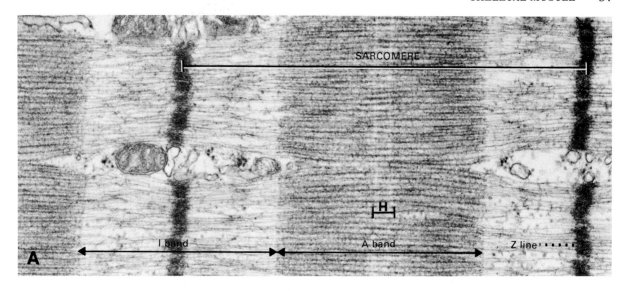

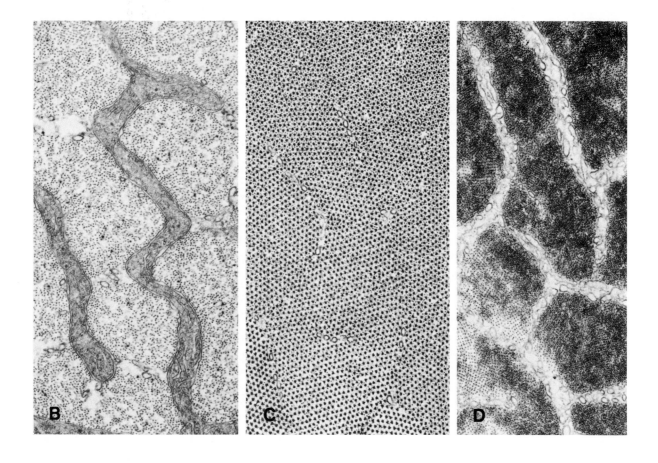

Myosin Molecule

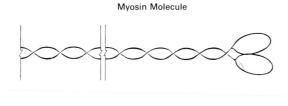

Thick Filament

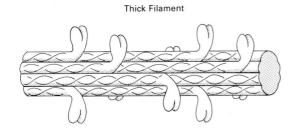

Thin Filament

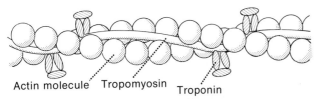

Actin molecule   Tropomyosin   Troponin

FIG. 3-4. Schematic representation of the molecular structure of myofilaments. For explanation see text.

proteins and a variety of substances which are involved in metabolic processes of the muscle cell.

Myofibrils and Myofilaments

The myofibrils are cylindrical structures, 1–2μm in diameter, and run the entire length of the muscle fiber (see Fig. 3–1). They are composed of two types of longitudinally disposed filamentous subunits, the thick and thin myofilaments. The **thick filaments** are made primarily of the protein *myosin* and the **thin filaments** are composed chiefly of the protein *actin* associated with two other proteins, *tropomyosin* and *troponin*. The interaction and sliding of the two types of filaments in relation to one another forms the basic mechanism of muscle contraction.

Thick and thin filaments are around 1.6 and 1.0μm long, respectively, each type being stacked in precise arrays. The overlapping arrays of myosin and actin filaments define the bands visible in the myofibrils (Figs. 3–1, 3–2, 3–3).

The Banding Pattern. The aligned array of the thick filaments represents the **A band** (so named because in polarized light it behaves *anisotropically*). In the central zone of the A band (**H zone**), only myosin filaments are present, but these filaments interdigitate with the thinner actin filaments on either side of the H zone (Fig. 3–3). Transverse connections secure the midpoints of the myosin filaments to one another and this line of cross links is resolved as the **M line** in the center of the H zone.

The lighter band between adjacent A bands is occupied by the thinner actin filaments and is known as the **I band** (so named because in polarized light it behaves *isotropically*) (Fig. 3–3). Across the center of the I band the ends of actin filaments in one array are secured to filaments of the neighboring array by complex cross linkages creating the **Z line** which is more conspicuous than the M line. The serially repeating units of myofibrils between two Z lines are the **sarcomeres.**

When the muscle fibers shorten, the two sets of filaments slide into one another, reducing the widths of the I and H bands (or even completely obliterating them), while the width of the A band remains virtually unaltered. Thus muscle shortening takes place *not* by the shortening of individual filaments but by the sliding of units of fixed lengths, similar to the sliding of the pieces of a telescope. To appreciate this mechanism, it is necessary to understand the molecular configuration and three-dimensional arrangement of the myofilaments.

Molecular Structure of Myofilaments. Over 100 **myosin molecules** make up a thick filament. The myosin molecule is shaped rather like a golf club. Its straight "handle" or tail piece consists of two strands helically coiled *(light meromyosin)*. The globular head *(heavy meromyosin)* is actually bilobed. The tail pieces are aligned parallel to one another forming the backbone of the thick filament, while the globular heads protrude laterally. The protrusions are aligned spirally on the surface of the myofilament and are directed toward the actin filaments (Figs. 3–1, 3–4). In contraction the myosin heads play the more active part. They perform three functions: 1) bind adenosine triphosphate (ATP) at a specific site on the molecule, 2) act as an ATPase enzyme catalyzing the hydrolysis of ATP to adenosine diphosphate (ADP) plus inorganic phosphate (P_i), 3) interact with proteins of the thin filament forming *crossbridges*.

Actin molecules are a globular protein which are

aligned in two single strands that entwine helically and make up the actin filament (Fig. 3–4). A second protein, **tropomyosin,** is bound to the actin helix in the two grooves between its two monomers. At regular intervals a third globular protein, **troponin,** is present on the surface of the filament. The troponin molecule actually consists of three subunits. The tropomyosin-troponin complex is believed to perform two apparently contrasting functions: 1) inhibit crossbridge formation by hindering interaction of myosin heads with the actin molecules and 2) bind calcium ions which cancel out the inhibitory action and thereby promote crossbridge formation.

The Three-Dimensional Arrangement of Myofilaments.

A transverse section across the A band (Fig. 3–3) reveals that thick and thin filaments are distributed in an ordered pattern within the myofibril. Six actin filaments surround a centrally placed myosin filament in a hexagonal lattice. At high resolutions the laterally projecting globular heads of myosin molecules are also evident in such a plane. It is the prevailing view that when a myofibril shortens, the myosin filament slides, making and breaking contact between its spirally arranged lateral projections and the actin molecules of the six surrounding thin filaments. By this mechanism, further discussed below, the actin filaments are advanced along the myosin filaments producing more and more overlap between the arrays of thick and thin filaments.

Membrane Systems of the Muscle Fiber

The transverse tubules and the sarcoplasmic reticulum display a particular orientation to the sarcomere (Fig. 3–5). **T-tubules** penetrate among the myofibrils and aborize in a transverse plane that in human skeletal muscle corresponds to the junction of the A and I bands. T-tubules are not continuous with the sarcoplasmic reticulum but are intimately related to it. The sarcoplasmic reticulum is a regular repeating structure composed of longitudinally oriented tubules which surround the myofibrils. At the level of the A–I junction the tubules coalesce into a **terminal cistern** where they abut against the transverse tubules. Each transverse tubule is contacted by two terminal cisternae, one on either side. The T-tubule and two apposed terminal cisternae constitute the **muscle triads.** In human skeletal muscle there are two triads per sarcomere but in human cardiac muscle or amphibian skeletal muscle there is only one,

located at the Z line. The triads play a key role in muscle contraction. The action potential generated at the neuromuscular junction on the sarcolemma is propagated along the muscle fiber membrane and into the muscle fiber along the T-tubule system. The depolarization of the T-tubule membrane causes the release of calcium ions from the terminal cisternae, an event which initiates contraction.

MUSCLE CONTRACTION

The Molecular Basis of Contraction

During contraction, the sliding of the two sets of filaments occurs because of cyclic interaction between proteins on the thick and thin filaments. Strong bonds are established between binding sites on the bilobed myosin heads and binding sites on the actin molecules forming a complex called **actomyosin.** The high energy compound, **ATP,** which is actually bound to the myosin head, participates in this cyclic interaction in the way illustrated in Figure 3–6.

Actin binds strongly to myosin in the actomyosin complex ($1 \rightarrow 2$, Fig. 3–6). ATP dissociates this complex into actin and myosin with the ATP remaining bound on the myosin ($3 \rightarrow 4$, Fig. 3–6). Since myosin is an ATPase, the ATP on the myosin is hydrolyzed in a series of steps to produce ADP and inorganic phosphate (P_i). Several conformational changes occur in the myosin during these reactions. The steps between the formation of the hydrolysis products on the myosin and their dissociation contain at least one slow step. Thus myosin by itself is a poor ATPase. Actin appears to speed up this process by binding to the complex of myosin plus the hydrolysis products, and allows dissociation of the hydrolysis products to occur more rapidly ($2 \rightarrow 3$, Fig. 3–6). Actin thus makes myosin a better ATPase.

It is not known how the energy liberated by ATP is made available to provide a relative force between the two sets of filaments. However, the filaments appear to have a polarity such that the thin filaments are propelled toward the center of the thick filaments. During contraction the interactions take place many times at many different sites between myosin and actin filaments throughout the sarcomere. If the muscle is held at a constant length, interactions presumably occur a number of times at one site. If the muscle is allowed to shorten, the interactions take place consecutively at a number of sites along the filaments. When

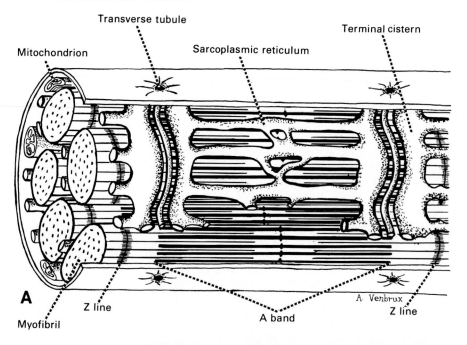

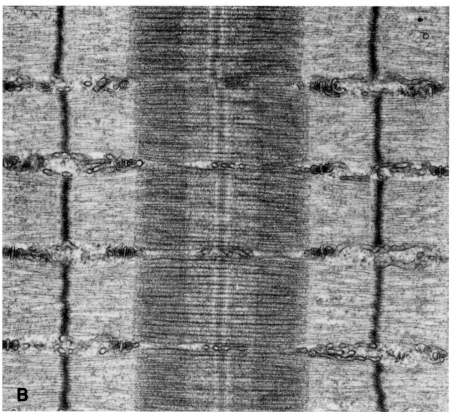

energy is liberated at each of the sites, presumably the projection angle of the myosin head becomes altered, permitting an advancement of the actin filament. Thereafter, new crossbridge formation becomes possible with the next actin molecule. Highly schematically, one could look at the projection of thick filaments as oars that connect with the thin filament and row the thick filament along with respect to the thin filament.

Electrical Events

In the intact body, muscle contraction is initiated by nerve impulses generated in motor neurons of the central nervous system and transmitted along axons to motor end plates where new impulses are set up on the muscle fibers. These impulses or action potentials spread along the sarcolemma and the system of transverse tubules triggering contraction of the fiber. An *impulse* is a transient change in the *potential difference* across the cell membrane of nerve and muscle. These electrical events are treated here only in a summary form; for more comprehensive discussion of the phenomenon, the reader is referred to the selected readings listed at the end of the chapter.

The Action Potential. If a microelectrode is inserted into an axon or a muscle fiber and a second electrode is applied near the outer surface, an electrical charge difference or voltage can be recorded *across* the cell membrane. This polarized state characterized by a potential difference *across* the cell membrane is typical of all resting cells and is known as the **resting potential.** The resting potential (70–90 mv), due to charges separated by the lipid/protein membrane which serves as an electrical capacitor, arises because the membrane actively transports ions, and because the membrane is selectively permeable to ions. Sodium (Na^+) is actively pumped out and potassium (K^+) is actively pumped in, establishing concentration gradients of these two cations between the exterior

and interior of the cell. The extracellular concentration of Na^+ is much greater than its concentration in the intracellular fluid, whereas the concentration gradient for K^+ is in the reverse direction. These concentration differences create the tendency for K^+ and Na^+ to diffuse in reverse directions. Because the resting muscle cell membrane is many times more permeable to the diffusion of K^+

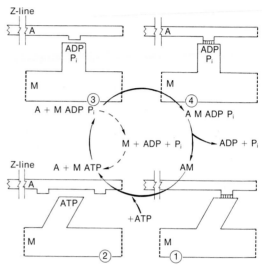

FIG. 3–6. A highly schematic diagram illustrating a possible model for coupling ATP hydrolysis by myosin (M) assisted by actin (A) to crossbridge interaction and movement of the thick (M) and thin (A) filaments (muscle shortening). The arrows show in summary the chemical reactions taking place in the hydrolysis of ATP to ADP and inorganic phosphate (P_i) catalyzed by myosin. They are as follows: steps 1–2, ATP dissociates actin and myosin; steps 2–3, myosin hydrolyzes the bound ATP. As shown by the **interrupted arrow** ADP and P_i dissociate slowly from myosin if Ca is not present (absence of Ca prevents interaction with actin). The free myosin then rebinds ATP, hydrolyzes it and rejoins the cycle at step 3; steps 3–4, actin binds to myosin with attached hydrolysis products; steps 4–1, actin binding allows the hydrolysis products to dissociate more rapidly than from myosin alone **(interrupted arrow).** The diagrams show schematically thick and thin filaments and crossbridge positions that might be associated with each of these chemical states, 1–4. State 3 corresponds to the resting state in muscle. Low Ca prevents the interaction of A and M · ADP · P_i. State 1 corresponds to rigor mortis. In this scheme, energy from the hydrolysis of ATP would be stored as conformational change in the crossbridge. This energy would be released as the bridge moves (state 4–1) while the bridge is attached, producing a relative sliding of the two filaments with respect to each other. (After Huxley HE, Chap 7 in Bourne GE: The Structure and Function of Muscle, Vol. 1) New York, Mederic Press 1972

◄**FIG. 3–5. (A)** Schematic, three-dimensional representation of the membrane systems in a segment of a human skeletal muscle fiber. **(B)** Electron micrograph of a segment of a muscle fiber showing the profiles of muscle triads located opposite the junctions of A and I bands. Note the sarcotubules most prominent in I band regions. Comparison of **A** and **B** will put the exaggerations of the schematic representation into perspective. Refer also to Figure 3–2. (Courtesy of B. R. Eisenberg, A. M. Kuda and J. Ultrastruct. Res.)

than to Na^+, the net result is a tendency for K^+ to diffuse out of the cell making the inside negative with respect to the outside. Consequently, the resting potential of the membrane is manifest by positive charges on the outside and negative charges on the inside of the cell membrane.

A small decrease in the internal negativity (depolarization) of the cell to threshold will set off the action potential. The action potential is produced by a depolarization because the sodium channels of the cell membrane open transiently in response to this change in membrane potential. The opening of these channels allows entry of sodium ions, which tends to decrease further the internal negativity of the cell. This further depolarization in turn tends to open more sodium channels. Thus a regenerative cycle is set up, resulting in a rapid decrease in the internal negativity of the cell, which becomes manifest as the action potential. The action potential is a brief depolarization because the sodium channels are open only transiently. In some excitable cells, potassium channels also open to allow K^+ to exit, helping to repolarize the cell. These changes in membrane permeability which account for the action potential are diagrammed in Figure 3–7.

Propagation of the Action Potential. Now that the generation of an action potential at one point on a nerve or muscle cell has been described, the question arises, How does this action potential propagate from that point to the rest of the excitable cell? Propagation of the action potential along the nerve or muscle fiber occurs because the fibers are in an ionic medium; thus, the differences in membrane potential along the fibers cause ions to flow, which tends to minimize the potential. Charges will flow between resting and active regions of the axon or muscle fiber, and, therefore, the resting regions will experience a depolarization, tending to bring them to the threshold. In this manner the action potential spreads along the nerve or muscle fiber.

Motor axons are myelinated and the action potential appears to jump from one node of Ranvier to the next, whereas in the muscle fiber the impulse spreads without interruption from the motor end plate along the sarcolemma to both ends of the muscle fiber. Transmission of the impulse from the terminal branches of axons to muscle fibers takes place by a chemical transmitter which is released at neuromuscular junctions, specialized structures known as **motor end plates** or the **myoneural junction.**

Neuromuscular Transmission

The Motor End Plate. The terminal branch of the motor axon, having lost its myelin, is covered over by the remaining Schwann cell (teloglial cell) like a lid, leaving the bulbous axon terminal directly exposed to a specialized, recessed area of the sarcolemma (Fig. 3–8). The Schwann cell, axon terminal, and sarcolemma constitute the motor end plate.

The axon terminal contains mitochondria and numerous vesicles in which the chemical transmitter **acetylcholine** is believed to be stored (Fig. 3–8D). The axolemma remains separated everywhere by a 300–500 A wide gap from the sarcolemma which retains its glycoprotein covering throughout. This subneural sarcoplasmic membrane or plate forms a trough into which the axon terminal is recessed. In addition, the plate is thrown into numerous minor folds, greatly increasing its surface area and creating a large number of subneural clefts. Mitochondria abound in the subjacent sarcoplasm.

The Chemical Transmitter. Depolarization of the axon terminal due to the arrival of an action potential causes the release of acetylcholine from a number of vesicles (around 300) into the gap of the end plate, permitting its diffusion toward the subneural plate to which it becomes bound by special receptors. The presence of Ca^{++} ions is necessary for acetylcholine release to occur from the axon terminal. This Ca^{++} enters the nerve terminal from the extracellular fluid. The interaction of acetylcholine with the receptors leads to depolarization of the subneural sarcolemma and this depolarization is called the **end plate potential.** When threshold level is reached an action potential is generated which will then be propagated in both directions toward the ends of the muscle fiber.

Some of the acetylcholine that is released binds reversibly to the receptors, but the free acetylcholine can be hydrolyzed by **acetylcholine esterase,** an enzyme present in the gap. Acetylcholine can also diffuse out of the end plate gap. Removal of acetylcholine from the receptors and elimination from the end plate gap by hydrolysis or diffusion terminates the end plate potential. These events happen rapidly enough in normal motor end plates that one action potential in the nerve terminal produces only one action potential in the muscle fiber.

Disorders of Neuromuscular Transmission. Two diseases illustrate the effect of disorders

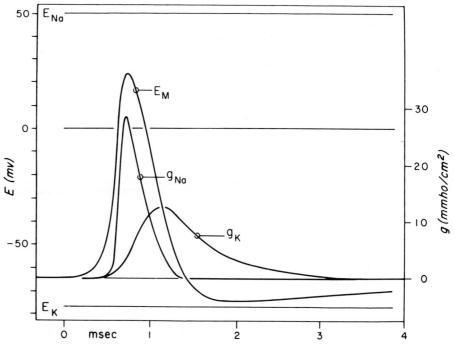

FIG. 3–7. Calculated time courses of the propagated action potential and underlying conductance changes from measurements on a squid axon. The curve labeled E_M is the action potential with E_M being the membrane potential. g_{Na} is the Na conductance and g_K the potassium conductance. Note the great increases in g_{Na} and g_K and the delayed onset of g_K. Notice that the depolarization precedes the g_{Na} increase (opens Na channels), but that g_{Na} decreases before repolarization (Na inactivation). The increased g_K occurs at about the same time as the repolarization. (Hille B, Chap 4 in Brookhard JM, Mountcastle VB, Kandel ER, Geiger SR (Eds): Handbook of Physiology, Vol. I. Bethesda, American Physiological Society, 1977); originally from the work of Hodgkin and Huxley, 1952.

in neuromuscular transmission; myasthenia gravis and the myasthenic syndrome. Both present clinically as weakness but the weakness develops in contrasting patterns in the two conditions.

In **myasthenia gravis,** muscles become increasingly weak with repeated attempts at using them. For instance, the sustained effort of keeping the eyes open leads to increasing weakness of the muscles that elevate the eyelids until they fail, resulting in ptosis. The condition is believed to be due to circulating antibodies directed against the acetylcholine receptors of the subneural sarcolemma. These antibodies bind to the receptors leaving but few available to acetylcholine. Thus in a motor end plate, less depolarization is produced by the normal quanta of the transmitter released from the axon. Because it takes some time to resynthesize acetylcholine, repetitive stimulation will tend to deplete the available acetylcholine supply and the depolarization produced by acetylcholine released by successive nerve impulses will become smaller and smaller and will not reach threshold for an action potential. Thus the weakness becomes more and more apparent.

In **myasthenic syndrome,** the muscle is weak at the outset and gathers strength as movement is repeatedly attempted. It has been shown in patients suffering from the syndrome that fewer prejunctional vesicles are released by activation of the axon terminal than in normal motor end plates. A single impulse, therefore, may release an insufficient amount of acetylcholine for inducing an action potential at the sarcolemma. Repeated impulses allow more Ca^{++} to enter the nerve terminal, increasing the number of quanta of the transmitter released per impulse into the subneural clefts to make initiation of an action potential in the muscle more probable. Repeated attempts of the movement will achieve this state at increasing numbers of motor end plates, and the contraction of the muscle will progressively gather strength.

In addition to these and other diseases a number of drugs block neuromuscular transmission (e.g., curare and curarelike substances). These agents are poisons and kill by paralyzing the muscles of respiration. They are also used as muscle relaxants during surgery and then ventilation of the lungs has to be provided mechanically.

Excitation-Contraction Coupling

In resting muscle the interaction of actin and myosin filaments necessary for muscle contraction is prevented. It is the prevailing view that the regulator protein tropomyosin-troponin complex associated with the actin filament hinders crossbridge formation between the myosin heads and the actin molecules. This inhibitory action is dependent on the *absence* of calcium ions in the

FIG. 3–8. A motor endplate shown schematically in **A, B,** and **C** and in an electron ▶ micrograph in **D.** In **A** the endplate is seen with the light microscope in a section along the longitudinal axis of the muscle fiber and in **B** in a surface view. An area such as outlined by the rectangle in **A** is shown in **D** and is schematically reproduced in **C.** In **D** note the endplate gap in the subneural trough and subneural clefts, the vesicles and mitochondria in the bulbous axon terminal, the glycoprotein coating of the sarcolemma and the numerous mitochondria in the sarcoplasm. (**A** through **C** Bloom W, Fawcett DW: A Textbook of Histology, 10th ed. Philadelphia, WB Saunders, 1975; **D** courtesy of Dr. D. E. Kelly)

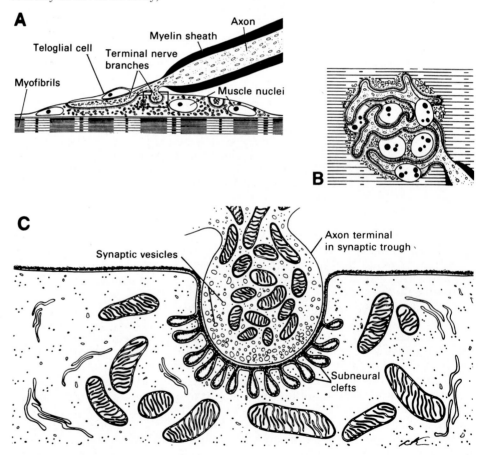

A

Axon
Myelin sheath
Teloglial cell
Terminal nerve branches
Myofibrils
Muscle nuclei

B

C

Synaptic vesicles
Axon terminal in synaptic trough
Subneural clefts

sarcoplasm, and becomes abrogated when calcium ions are made available. The activation of contraction requires an action potential which results in the entry of calcium ions into the sarcoplasm. Therefore, in the last analysis the control of contraction in skeletal muscle is achieved by the control of sarcoplasmic Ca^{++} concentration.

Control of Sarcoplasmic Ca^{++} Concentration.

Calcium is concentrated and stored by the sarcoplasmic reticulum through a "calcium pump" or transport system which avidly transfers Ca^{++} from the sarcoplasm into the sarcotubules. Hydrolysis of ATP is required for this process.

Depolarization of the sarcolemma in the T-tubule system caused by the action potential spreads down the T-tubule from the surface into the interior of the muscle and induces the release of Ca^{++} from the terminal cisternae of the reticulum. The precise mechanism of this Ca^{++} release is not

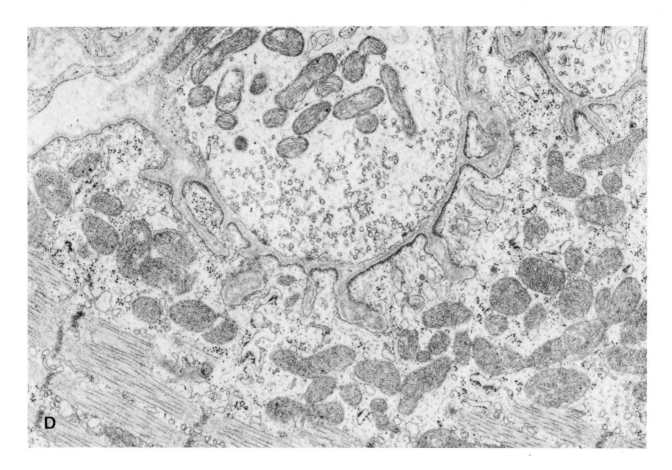

D

known at present. Nevertheless, the liberated Ca^{++} can now combine with troponin and crossbridge formation can proceed.

Activation of Crossbridge Formation. In relaxed muscle, tropomyosin is so situated on the actin helix that it "blindfolds" the binding sites on the actin molecules thereby sterically hindering combination with matching binding sites on the myosin heads. When Ca^{++} ions become available in the sarcoplasm, they combine with troponin located at regular intervals along tropomyosin, causing the latter to "roll" into a position in its groove which uncovers the binding sites on the actin molecules (Fig. 3–9). The myosin heads can now contact these sites and the crossbridge can be formed.

As discussed earlier, the crossbridges will be made and broken through the combined action of actin, myosin, and ATP, while the actin filament is moved along by the energy liberated by the hydrolysis of ATP on myosin. Ca^{++} dissociates from troponin and the binding sites become covered once more by the regulator proteins. The dissociated Ca^{++} will be taken up by the sarcoplasmic reticulum. To maintain the muscle in contraction these events need to be repeated through incoming nerve impulses leading to repeated Ca^{++} release and a maintained sarcoplasmic Ca^{++} level.

This scheme of Ca^{++} activation through troponin does not apply to all muscles. Some muscles do not contain troponin and are activated by Ca^{++} binding to the thick filaments. Other muscles (e.g., smooth muscle) may be controlled by Ca^{++} through phosphorylation of myosin. In all cases Ca^{++} appears to trigger an event which allows interaction of crossbridges.

Hypocalcemic Tetany

A decline in the free serum calcium concentration can bring on a condition called hypocalcemic tetany. Hypocalcemia can be produced by a number of diseases and conditions, such as hypoparathyroidism, hyperventilation, vitamin deficiency, excessive loss of fat in the stools, or faddish diets. All lead to symptoms involving hyperexcitability of nerves and muscles. The symptoms include carpopedal spasms (extreme flexion of wrist or ankle), Chvostek's sign (contraction of facial musculature in response to mechanical stimulation of a facial nerve), laryngeal spasms, and emotional hyperirritability or convulsions. How does a fall in free serum calcium cause these symptoms?

Calcium plays a major role in at least three of the processes necessary for adequate control of muscular contraction. These processes are neuromuscular transmission, excitation-contraction coupling, and control of the excitability of the cell membrane in nerve and muscle. In neuromuscular transmission and excitation-contraction, calcium is a facilitator. At the neuromuscular junction, Ca^{++} is necessary for transmitter release. In the muscle,

FIG. 3–9. Schematic representation of how Ca^{++} controls actin and myosin interaction in some muscles. On the left, in the absence of Ca^{++}, tropomyosin hides the binding site from myosin and the muscle is relaxed. On the right, in the presence of Ca^{++}, the tropomyosin moves into the groove exposing the binding site, allowing interaction, and the muscle contracts.

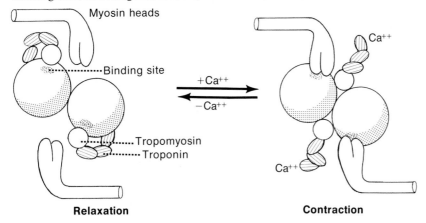

excitation causes release of calcium from the sarcoplasmic reticulum which allows the contractile proteins to interact. Therefore, it might be expected that low calcium levels would lead to either block of transmission at the neuromuscular junction or block of excitation-contraction coupling within the muscle. These are opposite to the increased tendency for muscle contractions observed in patients with hypocalcemic tetany. The solution of the paradox has to be sought in the third effect of calcium which is exerted on the cell membrane. Calcium directly affects the excitability in such a manner that a decrease in serum calcium leads to hyperexcitability of the cell membrane. This effect becomes manifest before neuromuscular transmission or excitation-contraction coupling could be affected, and it is the cause of the hyperexcitability seen in hypocalcemic tetany.

Although calcium can affect all three phenomena, the levels of free calcium on which these phenomena rely are different in the three cases. As the ionized level of calcium in the serum is decreased from its normal value of near 1.2 mM (total calcium is about 2.5 mM), the first property to be affected is membrane excitability. Membranes become more excitable. The tendency to tetany increases as the free level of calcium falls below 1 mM. If the level of free (ionized) calcium is reduced still further, blockage will occur at the neuromuscular junction due to the inability of nerve terminal depolarizations to release sufficient transmitter. Finally, as the ionized calcium level is reduced below 0.1 mM, excitation-contraction coupling in the muscle will be blocked. Excitation-contraction coupling in skeletal muscle is insensitive to free calcium because the calcium level in the sarcoplasmic reticulum in skeletal muscle is insensitive to extracellular calcium. (This is not true in cardiac muscle where cardiac contractility depends strongly on free Ca^{++}.) Thus, although theoretically lowering the serum calcium could affect a number of sites in the motor unit, membrane excitability of both nerves and muscles is affected first in hypocalcemia, and this explains all the observed manifestations of hypocalcemia.

The mechanism of increased membrane excitability due to hypocalcemia can be explained by the relationship which exists between extracellular calcium and the increase in sodium permeability of the membrane brought about by membrane depolarization. Figure 3–10 illustrates this. At a given membrane potential, the sodium permeability that can be turned on by depolarization is higher with low serum calcium than it would be

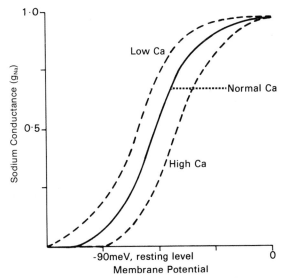

FIG. 3–10. Effect of extracellular Ca^{++} on the relationship between the membrane potential and the maximal g_{Na} achieved by a depolarization to that potential. The curve is shifted to the left as extracellular Ca^{++} is decreased. For depolarizations above the resting potential, a greater sodium conductance (g_{Na}) is achieved at the lower Ca^{++}, resulting in greater excitability.

with normal serum calcium. The membrane "thinks" it is more depolarized than it is. Normal excitability of nerves and muscle cell membranes is caused by the fact that depolarization causes an increase in sodium permeability (or conductance) leading to entry of sodium into the cell, which, in turn, results in further depolarization, and so forth (see page 41, The Action Potential). Thus, shifting this relationship between sodium permeability and membrane potential makes the membrane more excitable.

MECHANICAL PROPERTIES OF MUSCLE

The foregoing section dealt with the contractile units of skeletal muscle, the response of which to an activating stimulus was momentary contraction followed by relaxation. The performance of muscles in the intact body is infinitely more complex than this simple on-or-off response. It is the purpose of this section to analyze the basic mechanical properties of muscles which explain their behavior when they are activated in the body.

It is necessary first to define a few simple terms

and concepts. Contraction of a muscle fiber generates **force.** Muscle force and tension are used synonymously. There is tension in the muscle as it produces force. If the muscle length is held constant the contraction is **isometric.** If the muscle length is allowed to change, the muscle force will equal the weight (load) as the muscle contracts and this contraction will be termed **isotonic.** If the load is less than the isometric force that the muscle can produce, the muscle will shorten and lift the load. If the load is greater than the isometric force, the load elongates the actively contracting muscle which resists this lengthening.

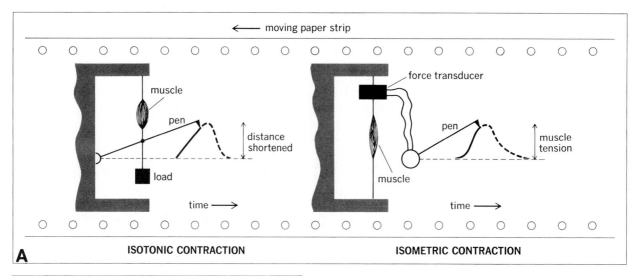

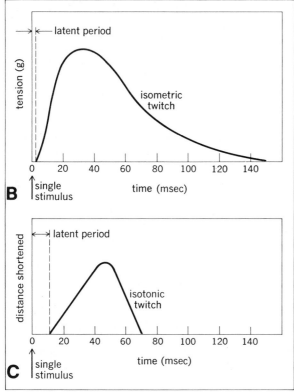

FIG. 3–11. Isotonic and isometric muscle contraction. **A** shows the method of recording. The mechanical response of the muscle to a single stimulus of approximately 1 msec duration is a biphasic twitch whether the exchange is recorded as tension **(B)** or as shortening **(C).** (Vander AJ, Sherman JH, Luciano DS: Human Physiology, 2nd ed. Copyright © McGraw-Hill, New York, 1970. Used with permission of McGraw-Hill Book Company)

Slow and Fast Twitch Muscles

The Muscle Twitch.   The response of a muscle fiber or of a whole muscle to a single electrical stimulus delivered either directly to the muscle or to its motor nerve is a brief contraction or a twitch which can be observed or recorded by measuring either the shortening of the muscle (isotonic contraction) or the increase in muscle tension if the muscle is held isometrically. Figure 3–11 illustrates the recording of a muscle twitch.

There are fast and slow twitch muscles in the body and the duration of the muscle twitch varies from muscle to muscle but is characteristic for given muscles of an individual. For instance, in muscles responsible for eye movements (e.g., internal rectus) the muscle twitch lasts approximately 10 msec, whereas in a large leg muscle such as the soleus, it is about 100 msec. In both slow and fast twitch muscles an action potential lasts only 1 to 2 msec, resulting in a more prolonged rise in sarcoplasmic Ca^{++} concentration which in turn triggers an even slower mechanical event, the muscle twitch. The duration of this twitch is determined by the properties of individual muscle fibers which can be classified into slow twitch (type I) and fast twitch (type II) fiber types.

Type I and Type II Fibers.   Slow and fast twitch fibers can be distinguished morphologically and histochemically (Fig. 3–12). Type I or slowly contracting fibers are of small diameter, have wide Z lines, are relatively rich in myoglobin, and their mitochondria are large, numerous, and complex, whereas type II fibers are more rapidly contracting, may be of large diameter, contain much stored glycogen, and vary greatly in amount of myoglobin and number of mitochondria. Because of the abundance of mitochondria, slow fibers have a high content of oxidative enzymes and stain strongly for succinic dehydrogenase. On the other hand, myofibrillar ATPase activity is higher in fast fibers because the speed of the fiber is determined by the rate at which ATP is split, causing movement of the crossbridges. Different rates of ATP splitting can be demonstrated in slow and fast fibers by a staining reaction with myosin ATPase, a method for distinguishing between the two fiber types (Fig. 3–12). Some investigators further subdivide the type II fibers on the basis of content of oxidative enzymes, but this may just be a continuum influenced by activity.

The proportions of type I and type II fibers vary substantially from muscle to muscle, and in man there are no pure muscles. However, all motor units are pure, consisting exclusively either of fast or of slow twitch fibers. The speed of a muscle depends on the relative preponderance of slow or fast motor units.

It has been proven in animals which possess muscles composed purely of fast or slow fibers that the motor neuron is the crucial determining factor of fiber type. If the motor nerves to a slow and to a fast muscle are cut and a cross anastomosis is established between the cut ends, letting the fast nerve grow down to the slow muscle and the slow nerve to the fast muscle, it will soon be found that under the influence of the respective motor nerves, the muscle has changed its type. There will be changes in the speed of contraction and in the morphology and histochemistry of the muscle fibers. The muscle's metabolism, on the other hand, can be controlled and changed by the level of activity; in other words, by exercise and training. This will be discussed further in relation to energy metabolism of muscle.

Summation of Tension

If a second stimulus is applied to a muscle before the twitch elicited by a preceding stimulus had subsided, a second contraction will be superadded on the response that is already in progress. Relaxation will be delayed and the tension will increase above that observed during the first twitch (Fig. 3–13). This will be the case even if the two successive stimuli were equal and each elicited a maximal response from the muscle when applied separately. This property of skeletal muscle is known as **summation.** The phenomenon can be defined as the ability of the muscle to summate mechanical responses to repeated, discrete stimuli with the mechanical response to a preceding stimulus.

If the stimulus consists of a volley of impulses, the muscle will respond with sustained tension which may oscillate at the frequency of the imposed stimulation. As this frequency becomes higher a sustained, maximal mechanical response will be elicited. This maximal response is called **tetanus** (Fig. 3–14). The tension attained during tetanus is always greater than or equal to the tension generated during a single twitch.

The frequency of the stimulus necessary for eliciting a maximal, tetanic response depends upon the speed of the muscle. For instance, in the slow soleus as few as 30 stimuli per second will produce tetanus, while in the internal rectus of the eye, stimulation frequency has to be raised to 350 per second.

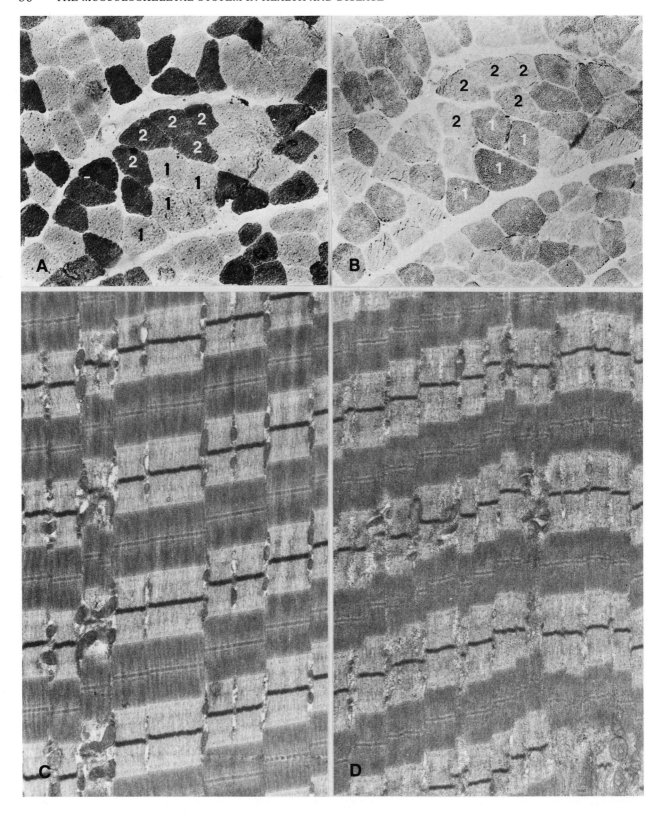

Mechanisms of Summation of Tension. Two factors contribute to the increasing tension that develops in muscle during stimulation culminating in tetanus.

1. Repeated stimuli or action potentials will cause repeated release of Ca^{++} from the terminal cisternae of the sarcoplasmic reticulum, and the average calcium concentration will rise steadily in the sarcoplasm. This progressive increase activates more and more crossbridges, sites at which muscle tension is generated.

2. Tension generated by the myofilaments is transmitted to the object upon which the muscle is acting via a series of elements that possess varying degrees of inherent elasticity. These elements, known collectively as the *series elastic element of muscle* consist of the muscle crossbridges, the sarcoplasm, sarcolemma, endomysium, myotendinal junction, and tendon. Collectively, they act as a spring interposed between the object and the force. The muscle will not attain its maximum active force until the series elastic element is stretched, a state reached in tetanus. Whereas in a single twitch, muscle tension subsides after only partial stretching of the elastic element.

◄**FIG. 3-12.** Type I (slow twitch) and type II (fast twitch) fibers from human skeletal muscle. **(A)** and **(B)** Serial cross sections through normal human muscle. Photomicrographs from frozen sections reacted for myofibrillar ATPase at pH 9.4 **(A)** and for NADH-tetrazolium reductase **(B).** NADH-tetrazolium reductase (synonyms NADH-dehydrogenase, NADH-diaphorase in old terminology) gives an indication of the tissue's ability to support oxidative metabolism. Tetrazolium can intercept electrons at some point along the electron transport chain. The tissue is soaked in both tetrazolium and NADH. The NADH-tetrazolium reductase removes the H from NADH and reduces the tetrazolium to produce a dark colored product. Muscles with higher capacity for oxidative metabolism have greater ability to reduce NADH and also transfer electrons down the electron transport chain and so give a darker color with this treatment. Type I fibers are light with the ATPase and dark with NADH-tetrazolium reductase, marked 1; type II fibers have the reversed staining pattern, marked 2. (× 320) **(C)** and **(D)** Electron micrographs of longitudinal sections of human muscle. **(C)** Type I fiber with high mitochondrial content, thick Z band, and sparse sarcoplasmic reticulum. **(D)** Type II fiber with low mitochondrial content, narrow Z band, and extensive sarcoplasmic reticulum. (Courtesy of Dr. Brenda R. Eisenberg) (× 10,000)

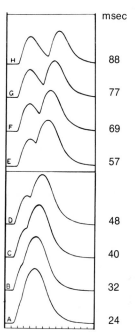

FIG. 3-13. Summation of muscular contraction by double stimulation. Isometric records of the medial head of the gastrocnemius muscle responding to two supramaximal stimuli to the motor nerve in succession. Ordinate: Tension in arbitrary units. Abscissa: time in 20 msec time mark. Intervals in msec between stimuli are indicated along the right margin for tracings A–H. (Ruch TC, Patton HD: Physiology and Biophysics, 9th ed. Philadelphia, WB Saunders, 1965)

Length-Tension Relationship

The length of the muscle has a profound effect upon the force the muscle produces. In the **resting state,** muscles in the body have a certain degree of elastic tension in them illustrated by the fact that when their tendon is cut they retract to a shorter length. A load applied to a relaxed muscle will stretch it beyond its resting length, increasing elastic tension within the muscle. In addition, there will be an increase in stiffness. Thus, the muscle behaves like an elastic structure not unlike a spring. This property is due mainly to the muscle's connective tissue stroma which bears much of the load when the muscle is stretched passively.

The tension developed by *isometrically contracting* muscle bears a precise relationship to the length at which the muscle is being held (Fig. 3–15). There is an optimal length for force development. At this length a single muscle fiber produces 2–4 kg force per cm² cross sectional area.

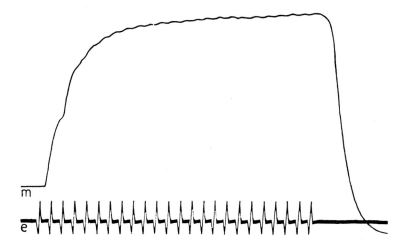

FIG. 3–14. The maximal mechanical response of the cat extensor digitorum longus muscle. Mechanical tension (m) is recorded together with electrical activities (e) in the muscle. The action potentials remain discrete, but tension is maintained continuously. Rate of stimulation 67 per sec. There are 15 msec intervals between each action potential. (Ruch TC, Patton HD: Physiology and Biophysics, 9th ed. Philadelphia, WB Saunders, 1965, after Creed et al: Reflex Activity of the Spinal Cord. Oxford, Clarendon Press, 1932)

If all the muscles of the body were aligned parallel, the maximum force they could exert would lift a 25-ton weight. During running, the force of the gastrocnemius equals up to six times the body weight. Thus muscles generate large forces when operating near their optimal length. This optimal length is near their resting length in the living body.

Mechanisms of Length-Tension Relationship. The length-tension relationship can be explained by correlating the length of a sarcomere with the length-tension curve recorded for a single muscle fiber (Fig. 3–16). When the sarcomere is stretched to maximum length, there is no overlap between actin and myosin filaments (1, in Fig. 3–16). No tension can be generated because crossbridges cannot be formed in this position between the filaments. At shorter and shorter sarcomere lengths, the tension generated by the muscle fiber increases as there is more and more overlap between actin and myosin filaments; maximum tension being reached at the point of maximum overlap (2, 3, in Fig. 3–16). The number of possible sites for crossbridge formation and force generation are maximum in this position. At shorter sarcomere lengths the tension declines rapidly as the opposing sets of actin filaments become telescoped into one another and the myosin filaments contact and distort the Z line (5, 6, in Fig. 3–16). Another contributing factor is that there may be less Ca^{++} released from the sarcoplasmic reticulum at shorter sarcomere lengths.

Speed and Load Relationship

It is common experience that a lighter weight can be lifted more rapidly than a heavy one. Measurements in human muscles have established that the initial speed of shortening of a tetanically stimulated muscle will be smaller if the load is large. For a given load the contraction speed varies from muscle to muscle but it can be as fast as 20 muscle lengths per second, which in the case of the quadriceps is approximately 15 mph.

This speed-load relationship can be readily explained in terms of the sliding filament model of contraction. One way to explain this is as follows: The force or tension generated depends on the number of interaction sites between actin and myosin filaments. Since the probability of interaction between two sites depends on the amount of time they spend in the vicinity of one another, at higher shortening velocities there is less probability for interaction than at slower velocities. Less interaction means that less force can be exerted and a smaller load lifted. If the load is large, more interactions are needed between the filaments to generate a larger force, and the slower movement of the filaments predisposes to this.

ENERGY METABOLISM OF MUSCLE

Muscles do work and for this they rely on several sources of energy stored mainly in the muscle fiber. When the energy supply of muscle is exhausted, muscle fatigue results and the muscle will be unable to contract again and perform work until its energy sources are replenished. The susceptibility to fatigue varies in different muscles and is related to the capacity of the muscle to generate sources of energy. This capacity is developed to different degrees by type I and type II fibers. Whether a muscle becomes fatigued slowly or rapidly is largely determined by the relative proportion of slow and fast fibers that constitute it, and by the relative development of oxidative metabolism.

Sources of Energy

ATP is the immediate source of energy in muscle and it directly furnishes the driving force of contraction. All other forms of stored chemical energy have to be converted to ATP before the muscle can ultilize them. The processes of conversion are so rapid that a fall in ATP concentration cannot be detected in contracting muscle despite the fact that the amount of ATP directly available is very limited at all times. Energy sources for replenishing ATP consist of 1) creatine phosphate; 2) anaerobic metabolism of glycogen through glycolysis; and 3) oxidative phosphorylation. These are the energy sources which will diminish during work performed by the muscle, and it is the

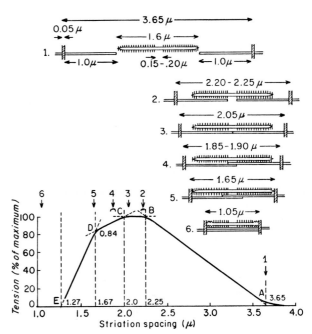

FIG. 3-16. The relationship between isometric tetanic tension and sarcomere length in frog skeletal muscle fibers. The landmarks of the relation are designated A–E. B and C correspond to the plateau, D the sharp bend in the curve at short sarcomere lengths, and A and E the extremes of the curve where active tension is near zero. The intercepts of the vertical dashed lines with the abscissa indicate the sarcomere lengths associated with the landmarks. The numbers on the curve correspond to sarcomere lengths at which the filaments are in the positions shown in the diagrams above the curve. Dimensions on the filaments are best estimates on the basis of existing data. (Modified from Gordon, Huxley, Julian: J Physiol 184:170, 1966)

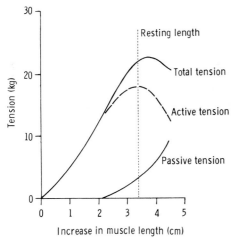

FIG. 3-15. Length-tension diagram for skeletal muscle. The passive tension curve measures the tension exerted by the muscle at each length when it is not stimulated. The total tension curve represents the tension developed when the muscle contracts isometrically in response to a maximal stimulus. The active tension is the difference between the two. (Drawn from data on human triceps muscle, Report to the NRC, Committee on Artificial Limbs, on Fundamental Studies of Human Locomotion, and Other Information Relating to Design of Artificial Limbs, Vol 2. University of California (Berkeley), 1947; reproduced with permission from Ganong WF: Review of Medical Physiology, 9th ed. Copyright by Lange Medical Publications, Los Altos, 1979.)

depletion of these secondary sources of energy that leads to fatigue.

Since ATP not only furnishes the energy for contraction and for the active movement of cations but also regulates contraction by dissociating crossbridges between myosin and actin filaments when ATP itself binds to myosin, the buffering effect of the secondary energy sources ensures, through the provision of a practically constant ATP concentration, that the myofilaments do not remain permanently affixed to one another. Were this to happen the muscle would be irreversibly contracted because the crossbridges could not be broken due to lack of ATP. Such a state is known as **rigor.**

When energy is released by the muscle, ATP is hydrolyzed to ADP and P_i. The reassociation of these hydrolysis products into ATP through oxidative phosphorylation and glycolysis is a slow process involving many enzymes. Therefore, the muscle has to rely on a more rapidly mobilizable source for ATP reconstitution. This source is **creatine phosphate,** which, like ATP itself, is a high energy phosphate compound. A muscle enzyme, **creatine phosphokinase,** catalyzes the transfer of the high energy phosphate from creatine phosphate to ADP, rapidly generating ATP.

Creatine phosphate, in turn, will be reconstituted from ATP derived from the breakdown of stored glycogen, or other substrates that reach the muscle via the circulation. However, during sustained activity the muscle can derive high-energy phosphate bonds from the glycolysis of glycogen in the absence of oxygen. If oxygen is supplied plentifully, ATP synthesis is achieved by oxidative phosphorylation through the citric acid cycle. During intensive exercise the oxygen supply to the muscle may not be able to keep pace with the need for oxygen and then glycolysis will proceed anaerobically via the conversion of hexose to pyruvates and to lactic acid, rather than to CO_2 and H_2O. This anaerobic metabolism of glycogen also liberates energy available for ATP resynthesis, albeit the liberated energy is many times smaller than in the oxidative process (Table 3–1). In this way the supply of oxygen becomes the limiting factor, in the last analysis, to sustained, intensive, muscular exercise. Type I muscle fibers richly supplied by capillaries and generously endowed with mitochondria, oxidative enzymes, and myoglobin which binds O_2 and can serve as an O_2 store, will resist fatigue better than muscle fibers that are not so privileged.

Energy Metabolism and Exercise

Muscles required for prolonged low frequency activity depend on a continuous supply of energy. Such is the case with the muscles active in maintaining posture. In these muscles slow motor units made up of type I fibers predominate. Consequently, postural muscles are more resistant to fatigue than muscles used for short bursts of intensive activity. In the latter, fast motor units consisting of type II fibers are dominant.

The purpose of endurance exercise or training is to increase the fatigue resistance of type II fibers. It is clear from experience that changes do occur in muscle as a consequence of training. The changes include hypertrophy and an increase in sarcoplasmic volume and the number of myofibrils as well as an increase in mitochondria and capillary supply to the muscle fibers. All these factors enhance oxidative phosphorylation in the muscle and through this, achieve an improved fatigue resistance. On the other hand, the speed of the fiber will not change as this is determined by its motor neuron.

In disuse, muscles lose mitochondria, sarcoplasmic volume, and myofibrils, which explains the weakness and loss of muscle bulk observed after immobilization of limbs. The fibers initially affected by disuse atrophy are type II fibers.

TISSUE TURNOVER AND REGENERATION IN MUSCLE

Skeletal muscle is derived from mesenchyme and, in particular, from the myotomes, which represent

TABLE 3–1.   Sources of Energy Stored in a Muscle Fiber

Energy stored as	Utilized through	Initial quantity	Duration of isometric tetanic contraction supported by each energy source (in sec.)
ATP	ATP → ADP + P$_i$	3 mM	2
CP	CP + ADP → ATP + C	20 mM	15
Glycogen	glycolysis	100 mM	120
Pyruvate from glycogen above	Oxidative phosphorylation	hexoses 200 mM	3000 (50 min.)

a portion of the somites (Chap. 12). Mesenchymal cells differentiate into myoblasts, many of which subsequently fuse together to form multinucleated myotubes. Each myotube develops into a muscle fiber. Once fusion occurs the cells loose their potential for proliferation and their life span is presumably as long as that of the individual. The total number of muscle fibers appears to be established at around birth. Growth of skeletal muscle tissue takes place by increase in the number of myofibrils and in sarcoplasmic volume. The enlargement of muscles as a result of sustained physical exercise is also an expression of cellular hypertrophy and not of increased cellularity.

In skeletal muscle, cellular turnover or cell renewal does not usually occur. The nuclei in muscle fibers contain the diploid amount of DNA and neither mitosis nor amitotic division is observed. Turnover does occur at the molecular level, for instance a myosin molecule has a half life of 6–7 days. It is not at all clear how such a molecule which is part of a complex filament structure might be replaced.

It is often stated that skeletal muscle does not regenerate. This erroneous belief comes from clinical studies of muscle injuries in which the large amount of scar tissue formed seriously limits any possibility of proliferation by cells other than fibroblasts. It has been known for many years that skeletal muscle does regenerate under experimental conditions (limb amputations in amphibia, crush and cold injuries in mammals), some of which mimic quite closely the types of injuries seen in clinical practice. Presumably, if scar tissue formation could be controlled, some regeneration of muscle could also be anticipated in man.

The mechanisms of regeneration have not been completely explained and at present two conflicting theories have been proposed. One theory holds that, in an injured fiber, the nuclei somehow organize a new cell around themselves, proliferate, and their progeny fuse to form new muscle fibers. The second theory holds that some primitive cells, known as **satellite cells** persist in skeletal muscle and retain their stem cell potential for generating muscle cells. Upon injury these reserve muscle precursors respond by dividing and giving rise to new myoblasts which then fuse to form muscle fibers. Recent experiments using cell labeling techniques *in vivo* espouse the idea that satellite cells are indeed reserve cells for muscle regeneration.

SUGGESTED READING

Bourne GE (ed): The Structure and Function of Muscle, 2nd ed. New York, Academic Press, 1972–1973
Numerous, comprehensive review articles contributed by leading workers in structural, physiological and biophysical aspects of muscle, collected in four volumes. Especially notable are the articles by
a. *Huxley HE: Molecular basis of contraction in cross-striated muscle (Vol 1)*
b. *Peachey LD, Adrian RH: Electrical properties of the transverse tabular system (Vol 3)*
c. *Nachmanson D: Neuromuscular junction: the role of acetylcholine in excitable membranes (Vol 3)*
d. *Needham DM: Biochemistry of muscle (Vol 3)*

Carlson FD, Wilkie DR: Muscle Physiology. Prentice-Hall, 1974
This is a reasonably advanced text on muscle physiology, covering almost all aspects of muscle contraction. It is particularly strong in the area of mechanics and energetics.

Drachman DB: Myasthenia gravis. N Engl J Med *298(3)*:136, 186, 1978
This reference is an excellent review of what is known about the physiological basis of myasthenia gravis.

Goodgold J, Eberstein A: Electrodiagnosis of Neuromuscular Diseases. Baltimore, Williams & Wilkins, 1972
This book has brief reviews of nerve excitability, neuromuscular transmission and muscle contraction, as well as going into the origin of the electromyogram. It has a much more extensive treatment of the use of EMG in diagnosing neuromuscular diseases.

Hille B: Ionic basis of the resting and action potentials. In Brookhard JM, Mountcastle VB, Kandel ER, Geiger SR (eds): Handbook of Physiology. Vol I, The Nervous System. Bethesda, American Physiological Society, Philadelphia, Williams and Wilkins, 1977
This is an excellent comprehensive coverage of excitability, giving an up-to-date presentation of the material at a fairly detailed level. It begins at a relatively elementary level but develops the material in great detail.

Hoyle G: How is muscle turned on and off? Sci Am *222*:84, 1970
A stimulating exposition of the hypothesis that the flow of calcium ions in response to a nerve signal gives rise to contraction and that the withdrawal of ions results in relaxation.

Katz A: Physiology of the Heart. New York, Raven Press, 1977
Although this book concentrates on the physiology relative to heart muscle, it is an excellent review of muscle contraction in general. This book is particularly strong on the molecular aspects of contraction and the control of contraction.

Katz B: Nerve, Muscle, and Synapse. New York, McGraw-Hill, 1966
This is a good, well-written review in the area of excitability and neuromuscular transmission. It is a little out of date now, but still provides excellent basic coverage of both excitability and neuromuscular transmission. The section on muscle is quite abbreviated.

Kuffler SW, Nichols JG: From Neuron to Brain. Sinauer Associates, Sunderland, Mass, 1976
As the title indicates, it is the coverage of material from excitability at the neuron level to synaptic transmission to brain function. It is a well-written text, and is up to date on the areas covered.

4
Muscle Action and Its Control

CORNELIUS ROSSE

How our muscles perform the specific tasks we expect of them is a complex and incompletely understood question. The mechanisms of which we have some knowledge are best considered by dealing separately with

1. Sense organs of muscle and tendon
2. Segmental afferent input to motor neurons
3. Local or spinal reflexes which control muscle action
4. The suprasegmental centers located in the brain which, through descending pathways, exert an influence over the segmental spinal reflex centers

The motor neurons represent the final common pathway in muscle activation and all mechanisms, segmental or suprasegmental, capable of modifying muscle contraction operate by exciting or inhibiting these cells. Before considering these mechanisms it will be necessary to clarify in anatomic terms the types of actions muscles can engage in when called upon in the intact body.

THE ACTION OF MUSCLES IN THE BODY

Fixed and Moving Points of Muscle Attachment

Movement of one bone in relation to another takes place at a joint, and it is produced actively by the isotonic contraction of muscles which cross the joint. As the contracting muscle shortens, it approximates its site of insertion to its site of origin. When the muscle is twisted or spiralized, its shortening also brings the line of its insertion into one and the same plane with the line of its origin, imparting a spin to the moving bone. The muscle's site of **origin** remains fixed while its site of **insertion** describes an arc in any given movement, whether or not there is an element of spin.

Fixed and moving points of the muscle's attachment may be reversed due to the stabilizing action of a different set of muscles or external forces. For instance, the *usual* action of the pectoralis major is to adduct the arm against the rib cage. In this movement the muscle's attachment to the sternum and the ribs represents its origin, and its attachment to the humerus its insertion. However, when a patient in respiratory distress leans on both elbows, the two humeri become stabilized, serving now as the site of origin for the pectoralis major muscles and the contracting muscles now will lift the ribs, assisting in respiratory movements by expanding the rib cage. In these two instances, origin and insertion have been reversed. This principle is important when normal and deranged movements are analyzed. However, in anatomic terminology the muscle's point of attachment that remains fixed during its *usual* or *habitual* action is spoken of as its origin, and its attachment site that moves under the same circumstances is regarded as its insertion. Accordingly, the pectoralis major is said to originate on the sternum and ribs and to insert on the humerus.

Prime Movers and Antagonists

Many muscles cross more than one joint and when they contract movement will occur at all the joints crossed by the muscle or its tendon. At each joint the resulting movement depends on the shape of the articular surfaces and on the relation of the muscle's line of pull to the axes of the joints. In order to produce the desired result, movement at some of the joints may have to be prevented. Therefore, **when a movement is carried out, a combination of muscles is called into action.** The muscle or muscles in this combination responsible for initiating and maintaining the desired movement are known as the **prime movers.** The muscle or muscles capable of directly opposing this movement or ini-

57

tiating the converse movement are known as the **antagonists.** For instance, if flexion of the fingers (interphalangeal joints) is desired, the prime movers will be the flexor digitorum superficialis and flexor digitorum profundus muscles, and the antagonists, the digital extensors (extensor digitorum and interossei).

It has been established by electromyography that the antagonists remain inactive while the prime movers do their work and the resistance offered by the antagonists to prime mover force is due to their viscosity and elasticity. The relaxed antagonists are stretched by the contracting prime movers and during the active phase of the movement contraction of the antagonists in response to the stretch is reflexly inhibited. The mechanism for this inhibition will become clear later.

Gravity as the Prime Moving Force. When the prime moving force is generated not by muscle action but by gravity, the movement will be controlled paradoxically by muscles capable of producing the converse movement, that is by the antagonists. For instance, if the forearm resting on the elbow is allowed to fall passively to the table, the prime moving force responsible for this elbow extension is provided by gravity. Control over this movement is exerted by the antagonists, that is, by the elbow flexors. The weight of the forearm subjects the elbow flexors to a sustained stretch, in response to which tension is generated in the muscles. Under voluntary control the flexors will elongate while contracting, the elbow will extend and the forearm will come to the table at the desired rate.

This mechanism is particularly important in the maintenance of upright posture. All antigravity muscles function in response to the stretches they are subjected to by the force of gravity. Gravity must be taken into consideration in the clinical assessment of all normal and abnormal movements.

Stabilizers and Synergists

The site of a muscle's origin has to be immobilized, and in the limbs, which consist of a series of joints, this is accomplished as a rule by muscle action. Prime movers and antagonists contract in unison functioning as **fixation** or **stabilizer muscles.** For instance, during push-ups the scapula and the shoulder joint will be stabilized by the contraction of surrounding muscles to provide a firm base for the contracting elbow flexors and extensors which

work against gravity at a controlled rate. The stabilizers are called into action as part of the total movement without any specific command.

Not only has the muscle's origin to be stabilized but the unwanted components of its action have to be cancelled out if the muscle crosses more than one joint or if its unrestrained pull produces more than one type of movement at a single joint. The elimination of unwanted movements is done by **synergists.** As their name implies, synergists assist the prime movers in exerting an action in such a manner that by working together a movement is produced which neither muscle could bring about by itself. The example of finger flexors quoted previously illustrates the principle. The digital flexors originate in the forearm, and when they contract, flexion of the wrist as well as of the interphalangeal joints will occur unless wrist movement is eliminated by synergists. Extensor muscles of the wrist contract reflexly when finger flexion is attempted, and the wrist will be noticeably extended to facilitate a powerful grip by the flexing fingers.

Spurt and Shunt Action of Muscles

The force generated by prime mover contraction can be resolved into two vectors (Fig. 4–1). One vector acts *across* the moving bone and causes the point of insertion to swing through an arc, while the other vector acting *along* the moving bone forces the two articulating bones against each other. The two force components have been called **spurt** and **shunt** action of a muscle, respectively. If a muscle originates far from a joint and inserts near it, its pull across the moving bone will be greater than along it, and such a muscle is considered a spurt muscle. On the other hand, if a muscle originates close to a joint and inserts far from it, its pull along the moving bone will be greater than across it, and such a muscle is regarded as a shunt muscle. Among flexors of the elbow the brachialis and biceps are spurt muscles while the brachioradialis is a shunt muscle.

The importance of spurt muscles is self-evident, and they are primarily recruited to execute the desired movement. The need for shunt muscles can be appreciated by considering that 1) spurt muscles impart a centrifugal force to the bone that moves on a curved articular surface causing it to tend to fly off at a tangent to the articular surface, and 2) spurt muscles may move the bone into such a position that their force vector acting along the bone will tend to dislocate the joint (Fig. 4–1). The brachioradialis, functioning as a shunt muscle at

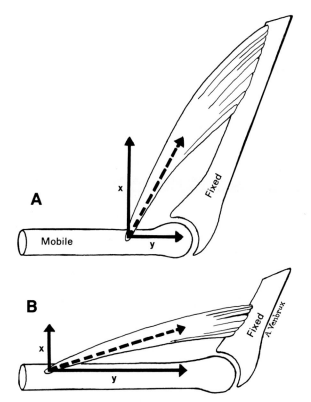

FIG. 4–1. Spurt and shunt action of muscles. The force generated by contraction of the muscle **(interrupted arrow)** can be broken down into two vectors, x and y. Spurt action is due to vector x acting across the mobile bone while shunt action is due to vector y acting along the mobile bone. The muscle shown in **A** is a spurt muscle (x > y), the muscle in **B** is a shunt muscle (y > x). (Modified from Warwick R, Williams PL (eds): Gray's Anatomy, 35th ed. Philadelphia, WB Saunders, 1973)

the elbow, can be expected to be active during rapid movements whatever the direction of the swing. It has, indeed, been confirmed by electromyography that the muscle contracts during rapid elbow flexion and extension. Thus, during movement, the shunt action of muscles contributes to maintaining joint integrity. In those positions of the joint where the ligaments are lax, shunt muscles guard against dislocation.

Versatility of Muscle Action

It will be appreciated that a single muscle can act in a variety of ways. As a prime mover, a muscle may flex one joint and extend the other, as the hamstrings, for instance, flex the knee and extend the hip. In converse movements the same muscle functions as an antagonist, and in other circumstances it will participate in a movement as a fixator or synergist. The same muscle may function as a spurt or shunt muscle at the same joint depending on which of its attachments is stabilized to serve as its origin. With the foot off the ground, the hamstrings flex the knee by their spurt action, acting at the same time as shunt extensors at the hip. On the other hand, when a foot is planted, the same muscles become shunt flexors at the knee and spurt extensors at the hip. In some instances, the muscle contracts isometrically; in others, isotonically. In the latter case, it may shorten or lengthen as it counteracts the load.

For a muscle to perform in such a versatile way it must be endowed with a sophisticated sensory apparatus and with mechanisms for feedback to the motor neurons and to higher centers of coordination in order to be able to contribute appropriately to the execution of a voluntary act.

SENSORY MECHANISMS IN MUSCLE AND TENDON

The so-called motor nerve of a muscle contains, in addition to the axons of motor neurons, a substantial number of *sensory* or *afferent* nerve fibers whose cell bodies are located in dorsal root ganglia (Fig. 4–2). Many of these sensory fibers are concerned with pain and they terminate as free endings on the perimysium and endomysium, in fat present among the muscle fibers, or in relation to blood vessels. A few sensory fibers terminate in pacinian corpuscles or in similar, club-shaped receptors concerned with pressure sensation. Pressure receptors are abundant in the joint capsule, ligaments, and periarticular tissues, and the proprioceptive impulses generated in them contribute to our consciousness about the position of our limbs. Such receptors, however, are scarce in muscle and tendon, and they are essentially of no importance in the control of muscle contraction. The afferent fibers that are most important in sensory feedback from the muscle originate from specialized structures which are unique to muscle and tendon. These are the **muscle spindles** and the **Golgi tendon organs.** Muscle spindle afferents detect muscle length and are referred to as **stretch receptors.** Golgi tendon organs sense tension, which can be produced by muscle contraction or by extreme stretching of the muscle-tendon unit.

There are important differences between afferents from the muscle spindle and the tendon or-

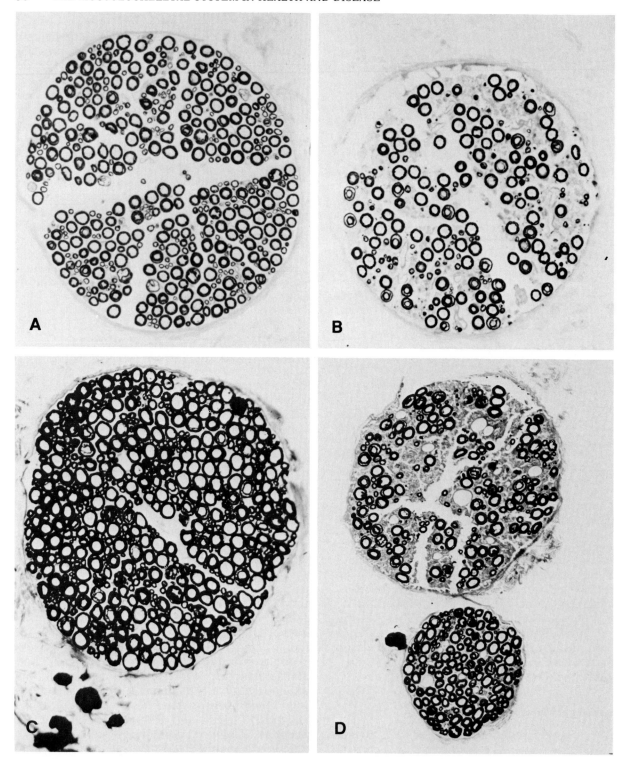

gan. Muscle spindle afferents have a low threshold to stretch of the muscle-tendon unit because they are located on compliant muscle fibers, whereas tendon organ afferents are embedded in more resilient collagen fibers and are much less sensitive to stretch. Muscle spindle afferents provide information both about changes in muscle fiber length and about the speed of changes in muscle length. Moreover, the most important impulses relayed from the muscle spindles to the spinal cord *excite* a reflex contraction of the same muscle (stretch reflex), whereas afferent impulses from tendon organs *inhibit* contraction of the muscle from which they originate. These differences are important in understanding the spinal reflexes which control muscle contraction, but this can only be accomplished if the structure and central connections of the stretch receptors are appreciated.

The Structure of Muscle Receptors

The Golgi Tendon Organ. The tendon organ consists of a small fasciculus of collagen fibers enclosed by a delicate spindle-shaped connective tissue capsule which is penetrated by one or two sensory nerve fibers, branches of the nerve that supplies the muscle (Fig. 4–3). The structures are embedded in the muscle's tendon at the myotendinal junction, and the encapsulated fibers of each are connected *in series* to about ten muscle fibers which belong to several motor units. Within the capsule, the nerve fibers terminate in numerous branches and are entrapped among fibers of the

---

◀ **FIG. 4–2.** Transverse sections of nerves from the hind limb of cats. The myelin sheaths of the nerve fibers are stained black. **(A)** Nerve to the popliteus muscle, normal. **(B)** Nerve to the popliteus muscle in the opposite limb of the same cat as in **A**. In this nerve only efferent fibers remain because the dorsal roots have been divided on this side experimentally 35 days previously, leading to degeneration of all afferent nerve fibers. **(C)** Normal nerve to the popliteus of another cat. **(D)** The large nerve is the nerve to the popliteus muscle in the opposite limb of the same cat as in **C**. In this nerve only afferent fibers remain because the ventral roots have been divided on this side 48 days previously, leading to degeneration of all motor nerve fibers. The adjacent small nerve is the interosseous nerve which is entirely sensory; consequently, division of ventral roots has not eliminated any nerve fibers from it. (Boyd IA, Davey MR, Andrew BL (ed): Control and Innervation of Skeletal Muscle. A symposium at Queen's College, Dundee, University of St. Andrew's, 1966, p 35)

collagen fasciculus. These nerve endings are presumably compressed and depolarized when the tendon is stretched by the contracting muscle, inducing the tendon organ to fire. The tendon organ is sensitive to tension. Exquisitely small tension produced by the contraction of those muscle fibers which terminate in the collagen fasciculi of the tendon organ will increase the discharge of afferent impulses. However, passive stretch of a relaxed muscle must be extreme before it causes enough increase in tension to induce firing by the tendon organ.

The Muscle Spindle. Muscle spindles are more complex than tendon organs. They are delicate, fusiform (spindle-shaped) structures interspersed among the fibers of skeletal muscle, their orientation is *parallel* with the muscle fibers, and their two poles are anchored to the endomysium and perimysium, although some spindles may span the entire length of the muscle attaching to its tendons of origin and insertion. When a muscle is passively stretched, the spindles will be put under tension, while contraction of the muscle will relieve the spindles of any tension.

A spindle consists of several (6–30) specialized muscle fibers, the **intrafusal fibers,** which are partially enclosed by a connective tissue capsule. The capsule is best developed over the equatorial region of the spindle and is filled with lymph. The spindles are surrounded by the regular, **skeletomotor** or **extrafusal fibers** that make up the bulk of the muscle and are responsible for generating the force exerted by the muscle. Capillaries and both sensory and motor nerve fibers penetrate the capsule, and both types of nerves terminate on the intrafusal fibers (Fig. 4–4).

The intrafusal fibers are striated muscle, but differ from extrafusal, skeletomotor fibers in that their equatorial zone is largely devoid of striations and is dilated by the accumulation of nuclei. In some fibers the nuclei occupy a central bag of sarcoplasm **(nuclear bag fibers)**, in others they form a chain in the core of the fiber **(nuclear chain fiber).** The nuclear bag is the region most susceptible to stretch, because due to the paucity of myofibrils it is presumably the most compliable part of the fiber. Nuclear chain fibers and the polar regions of nuclear bag fibers are presumably less compliable. These differences are reflected in the activity of different types of afferent nerve fibers and nerve endings associated with the respective regions.

Each spindle has a large **afferent fiber** (group Ia fiber), and branches of this fiber wrap both around

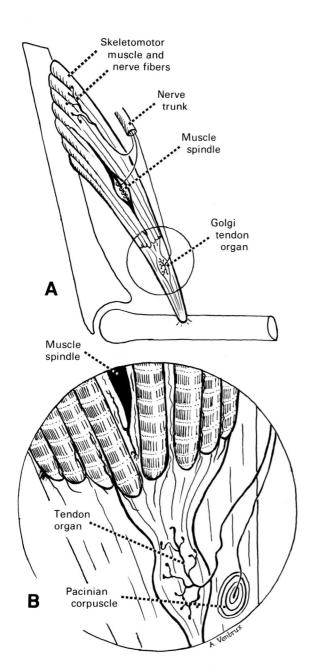

Skeletomotor muscle and nerve fibers

Nerve trunk

Muscle spindle

Golgi tendon organ

A

Muscle spindle

Tendon organ

Pacinian corpuscle

B

A. Venbrux

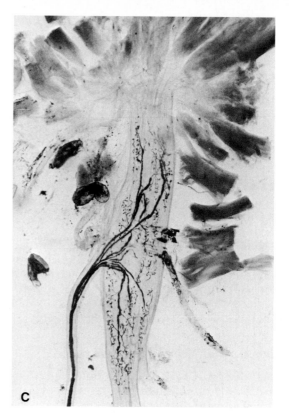

C

FIG. 4–3. **A** and **B** are schematic representations of the location of muscle spindles and Golgi tendon organs. The circled area in **A** is shown enlarged in **B**. Only one muscle spindle and one tendon organ are illustrated. The sizes of both are exaggerated in relation to the whole muscle. For the detailed anatomy of the muscle spindle see Figure 4–4. **C** is a microphotograph of a tendon organ which was dissected out of a tendon of a cat. The organ measures approximately 0.5 mm in length. Several of the teased muscle fibers have been retained which can be seen converging on the encapsulated, spindle-shaped receptor organ. The nerve, stained black by a silver stain, enters the equatorial region of the organ and its terminal branches are seen entwined among and around the delicate collagen fibers of the organ, which appear transparent. (**C**, Barker D, in Hunt CC (ed): Handbook of Sensory Physiology, Vol. III/2. Heidelberg, Springer-Verlag, 1974.)

FIG. 4-4. **A** is a schematic representation of a muscle spindle, the central portion of which is enlarged. The capsule has been cut open and only one nuclear bag and one nuclear chain fiber is depicted in the interior. A nerve pierces the capsule. The large afferent nerve fibers (white) terminate in annulospiral endings around the central zone of the muscle fibers, while the small afferent fibers (white) terminate in flower spray endings on the paracentral segments. Fusimotor or gamma efferent nerve fibers (black) terminate on both types of intrafusal fibers. Before entering the capsule the same nerve also gives alpha efferents to the extrafusal muscle fibers.

(B) Microphotograph of a muscle spindle teased from the ▶ peroneus brevis muscle of a cat and treated by a silver stain to demonstrate nerve fibers. In this spindle only afferent fibers are present because the ventral roots have been divided in this animal some time ago, leading to degeneration of the gamma efferents. The large nerve fibers terminating in annulospiral endings are readily distinguishable from the more delicate fibers which terminate in flower spray endings. A capillary is also visible. (**B**, Barker D, in Homma S (ed): Progress in Brain Research, Vol. 44. Amsterdam, Elsevier Scientific Publishing, 1976)

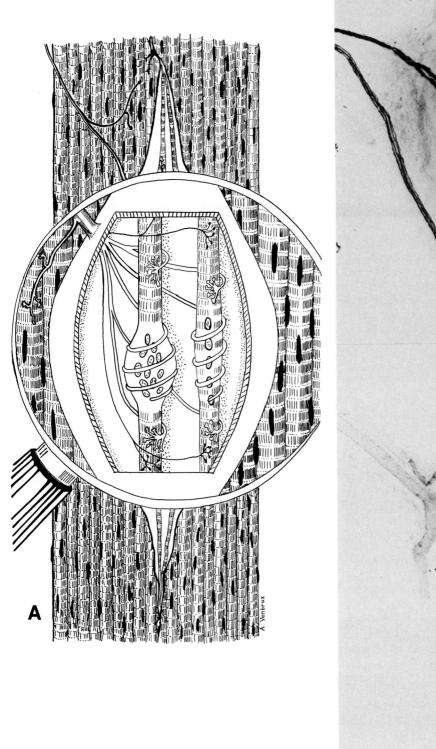

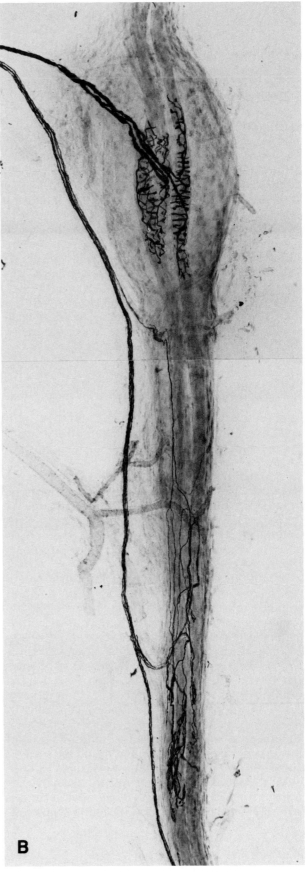

A

B

the nuclear bags and around the central zone of nuclear chain fibers. These endings are known as **primary** or **annulospiral endings.** Spindle afferents of smaller size (group II fibers) terminate primarily on the polar segments of nuclear chain fibers by so-called **secondary** or **flower spray endings.** Annulospiral endings of nuclear bags are sensitive to the velocity as well as the amplitude of stretch, while those on nuclear chain fibers reflect primarily the amplitude of stretch.

Intrafusal fiber contraction is brought about by the **motor nerves** that enter the spindle. Because of their smaller diameter these **fusimotor fibers** are also known as **gamma efferents.** They terminate by motor endplates on the polar segment of the intrafusal fibers (Fig. 4–4). When these segments contract, the central zone of the fiber where the primary sensory nerve endings are located will become stretched. Extrafusal or skeletomotor muscle fibers are supplied by axons of larger diameter which are known as **alpha efferents** or **skeletomotor nerve fibers.**

Activation of Stretch Receptors

Passive stretching of a muscle increases the length in its extrafusal and intrafusal fibers, the annulospiral endings in the spindles become depolarized, and action potentials are transmitted to the spinal cord along the spindle afferents (Fig. 4–5). The central zone of the intrafusal fibers may also be stretched by contraction of the two polar segments of the fiber. This takes place concurrently with skeletal motor contraction (alpha-gamma coactivation) during voluntary action of a muscle, a phenomenon discussed later.

The discharge frequency of annulospiral receptors is proportional to the rate of stretch and provides information about the *speed* of passive stretching or the speed of muscle contraction. A sustained plateau of discharge from these receptors is indicative of the *magnitude* of stretch. Once threshold excitation is reached in flower spray endings these receptors will also partake in the monitoring of muscle lengths. They adapt more slowly to the stimulus than do annulospiral endings and their response is tonic rather than phasic. Annulospiral endings on nuclear chain fibers and flower spray endings are well adapted for sensing the magnitude of stretch in postural muscles subjected to sustained loading, while the sensitive annulospiral endings on nuclear bag fibers are well suited to give a dynamic response, the type of in-

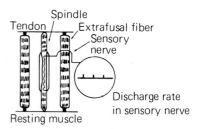

Resting muscle

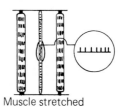

Muscle stretched

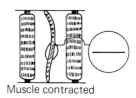

Muscle contracted

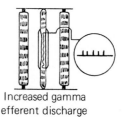

Increased gamma efferent discharge

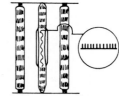

Increased gamma efferent discharge - muscle stretched

FIG. 4-5. The effects of stretching, contraction, and gamma efferent activation on muscle spindle discharge. (Reproduced with permission from Ganong WF: Review of Medical Physiology, 9th ed. Copyright by Lange Medical Publications, Los Altos, 1979)

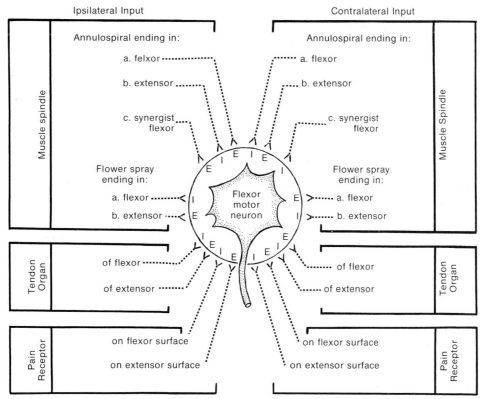

Ipsilateral Input

Contralateral Input

FIG. 4–6. Some of the segmental afferent input converging on a typical spinal motor neuron. The influence of each input is indicated as excitatory (E) or inhibitory (I). The example chosen is a flexor motor neuron. A corresponding diagram of inputs to an extensor motor neuron would be identical except that the influence of multisynaptic paths fed by pain receptors would be reversed. With the exception of annulospiral afferents from the ipsilateral flexor muscle, all inputs are multisynaptic. (Based on Ruch TC, Patton HD: Physiology and Biophysics, 9th ed. Philadelphia, WB Saunders, 1960)

formation required for sensing rapid phasic movements of the limbs.

The sensitivity of muscle spindles can be increased by the firing of gamma efferents (Fig. 4–5). If gamma motor neurons are activated by impulses from higher centers, the spindle afferents will be sensitized to stretch because the contraction of the poles of the intrafusal muscle fibers places some stretch on sensory afferents. On the other hand, if alpha motor neurons are selectively activated, stretch will be removed from the muscle spindles by contraction of the extrafusal fibers (Fig. 4–5). Then the muscle spindles will be silenced, but the Golgi tendon organs will be excited, because the tension generated stretches the muscle's tendon.

It will be explained in connection with spinal reflexes that action potentials generated in an-

nulospiral endings deliver excitatory postsynaptic potentials to motor neurons. The synaptic connections of flower spray afferents are less precisely understood. Some may inhibit the motor neurons serving the extrafusal fibers of the muscle while others may excite motor neurons of synergists and inhibit those supplying the antagonists.

SEGMENTAL AFFERENT INPUT TO SPINAL MOTOR NEURONS

Afferent impulses arising from muscles or from other receptors in skin or deeper tissues are relayed to the spinal cord via the central processes of unipolar neurons situated in dorsal root ganglia. Some of this sensory input is transmitted to the brain where it may or may not reach consciousness, but much of it is relayed immediately to the motor neurons located in the same segment of the spinal cord as the entering dorsal root. This local synaptic input is largely responsible for determining the activity of spinal motor neurons and hence the activity of the muscles that serve a particular joint. Such reflex arcs limited to discrete segments form the basis of the local or segmental control of muscle contraction, and this will be discussed in the following section. Whether muscles behave as prime movers, antagonists, or syngerists in such reflex action depends largely on the type of synaptic connections that the afferents of various peripheral receptors establish with motor neurons within appropriate segments of the same (ipsilateral) or the opposite (contralateral) halves of the spinal cord (Fig. 4–6).

The only types of afferents which synapse directly with motor neurons are the large muscle afferents of the annulospiral endings (group Ia spindle fibers), and their effect on the motor neuron is always excitatory. This monosynaptic reflex arc constitutes the basis of the stretch reflex and is confined to the same side and the same segments of the cord as the afferent input. Other types of afferent input, for instance, from pain receptors, Golgi tendon organs, or from flower spray endings of the muscle spindle, are relayed to motor neurons via one or more interneurons and synapses. The postsynaptic potentials generated by some of the interneurons are excitatory to the motor neurons, while others are inhibitory. It is via such multisynaptic pathways that all impulses are relayed to the contralateral half of the spinal cord and also to adjacent segments above and below. A single afferent fiber that branches and synapses with excitatory and inhibitory interneurons may, therefore, simultaneously excite or inhibit appropriate groups of muscles. Via such a pathway the stimulus may also involve adjacent segments and recruit related muscle groups as synergists or fixators, and at the same time may inhibit the motor neurons of the antagonists.

The effects of some of these impulses on a typical motor neuron are summarized in Figure 4–6. Each motor neuron is subjected to a multitude of influences, and the balance of these determines at any one time the membrane potential and, therefore, the excitability of the cell. The motor neuron, the final common pathway for muscle activation, integrates these local messages with influences which reach it from higher centers via descending pathways.

Reciprocal Innervation

In general, impulses capable of exciting or inhibiting motor neurons of a particular muscle exert at the same time the opposite effect on the motor neurons which supply the antagonists of that muscle (Fig. 4–7). This reciprocal circuitry, known as **reciprocal innervation,** subserves a basic physiologic principle in muscle action: a volley of impulses that generates contraction in one muscle by exciting the motor neurons, as a rule turns off the motor neurons that supply the opposing muscles. By this principle, conflict between prime movers and antagonists is avoided.

Such reciprocity extends to motor neurons in the contralateral half of a segment. A volley which excited flexor motor neurons and inhibited extensor motor neurons in the right half of a segment when relayed to the left by interneurons, as a rule generates postsynaptic potentials that will be excitatory to extensor motor neurons and inhibitory to their flexor counterparts. When fixation of a joint is required by coordinated contraction of prime movers and antagonists, suprasegmental motor centers intervene and appropriately modify the balance of synaptic input to the respective groups of motor neurons. By this mechanism cocontraction of various muscle groups becomes possible.

REFLEXES IN CONTROL OF MUSCLE ACTION

The Stretch Reflex or Myotatic Reflex

A load applied to a muscle stretches it, and the muscle responds reflexly by *sustained contraction* which is maintained until the load is removed or the muscle becomes fatigued. The greater the load the more the muscle is stretched, and its contraction will be the more powerful. Experiments on decerebrate animals and humans make it clear that such adjustments in muscle tone occur as spinal reflexes and do not require intervention from the brain. Postural muscles are subjected to sustained stretch by the force of gravity, and when the center of body mass is displaced, as it is during bending over or lifting a heavy object, the muscles adjust their contraction automatically without a conscious attempt to maintain balance.

This phenomenon is based on the stretch reflex or myotatic reflex, which functions as a feedback mechanism between the muscle spindle and the motor neurons that innervate the same muscle.

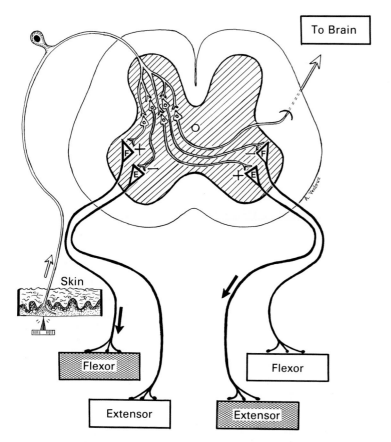

FIG. 4-7. A highly schematic representation of reciprocal innervation. Only one interneuron is shown between a terminal branch of the afferent nerve fiber and a motor neuron, but in reality multiple such interneurons exist. (E = extensor motor neuron; F = flexor motor neuron; + = excitatory postsynaptic potential; − = inhibitory postsynaptic potential). In the instance illustrated, the afferent impulse is provoked by a pain stimulus applied to the skin. Such a stimulus results in a flexion or withdrawal reflex (excitation of flexor and inhibition of extensor motor neurons) and also in a crossed extension reflex.

The stretch depolarizes the receptors in a number of muscle spindles inducing the relay of asynchronous impulses to the spinal cord via the spindle afferents (Fig. 4–8). Alpha motor neurons in the ventral horn will be excited asynchronously, the consequent skeletomotor contraction will counteract the stretching force and will unload the spindles. Silencing of spindle receptors terminates motor neuron discharge and leads to extrafusal fiber relaxation. If the load or stretch is reapplied, however, a cohort of spindles will again be stimulated, reactivating the stretch reflex. Because of the asynchrony and rapid conduction of impulses along this monosynaptic reflex arc, the muscle appears to respond to the sustained stretch by a smooth sustained contraction.

The stretch reflex is extensively utilized during the normal action of muscles. This reflex is also important clinically because assessment of a muscle tone essentially tests the stretch reflex. Slow and deliberate passive flexion and extension of joints by the examiner activates the stretch reflex in the appropriate muscle groups (Fig. 4–8). The resistence offered by the muscle to this passive movement is known as **muscle tone,** and it represents the summation of intrinsic elastic tension and the active contraction forces that develop in the muscle as a consequence of the stretch reflex. Muscle tone is further discussed in Chapter 27.

The Tendon Jerk

When the stretch applied to a muscle is momentary and sudden rather than sustained, the response elicited will be a brief twitch rather than a sustained contraction. In eliciting a tendon jerk the sudden stretch is provoked by sharply tapping the tendon of a slightly stretched muscle. Normally, the reflex twitch contraction observed as the jerk is confined to the muscle whose tendon was hit. The tendon jerk is a special and artifactual example of the stretch reflex. A large number of muscle spindle receptors are depolarized simultaneously and instead of the asynchronous pitter-patter afferent input characteristic of the regular stretch reflex, a volley of impulses will be relayed to the motor neurons *synchronously,* leading to synchronous alpha efferent activation and extrafusal fiber contraction. This motor activity will not be sustained because following the twitch the stretch receptors will be silenced and will not be reactivated.

The tendon jerk is useful clinically because it demonstrates for a given muscle the integrity of the components of the stretch reflex. These components are the muscle spindles and their afferents, a specific segment of the spinal cord, alpha motor neurons, their axons in the muscle's motor nerve, the neuromuscular junction, and extrafusal muscle fibers. In addition, the amplitude and speed of the tendon jerk give some information about other segmental and supraspinal influences on the motor neurons. Thus, in eliciting tendon jerks, information may be deduced both about the segmental components of the reflex (if any of these are abnormal, tendon jerks will usually be *depressed*) and about suprasegmental control of the inputs to the motor neurons. Some of the latter must be inhibitory to account for the fact that with damage to the descending nerve tracts the tendon jerks may be *exaggerated*. Although tendon jerks are part of the routine clinical evaluation of the musculoskeletal and nervous systems, it must be borne in mind that because of the mass response provoked, the tendon jerk is relatively crude, and it detects only gross derangement of the factors which influence the stretch reflex. Unlike the stretch reflex, the tendon jerk plays little or no part in the control of normal muscle action in the body.

The Inverse Myotatic or Clasp-Knife Reflex

As explained above, the more a muscle is stretched, the more powerful will be its contraction. The stretch receptors in tendon organs provide an inhibitory mechanism for limiting this response in order to guard against tissue damage which might be incurred by the forces generated via the all too eager stretch reflex. Once the tension mounts to the threshold of the tendon organs, muscle contraction will be reflexly inhibited (autogenic inhibition). The effect being the inverse of the myotatic or stretch reflex.

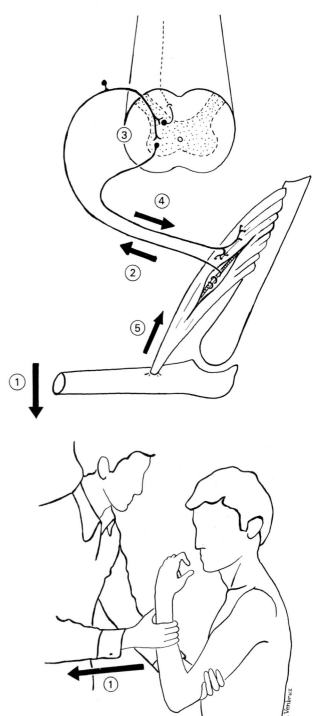

FIG. 4-8. Schematic representation of the stretch reflex. 1. Passive extension of the elbow by the examiner stretches the flexor muscle (e.g., brachialis). 2. Some of the spindle afferents are excited. 3. Excitatory postsynaptic potentials are generated and some of the alpha motor neurons depolarized. 4. Efferent impulses induce extrafusal fiber contraction. 5. Resistance is offered to the stretching force (force exerted by the examiner) due to contraction of the muscle.

This phenomenon was originally observed experimentally in the decerebrate cat in which antigravity muscles exhibit spasticity or increased muscle tone and may also be demonstrated in muscles of spastic patients. If a muscle of a spastic patient is stretched by bending a joint passively, muscle tension will increase further due to the stretch reflex until at a certain threshold the muscle suddenly relaxes and the joint gives way like a spring-loaded jackknife (clasp-knife reflex). This sudden relaxation is brought about by inhibition of motor neurons through depolarization of tendon organ afferents. The spastic muscle provides an extreme example but the inverse myotatic reflex probably is called into operation also during normal muscle action where it may be one of the mechanisms for inhibiting muscle contraction.

Nocifensive Reflexes

Noxious or harmful stimuli applied to the skin or to deeper structures (e.g., periosteum) elicit defensive or **nocifensive reflexes** by inducing muscle contraction. These spinal reflexes can be observed in a decerebrate animal or man just as well as in the conscious state. A limb reflexly withdraws from an irritating stimulus usually by the contraction of flexor musculature (**withdrawal or flexion reflex**) (Fig. 4–7). In accord with the principle of reciprocal innervation, during a flexion reflex extensor motor neurons are inhibited. The contralateral limb may also be involved in the reflex, but here the extensor musculature will be activated in what is called the **crossed extension reflex** (Fig. 4–7).

The first line defense subserved by the flexion-crossed extension reflexes becomes evident if we consider what happens when one steps bare foot on a thumb tack. The leg will be withdrawn immediately by dorsiflexion of the ankle, flexion of the knee and hip, while the opposite leg will be extended to support the body weight which now falls entirely on it. Such a wide spread response is comprehensible on the basis of the multisynaptic connections established by incoming sensory fibers with different groups of motor neurons.

Alpha-Gamma Coactivation

In the reflexes discussed so far, skeletomotor muscle fiber contraction depended on afferent impulses relayed to motor neurons from receptors situated in muscles, skin, or in other tissues. Such reflex contraction is self-limiting in that it eliminates the synaptic drive of motor neurons. Clearly, mechanisms must exist which permit sustained muscle activity in the absence of stimuli to the skin or muscle. For instance, phasic movements of the limbs executed under voluntary initiative and control are not directly dependent on peripheral stimulation. Voluntary action of muscles is governed by the brain, but it includes the segmental reflex centers and, in particular, the circuits of the stretch reflex. Voluntary muscle contraction involves the **gamma loop** which entails the *coactivation* of gamma and alpha efferents.

Descending impulses carrying the command for initiating a voluntary movement depolarize both alpha and gamma motor neurons. Alpha motor neuron discharge generates the force required for the movement but the coactivation of gamma efferents is advantageous for 1) sustaining the movement via facilitation of alpha motor neurons and 2) for maintaining the muscle's sensitivity to stretch throughout contraction.

The intrafusal fiber contraction resulting from gamma efferent discharge maintains the annulospiral spindle receptors under stretch, despite the fact that the extrafusal fibers are shortening. The provoked spindle afferent discharge facilitates the alpha motor neurons and thereby contributes toward sustaining contraction. Because of this alpha-gamma linkage or gamma loop the spindles shorten with the muscle. Continuous gamma efferent activity throughout contraction serves furthermore to maintain spindle sensitivity to any lengthening force (stretch) imposed on the muscle during contraction. This mechanism provides for reflex adjustment of alpha motor neuron discharge throughout the voluntary movement.

THE SUPRASEGMENTAL CONTROL OF MUSCLE ACTION

In man motor centers located in the brain dominate spinal reflexes and control the specific muscle groups associated with discrete joints. The cardinal members of this **suprasegmental motor system** are the cerebral cortex, certain brain stem nuclei (red nucleus, vestibular nuclei, reticular formation), the basal ganglia, and the cerebellum. Figure 4–9 illustrates schematically the relationship of these centers to the segmental spinal motor neuron pool and to one another. The major anatomic components of the suprasegmental motor system are illustrated schematically, with related parts of the

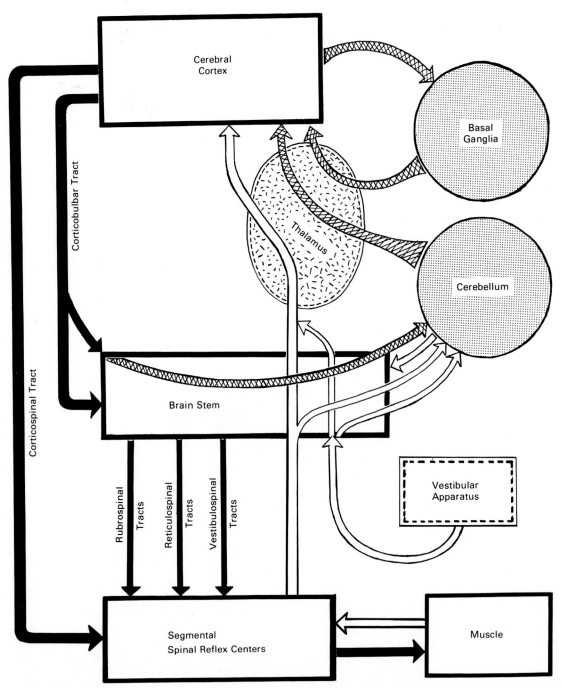

FIG. 4-9. Simplified diagrammatic representation of the relationships between various components of the suprasegmental motor system and the segmental spinal reflex centers. The main descending tracts are shown in solid black and ascending or afferent pathways to the cortex or cerebellum are shown in white. The interconnections of the cerebral cortex, cerebellum, and basal ganglia are indicated by crosshatched arrows.

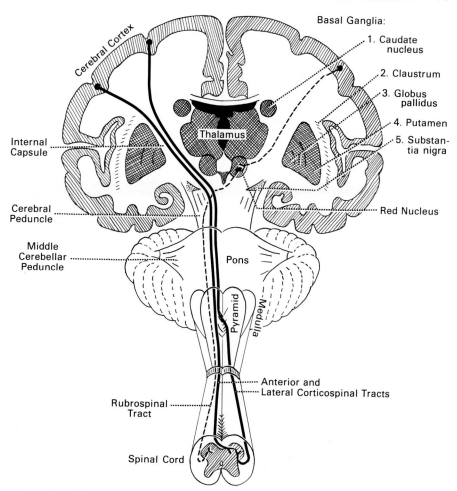

FIG. 4–10. Schematic representation of the anatomy of the suprasegmental motor system. The cerebral hemispheres are shown in a coronal section, while the pons, medualla oblongata, cerebellum, and spinal cord are in surface view. The course of the corticospinal tracts (**solid lines**) and the corticorubrospinal tracts (**interrupted lines**) is illustrated. The lateral corticospinal tract crosses to the opposite side in the pyramidal decussation, the anterior tract only shortly before terminating in the ventral horn. The rubrospinal tract crosses to the opposite side in the midbrain.

brain, in Figure 4–10. Only a summary review of this system is appropriate in the chapter; more comprehensive accounts must be sought in the references. The purpose of this review is to integrate suprasegmental motor centers with the entire motor apparatus and to give some basis to the discussion of deranged motor behavior which is the concern of Chapter 27.

The cerebral cortex projects directly to the segmental spinal motor neuron pool via the **corticospinal tracts** (Fig. 4–9). The cortex also projects to the nuclei of the brain stem **(corticobulbar tract)**, to the basal ganglia, and via the brain stem to the cerebellum. Apart from the corticospinal tracts, the segmental spinal reflex centers receive suprasegmental input only from the brain stem nuclei. Of these the **rubrospinal, vestibulospinal** and **reticulospinal** tracts will be discussed. The basal ganglia and the cerebellum feed back to the cerebral cortex by pathways which traverse or relay in the thalamus, and they also make connections with brain stem nuclei that send axons to the spinal cord (the latter connections are omitted from Fig. 4–9). Via these connections the basal ganglia and the cerebellum substantially modify and refine the influence of the cortex and of the brain stem on the spinal motor neuron pool.

The motor system can be influenced by all major sources of afferent impulses. The sources include: 1) the vestibular apparatus, 2) muscle, joint, and cutaneous receptors, 3) the visual system, and 4) the auditory apparatus. The cerebellum taps the major streams of incoming impulses, and processing them, it plays an important role in integrating the information derived from the periphery with the motor behavior dictated by the cerebral cortex. Only a fraction of the impulses that ascend to the brain are destined to inform our consciousness of the activity and position of our muscles, joints, and limbs. The rest of the sensory input drives the suprasegmental motor centers in a manner not yet completely understood, and it is essential for normal patterns of motor behavior.

The Influence of the Cerebral Cortex

The **motor cortex** has been defined as the precentral cortical area concerned with the major final output of nerve impulses responsible for voluntary movements. Clinicopathologic evidence and stimulation experiments localized the motor cortex to regions of the frontal lobe just anterior to the central sulcus. However, only 60 percent of the axons constituting the corticospinal and corticobulbar tracts issue from neurons located in the motor cortex; the remainder originate in the parietal lobe, posterior to the central sulcus. In the substance of the hemispheres, the axons traverse two fan-shaped laminae of white matter known as the **internal capsule,** and on reaching the brain stem they surface on the ventral aspect of the midbrain where they contribute to the bulk of the **cerebral peduncles.** With few exceptions, it is characteristic of the corticospinal and corticobulbar fibers to cross to the contralateral half of the brain stem or spinal cord before synapsing with motor neurons or interneurons. The majority of corticospinal fibers, identifiable on the surface of the medulla oblongata as the bulging **pyramids,** decussate at this level and continue distally as the **lateral corticospinal tract,** while the remainder known as the **anterior corticospinal tract** will cross only shortly before reaching the segmental neuron pool of their destination in the spinal cord (Fig. 4–10).

The **corticobulbar fibers** terminate either in motor neuron pools concerned with the innervation of striated muscle in the head and muscles of

similar derivation in the neck, or they relay to other brain stem nuclei which either project to the cerebellum (nuclei in the pons) or to the segmental spinal reflex centers via the rubrospinal and reticulospinal tracts. The latter two provide alternative pathways for cortical influence to the spinal reflex centers (Figs. 4–10, 4–11).

Among the **corticospinal fibers** only the largest axons make direct, monosynaptic connections with motor neurons, and these synapses are excitatory. Such large axons derived from so-called Betz cells of the motor cortex represent but a few percent of all corticospinal fibers, and they terminate predominantly on motor neurons concerned with the distal muscles of the limbs used in precisely controlled fine movements. Most corticospinal fibers are of smaller diameter and they influence more widespread motor neurons pools by relaying through interneurons. Because corticospinal fibers can activate both excitatory and inhibitory interneurons, this multisynaptic pathway enables the same descending impulse to excite one group of muscles and to inhibit their functional antagonists simultaneously. Thereby the suprasegmental command overrules the segmental postural reflexes, liberating the muscles for voluntary performance. As discussed in relation with alpha-gamma coactivation, both fusimotor and skeletomotor neurons are influenced by the descending impulses.

Not all corticospinal fibers are concerned with voluntary movements, nor are corticospinal fibers the only pathway through which the segmental reflex centers can be influenced. Fine motor control will be lost in a limb if the area of the motor cortex specifically concerned with that limb is destroyed, but all movement may not be lost. Likewise, partial or complete interruption of the descending tract in the internal capsule, cerebral peduncle, pyramid, or spinal cord does not necessarily lead to total loss of movement in the part affected. Depending on their precise location, such lesions may produce profound changes in muscle tone which may be more debilitating than the loss of voluntary control.

The Influence of the Brain Stem

The corticospinal tracts descend through the brain stem and are joined by the **rubrospinal** and **reticulospinal tracts** which originate from the red nucleus of the midbrain and from nuclei in the reticular formation of the pons and the medulla oblongata (Figs. 4–10, 4–11). All these nuclei receive corticobulbar afferents and the tracts that descend from them provide alternative pathways for cortical control of the spinal segmental reflex centers. These tracts are largely intermingled in the spinal cord with corticospinal fibers, and their influence on the motor neuron pool is quite similar to that of the more direct fibers.

The **vestibular apparatus,** located in the inner ear and concerned with the special sense of equilibrium, head positioning, head acceleration, and deceleration, projects to the segmental spinal reflex centers through the brain stem. Two **vestibulospinal tracts** originate in vestibular nuclei of the brain stem which are under the direct influence of the vestibular nerve and the cerebellum (Fig. 4–11). These tracts remain predominantly ipsilateral and they project mainly to the segmental motor neuron pool of the axial musculature but can also affect motor neurons of limb muscles. The multisynaptic pathways are excitatory to spinal extensors and inhibitory to spinal flexors.

Vestibular impulses are relayed to the cerebral cortex as well as to the cerebellum, but the vestibular system operates largely at a subconscious level, and is responsible for postural reflexes. Discussion of these reflexes is beyond the scope of this book. It should, however, be noted that the cerebral cortex and the cerebellum override and modulate postural reflexes and integrate them into voluntary motor behavior.

The Influence of Basal Ganglia

Large masses of gray matter located in the substance of the cerebral hemispheres and in the rostral part of the brain stem are known collectively as the **basal ganglia.** The members of this complex are interconnected and include the **caudate nucleus, the putamen, globus pallidus, claustrum, subthalamic nucleus,** and **substantia nigra** (Fig. 4–10). None of the basal ganglia project to spinal reflex centers, but it is known that the motor activity of the cerebral cortex is modulated by them via a circuit that includes certain nuclei of the thalamus through which cerebellar input to the cortex also passes. Certain brain stem nuclei also appear to be modulated in some way by the basal ganglia. The excitatory and inhibitory influences exerted on the cortex are so complex that their physiology does not yet fall into a clearly understood pattern. When various nuclei of the basal ganglia are damaged, the resulting motor behavior disturbance is characterized sometimes by uncontrolled movements such as tremor, ballismus, and choreiform

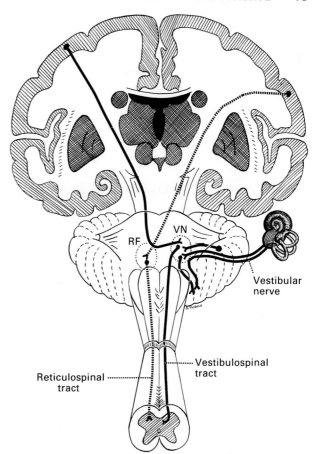

FIG. 4–11. Reticulospinal and vestibulospinal tracts with some important connections of the respective brain stem nuclei. Some components of the corticobulbar tracts relay to nuclei of the reticular formation (RF) located in the brain stem. From these nuclei originate the reticulospinal tracts. Vestibular nuclei (VN) receive afferents from the vestibular apparatus, the cerebellum, and also from the cerebral cortex. They project to the spinal cord via the vestibulospinal tracts, to the cerebellum via the inferior cerebellar peduncle, and to the cerebral cortex (not shown). The reticular formation and the vestibular nuclei are more extensive and diffuse than it is possible to illustrate in such a simplified diagram.

movements. Damage to other basal ganglia may result in changes in muscle tone or general hypokinesia (reduced movement). These abnormalities are discussed in Chapter 27.

The Influence of the Cerebellum

The primary function of the cerebellum is to coordinate movement and to control its precision both

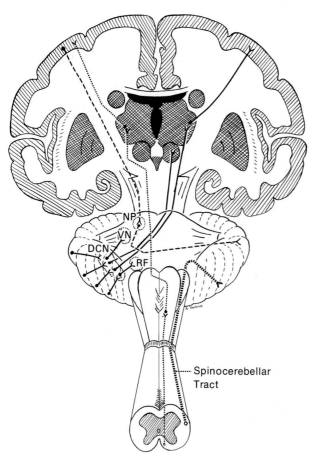

Spinocerebellar
Tract

FIG. 4–12. A summary of the connections of the cerebellum. Proprioceptive impulses are relayed from the spinal cord directly to the cerebellum via the spinocerebellar tracts **(heavy interrupted line).** Of the two spinocerebellar tracts only the ventral tract is illustrated; the dorsal tract, of similar function and destination, follows a slightly different course in the brain stem. Proprioceptive impulses travel also in the dorsal columns of the spinal cord **(light interrupted line),** and on their way to the cerebral cortex relay in the medulla and thalamus. Corticopontine fibers **(long interrupted line)** relay in the nuclei pontis (NP), and cerebral influence reaches the cerebellar cortex via pontocerebellar fibers in the middle peduncle. Input from the vestibular nerve to the cerebellar cortex is illustrated in Figure 4–11. Efferent impulses **(solid line)** arising from the cerebellar cortex relay in several deep cerebellar nuclei (DCN)—here shown schematically as one nuclear mass—and the efferents of these nuclei reach the vestibular nucleus (VN), the reticular formation (RF), the red nucleus, and thalamus whence they are transmitted to the cerebral cortex. No attempt is made in this schematic drawing to localize the origin and termination of the various tracts to specific parts of the cerebellum.

in time and space. This large part of the brain may be resected without any evident impairment of sensory perception, intellectual faculties, or significant loss of muscle power, but precision and smoothness of movement will be lost.

The cerebellum consists of a narrow median ridge, the **vermis,** and two large lateral **hemispheres,** which like the hemispheres of the cerebrum, possess an outer **cortex** of gray matter and more deeply seated **nuclei** embedded in a central core of white matter. A more detailed description of cerebellar anatomy is not appropriate for the purposes of this chapter. Suffice it to state in broad terms that the cerebellum is appended to the brain stem by three pairs of large fiber bundles, the **superior, middle,** and **inferior cerebellar peduncles** through which information is relayed to and from the cerebellum.

The bulk of the afferent input to the cerebellum is derived from three major sources capable of profoundly influencing movement (Figs. 4–9, 4–12): 1) the vestibular apparatus and vestibular nuclei of the brain stem, 2) stretch receptors of muscle and tendon and proprioceptive afferents from joints and periarticular tissues, which ascend to the brain stem via the spinocerebellar tracts in the spinal cord, 3) the cerebral cortex, via the corticobulbar tract and nuclei of the pons. The cerebral cortex, of course, receives proprioceptive input from the dorsal column tracts of the spinal cord which relay in the brain stem (gracile and cuneate nuclei) and the thalamus. This input modulates the influence of the cerebral cortex on the cerebellum. These three major channels of afferent impulses project directly to the cerebellar cortex, and it is here that they are processed and integrated through a rather complex circuitry. The output of the cerebellar cortex is first relayed to the deep cerebellar nuclei and the efferents of these neurons project either to the vestibular and reticular nuclei of the brain stem where they influence the descending vestibulospinal and reticulospinal tracts, or they ascend to the red nucleus and motor cortex via the thalamus where they modulate the impulses that descend to spinal motor neurons along the corticospinal and rubrospinal tracts (Figs. 4–9, 4–12).

The areas to which vestibular, spinal, and cerebral impulses project are fairly well defined on the cerebellar cortex, as are the specific cerebellar nuclei which dispatch efferent impulses to the brain stem and to the cerebral cortex. In contrast to cerebral modulation of movement, it is characteristic of the cerebellum that one of its hemispheres influences movement on the ipsilateral side of the body, and this influence on the spinal motor neuron pool is exerted indirectly via corticospinal and bulbospinal descending tracts. Disturbances of cerebellar function, or the removal of cerebellar influence from the motor centers becomes evident when muscles are being used, contrasting in this respect with abnormalities of the basal ganglia. Cerebellar dysfunction is manifest, for instance, by the loss of coordination between prime movers, synergists, and antagonists, by the breakdown of complex movements into their component units, by overshooting and undershooting in limb movements, and by intention tremor. These abnormalities are discussed again in Chapter 27.

Suprasegmental Influence on Muscle Tone

In the last analysis, muscle tone depends on the activity of alpha motor neurons. In the normal muscle, dynamic tone is generated by the tonic stretch reflex through afferent input from the muscle spindles. The sensitivity of the spindles is increased by gamma motor neuron activity. This mechanism is mediated by the following circuit: gamma motor neuron discharge → intrafusal fiber contraction → excitation of spindle stretch receptors → alpha motor neuron discharge → skeletomotor fiber contraction (i.e., muscle tone). Suprasegmental influences may alter the activity of both gamma and alpha motor neurons and thereby change muscle tone. This explains how under stressful situations muscle tone may be increased in normal individuals and spinal reflexes may become more brisk than in a "relaxed" state. Available physiologic and clinicopathologic data are as yet inadequate for synthesizing a unified, simple concept of how the different descending tracts affect the balance of synaptic input to motor neuron pools of functionally distinct muscle groups. It is well known, however, that interruption of descending pathways in the internal capsule leads not only to contralateral paralysis, but such a lesion also increases the tone of antigravity muscles and of upper limb flexors on the side contralateral to the lesion. This is a common syndrome in patients who suffer a stroke. The spasticity is believed to be due to interruption of neuronal pathways which inhibit other motor centers, and as a consequence the excitatory influence of these centers is exaggerated on the spinal motor neuron pool. In the example quoted, muscle spasticity is thought to be due to the unrestrained excitatory activity of the reticulospinal and vestibulospinal tracts, because the lesion in the internal capsule removes cortical inhibition from the brain stem nuclei. Disruptions of connections between the basal ganglia and the motor cortex cause excessive muscle tone which in this case is known as rigidity. Rigidity develops because the inhibitory influences of the basal ganglia are abolished by such lesions. Chapter 27 discusses abnormalities of muscle tone that result from suprasegmental disorders.

SUGGESTED READING

Granit, R. The Basis of Motor Control. New York, Academic Press, 1970
A comprehensive monograph integrating the activity of muscles, alpha and gamma motor neurons and their control systems.

Kottke, F. J. Reflex patterns initiated by the secondary fiber endings of muscle spindles. A proposal. Arch. Phys. Med. Rehabil. 56:1, 1975
The author describes regional responses to stretch stimuli in spastic patients and suggests that these are mediated through flowerspray receptors of muscle spindles.

Lockhard, R. D. Anatomy of muscles and their relation to movement and posture. In Bourne, G. H. (ed): The Structure and Function of Muscle, Vol. 1, Part 1, 2nd ed., New York, Academic Press, 1972, p. 1
An interesting discussion of the design and gross structure of muscles in the human body correlated with the various types of actions individual muscles or muscle groups can perform.

MacConnaill, M. A., and Basmajian, J. V. Muscles and Movements. Baltimore, Williams & Wilkins, 1969
A readable and interesting book. Its first half deals with the theory and mathematical analysis of muscle action, and in its second half treats specific muscle groups and movements with an interesting approach.

Patton, H. D., Sundsten, J. W., Crill, W. E., and Swanson, P. D. Introduction to Basic Neurology. Philadelphia, W. B. Saunders, 1976
Chapters "Spinal Reflex Pathways," "Reflex Behavioral Patterns," "Suprasegmental Control of Movement," "The Basal Ganglia," and "The Cerebellum" present well written, concise accounts of neuromuscular physiology and motor behavior highly pertinent to the present chapter.

de Reuck, A. V. S., and Knight, J. (eds): Myotatic, Kinesthetic and Vestibular Mechanisms. Ciba Foundation Symposium, Boston, Little, Brown, 1967
An excellent collection of papers by leading workers in the field. The chapter by D. Barker is particularly relevant.

Willis, W. D., and Grossman, R. Y. Medical Neurobiology. St. Louis, Mosby, 1973
Well-illustrated book dealing with neuroanatomical and neurophysiological principles basic to clinical neuroscience.

5
Joints

CORNELIUS ROSSE, PETER A. SIMKIN

The joint with its associated structures represents the functional unit of the musculoskeletal system. **A joint, or articulation, is a union of two or more bones.** The mode of construction of this union varies greatly and reflects the function required of the joint. The function of joints is to secure the union of the articulating skeletal pieces and to permit, even facilitate, their movement in relation to one another. Joints are the bearings of the body machine.

CLASSIFICATION AND DEVELOPMENT OF JOINTS

Joints may be classified according to several criteria but none of the proposed classifications is entirely satisfactory or consistent. In the great majority of mammalian joints, free articular surfaces slide, spin, or roll upon one another, there being no other tissue interposed at all between the mating surfaces. Movement in such joints is facilitated by a lubricant, synovial fluid, and such joints are known as **synovial joints. In nonsynovial joints** there are no free surfaces and connective tissue of considerable strength is interposed between opposing surfaces of bones. Such an arrangement largely precludes movement of the skeletal pieces though some angulation and distraction may be possible. When the intervening tissue is fibrous tissue, the joint is called a **fibrous joint,** and when it is cartilage, a **cartilaginous joint.**

In terms of the definition given, an epiphyseal plate should also be regarded as a joint, in which hyaline cartilage unites two bones. Hyaline cartilage between bony pieces invariably ossifies; these so-called *primary cartilaginous joints* serve only for the purpose of growth and may be disregarded in the present discussion. On the other hand, fibrocartilage interposed between bones does func-

tion as a joint, and usually remains functional throughout life. Such fibrocartilaginous (or *secondary cartilaginous*) joints are known as **symphyses.**

Joints have also been classified as **immovable, slightly movable,** and **freely movable,** on the basis of the amount of movement possible. These so-called *functional* categories have been equated with fibrous, fibrocartilaginous, and synovial joints, respectively, although exceptions must be made to this generalization. It is helpful to consider the characteristics of some of these joints together with their development.

Development

The development of joints is governed by genetic factors but appropriate mechanical forces are also required *in utero* and throughout life for the attainment and maintenance of normal joint anatomy. When joints are unable to move, as in congenital paralytic neuromuscular disorders, the synovial cavity and other articular structures fail to develop. Likewise, a joint immobilized or denied normal usage will degenerate and will become replaced by poorly organized connective tissue.

As discussed in Chapter 2, the primordia of bones develop in embryonic connective tissue or mesenchyme and, with the exception of membrane bones, ossification is preceded by cartilage formation (Fig. 5–1). The layer of mesenchymal cells which will become the perichondrium and later the periosteum continues across the gap between the primordial bones, enclosing some mesenchyme between them. This mesenchyme, referred to as the **interzonal mesenchyme,** represents the primitive joint and has the potential to develop in a variety of ways.

In **nonsynovial joints** the interzonal mesenchyme differentiates into fibrous tissue or fibrocar-

77

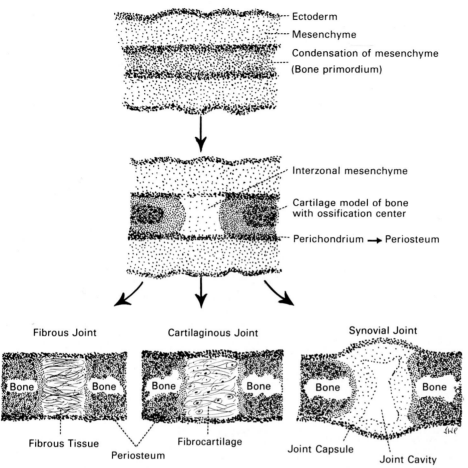

FIG. 5-1. Schematic representation of the embryologic development of different types of joints. For description see text.

tilage. **Fibrous joints** develop between the bones of the skull, exemplified by the **sutures** and by the union of the teeth and their sockets. Fibrous joints do not develop outside the skull with the single exception of the distal tibiofibular joint or syndesmosis. During growth the sutures permit the expansion of the brain and up to the age of two, some bones of the cranium remain palpably separated. The intervening gaps known as **fontanelles** are bridged by the fibrous tissue of the widely open sutures. With the cessation of growth, fibrous joints are rendered immovable. The tibiofibular syndesmosis, the only fibrous joint of the appendicular skeleton, permits some movement between the two bones throughout life but its chief function is to prevent separation of the tibia and fibula at the ankle joint.

Fibrocartilaginous joints or **symphyses** are found between the bodies of the vertebrae (inter-

vertebral disks), the two pubic bones (pubic symphysis), and between the manubrium and sternum. All these bones are formed in hyaline cartilage and a layer of this tissue is retained on the joint surfaces. Collagen fiber bundles of the intervening fibrocartilage penetrate the hyaline cartilage on each side and are anchored in subchondral bone. Symphyses are only slightly movable. The considerable range of movement possible in the vertebral column is due to the summation of relatively minor angulations between consecutive vertebrae. The fibrocartilage anchors the articulating bones securely to one another and is ideally suited for withstanding compression and shearing forces.

The development of **synovial joints** differs from that of nonsynovial joints in that the interzonal mesenchyme liquifies between the articulating surfaces, generates a **joint cavity,** and thereby renders the articular surfaces *free.* Such a joint is well adapted for movement and represents the most highly evolved articulation in phylogeny. In man, with the two exceptions already noted (tibiofibular syndesmosis and the pubic symphysis), all joints of the appendicular skeleton are synovial. In the axial skeleton there are synovial joints between the arches of consecutive vertebrae, between the skull and the first two cervical vertebrae, and at the junction of the ribs with the vertebrae and with the sternum. Although synovial joints are, as a rule, capable of free motion, the possible range of movement varies greatly in different joints in accord with their requirements for function and stability.

In synovial joints as in symphyses, the articular surfaces are covered by hyaline cartilage, but in synovial joints this tissue acquires the specialized architecture of articular cartilage. Peripheral portions of the interzonal mesenchyme differentiate into two types of tissue. Layers of cells facing the joint cavity develop into the synovial membrane. More peripheral cells together with those derived from the periosteum bridging the gap between the articulating bones, develop into the joint capsule and its associated ligaments. These cells transform into dense fibrous tissue and represent one of the factors that furnishes stability to the articulation. In certain synovial joints the interzonal mesenchyme also forms fat pads and fibrocartilaginous structures. The latter include labra or lips formed around the hip and shoulder sockets, and articular disks which partly or completely divide the joint cavity and improve the fit of the mating surfaces.

THE SYNOVIAL JOINT

Continuous interaction with the environment relies on movements that invariably involve multiple synovial joints. Of all joints synovial joints are the most numerous in the body and they are the most frequently affected by trauma and disease. To deal with these processes it is essential to understand the general anatomy, the component tissues, and the functional mechanics which govern movement in these joints.

General Anatomy

The anatomic features of a synovial joint are shown diagrammatically in Figure 5–2. Comparison with Figure 5–3 which is a photograph of a bisected synovial joint amply emphasizes the

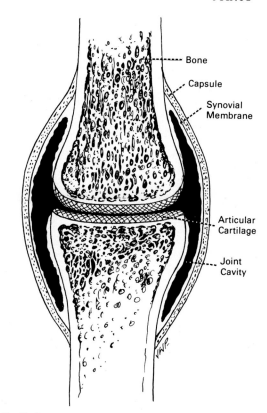

FIG. 5–2. Diagrammatic representation of the anatomic features of a typical synovial joint seen in a section cut across the middle of the joint. The extent of the joint cavity is exaggerated to show the anatomic arrangement of the synovial membrane more clearly.

exaggerations and distortions of schematic representations.

As a rule, synovial joints are completely enclosed by the **joint capsule,** and all structures inside this fibrous sleeve are regarded as intraarticular. In the majority of joints the capsule's attachment to bone is close to the margins of the articular surfaces, although it is some distance away in some large joints of the limbs (shoulder and hip). On the long bones the capsule may attach to the epiphysis or metaphysis, enclosing fairly extensive nonarticular bony surfaces within the joint. In some instances, the epiphyseal line is partly or completely intraarticular.

The **articular surfaces** or facets are reciprocally curved, though complete congruity does not exist between them. The extent of interlocking between the surfaces is considerable in some joints (hip, elbow) while in others it is much less striking (knee, radioulnar joints). The fit of the mating ar-

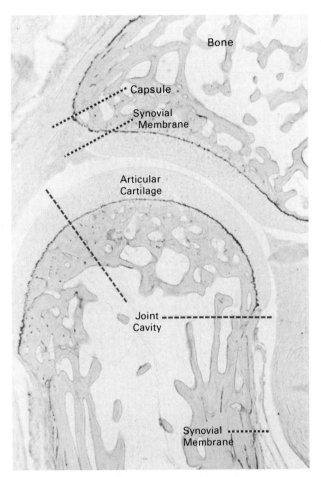

Bone

Capsule

Synovial
Membrane

Articular
Cartilage

Joint
Cavity

Synovial
Membrane

FIG. 5–3. Microphotograph of the interphalangeal joint of a finger. The joint has been sectioned sagittally to correspond to the schematic drawing in Figure 5–2. The spongy bone is more dense in the subchondral area. A black line represents the deepest, calcified zone of articular cartilage and clearly demarcates this tissue from subchondral bone. Folds of the synovial membrane bulge into the spaces between the diverging articular surfaces. The relationship of the membrane to intraarticular portions of the phalanx not covered by articular cartilage is clearly shown in the lower half of the photograph. (Courtesy of the Arthritis Foundation)

ticular surfaces is improved somewhat by the annular fibrocartilaginous lip or **labrum** attached around the socket-shaped facet in the shoulder and the hip joints.

The **synovial membrane** lines the capsular sleeve (it is bound to it) and attaches around the edges of the articular surfaces. The membrane invests nonarticular bony surfaces in the joint cavity as well as fat pads, tendons, and ligaments. Fat pads

are always between the capsule and the synovial membrane, and tendons and ligaments traversing the joint (e.g., in shoulder and in knee joints) are ensheathed by the membrane. These structures, though intraarticular, are not bathed by synovial fluid, which fills the synovial cavity. Only articular surfaces, labra, and articular disks are in direct contact with synovial fluid.

Several joints contain fibrocartilaginous disks. The circumference of these **articular disks** fuses with the capsule, and they are usually anchored also to one or both articulating bones (knee, wrist joints). They are never loose in the joint and may receive the insertion of muscles. Though the center of the disks may become worn through, they normally divide the joint into two compartments and are interposed like a shelf or pad between the articulating surfaces (temporomandibular, sternoclavicular, acromioclavicular, and ulnocarpal joints). An exception to this is the knee where the disks are incomplete, crescent-shaped, and are known as *menisci*. While the function of the disks is not precisely known, it is assumed that they act as shock absorbers, aid a more even distribution of weight and synovial fluid, and improve the fit of articular surfaces. They are characteristic of those joints where gliding movements occur in combination with angular and rotational displacements. The menisci of the knee may be resected without obvious impairment of function, but they usually regenerate sometime after resection. Less is known about articular disks of other joints.

Component Tissues

Articular Cartilage. Articular cartilage differs from hyaline cartilage elsewhere in the body in that it is not covered by perichondrium, does not ossify, and its collagen fibers form a three-dimensional network adapted to load bearing and to maintaining the integrity of a smooth surface. This surface is highly wear resistant and almost friction free. Due to the capacity of collagen fibrils to bind proteoglycans into a highly resilient, water-filled, structural gel, articular cartilage is able to resist and to distribute into subchondral bone the enormous compressive forces developed by muscle action and gravity.

The *deepest zone* of articular cartilage is calcified, and over an undulating surface of ridges and grooves it is continuous with subchondral bone (Figs. 5–3, 5–4). Scanning electron microscopic studies of suitably digested, unfixed, human articular cartilage have confirmed that individual collagen fibrils originate in the trabeculae of subchondral bone. These fibrils become grouped into larger bundles at the interface of calcified and uncalcified cartilage (tide mark) and then run radially toward the surface crossing each other in the *middle zone* of the cartilage. This arrangement gives the impression of arcades (Fig. 5–4) which were originally described by Benninghoff in 1925. The collagen bundles open out into a felt-work of fibrils in the *superficial zone* and become oriented randomly but parallel to the surface, creating a protective or *armor layer*. The surface of human articular cartilage is quite smooth. However, the scanning electron microscope reveals humps on the surface of juvenile articular cartilage (Fig. 5–5A), in all possibility corresponding to chondrocytes in the armor layer which is more cellular in the child than in the adult. In the adult the humps are replaced by depressions or pits (Fig. 5–5B) which are probably due to the collapse of the armor layer into the underlying lacunae. It is not known whether or not such humps and pits are present *in vivo* before articular cartilage is processed for microscopy. When articular cartilage fails, flaking first occurs parallel to the superficial collagen fibers with subsequent progression to clefts which may penetrate the full thickness of the cartilage (see Chap. 24).

Chondrocytes are relatively sparse in articular cartilage. They are large and round in the deeper layers and continuously synthesize proteins and glycosaminoglycans. Toward the surface they are compressed and flattened. After the cessation of growth, mitotic figures are usually not seen. Chondrocytes are capable of resuming mitotic activity *in vitro*, however, when the pericellular matrix is dissolved, or when the cartilage undergoes degenerative changes *in vivo*.

Articular cartilage is avascular and devoid of nerves. For its nourishment, it largely depends on the movement of fluid in and out of its matrix. When load is applied, water is expressed from the cartilage. With subsequent decompression, water is imbibed. This fluid movement is thought to be important, not only in the metabolism of articular cartilage, but also in lubrication of the articular surfaces.

Joint Capsule. The joint capsule consists chiefly of interlacing collagen fiber bundles which provide strength but little elasticity. During movement the capsule tends to be thrown into accordionlike folds on one aspect of the joint, while it becomes taut on the opposite aspect, thus limiting the range of movement. The oblique course of the fiber bundles which criss-cross each other may also permit rotation of the bones, imparting an apparent elasticity to the capsule. The capsule may be as much as several millimeters thick and as a rule is directly reinforced by **ligaments.** Additional or **accessory ligaments** may also be found independent of the capsule, and can be either inside or outside the joint. In general, ligaments are found in the planes in which the joint requires greater stability, where they restrain motion in an undesirable direction. The simplest construction is seen in a hinge joint, where ligaments on either side (collateral ligaments) prevent side-to-side motion but do not hinder motion through the axis of the hinge.

Defects may exist in the capsule through which the joint cavity communicates with adjacent bursae (e.g., subscapularis bursa of shoulder joint), or through which muscles or their tendons enter or leave the joint (e.g., shoulder and knee joints). Fusion of tendons with the capsule may substantially reinforce it (e.g., rotator cuff of the shoulder joint) or the capsule may be partially replaced by a ten-

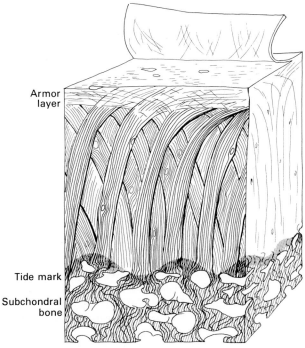

FIG. 5–4. Schematic view of the collagen fibrillar organization in human articular cartilage in a full thickness block from the surface to the deep subchondral bone. The most superficial lamina of the armor layer (lamina splendens) has been incised, peeled off, and reflected. (Redrawn from Minns RJ, Steven FS: J Anat 123:437, 1977)

Armor layer

Tide mark

Subchondral bone

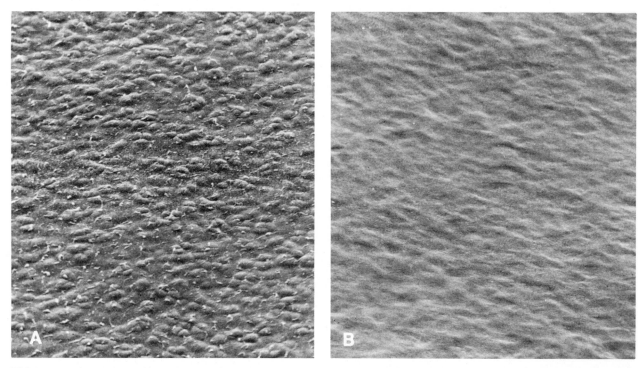

FIG. 5–5. The surface of human articular cartilage seen with the scanning electron microscope. **(A)** Femoral condyle of a 7-year-old boy showing numerous humps and flocculent precipitate of synovial fluid. (× 230) **(B)** Femoral condyle of a 34-year-old man showing pits characteristic of adult cartilage. (× 120) (Courtesy of Dr. F. N. Ghadially and **A** also of J Anat, 124:425, 1977)

don with which it fuses (e.g., quadriceps tendon and its sesamoid bone, the patella in the knee).

Synovial Membrane. The synovial membrane or **synovium** is a delicate, continuous lining of vascular connective tissue. Two layers can be distinguished in the membrane: 1) the **synovial intima** facing the joint cavity which consists of synovial cells embedded in matrix and 2) the **subintima,** highly vascular, loose connective tissue in which the amount of fat cells, collagen, and elastic fibers varies from place to place. Although synovial joints are often spoken of as serous cavities, the synovial membrane is not equivalent to coelomic serous membranes such as the peritoneum or pleura.

Synovial cells do not form a continuous epithelium and a basement membrane is lacking. The intima may be 1–4 cells deep or the synovial cells may expose the matrix in places directly to synovial fluid. Two types of synovial cells may be distinguished by electron microscopy but transitional forms between the two also exist. One type of cell has extensive rough surfaced endoplasmic reticulum and is responsible for secreting

hyaluronic acid, the important component which renders synovial fluid viscous. The other cell type appears to be primarily involved in pinocytosis and phagocytosis.

The synovial microvasculature consists of a rich bed of capillaries. Small solutes exchange rapidly across these microvessels and the over-all exchange is limited principally by passive diffusion through the interstitial tissue interposed between the synovial cavity and the capillaries. The subintimal loose connective tissue also contains lymphatics, free lymphocytes, mast cells, monocytes and macrophages. Under pathologic conditions, the latter play an important role in removing particulate matter (including blood cells) from the joint cavity.

Macroscopically, the synovial membrane is pink, smooth, and shiny. It is thrown into folds and presents villous projections on its surface. After synovectomy, the synovial membrane rapidly regenerates from the connective tissue on the inner aspect of the capsule. Indeed, synovial membrane may arise from loose connective tissue anywhere in the body. The structure of synovial membrane in bursae and tendon sheaths resembles that found in synovial joints.

Synovial Fluid. The synovial cavity is normally collapsed and in most joints exists only as a potential space. The space visible between the articulating ends of bones on x-rays is often spoken of as the *joint space*. However, this space is occupied by articular cartilage which is transparent to x-rays (Chap. 8). Synovial fluid moistens and lubricates the articular surfaces, the synovium, and the intraarticular disks. This film of fluid fills the cavity but normally its volume is too small to form pools. Therefore, attempts to aspirate fluid from normal joints are usually unsuccessful except in the knee, from which up to 3 ml of fluid may be obtained on occasion, because this joint is particularly large and complex.

The fluid itself is a filtrate of plasma. It contains electrolytes and other small molecules at concentrations essentially the same as plasma but with a much lower level of total protein (less than 2 g/100 ml). Almost all of the protein normally present is albumin and other small proteins. Larger molecules such as fibrinogen and certain components of the complement are present only in trace amounts, thus normal fluid does not clot and has low levels of hemolytic complement activity. The most distinguishing characteristic of synovial fluid is the presence of hyaluronate molecules. These large, polymeric, glycosaminoglycan molecules make the fluid viscous and slimy.

Synovial fluid provides nourishment to articular cartilage and to articular disks. Through the exchange of molecules between synovial microvasculature and these tissues, it is also responsible for clearing their metabolites. Synovial fluid serves as a lubricant not only for the articular bearings (cartilage on cartilage) but also for the folding and unfolding of synovium over temporarily free articular surfaces. It contributes to joint stability through its surface tension, behaving essentially as an adhesive.

Blood and Nerve Supply

An anastomotic plexus of blood vessels *(periarticular anastomosis)* and nerves surrounds the capsule on the exterior, and branches of these plexuses penetrate the capsule (see Fig. 7–5). The periarticular anastomosis is fed by branches of arteries passing the joint and is the source of blood to the capillary bed in the synovial membrane and also to the epiphyses.

Joint pain and the awareness of the precise position of the limbs (proprioception) amply testify to the rich innervation of joints and associated structures. Articular nerves are composed of **somatic sensory fibers** (pain, pressure, vibration sense, temperature, and proprioception) and of **autonomic vasomotor fibers.** The nerves are distributed to the fibrous capsule, the ligaments, the synovial membrane, and the periosteum. Articular cartilage is devoid of nerve supply. Practically all nerves in the synovial membrane are thought to serve a vasomotor function. Proprioceptive and pain impulses generated in the capsule and ligaments play a major role not only in informing us of the position of our limbs but in influencing reflex contraction and inhibition of muscles that act on the joint. **As a rule, each joint is supplied by branches of all nerves which innervate the muscles producing movement at that joint.** In most joints, the aspect of the capsule stretched by the contraction of one muscle is supplied by the nerve innervating the antagonists of that muscle. This relationship is likely to be an important factor in preventing overstretching the capsule.

The afferent impulses arising in joints are generated by several types of receptors. These nerve endings include lamellated Ruffini and paciniform corpuscles concerned with proprioception and free nerve endings sensitive to pain. In addition, tendon organs (Chap. 4) are present in some ligaments. When the nerve supply is lost, the joint rapidly undergoes degenerative changes, suggesting that the innervation of joints is an important factor in maintaining their normal structure.

MOVEMENTS IN SYNOVIAL JOINTS

The simplest movement possible between two articulating surfaces is *sliding* or gliding—one bone moving bodily across the surface of the other. If the surfaces are fairly flat, gliding may take place in any direction, but angular or rotational displacements will essentially not occur between the articulating bones. Because of the flatness of the surfaces such joints are known as **plane joints.** Many articulations between the bones of the carpus and tarsus (intercarpal and intertarsal joints) as well as between the arches or vertebrae are of such type.

The effective use of the limbs and movements of the head rely on joints in which the articular surfaces present pronounced curvatures, which may be considered as segments of spheres, ellipsoids, cones, and cylinders. The lack of complete con-

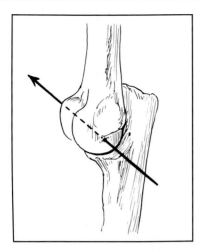

FIG. 5–6. Hinge joint (elbow).

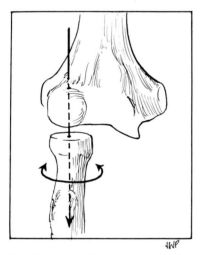

FIG. 5–7. Pivot joint (superior radioulnar joint).

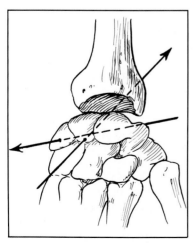

FIG. 5–8. Ellipsoid joint (radiocarpal joint).

gruity as well as disproportion in size between the mating surfaces permits some *rolling* (or rocking) and *spinning* of one bone upon the other. In most joints, the movement of greatest amplitude is achieved by one bone sliding on the other, the axis of motion being placed at the center of the arc defining the convex member of the pair. As a consequence, the end of the moving bone distal to the articulation describes arcs. Traditionally, such movements have been explained with reference to the *axes* placed through the center of the curved articular surfaces. The number of such possible axes around which movement may be produced *independently* and actively, determines the *degrees of freedom* in a joint.

The varieties of synovial joints and their characteristic movements are most satisfactorily explained on an elementary level by retaining this traditional concept of joint axes and classifying the joints accordingly. It is important, however, to carry the analysis of movements a step further and consider the mechanics of joints in the light of more recently developed concepts of kinesiology. The subsequent section will concern itself with such an analysis, while for the present synovial joints will be discussed according to joint axes and the types of movements their anatomy permits.

Varieties of Synovial Joints and Their Movements

Those joints in which one or more articular surfaces are perceptibly curved may be classified as uniaxial, biaxial, and polyaxial. These varieties of joints possess one, two, or three degrees of freedom, respectively.

Uniaxial Joints. Movement is possible around only one axis. This axis may be transverse across the articular surfaces, in which case the joint is regarded as a **hinge joint** (Fig. 5–6); or the axis may lie longitudinally along the shaft of the bone, in which case one speaks of a **pivot joint** (Fig. 5–7). The humeroulnar joint at the elbow and the interphalangeal joints of the hand and feet are hinge joints; the radioulnar and the atlantoaxial joints are pivot joints.

The movements permitted in a hinge joint are flexion and extension. **Flexion** occurs when the angle between the adjoining bones is decreased, as when the elbow is bent forward. **Extension** occurs when the angle between the adjoining bones is increased, as when the arm is straightened at the elbow. Both movements take place in one and the same plane.

Only one movement is permitted in a pivot joint, rotation. **Rotation** occurs when a bone spins around a central longitudinal axis without undergoing any displacement from that axis. This is equally true of the radius which rotates in a stationary osseoligamentous ring (p. 207), and of the atlas, which, as a ring, rotates around the stationary odontoid process (see Fig. 9–6).

Biaxial Joints. Movement is possible around two axes, which lie at approximately 90° to one another. Ellipsoid and saddle joints fall into this category.

In an **ellipsoid joint,** a convex ellipsoid surface is received into a concave ellipsoid surface, like an egg resting in a spoon. One axis is along the long diameter and the other along the short diameter of the articular surfaces (Fig. 5–8). The wrist joint and the metacarpophalangeal joints are shaped in this manner. Movement on the long axis produces flexion and extension in one plane, while on the short axis, abduction and adduction take place in another plane. **Abduction** is movement away from the median plane and **adduction** is movement toward it. For finger movements the reference line is the middle finger.

In a **saddle joint** (Fig. 5–9) the articular surfaces are saddle-shaped as, for example, in the carpometacarpal joint of the thumb. The same movements are possible as in an ellipsoid joint. In the anatomic sense, ellipsoid and saddle joints do not permit independent or active rotation of the bones, but **circumduction,** the harmonious combination of flexion-abduction-extension-adduction, gives the impression of rotation as the bone circumscribes a conical space.

Polyaxial Joints. Movement is possible around innumerable axes, exemplified by the ball-and-socket joint. In a **ball-and-socket joint** (Fig. 5–10) the articular surfaces are reciprocal segments of a hypothetical sphere, as, for example, in the shoulder and hip joints. All the types of movements described so far are possible at a ball-and-socket joint, including rotation and circumduction.

Mechanics of Movement

The foregoing consideration of movements, though helpful, does not reflect the true behavior of joint surfaces. More accurate concepts in the mechanics of joint movement are useful in understanding such complex joints as the shoulder, hip, and knee. The following discussion anticipates the analysis of movement at these joints, and their movements are dealt with in the appropriate chapters.

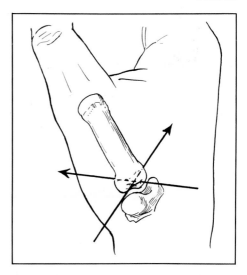

FIG. 5–9. Saddle joint (carpometacarpal joint of the thumb).

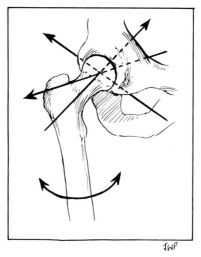

FIG. 5–10. Ball-and-socket joint (hip). Only three of the innumerable axes are shown.

The Nature of Articular Surfaces. As already implied, articular surfaces are geometrically imperfect, and in all varieties of synovial joints, including plane joints, the surfaces are composites of several convex or concave ovoids. The radii of these ovoids, of course, vary greatly from joint to joint. In the majority of joints, convex or male ovoid surfaces articulate with concave or female ovoids and there is considerable disparity in size and curvature between the male and female surfaces in any given joint. In other joints, each surface is composed of ovoids convex in one plane and concave in the other (sellar or saddle-shaped surfaces), and the larger of these is considered the male. In all but

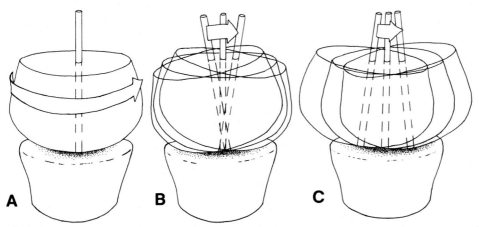

FIG. 5-11. Spin **A,** roll **B,** and slide **C,** the three basic types of movement possible between a pair of male and female articular surfaces in a synovial joint. In the example illustrated, the male surface moves over a stationary female surface. A moving female surface on a stationary male surface would be likewise free to spin, roll, or slide. Usually these movements occur in combinations. (Redrawn from Warwick R, Williams PL (eds): Gray's Anatomy, 35th ed. Philadelphia, WB Saunders, 1973)

one position of a joint, contact between the surfaces is restricted to a small area only, which is due to the incongruity of the mating pair. The male ovoid, as a rule, has a smaller radius than the female. This arrangement is decidedly unstable and greatly enhances the tendency for movement. Movement is further facilitated by the lubricating properties of synovial fluid which fills the wedge-shaped spaces between the divergent surfaces around the restricted area of contact.

Basic Types of Movements. All the types of movements discussed in the previous section are the outcome of three basic displacements. These displacements are: a **spin,** a **roll,** and a **slide.** The definitions of these movements are explicit in Figure 5-11. It should be evident that in view of the permutable relationship between the articular surfaces, and because of the composite nature of forces that act on the bones, pure spins and pure rolls are rather unusual events. As a rule, spins and rolls of a bone in all varieties of joints are accompanied by sliding. At the same time, it must be appreciated, though it is not intuitively obvious, that when a bone is moved on a curved surface by a succession of slides whose paths make angles with one another, the bone will inevitably undergo a spin. In other words, using the anatomic terminology, the bone will be rotated even though an active force required for independent rotation (for pure

spin, that is) has not been called into operation. The geometric and mathematic proof of this will not be developed here, but this principle of **conjunct rotation** should become comprehensible with reference to Figure 5-12 and to the description of shoulder abduction discussed in Chapter 13.

Loose Pack and Close Pack Positions. The joint is said to be in **loose pack** when the movements described above are permitted. The contact of articular surfaces is assured by atmospheric pressure, surface tension of synovial fluid, and by the tone of the muscles that surround the joint, while the joint capsule and ligaments are relatively loose. In loose pack it is possible to distract the surfaces, and it is in these positions that the joint is most liable to dislocation. A position can be reached, however, in all joints where, instead of a limited area, there is extensive contact between the articular surfaces with maximal congruence of their male and female surfaces. Such a situation obtains at one extreme of habitual movements (abduction of the shoulder, extension of the hip, knee, and interphalangeal joints), and the joint is then said to be in **close pack.**

In most joints, the position of close pack is attained by conjunct rotation during the final phase of a slide. This slide may or may not be accompanied by rolling. Due to the twist imparted by this rotation, the capsule and ligaments become maximally spiraled and taut. As a consequence, the articular surfaces will be tightly compressed and cannot be distracted; the two bones in essence become one. Further movement due to muscle contraction is reflexly inhibited by the activation of mechanoreceptors in the stretched capsule and ligaments. In close pack, the joint is "locked" or "screwed home," and it has to be unlocked or unscrewed by a force vector which reverses the conjunct rotation before the joint can return into loose pack. In close pack the joint is least liable to dislocation, but when excessive force is applied the joint surfaces are particularly prone to trauma and the capsule and ligaments to tearing.

From a functional point of view, the close pack position is especially important in those joints which transmit the weight of the body in the standing position. Close pack furnishes stability to these joints with the minimum expenditure of muscular energy. At the hip, knee, and ankle, attainment of close pack is assisted by the force of gravity (Chaps. 17 and 18).

JOINT LUBRICATION

The lubrication of cartilage on cartilage has been extensively studied. In terms both of durability and efficiency, human joints far exceed the specifications for any man-made bearings of similar design. Possible mechanisms responsible for this superior performance, however, have proven difficult to elucidate. It is clear that the system is complex, and most investigators now agree that it incorporates features both of boundary and of fluid film lubrication. The boundary component consists of a renewable coating of glycoprotein molecules which covers the surface of articular cartilages. The fluid or *squeeze film component* is a layer of synovial fluid interposed between the surfaces. As this fluid is compressed during joint motion, water is squeezed from it and it becomes progressively more gellike, hence more difficult to express. Both of these mechanisms serve to prevent contact between the high points of articulating cartilages. In addition, important contributions are also made by the elasticity and porosity of cartilage which allow water to be expressed and reimbibed during compression and decompression of contact areas. Although most investigators of joint mechanics concur with these explanations, points of controversy remain, for instance those concerning the possible role of hyaluronic acid in joint lubrication mechanisms. Unfortunately, these explanations have not yet resulted in more

effective prevention or treatment of the increased friction and wear observed in various joint diseases.

The lubrication of synovium on cartilage may be an equally important factor in joint mechanics, though it has been studied less than the cartilage on cartilage bearing. Extensive areas of the articular surfaces are always in contact with synovium in the majority of joints. This is true in hinge joints (elbow, knee), ellipsoid joints (metacar-

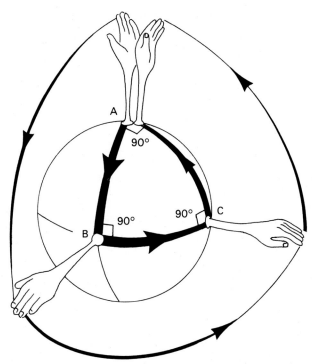

FIG. 5-12. Graphic explanation of the spin or *conjunct rotation* which accompanies a succession of slides occurring between two reciprocally curved articular surfaces. A model arm carrying a hand is moved on the surface of a sphere from point A → B → C → A along the shortest possible paths connecting the consecutive points (i.e., along chords). It is clear from the position of the thumb and the plane of the palm that the succession of slides results in 90° rotation of the arm by the time it is returned to position A. In this instance each angle of the triangle enclosed by chords AB, BC, and CA measures 90°, giving a total of 270°; that is more than 180° because the triangle is on a convex rather than flat surface. The amount of conjunct rotation or spin is always equal to the sum of the three angles minus 180°; in this case 270° − 180° = 90°. For further explanation see text. (Redrawn from Warwick R, Williams PL (eds): Gray's Anatomy, 35th ed. Philadelphia, WB Saunders, 1973)

pophalangeal joints), and ball-and-socket joints (shoulder) where the convex articular surfaces are considerably larger than the concave surfaces. As the joint is used, the highly vascular, innervated synovial tissue must fold and slide easily out of the way without being pinched. The free use of normal joints without intraarticular pain or bleeding provides ample testimony to the effectiveness of this *second system of joint lubrication*. Although its mechanism as yet is unclear, there is evidence that hyaluronic acid may be more important here than in the lubrication of cartilage on cartilage.

FACTORS OF JOINT STABILITY

The importance of loose and close pack positions of a joint with regard to its stability was discussed previously. Considerable forces may be transmitted through joints even when they are in loose pack. Adaptation of joint anatomy assures integrity also under these circumstances.

There are three main factors which provide stability to a joint: 1) the shape of the articular surfaces, 2) ligaments (including the capsule), and 3) muscles.

The relative importance of these factors varies in different joints. For instance, stability to the hip joint is provided mainly by the deep bony socket into which the head of the femur fits. In the shoulder joint the socket is shallow, and therefore muscles are the most important factor in joint stability. On the other hand, the knee in the standing position relies primarily on its ligaments for stability. In the treatment of joint injuries the relative importance of these three factors must be considered for each joint.

Atmospheric pressure and surface tension of synovial fluid also contribute significantly to the maintenance of joint stability, especially in loose pack positions. Their importance may be readily demonstrated by the common phenomenon of knuckle cracking. The relaxed, extended third finger may normally be moved through at least 30° of abduction and adduction at the metacarpophalangeal joint, thus demonstrating that the joint is in loose pack and its collateral ligaments are not taut. The joint, however, cannot be distracted until the traction reaches about 10 kg force, when the joint cracks. At that time the articular surfaces suddenly separate and a small bubble of gas appears within the joint cavity which may be demonstrated radiographically. In this phenomenon, the distraction force acting across the joint is opposed both by atmospheric pressure and by the surface tension of the synovial fluid. The latter acts as an adhesive to maintain the apposition of the articulating surfaces. When these forces are overcome, the intraarticular pressure falls suddenly to a level so far below atmospheric pressure that gas is released from the waterphase and an audible crack occurs. The instructive message of this example lies in the relatively large force required to distract such a small joint. In larger joints, the stabilizing forces contributed by surface tension and atmospheric pressure must be proportionately greater. However, these forces are exceeded by the forces generated by muscle action, and without ligamentous or muscular support joints cannot perform the functions required of them.

SUGGESTED READING

Barnett, C. H., Davies, D. V., and MacConaill, M. A. Synovial Joints. London, Longmans, 1961
An interesting and well-written book interrelating structure, mechanical considerations and function of synovial joints.

Gardner, E. The anatomy of the joints. American Academy of Orthopaedic Surgery, Instructional Course Lectures 9:149–170, 1952
In three sections the author presents an interesting account of the development, nerve supply and synovial tissue of joints. Extensive bibliography.

Ghadially, F. N., Moshurchak, E. M., and Thomas, I. Humps on young human and rabbit articular cartilage. J. Anat. 124:425, 1977
The authors discuss the various factors which may influence the appearance of articular cartilage when viewed by scanning electron microscopy.

MacConaill, M. A., and Basmajian, J. V. Muscles and Movements. Baltimore, Williams & Wilkins, 1969
The first five chapters deal with the basic types of movements at joints illustrated by many good examples. The appendix presents the geometry and algebra of articular kinematics.

Minns, R. J., and Steven, F. S. The collagen fibril organisation in human articular cartilage. J. Anat. 123:437, 1977
An interesting documentation of collagen fibril architecture in articular cartilage.

Sokoloff, L. (ed). The Joints and Synovial Fluid. New York, Academic Press, 1978
An excellent treatise on joints. The different chapters written by experts in the field give the most up-to-date information on the embryology, fine structure, innervation, lubrication and immunobiology of joints.

Torzill, P. A. The lubrication of human joints: a review. In Fleming, D. G., and Feinbert, B. N. (eds): CRC Handbook of Engineering in Medicine and Biology. Cleveland, CRC Press, 1976, pp. 225–251
A comprehensive and highly readable review of the systems responsible for lubrication of normal human joints.

Warwick, R., and Williams, P. L. (eds). Gray's Anatomy. 35th ed. Philadelphia, W. B. Saunders, 1973
The introductory sections to Chapter 4: Arthrology, give an excellent, lucid and concise description of joint anatomy and kinesiology. The illustrations are very helpful.

6
Reaction to Injury in the Musculoskeletal System

ABNER GOLDEN

The tissues of the musculoskeletal system can manifest the same kinds of pathologic processes which occur elsewhere in the body, such as congenital malformations, infections, disorders mediated by immunologic mechanisms, disturbances of vascular supply, trauma, abnormalities of metabolism, regressive changes, and neoplasms. The goal of this chapter is to consider concisely the more important and more common disorders to which the musculoskeletal system is subject, and to illustrate how universal tissue reactions to injury are modified by the unique structural characteristics of bone, skeletal muscle, and synovial joints. A brief description of the events of inflammation and tissue repair is followed by discussion of such examples as fracture repair, osteomyelitis, certain other disorders of bone, polymyositis, muscle atrophy, degenerative joint disease, infections of synovial joints, and rheumatoid arthritis. Primary neoplasms of the musculoskeletal system are relatively uncommon, and they are discussed in Chapter 29. Each of the major disease entities will be treated more comprehensively in separate chapters later in the book.

THE INFLAMMATORY REACTION

The inflammatory reaction, common to all vertebrates, consists of a medley of biologic events, usually triggered by cell injury and death. Optimally, the inflammatory response results in the healing of injury, the replacement of damaged and destroyed tissue, and restoration of function. These events, though overlapping, can be separated sequentially into 1) altered vascular permeability that permits increased passage of plasma into an area of injury, 2) migration of circulating leuko-cytes from the vascular compartment to interstitial loose connective tissue, 3) phagocytosis and enzymatic digestion of dead cells and tissue elements, 4) regeneration of parenchymal cells, when this is possible, or 5) proliferation of fibroblasts and capillaries with eventual scar formation. Tissue injury may be inflicted mechanically (trauma, heat) or by microorganisms. It may, however, be induced also by the activation of complement in immunologic reactions, by the release of substances from circulating leukocytes when they gain access to the extravascular compartment, and by vasoactive materials stored in tissue mast cells.

Altered vascular permeability is largely confined to postcapillary venules. An immediate, but transient, increase in permeability results from the release of histamine in an area of injury. A delayed and more prolonged effect occurs with activation of a variety of substances, including vasoactive amines, kinins, leukokinins derived from lysosomal enzymes in polymorphonuclear leukocytes, cleavage products of complement, prostaglandins, and basic peptides contained in leukocytes. Many factors contribute to the **migration of circulating granulocytes** and **monocytes** through cell junctions of postcapillary venules. Polymorphonuclear leukocytes are attracted by factors derived from bacteria, collagen breakdown products, certain components and cleavage products of complement, and substances released by leukocytes themselves. Monocytes are somewhat more sluggish, but respond to the presence of certain antigen-antibody complexes, fragments of complement, soluble substances released by bacteria, products of sensitized lymphocytes exposed to antigen, and substances released at the time of lysis of polymorphonuclear leukocytes. Lymphocytes may travel through endothelial cells rather than between them, particularly in response to factors released by sensitized lymphocytes exposed to specific antigens. **Phagocytosis** is performed by granulocytes and monocytes. It is greatly facilitated by the coating action of natural and acquired opsonins, among them immunoglobulins and factors derived from complement. Phagocytic leukocytes, particularly polymorphonuclear leukocytes, but also monocytes, may release lysosomal enzymes that can increase tissue injury, and, hence, augment and prolong the inflammatory reaction.

Following the digestion and removal of necrotic tissue, there is *regeneration* of parenchymal cells, when this is possible, or proliferation of capillaries and fibroblasts **(granulation tissue)**, leading eventually to scar formation. There is often an admixture of the two processes, particularly when tissue injury is extensive, and destruction is such that regeneration is unable to reconstitute normal structure.

Acute and Chronic Inflammation

The sequence of events that comprises the inflammatory reaction is remarkably constant, regardless of the site or cause of injury. Marked quantitative variations do occur, however, and reflect the relationship between the host defense mechanisms and the intrinsic properties of the agent causing tissue injury. Thus, for example, when rapid, extensive injury is followed by prompt control of the injurious agent, early phases of the inflammatory reaction predominate and healing will be rapid. This is **acute inflammation.** On the other hand, if an agent has restricted capacity to injure tissue and defense mechanisms against it are only partially successful in confining and destroying it, the later phases of inflammation predominate. These are characterized by mononuclear cell infiltration of the site of injury, granulation tissue formation, and fibrosis. Such a process is **chronic inflammation.** Chronic inflammation occurring in a localized area results in **granuloma** formation in most tissues.

Variations in the inflammatory reaction are also dictated by characteristics peculiar to certain tissues and organs. These characteristics include the tissue's capacity for regeneration, its susceptibility to the injurious effects of certain immunologic phenomena, adequacy of blood supply, rigidity of its architecture, or its resistance to phagocytosis and enzymatic digestion. Bone and some joint tissues have great capacity for regeneration following

acute injury, while skeletal muscle has at most very limited regenerative capacity. Therefore, many muscle injuries are followed by scar formation. Synovial tissues are particularly subject to immunologically mediated injury. The rigid structure of bone resists expansion, hence edema during the early inflammatory response causes vascular compression leading to extensive ischemic necrosis of bone and bone marrow.

The pluripotentiality of the connective tissue cells of the musculoskeletal system may become apparent in the healing of injuries. Although normally these cells are differentiated to function as fibroblasts, osteoblasts, or chondroblasts, connective tissue proliferation following injury may result in an inappropriate admixture of hyaline cartilage, fibrocartilage, bone, and fibrous and synovial tissue. This is dramatically apparent in the disorder myositis ossificans.

BONE

Reaction to injury in bone can be illustrated by the healing of a fracture and by bacterial infection of bone.

Fracture Repair

Following fracture of a bone, there is hemorrhage between the broken ends, beneath the periosteum, and in the surrounding musculature, followed by formation of a fibrin clot. Infiltration of polymorphonuclear leukocytes, and, later, mononuclear cells, occurs in response to the injury. Within a few days, granulation tissue is formed, derived from connective tissue elements of the bone marrow, endosteum, periosteum, and surrounding muscles. This granulation tissue soon shows signs of organization and primordial skeletal tissue is deposited in it. In a week or ten days there is differentiation of connective tissue cells to form osteoblasts and often chondroblasts. A recapitulation of both mesenchymal and endochondral bone formation then forms a provisional **callus** which reunites the fracture and forms a sleeve around the fracture site. There is extensive formation of woven bone, and the callus begins to show maximum radiodensity in two or three weeks (Fig. 6–1). Thereafter progressive remodeling occurs, and after months or even years there is total reconstitution of normal lamellar bone architecture in accordance with functional requirements.

Bacterial Infection of Bone

Bacterial infection of bone, or osteomyelitis, is most often caused by *Staphylococcus aureus* or *S. albus,* and illustrates the difficulty in healing of some injuries of bone. Osteomyelitis, predominantly a disorder of children, generally begins at the metaphysis of long bones, the area of highest vascularity. The initial injury in this area results in severe inflammation of the marrow sufficient to obstruct and thrombose blood vessels, thereby producing further ischemic destruction of bone and marrow. There is spread of infection through devitalized tissue and via blood vessels to the bony shaft and to the cortical surface, where the periosteum becomes lifted from the cortex by exudate and pus. Dead bone is gradually separated from viable tissue, forming a **sequestrum.** This necrotic bone is surrounded by large numbers of polymorphonuclear leukocytes and monocytes, and becomes perforated by sinuses and invaded by osteoclastic cells. Meanwhile, new bone formed beneath the periosteum tends to enclose and wall off the area of injury (Fig. 6–2). Healing may take place gradually, with resorption or exteriorization of dead bone. If osteomyelitis is not treated early and adequately, extensive necrosis of bone will continue and the failure to destroy the invading microbial organisms perpetuates the injury, leading to chronic infection characterized by the persistent exudation of dead polymorphonuclear leukocytes and monocytes in the form of pus. The pus may continue to drain along sinus tracts through bone and soft tissues, and this will be accompanied by reparative fibrosis as well as new bone formation.

Miscellaneous Disorders

The bone marrow is a frequent site of involvement in various systemic infections, particularly tuberculosis and other granulomatous disorders. The marrow is also a frequent site of tumor metastases. Some metastatic lesions result in destruction of bone. Others, particularly metastases from adenocarcinomas of the prostate and breast, stimulate production of new bone surrounding the tumor deposits, manifest by increased bone density on x-rays. Some neoplasms produce an *osteoclast activating factor* that leads to extensive bone resorption in the absence of altered parathyroid function.

The epiphyses of bones are peculiarly subject to **aseptic necrosis** or infarction, which is usually due to interference with the epiphyseal blood sup-

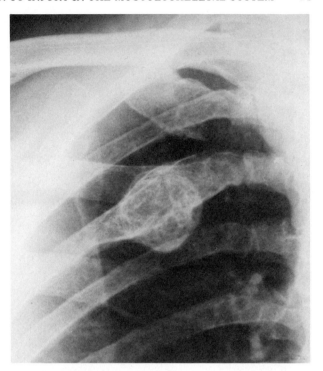

FIG. 6–1. Healing fracture of posterior aspect of fourth rib. A large callus has formed about the fracture site, and is being remodelled into mature cortical and trabecular bone. (Courtesy of Dr. Olcay S. Cigtay)

ply. Blood supply may be lost secondary to fracture, infection, or disease of the marrow, or the mechanism may be unknown. Aseptic necrosis is also known to occur in patients maintained on prolonged corticosteroid therapy.

MUSCLE

The replacement of injured or necrotic muscle fibers is greatly limited, and extensive injury to muscle usually results in fibrosis and scar formation. Effective regeneration does occur, however, when injury to the fiber is limited to one or more sarcomeres, and the endomysial sheath remains intact. Such injury is associated with the appearance of clusters of large sarcolemmal nuclei, swelling of the sarcoplasm which is basophilic due to a high content of ribonuclei acid, and the formation of new fibrils. These changes are believed to reflect regenerative activity. At a later time, new nerve fibers may grow into such an area of regeneration and new motor end plates may be formed.

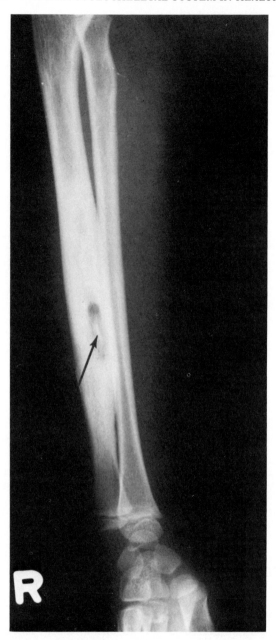

FIG. 6–2. Chronic osteomyelitis in a 9 year old boy. The sequestrum (arrow) is seen lying in an area of radiolucency. The surrounding area of widening and increased density constitutes the involucrum. (Courtesy of Dr. Arthur Lieber)

Muscle diseases of infectious origin are uncommon and include some parasitic, viral, and bacterial infections. The effect of these disorders on the integrity of muscle is generally mild, since the lesions are either segmental or are so widely distributed that functional impairment is minimal.

A more common type of injury to skeletal muscle results from a variety of immunologic mechanisms involving either circulating antibodies or cell-mediated immunity. In some disorders, muscle fibers themselves become injured and destroyed. In others, muscle is affected as a consequence of injury to such supporting structures as blood vessels, collagen, or motor end plates. The destructive results of these immunologic injuries derive from their chronicity and their tendency to recur. In **polymyositis,** there is degeneration and necrosis of muscle cells together with interstitial inflammation. Although there are attempts at regeneration, repeated injury produces atrophy and scarring with shortening and rigidity of muscles, leading to deformities and profound weakness.

Atrophy of muscle fibers consists of a progressive loss of myofilaments. When this is a diffuse and protracted process, as in some distal motor neuropathies or muscular dystrophies, there is an increase in the number of interstitial fat cells, and gradual replacement of entire muscles by adipose tissue. Loss of scattered fibers may result in hypertrophy of uninjured cells, manifested by an increased number of myofibrils.

JOINTS

In traumatic and other injuries the primary target may be any one of the three component tissues of synovial joints, but all of them may become affected secondarily. Mechanical injury to ligaments or the joint capsule and the paralysis of surrounding muscles interfere with joint stability and subject the joint to repeated trauma, sooner or later leading to degeneration of cartilage. Primary degeneration of cartilage also occurs and is usually a simple wear and tear phenomenon, although such enzymes as collagenases may also play a role. Degeneration of cartilage, whether primary or secondary to loss of joint stability or due to the stress of excessive weight-bearing, eventually leads to **degenerative joint disease** or **osteoarthritis.** In most instances the inflammatory reaction is sparse. In time there is disruption of the articular surfaces, sclerosis of underlying bone, and bone proliferation at the margins of the joint with osteophyte or *spur* formation.

Extensive injury to synovial and capsular tissues can result from abnormalities of the joint fluid, infections, and immunologic injuries. Regardless of the mechanism of injury, the establishment of a significant inflammatory reaction may be followed by the release of proteases and collagenases from leukocytes and, if persistent or recurrent, scarring and deformities will develop due to involvement of all joint tissues.

Abnormalities of joint fluid may result from repeated hemorrhage, as in **hemophilia,** or from the presence of crystals in patients with **gout** and **pseudogout.** The abnormal fluid is chemotactic to leukocytes and by this mechanism induces inflammation.

Infectious arthritis is almost always bloodborne. Destructive changes may occur early, due to release of enzymes during a brisk inflammatory reaction, but prompt elimination of the infecting microorganisms usually permits regeneration and reconstitution of a normal joint.

Rheumatoid arthritis is the most destructive and disabling of the principal joint diseases. Its pathogenesis has not been elucidated and the following account is a plausible hypothesis of how the injury to joint tissue may be incurred. The injury is immunologically mediated, and is in a large part related to the capacity of synovial membrane to function much as lymphatic tissue in a local immune response. An initial injury to the joint, perhaps viral, leads to the local formation of gamma globulin antibodies. These become antigenic in the joint fluid due to aggregation or denaturation, and stimulate the production in the synovial membrane of IgM or IgG antiglobulin antibodies, or rheumatoid factor. Antigen-antibody complexes are formed in the joint cavity. They bind complement, and the attendant release of chemotactic factors induces an inflammatory reaction with massive infiltration of polymorphonuclear leukocytes. Enzymes released from these cells injure cartilage and the synovial lining. There is deposition of fibrin, and granulation tissue grows over the injured structures. Cartilage deprived of its normal relationship to joint fluid undergoes further degeneration, and granulation tissue gradually fills the entire joint cavity. The result is progressive scarring with fibrous or bony fusion of the articulating bones.

SUGGESTED READING

Currie, S., Saunders, M., Knowles, M., and Brown, A. E. Immunological aspects of polymyositis. Q. J. Med. *40*:63, 1971
Evidence supporting an immunological pathogenesis of polymyositis is reviewed together with observations on lymphocyte stimulation by muscle antigen.

Radin, E. L. Mechanical aspects of osteoarthrosis. Bull. Rheum. Dis. *26*:862, 1975
A brief consideration of a mechanism of injury to articular cartilage that may lead to chronic degenerative joint disease.

Ryan, G. B., and Majno, G. Acute inflammation. Am. J. Pathol. *86*:183, 1977
A thorough review of the mechanisms involved in the vascular and cellular events of the inflammatory reaction, and of its systemic effects.

Williams, R. C., Jr. Rheumatoid Arthritis. Philadelphia, W. B. Saunders, 1974
An excellent presentation of the pathology and clinical manifestations of this disease. Chapter 10 considers the role of immune mechanisms in pathogenesis and Chapter 11 discusses rheumatoid factor.

7
Introduction to Anatomy and Examination of the Patient

CORNELIUS ROSSE,   D. KAY CLAWSON

In order to understand how the musculoskeletal system functions and how and why this function is disturbed by trauma and disease, one must learn to integrate anatomy, physiology, pathology, and physical examination, which is essentially an assessment of functional anatomy in the living.

Anatomy forms the basis for comprehending the function of the musculoskeletal system. A knowledge of the three-dimensional arrangement of various structures is gained from the dissected cadaver, and this knowledge should be transferred to the living body, where the function of these structures can be assessed.

Chapters 9–19 attempt such an integration and present the regional anatomy together with physical examination. This chapter serves as an introduction to such an approach, and deals with the use of terminology for describing normal and disordered anatomy, discusses the anatomic division of the skeleton, and introduces examination of the patient. The last chapter of the book presents a comprehensive screening examination of the musculoskeletal system, building on the subject matter of the chapters which dealt with the regions and the diseases of the system.

TERMINOLOGY

The use of precise terminology is necessary for accurate description as well as for communication without misunderstanding. Positions and directions are described in relation to the **anatomic position** in which the body is standing erect with the arms at the sides and palms facing forward (Fig. 7–1).

The **median plane** bisects the body into right and left halves. Any plane parallel with it is a **sagittal plane. Medial** describes a position nearer to the median plane, and **lateral** a position farther from it. In the limbs, other terms may be used synonymously with the latter two. In the upper limb, **ulnar** and **radial** designate medial and lateral respectively; in the lower limb, **tibial** and **fibular** (or peroneal) may be used in the same context.

A structure nearer to the front of the body is said to be **anterior** or **ventral** while a structure nearer to the back of the body is **posterior** or **dorsal.** In the case of the hand, **palmar** is often used synonymously with anterior. The **dorsum of the foot** faces upward while its **plantar** surface is the sole of the foot.

A **coronal plane** bisects the body at right angles to the median plane into anterior and posterior portions. A **transverse plane** bisects the body at right angles to the median plane into upper and lower parts. **Superior** means lying above and **inferior,** lying below. In the limbs, the terms **proximal** and **distal** are used to designate nearer and farther from the root of attachment of the limb.

The terminology used to describe various movements is presented in Chapter 5.

The most common terms used for describing abnormal deviations from the anatomic position (for example, deformities) are valgus and varus. In **valgus,** the distal segment of the limb is displaced away from the midline. In other words, the angle of deformity points toward the midline (for example, knock knees) (Fig. 7–2). In **varus,** the distal segment of the limb is displaced toward the midline. In other words, the angle of deformity points away from the midline (bowlegs) (Fig. 7–2). Other terms specific to regional deformities will be described in the appropriate chapters.

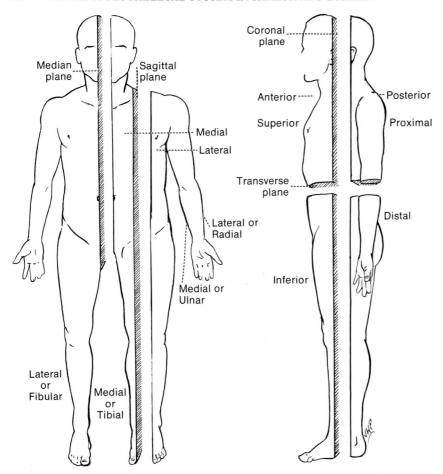

FIG. 7-1. Schematic representation of the body illustrating the anatomic planes and terms describing the position of different parts relative to one another. For description, see text.

THE SKELETON

Axial and Appendicular Skeleton

The **axial skeleton** consists of the skull, the vertebral column, the sternum, and the ribs. The bones of the limbs constitute the **appendicular skeleton.**

The bones of the axial skeleton are flat or irregularly shaped and are built of cancellous or spongy bone invested by a cortex of compact bone (Fig. 7–3). The majority of bones in the appendicular skeleton are long bones, made up of a shaft or **diaphysis,** which contains the medullary cavity, and two expanded ends, the **epiphyses** (Fig. 7–4). The epiphysis at each end extends from the articular cartilage to the epiphyseal plate and contains cancellous bone. In the majority of bones it re-

ceives the attachment of the joint capsule. The diaphysis begins to ossify from a primary center very early in intrauterine life, while the epiphyses ossify from secondary centers which appear at various times in different bones around and after birth. The **metaphysis** is the growing end of the diaphysis and is adjacent to the growth plate (Chap. 2). It is useful to retain the terms epiphysis and metaphysis even after bony union has occurred. In mature bones the metaphysis is that segment of the shaft which adjoins the epiphysis (see Fig. 2–12).

Primary and secondary ossification centers occur also in bones of the axial skeleton. The time of fusion is fairly precise and characteristic for each bone. The last growth plate is obliterated at the age of 21 to 22 years, but in the majority of

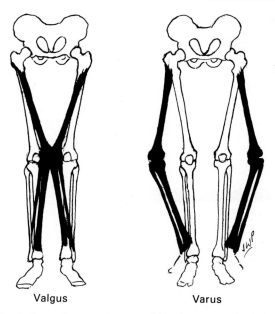

FIG. 7-2. Valgus and varus deformities at the knee.

Valgus   Varus

metaphysis, which are filled with spongy bone. Blood-borne tumor cells (metastases) and bacteria sequester primarily to highly vascular bone both in the appendicular and axial skeleton. Because of the high rate of blood flow, the metaphyses of growing bones are the most frequent sites of osteomyelitis.

Nerve fibers are mainly distributed to the periosteum, though a few enter the bone itself along with the arteries (Fig. 7-5). They are predominantly **sensory** (pain, pressure, vibration sense), but autonomic **vasomotor fibers** are also present. Bone pain due to trauma is usually periosteal in origin, but an expanding lesion such as a neoplasm within the bone can cause characteristic persistent and severe pain, even without periosteal involvement

EVALUATION OF THE PATIENT

Functional integrity in the musculoskeletal system may be viewed as the physical expression of health or disease, for several or all parts of this system are activated when the patient physically interacts with the environment. Consequently, physical illness primarily affecting other organ systems of the body may manifest itself through disturbance of musculoskeletal function. This account, however, of necessity is confined to the examination of the musculoskeletal system alone, realizing fully that such a limited approach is unrealistic in clinical medicine. To detect health or disease within the musculoskeletal system, the patient should be approached with a routine which forms the basis of general clinical practice. This classic approach consists of 1) history taking, 2) physical examination, and 3) laboratory investigations. A simple and abbreviated account is presented in this section with emphasis on aspects pertinent to the musculoskeletal system.

History Taking

Obtaining a history of the patient's complaints provides the most important clues for diagnosing musculoskeletal disease. In cases of severe trauma, institution of lifesaving measures takes precedence, but unless life is in danger, a precise account of the circumstances of injury and the evolution of the illness will be instrumental in determining which anatomic structures might be attacked. The severity of the patient's complaints dictates the caution necessary for proceeding with the examination. The patient's complaints are known as the

bones fusion generally takes place between the ages of 14 and 18. Fusion occurs earlier in the female than in the male.

Blood and Nerve Supply of Bones

The shaft of a long bone receives its major blood supply from a **nutrient artery** which enters the diaphysis through a foramen. Before it enters the bone, the artery gives branches to the periosteum, and then it is distributed to compact bone along the haversian canals and to the medullary cavity (Fig. 7-5). In addition, the periosteum receives smaller arteries from the attached muscles. These arteries anastomose with the branches of the nutrient artery and enter the compact bone through small foramina running transversely to the haversian system (Volkmann's canals). The epiphysis and metaphysis receive blood from yet a different source. This is the **periarticular plexus** represented by the anastomosis that surrounds the attachment of the joint capsule to bone. Prior to the fusion of the growth plate, there is very little anastomosis between the vascular network of the epiphysis and metaphysis. For an adequate blood supply of the bone, at least two of these three arterial systems must be intact. Ischemia leads rapidly to death of the bone.

The diaphysis consists chiefly of compact bone and is less vascular than the epiphysis and

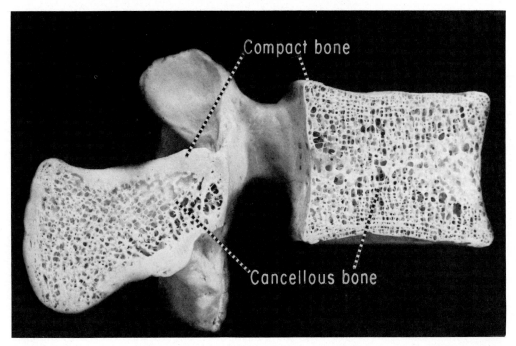

FIG. 7–3. Section across a vertebra. Cancellous bone is invested by compact bone or cortex, which is very thin over the body of the vertebra but is thicker over the spinous process.

symptoms. The following symptoms are of special importance in musculoskeletal disease: pain, weakness, limitation of movement, stiffness, deformity.

The location, onset, and character of each of these symptoms should be ascertained. The course of development of these symptoms from the time of their onset to the time of examination can provide important clues for the diagnosis. Assessment of the overall functional disability and the extent of interference with daily routine and social and vocational activities is an important aspect of history-taking. When the detailed history of the local symptoms has been obtained it is important to inquire about symptoms in other organ systems and also about previous illnesses. Such information may contribute to the diagnosis of musculoskeletal diseases or it may indicate whether or not the patient's musculoskeletal complaints are secondary to disease in other systems.

Pain. Patients can localize pain more or less precisely to individual bones or their parts, to joints, and to muscles or tendons since all these structures are supplied by somatic sensory nerves. The pain may be felt over a diffuse area, especially when its cause is deeply seated or removed from the site where the pain is felt (referred pain). When a superficial structure is involved, the patient may indicate the painful spot precisely with a finger.

Bone pain unless due to a bruise (subperiosteal hematoma) or fracture (which in some pathologic conditions may occur without any history of trauma), is deep and boring in character, often very intense, is not related to movement, and may keep the patient awake at night. Relief usually cannot be obtained without potent analgesic drugs. **Joint pain** is felt in and about the joint; in some diseases it may be exquisite. Movement always exacerbates it while rest and warmth relieve it. But in rheumatoid arthritis movement may relieve the pain and stiffness. The pain develops gradually in some conditions, in others its onset may be dramatic and sudden, and it may shift from one joint to the other. Weight bearing on a surface denuded of articular cartilage due to its degeneration will produce dull, deep-seated pain and is relieved by rest. Tears or sprains of the capsule, ligaments, and intra-articular disks can be extremely painful and are made worse by movement, and the injured structures can usually be diagnosed by physical examination and by ascertaining the mechanism of injury.

Muscle pain commonly develops as a result of

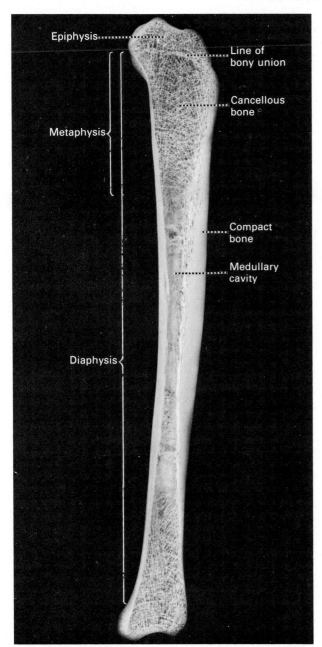

Epiphysis

Line of
bony union

Cancellous
bone

Metaphysis

Compact
bone

Medullary
cavity

Diaphysis

FIG. 7-4. Longitudinal section across a long bone of the appendicular skeleton (tibia) to show its different regions.

excessive or unusual exercise, but it generally imposes no disability and subsides within a day or two. Cramps are involuntary tetanic contractions which may develop during exercise or at rest, last only for a brief period of time, and are usually so painful that movement of the affected part is prevented. They can occur without apparent cause, but may be associated with vascular or muscle disease. More significant is the pain which develops in muscles in the course of their normal use and is immediately relieved by rest. This type of pain, most common in the calf and thigh muscles, suggests inadequate blood supply and demands thorough investigation. The pain of torn muscle or tendon fibers is generally related to excessive exertion and may involve the whole thickness of the muscle or tendon, or only individual fibers scattered throughout either structure. Pain is progressive and will not remit if the muscle is involved in an inflammatory process. Inflammation of synovial sheaths investing tendons gives precisely localized, often intense, pain, which in the early stages of the condition is made worse by movement and is relieved by rest. When persistent muscle pain, unrelated to exercise or injury, is associated with weakness, muscle disease must be suspected.

Dull, poorly localized pain may be **referred** to muscles and joints devoid of any disease or injury. Such referred pain may be due to compression of the nerves that supply the painful muscle or joint, or to disease in a distant structure served by the same nerves or spinal cord segments as the painful regions.

Weakness. It is important to distinguish muscle weakness from generalized fatigue and malaise. The inability to perform certain tasks will suggest the anatomic distribution of the muscles affected. Muscle groups may be involved symmetrically on the two sides of the body; the weakness may be more pronounced in peripheral or in proximal muscles of the limbs. The weakness may develop as the muscle is used repetitively or the muscle may gather strength with use. The patient may also have noted wasting or an associated stiffness in the affected muscles.

Limitation of Movement and Stiffness. Apart from pain and weakness, movements may be limited by abnormalities of the articular surfaces or by fibrosis and scarring of the joint capsule, ligaments, and muscles **(contractures).** In each instance the patient may complain of stiffness, and this has to be distinguished from increased tone or spasticity in the musculature. Contractures may

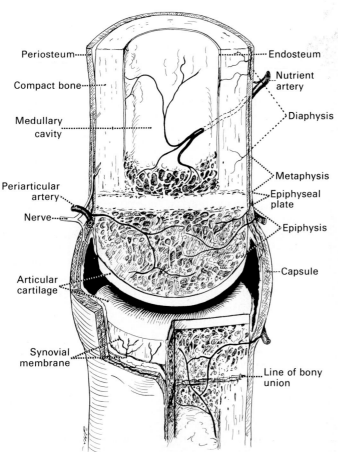

FIG. 7-5. Blood and nerve supply to bone and to a synovial joint. The upper bone is shown before, and the lower bone after, obliteration of the growth plate cartilage. The blood vessels which enter the periosteum from the attached muscles have been omitted from the drawing.

produce **deformity** and this may be the primary presenting symptom as it may be with congenital malformations and benign neoplasms.

Physical Examination

Physical signs are the observations and findings of the examiner which are elicited by the systematic process of inspection, palpation, percussion, and auscultation. The last two usually do not play any significant part in the routine examination of the musculoskeletal system except in the spine, where percussion is a reliable test for vertebral lesions. However, in addition to the above, it is especially important to test passive and active range of motion of joints, joint stability, muscle strength, and integrated function.

Evaluation of the musculoskeletal system is not complete without testing the motor and sensory components of the nervous system.

The examination of the musculoskeletal system is performed at two levels: general overview and local examination.

General overview of the system consists of inspection of posture, gait, and ordinary physical activities (for example, removal of clothes, getting onto the examination table).

The posture should be observed in the front, back, and side view, paying particular attention to the curvatures of the spine, the level of the shoulders and of the pelvis, the symmetry of the scapulae, and the buttock creases.

During walking, stride length should be equal, the trunk should remain straight, the pelvis should be level, and the arms should swing symmetrically. Deviations from the normal should be noted in relation to the phase of the gait and their cause should then be investigated by **local examination** (inspection, palpation, and assessment of range of motion, muscle function, and integrated function).

Inspection. **Symmetry** of the two sides in contour

and size should be observed in the general overview and in the local examination. Differences should be measured. The cause of any asymmetry must be determined. **Wasting, masses,** nodules, swellings, **deformities,** and change in **skin color** should be noted and related to the patient's symptoms.

Palpation. The symptoms of the patient and the physical signs noted in the course of inspection should be supplemented by palpation.

The origin of pain may be localized to anatomic structures by eliciting **tenderness** over them. Tenderness is pain produced by the pressure of the examining finger. Differences in **skin temperature** and **skin texture** should also be noted.

Assessment of **bone continuity** by palpation is important in diagnosing fractures, particularly in swollen parts and in the unconscious victims of trauma. **Abnormal mobility** and **crepitus** (grating sensation of bone) are confirmatory signs of a fracture. Crepitus felt over joints indicates roughness of the articular surfaces.

The underlying cause of deformities, lumps, and swelling may be determined by feeling their **consistency.** For example, bone deformities are hard; soft tissue swelling due to edema pits; joint swelling due to effusion fluctuates and can be tested by transmission of fluid impulse.

Muscles should be palpated for tenderness and the presence of muscle spasm. **Muscle spasm** is sustained muscular contraction reflexly induced by pain.

In the limbs **arterial pulses** should be palpated and compared on the two sides, especially if ischemia or arterial compression is suspected. The speed of filling of the capillary bed can be tested by observing the return of pink color to the fingertips or toes after their momentary compression.

Assessment of Range of Motion. To assess **passive range of movement,** the examiner moves the joint, while the patient keeps his muscles relaxed. Limiting factors in normal range of movement are the shape of the articular surfaces, ligaments, and muscles. An impression of the normal range can always be obtained from the examiner's own joint, but whenever the time course of disease is being ascertained or treatment is being instituted, the range of movement should be measured in degrees with a simple instrument called the **goniometer.** The limiting factors should always be identified in a diseased joint. **Subluxation** (an incomplete dislocation) of a joint may lead to abnormal range of

movement and to instability. A joint tends to sublux in the direction of the anatomic lesion. By attempting to stress the stabilizing ligaments in each direction, the physician can test the **stability of the joint.**

Active range of movement is assessed by having the patient use his own muscles. When a joint is examined, it should be put through all the possible movements.

Assessment of Muscle Function. In a physical examination muscle mass, muscle tone, muscle strength, and the nature of muscle contraction need to be assessed.

Alterations in **muscle mass** are determined by comparison of the two sides through inspection and measurement. Diminished bulk of a muscle due to any cause is called **wasting** or **atrophy.**

The **tone of a muscle** is the resistance it offers to passive elongation or stretch (Chaps. 4, 27). It is tested by the examiner stretching a relaxed muscle by passively moving a joint (see Fig. 4–8). The tension developed in the muscle by the activation of the stretch reflex is summated with the muscle's intrinsic elastic tension, and these two forces together are interpreted clinically as muscle tone. Normal muscle tone can be appreciated through practice by moving the joints of normal individuals. **Hypotonia** is a reduction in normal muscle tone and **hypertonia** is an increase in normal muscle tone. Lesions of the lower motor neurons (anterior horn cells) and of peripheral nerves always produce hypotonia (see Chap. 26). Hypertonia is due to a disturbed balance of suprasegmental input to the lower motor neurons (see Chap. 27).

When a muscle becomes hypertonic from intrinsic elastic changes, a full passive range of motion is not achieved due to the resultant contracture.

In assessing **muscle strength** it is important to pay attention to **positioning** of the part tested in relation to gravity. If muscle strength appears to be impaired when the limb is moved against gravity, the test has to be repeated with the elimination of gravity.

Muscles can be tested and their tendons thrown into prominence when the examiner resists the movement they produce. A fairly accurate **grading of muscle strength** is possible with the following scoring system:

5–Normal power. The muscle can move the joint through the full range of movement against gravity and against full resistance applied by the examiner.

4–The muscle can move the joint through the full

range against gravity and against some resistance, but is unable to overcome normal resistance.

3–The muscle can move the joint through the full range of movement against gravity, but is unable to overcome any additional resistance.

2–The muscle can move the joint through the complete range only when gravity is eliminated.

1–Contraction of the muscle can be felt by the examiner's hand but it is of insufficient strength to produce movement even when gravity is eliminated.

0–Complete paralysis. No visible or palpable contraction.

In normal muscle, contraction and relaxation form a continuous and smooth process. In a variety of muscle diseases spontaneous, involuntary, irregular contractions of motor units occur which are visible on the surface of the resting muscle. This is called **fasciculation.** Irregularities of movement, lack of coordination, and tremor signify disturbances in the suprasegmental motor system (Chaps. 4 and 27).

Assessment of Integrated Function. Integration of function is assessed by requesting the patient to perform special tasks which test the coordination between different parts of the musculoskeletal system and between the musculoskeletal system and the nervous system.

Disturbances in integrated functions as well as abnormalities in muscle strength or muscle tone call for a thorough examination of the nervous system which is beyond the scope of this chapter. The testing of **deep tendon reflexes** (biceps, triceps, knee and ankle jerks) and of cutaneous perception of **light touch** and **pain** (pinprick) should be routinely performed in the course of local examination of the regions of the mucsuloskeletal system.

Laboratory Investigations

A diagnosis should be made based on the history and physical examination. Specific investigations may be selected to confirm or refine this diagnosis. The indications and contraindications have to be considered for each of the contemplated tests. The data provided by the confirmatory investigations have to be interpreted in the light of the history and the physical exam. The following types of investigations are most helpful and most commonly used in the diagnosis of musculoskeletal diseases: radiologic investigations, hematologic studies, blood chemistry and enzyme studies, examination of joint fluid, electromyography, nerve conduction velocity measurements, and biopsies. The value of these procedures is discussed with the various types of diseases in Chapters 8 and 21–29.

SUGGESTED READING

Delp, M. H., and Manning, R. T. (eds) Major's Physical Diagnosis, 7th ed. Philadelphia, W. B. Saunders, 1968
Good description of the approach to the patient in general. The book deals with all organ systems; Chapters 12 and 13 pertain to the musculoskeletal and nervous systems respectively.

Hoppenfeld, S. Physical Examination of the Spine and Extremities. New York, Appleton-Century-Crofts, 1976
An excellent, well-illustrated, comprehensive presentation of all tests and maneuvers for the regional examination of the musculoskeletal system.

8
Radiologic Evaluation of the Musculoskeletal System

ROSALIND H. TROUPIN

X-ray examinations provide an important supplementary tool in the evaluation of patients with suspected injury or disease of the musculoskeletal system. Subtle fractures, smoldering infections, potentially lethal tumors, and a wide variety of other bone and joint abnormalities often have characteristic radiologic findings. These changes may be gross or subtle; at times they serve only to support a reasonably firm clinical diagnosis; in other settings the x-ray findings provide clearcut answers to clinically confusing problems.

CLINICAL APPLICATION OF X-RAY STUDIES

Effective use of x-ray studies in clinical problem solving is dependent on several factors. The actual need for examination must be sensibly considered. Judgment is required to distinguish potentially significant clinical complaints from those that are trivial or tangential; x-rays are poor substitutes for supportive psychotherapy. Filming techniques should center directly over the area of concern, include proper projections to ensure three-dimensional portrayal, and utilize exposure factors providing optimum visualization of bone and soft tissue structures. Finally, the images must be analyzed meticulously using background knowledge of normal radiographic anatomy to recognize pathologic deviations.

The skill and persistence of the observer will determine whether important visual clues will be perceived or disregarded. Subtle or ambiguous preliminary findings can often be clarified by individually tailored special projections or examinations. Disclosure of an x-ray finding which is abnormal but not etiologically specific can identify the need for an additional clinical or laboratory examination. In order to understand the capabilities and limitations of x-ray studies in the musculoskeletal system, a few background facts are needed about x-ray image formation.

X-RAY IMAGE FORMATION

X-ray Production

X-rays are the very short wave-length representatives on the spectrum of electromagnetic radiation. A conventional x-ray tube is schematically diagrammed in Figure 8–1. Its essential elements are a cathode filament and a target anode enclosed in a sealed evacuated glass tube. When the temperature of the tungsten filament of the cathode is raised to white heat, electrons are boiled off. If a very high voltage is applied across the tube, the electrons will be accelerated from the hot cathode toward the positive anode and acquire high velocities. When these high speed electrons strike the target anode, x-rays are radiated and heat is produced. The glass vacuum tube must be housed in a mechanical structure which provides cooling, shielding from electrical shock, and absorption of all the radiation other than that deliberately emanating from the aperture. A shutter or cone device (collimator) then modifies the x-ray beam to the size and shape desired for a given examination.

Film Images and X-ray Tissue Absorption

X-ray film, like photographic film, has a clear celluloid or plastic base coated with a silver bromide emulsion which undergoes alterations in response

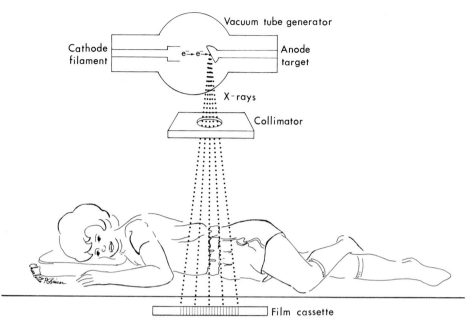

FIG. 8–1. Schematic diagram of x-ray generator and spatial relationships in clinical radiography.

to radiant energy. Chemical development then renders this visible as differential blackening and the resultant shadows or negatives are available for interpretation.

As the primary x-ray beam traverses a body part it will be absorbed to varying degrees dependent upon the density and volume of the tissue elements which it encounters. Figure 8–2A and B illustrate the independent effects of these two variables. High density bone will absorb more x-rays than adjacent soft tissues, fewer photons will be available to expose the film, and the resultant image will have a white area of **radiopacity.** Fat and gas have lower x-ray absorption, permitting more film blackening or **radiolucency.**

In conventional x-ray films, the absorption densities of many musculoskeletal tissues—muscle, cartilage, tendon, and even synovial fluid—are identical. Fortunately, fat is often present along tissue planes and between muscle layers, providing visibility by virtue of its lower absorption density. However, if the fat becomes infiltrated by water-density material such as blood, pus, edema, or tumor cells, these radiolucent boundaries become obliterated and radiologic abnormality becomes discernible.

A recent development, *computed tomography* (CT), uses computerized mathematical reconstruc-

tion of tissue density measurements to distinguish fine nuances of density among the soft tissues. Currently the expense and availability of this modality restrict its use to carefully selected clinical situations. One very important application of CT is to delineate the precise boundaries of soft tissue extension by a malignant bone tumor, in order to plan the margins of a surgical resection.

PLAIN FILM ANALYSIS

Basic proficiency in film interpretation is generally considered a clinical skill. However, beginning the development of this skill during preclinical training will greatly facilitate the study of the musculoskeletal system. An organized approach to collecting the visual data is essential, for ultimately it would be the patient who would suffer the consequences of disorganized or impulsive film analysis. The systematic approach requires that the x-ray image be studied in a sequential fashion, building interpretive habits which will eventually become automatic. Orientation, scrutiny of the soft tissues, assessment of the bone shape and surfaces, and finally study of internal bony structure, constitute a viewing technique that is intuitively logical as well as effective.

Orientation

An important first step should always be to verify that the films under consideration really belong to the patient in question and were not misfiled. Embarrassing and potentially dangerous errors can occur at this stage. It is also obviously essential to be certain which part of the body is being viewed and from what direction.

The technical adequacy of the film must be checked. An overexposed film will be too dark, with pertinent information burnt out. Some of the image can be salvaged by viewing the film with a high intensity light source. An underexposed film is too opaque and does not adequately penetrate dense tissue areas. That problem cannot be solved and the film needs to be repeated. In addition, structures can be blurred due to patient motion, or a variety of confusing clothing, technical, and processing artifacts may be present.

When one begins to study the film, it is usually more effective to actively seek out specific abnormalities rather than gaze in an undirected fashion at a film image.

Soft Tissues

On films of the limbs the skin, subcutaneous fat, and muscle are usually well demarcated, as well as the bone. Table 8–1 and Figure 8–3 give examples

TABLE 8–1. Soft Tissue X-ray Findings

X-ray appearance	Significant examples
Soft tissue swelling	Cellulitis, hemorrhage, edema
Calcification (Fig. 8–3A)	Metabolic or connective tissue disease, old trauma, parasites
Muscle atrophy	Paralysis, primary muscle disease, disuse
Opaque foreign body (Fig. 8–3B)	Gunshot wound, needle in foot
Gas in soft tissues	Open wound, gas-forming bacterial infection

of the types of potentially important findings which should be sought in the soft tissues.

External Features of Bones

Bone Shape. Each bone has its own characteristic shape and surface features. X-rays of the bones will be two dimensional representations of their distinctive size, shape, condyles, grooves, fossae, and ridges. X-rays will show if bones are congenitally malformed (Fig. 8–4A), if they have become deformed by trauma or softening, if they have been expanded by proliferating bone marrow (Fig. 8–4B), and so forth. The most frequently encountered example of a deviation from normal bone shape is a displaced fracture.

FIG. 8–2. Factors determining x-ray absorption. **(A)** Isodense step wedge showing that a greater thickness of tissue absorbs more energy and results in less blackening of the film. **(B)** Tissues of increased density absorb more radiation.

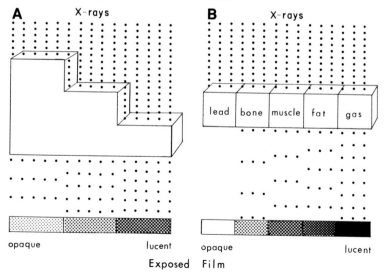

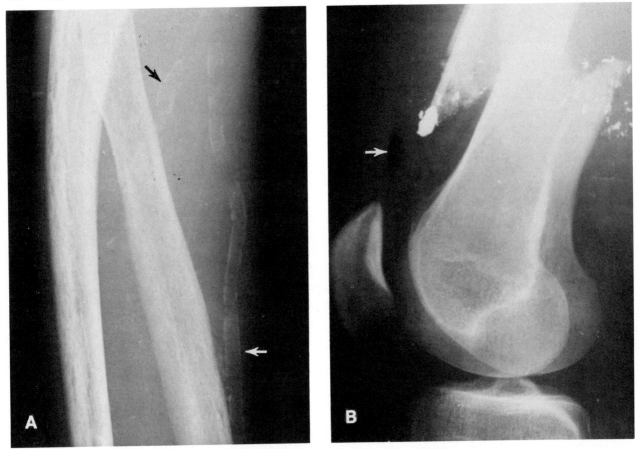

FIG. 8–3. **(A)** Soft tissue calcification. A patient with chronic renal failure showing extensive calcification through-out the arteries of the proximal forearm **(arrows)**. **(B)** Opaque foreign body. Penetrating gunshot wound resulting in fracture of the femur. Note multiple bullet fragments and bubbles of air **(arrow)** in the soft tissues.

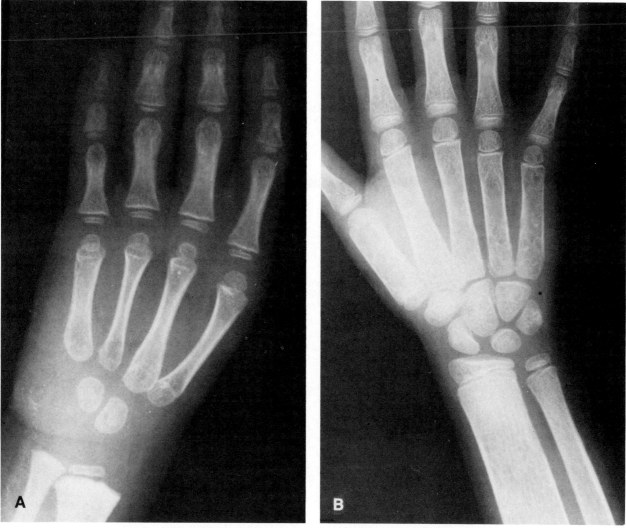

FIG. 8–4. Abnormalities in skeletal configurations. **(A)** Congenital skeletal malformation characterized by complete failure of the development of all bones associated with the thumb and/or carpal bones of the radial side of the wrist. **(B)** Diffusely expanded bones with thin cortices. Severe chronic anemia was causing compensatory hyperplasia and increased volume of bone marrow elements. Note rectangular shape of metacarpal diaphyses compared to tapered, tubulated normal shape in **A**.

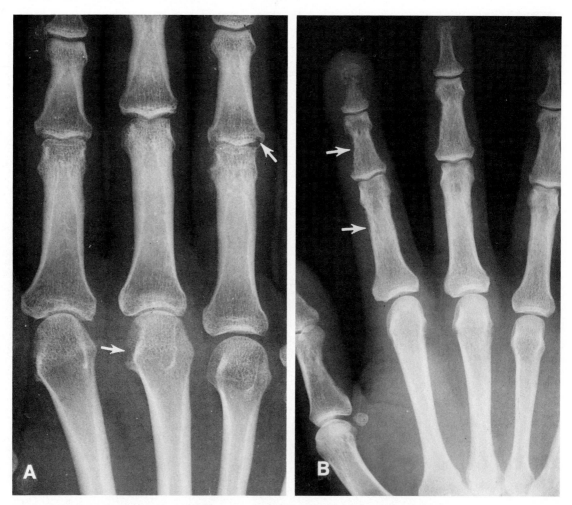

FIG. 8-5. Abnormalities along bone surfaces. **(A)** Rheumatoid arthritis showing focal erosions along joint margins **(arrows).** The cortical surfaces are otherwise intact. **(B)** Hyperparathyroidism. Diffuse smudgy erosions **(arrows)** along the phalangeal diaphyses. Note resorption of tips of distal phalanges. **(C)** Osteomyelitis of the humerus with periosteal new bone formation **(arrow)** appearing as thin dense

(continued)

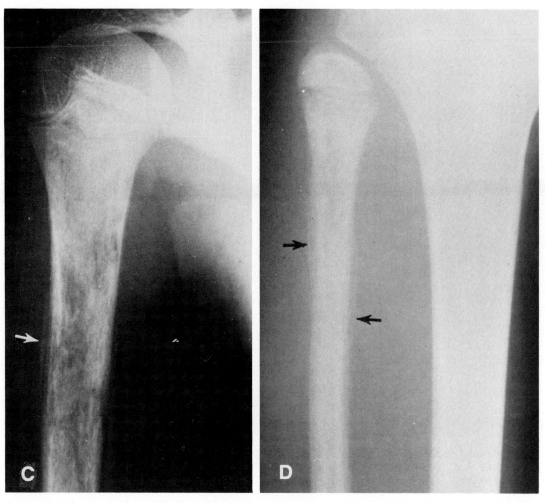

stripes paralleling the bone cortex. A permeative type of bone destruction is also evident within the shaft. **(D)** Malignant bone tumor. Periosteal new bone **(arrows)** is present along the fibula, in this instance because tumor cells dissecting under the periosteum have evoked a proliferative response from the periosteum. Contrast with normal tibial surfaces.

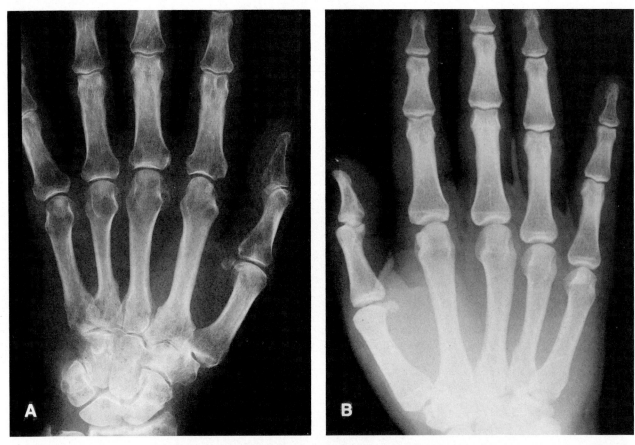

FIG. 8-6. Differences in bone mineral content. **(A)** The hand of a patient who suffered a shoulder injury several weeks ago. The entire upper limb was immobilized and the appearance of the hand reflects disuse demineralization. **(B)** Normal hand for comparison.

Bone Surfaces. Apart from the areas of cortical roughening normally seen at the site of tendon attachments, cortical surfaces should be smooth, white, and intact. Indistinctness implies abnormality and merits a closer look. Figure 8–5 is a composite of four situations where bone surfaces are abnormal; focal erosions in rheumatoid arthritis (Fig. 8–5A), diffuse cortical resorption in hyperparathyroidism (Fig. 8–5B), periosteal new bone formation due to underlying bone infection (Fig. 8–5C), and a similar periosteal reaction due to infiltrating malignancy (Fig. 8–5D).

Internal Structure of Bones

Diffuse Changes. There are quantitative radiographic methods which have been developed for measurement of bone mineral content in living patients, but they are not universally available. However, after looking at a few stacks of films, it is possible to develop a baseline and detect gross deviations of bone density from the normal. Figure 8–6 shows a moderately demineralized hand along with a normal one for comparison.

Focal Abnormalities. The x-ray appearance of a focal destructive bone lesion provides important clues to its biologic behavior. A lesion that is slowly growing will modify the shape of surrounding bones, and will often evoke a sclerotic reaction at its margin which is evident by an increase in density. Lesions lacking such modifications are more rapidly growing. The most aggressive, infiltrating processes are characterized by a poorly defined, permeative pattern of destruction. Figure 8–7 illustrates a spectrum of benign and malignant destructive bone lesions: multiple, slowly growing cartilage tumors (Fig. 8–7A), a benign tumor of fibrous tissue origin (Fig. 8–7B), metastatic carcinoma (Fig. 8–7C), and a primary bone malignancy (Fig. 8–7D).

SPECIAL EXAMINATIONS

Two x-ray views of a body part, made at right angles to one another, often provide all the information needed for resolving a given clinical problem. At other times, modifications and supplementary techniques are required to provide precise diagnosis for effective therapy. Some of these studies will reemerge in subsequent chapters; however, an overview is appropriate now for perspective.

Multiple Views

A single projection of a body part will show a complex summation shadow of all the structures traversed by the x-ray beam. In the *anteroposterior* or frontal projection of a knee for instance, it cannot be determined whether the patella is in front of, behind, or even within the femur (Fig. 8–8A,B). In addition, its anatomic detail is greatly obscured by the femur. A *lateral* projection will obviously localize the patella and give useful information about its configuration including its anterior and posterior surfaces (Fig. 8–8C,D). However, if there were really concern about structural integrity of the patella itself, in order to rule out fracture a tangential or axial view of it would be needed (Fig. 8–8E,F).

Serial Films

In many clinical circumstances, the evolution of x-ray changes over the course of a time interval will be the major consideration. X-ray evaluation of a healing fracture is a prime example of this (see Chap. 28). The goal of x-rays in this setting is to insure maintenance of proper anatomic relationships and to evaluate the status of healing.

Stress Views

In order to determine whether the ligaments are intact after a joint injury, the joint may be x-rayed in a position which would normally tighten or stress the ligament in question. Following a preliminary film to rule out a fracture, a stress film can be made, judiciously applying an appropriate deforming force. If, for example, the lateral ligaments at the ankle are in question, a film is made with the lower leg stabilized and the foot pushed medially, that is, inverted (Fig. 8–9). It is generally good practice to perform the same maneuver on the uninjured side to establish the baseline mobility for that individual.

Dynamic Studies

X-ray examinations in both still and cine format can be used to assess functional mobility as well as integrity of structure. Examples of this are illustrated in the chapters on the spine (cervical spine subluxation in rheumatoid arthritis) and upper limbs (motion at the wrist joint).

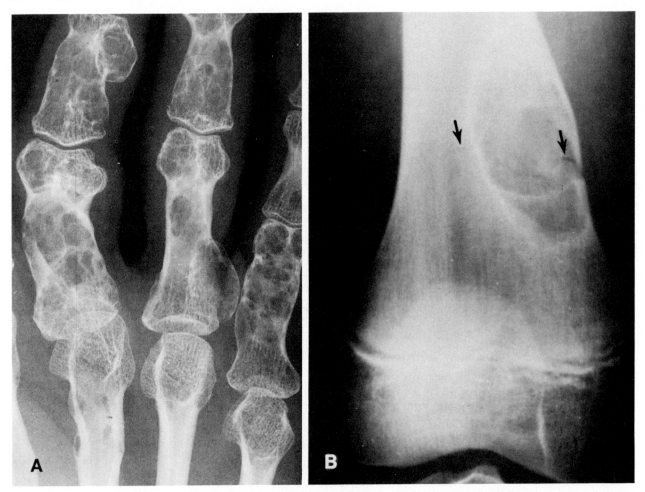

FIG. 8–7. Focal abnormalities of bones. **(A)** Multiple cartilaginous tumors (chondromas) have developed in the phalanges. They are slowly growing, causing well demarcated expansile thinning of the bones and consequent deformity. **(B)** Benign fibrous tumor (fibroma) in the femur showing eccentric location, sharp demarcation, and mild but definite cortical expansion. Note the pathologic fracture **(arrows)** which caused the patient to seek medical attention. **(C)** Widespread metastases to bone from a lung carcinoma. Defects are punched out without expansion or reaction by involved bone. This indicates very rapidly growing tumor implants. Externally visible deformities include soft tissue mass in middle finger, angulation of ring finger and shortening of fifth finger due to complete destruction of a phalanx. **(D)** Osteogenic sarcoma involving the femoral metaphysis in a child. The lesion shows a combination of destruction and sclerosis within the bone. Ossifying tumor tissue is breaking out through the cortex into soft tissues **(arrows).**

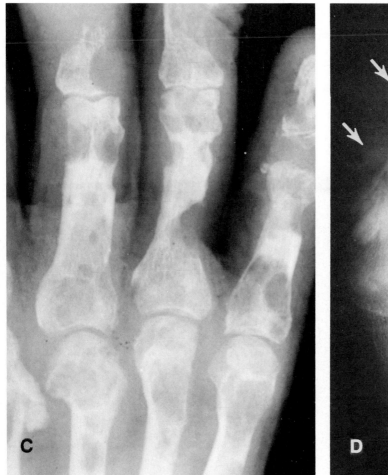

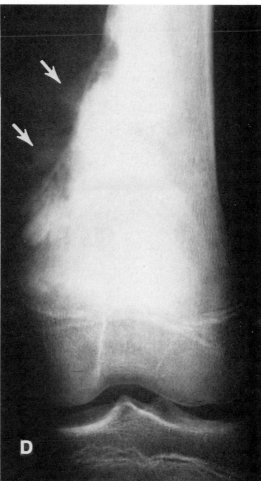

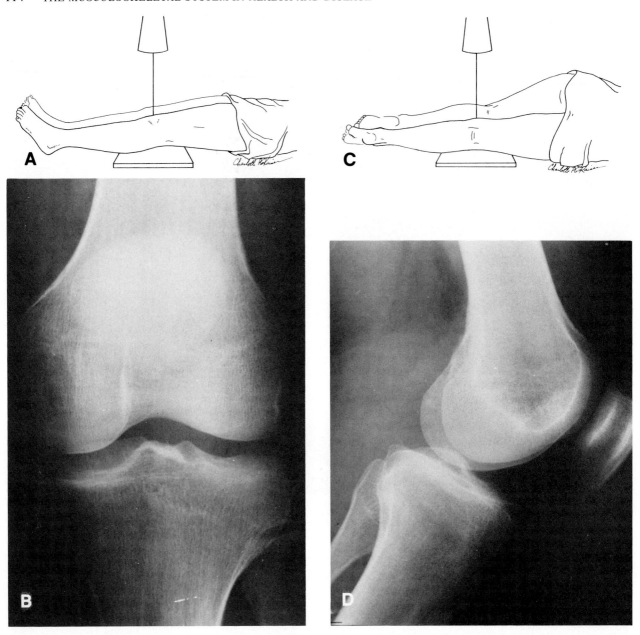

FIG. 8–8. Radiography of the knee—filming relationships and x-ray appearance in standard projections. **(A, B)** Anteroposterior (AP) projection. **(C, D)** Lateral projection. **(E, F)** Tangential patellar (sunrise) view.

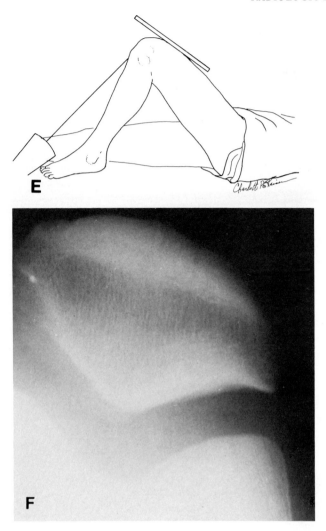

Tomography

It is sometimes impossible to achieve satisfactory visualization of a structure because of the complexity of overlapping shadows in every feasible projection. Tomography is a technique that employs reciprocal angular motion of the x-ray tube and film in order to blur out unwanted tissue planes and achieve an in-focus slice. An example (Fig. 8–10) compares the appearance of plain films and a tomogram in a patient with a lumbar spine fracture.

Arthrography

In order to delineate the nature and extent of a suspected intraarticular abnormality, arthrography may be performed, filming the joint in multiple projections after introducing contrast material and air into it. Plain films of joints are very informative in some situations, such as arthritis, however when the clinical question is one of a torn meniscus, focal erosion of articular cartilage, or a nonopaque intraarticular fragment, arthrography is needed. Figure 8–11 shows examples of normal and abnormal knee arthrograms with filming centered on the meniscus. Another arthrogram of the knee is shown in Chapter 18.

Arteriography

Intraarterial injection of opaque contrast material, followed by rapid sequential filming, provides

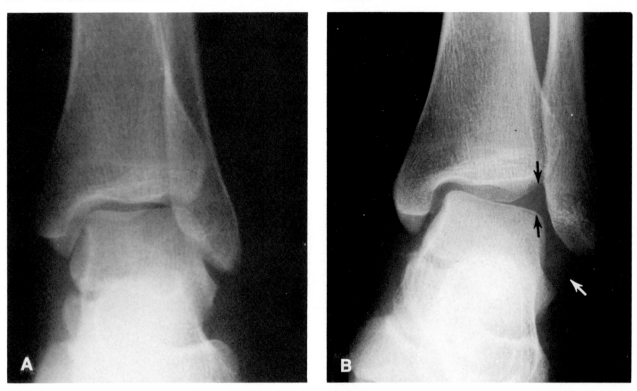

FIG. 8–9. Stress view of the ankle of a young patient who sustained an inversion injury. **(A)** Relaxed or baseline AP view showing apparently normal appearance of the bones. **(B)** Inversion stress view showing distraction in the lateral portion of the joint **(arrows).**

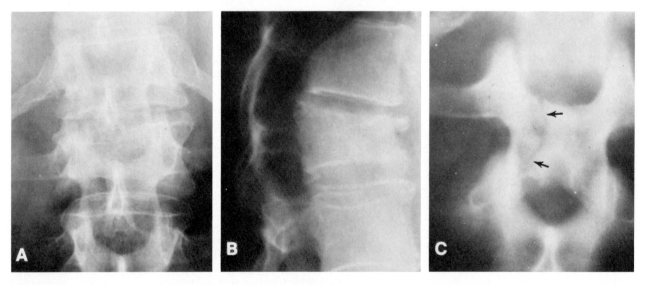

FIG. 8–10. Lumbar spine fracture illustrating the value of tomography. **(A)** AP and **(B)** lateral plain films demonstrate compression fracture of the L1 vertebral body. Compression deformity is most severe anteriorly and on the right. **(C)** Anteroposterior tomography. "Slices" through the vertebral body were merely confirmatory of the findings seen on plain films. However, a more posterior cut through the lamina shows an additional vertical fracture **(arrows)** through the posterior elements. This is a clinically more significant injury than would have been suspected on examination of the patient or on the plain films.

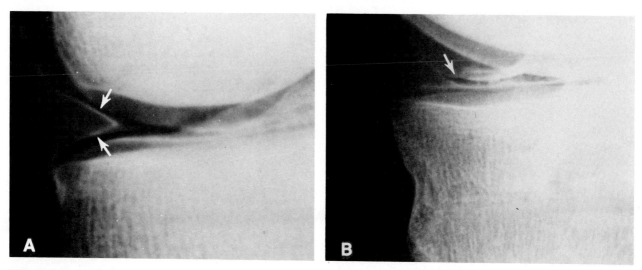

FIG. 8-11. Knee arthrography. Iodinated contrast material and air have been injected into the knee after sterile preparation and infiltration of a local anesthetic. Tightly coned down views are made, viewing the meniscus tangentially (medial meniscus in these illustrations) in multiple cross-sectional profiles. **(A)** Normal, intact medial meniscus. Its triangular shape **(arrows)** is outlined by the radiolucent air in the joint cavity. **(B)** Torn meniscus with air and contrast medium within the fissure of the tear **(arrow).**

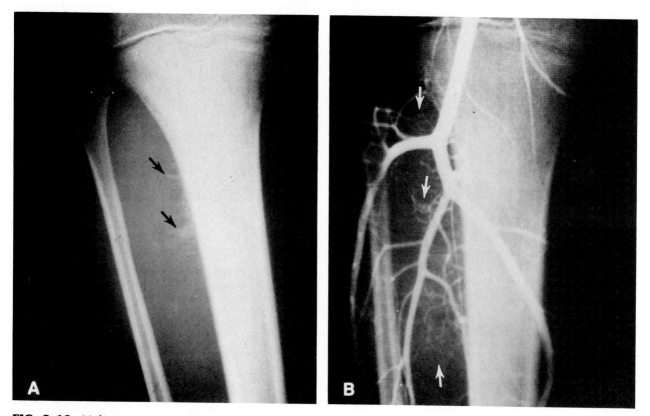

FIG. 8-12. Malignant tumor (Ewing's sarcoma) arising from the proximal tibia of a child. **(A)** Anteroposterior plain film. There is disruption of the tibial cortex laterally with linear calcifications (arrows) extending into soft tissues. Tumor bulk is suggested by the lateral displacement of proximal end of the fibula. **(B)** Femoral arteriogram shows opacification of popliteal artery and its branches. The main branches are stretched around the mass and there is abnormal hypervascularity **(arrows)** feeding the soft tissue component of the tumor.

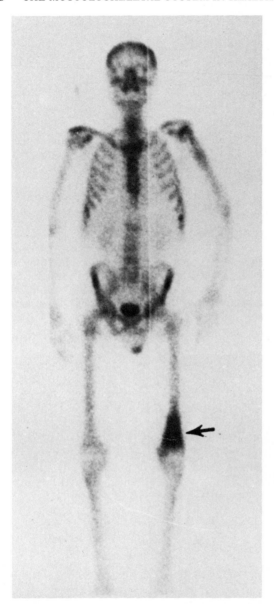

FIG. 8-13. Bone scan of a patient with recently diagnosed carcinoma of gastrointestinal tract. The presenting complaint was pain in the left leg. Radionuclide bone scan shows abnormal uptake in left femur **(arrow)**, left proximal humerus, and several ribs, indicating metastatic foci in both symptomatic and asymptomatic areas.

accurate delineation of the vasculature. Detection of arterial damage consequent to limb trauma or determination of the full extent of tumor spread in patients with malignancy are examples of the use of arteriography in musculoskeletal diagnosis (Fig. 8–12A,B).

Myelography

Contrast material injected by lumbar puncture into the subarachnoid space within the vertebral canal can provide detailed information on the condition of the spinal cord and nerve roots. There are characteristic configurations caused by lesions within the cord, subarachnoid space, and extradural regions. Herniated intervertebral disks are the most common of these lesions in clinical practice. Examples of myelograms are illustrated in Chapter 10.

Bone Scans

Radioactive isotopes have been developed which will preferentially go to bone, showing increased uptake in portions of the skeleton which are hypervascular or which have an increased rate of bone mineral turnover. A positive scan or *hot spot* is not etiologically specific, since identical images will be produced by tumor, infection, or trauma. The technique is very sensitive however and positive findings on scan will generally antedate the appearance of detectable x-ray abnormalities (Fig. 8–13).

SUGGESTED READING

Edeiken, J., and Hodes, P. J. Roentgen Diagnosis of Diseases of Bone, 2nd ed. Baltimore, Williams & Wilkins, 1973
   A comprehensive two volume reference work of skeletal radiology.
Squire, L. F., Colaiace, W. M., and Strutynsky, N. Exercises in Diagnostic Radiology. III. Bone. Philadelphia, W. B. Saunders, 1972
   Case presentations and problems in bone and joint radiology.
Troupin, R. H. Diagnostic Radiology in Clinical Medicine, 2nd ed. Chicago, Yearbook Medical, 1978
   An approach to radiologic problem-solving in multiple body systems.

9
The Vertebral Column

CORNELIUS ROSSE

The body of all vertebrate animals is built on a central axis known as the vertebral column. This backbone or spine consists of a series of bones called **vertebrae.** The vertebrae are firmly connected to one another by joints and ligaments, lending a considerable degree of springiness and flexibility as well as strength to the entire structure.

The vertebral column fulfills its principal function as a stiff but flexible axis. However, **regions** are discernible in it in which specific features of vertebrae and curvatures of the spine correlate with functions that are special to each region. The regions are the **cervical, thoracic, lumbar, sacral** and **coccygeal.**

In man, the vertebral column supports the head and the trunk in the erect position, and, via the pelvic girdle, transmits the weight of the body to the lower limbs. From the lower limbs it receives the propulsive impetus during locomotion. Thus it is continually subjected to a variety of forces. The rib cage is suspended on the vertebral column and the articulations between ribs and vertebrae permit the movements necessary for respiration. The vertebral column protects the spinal cord by enclosing it in the **vertebral canal.** From this canal issue all spinal nerves for the supply of the limbs and the trunk. The contents of the vertebral canal and the anatomic relationship between the spinal cord segments, spinal nerves, and the vertebrae are discussed in the following chapter. This chapter deals with the bony elements, joints, muscles, and movements of the vertebral column.

THE VERTEBRA

Vertebrae are made of cancellous bone (see Fig. 7–3), and in all regions of the spine they have two basic components: the **body** and the **vertebral arch.** The arch projects dorsally from the body, and the two enclose the **vertebral foramen** (Fig. 9–1). The bulk of the vertebra is represented by the body which is covered by hyaline cartilage on its superior and inferior surfaces. The contiguous surfaces are held together securely by **intervertebral disks.** The vertebral bodies and the disks progressively increase in height and in circumference in a caudal direction down to the sacrum. This is consistent with their function of bearing most of the weight.

The **vertebral arch** protects the spinal cord and the meninges housed in the **vertebral canal.** Each arch consists of two **pedicles** which strut posteriorly from the vertebral body and continue into the **laminae.** The two laminae meet in the midline (Fig. 9–1). The processes of the vertebra project from the vertebral arch. Two paired processes bear facets for articulations with neighboring vertebrae, while others serve for the attachment of muscles and ligaments. On each side, three processes are situated at the junction of the pedicle and the lamina. These are the **transverse process** and the **superior** and **inferior articular processes.** A **spinous process** points posteriorly at the union of the two laminae (Fig. 9–1).

X-Rays of Vertebrae

Despite the superimposition of several profiles, all parts of the vertebra can be identified on x-rays following a simple, disciplined approach. The approach is illustrated in Figure 9–2.

INTERVERTEBRAL JOINTS

Vertebrae articulate with one another by two types of joints: 1) a fibrocartilaginous joint or symphysis between vertebral bodies and 2) synovial joints between vertebral arches. A set of ligaments is associated with each type of joint.

119

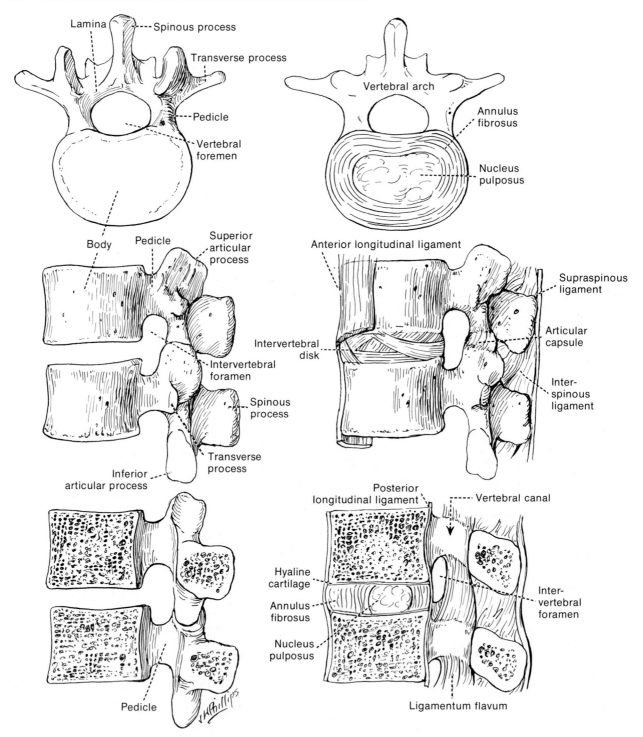

FIG. 9-1. The anatomy of the vertebra and the intervertebral joints with associated ligaments.

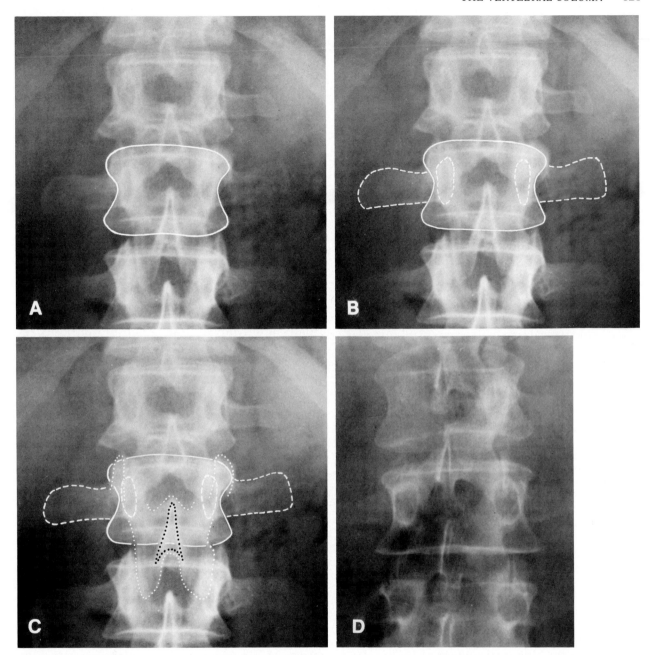

FIG. 9–2. A stepwise approach for identifying the anatomic parts of a vertebra on an anteroposterior x-ray film. **(A)** Outline the contour of the vertebral body. **(B)** Define the pedicles **(interrupted line)** and transverse processes. **(C)** Superimpose the profile of the laminae, superior and inferior articular process, plus the spinous process, which together resemble a butterfly **(dotted line). (D)** Several defects are present in the uppermost of these three lumbar vertebrae. The pedicle, the transverse process, and the superior and inferior articular processes are missing on the right side. They have been eroded by a malignant neoplasm situated in the intervertebral foramen. (Courtesy of Dr. Rosalind H. Troupin)

The Intervertebral Disk

The symphysis between vertebral bodies is the intervertebral disk. The structure of the disk is admirably suited for resisting displacement of vertebrae on one another while allowing some movement, and for withstanding and dissipating the forces that are transmitted along the vertebral column.

Each disk conforms in shape to the apposing surfaces of the adjacent vertebral bodies, and together the disks contribute one quarter to the height of the vertebral column above the sacrum. An intervertebral disk consists of a tough, peripheral fibrocartilaginous ring called the **annulus fibrosus** and of a more pliable, inner, gelatinous mass, the **nucleus pulposus** (Fig. 9–1).

The Annulus Fibrosus. On x-rays the disks appear as translucent spaces between the vertebral bodies (Fig. 9–2). The annulus is thicker anteriorly than posteriorly. Its bulk is made up of collagen fibers which run in roughly concentric lamellae. The fibers run obliquely between the vertebrae and are anchored in the hyaline cartilage that covers the superior and inferior surfaces of vertebral bodies. Their attachment is secured by calcification in the cartilage. In adjacent lamellae the fibers slant in opposite directions (Figs. 9–1, 9–3), thus generating a mechanism which permits and also limits rotation between vertebrae. In addition, this arrangement lends a certain degree of elasticity to this fibrous ring. When compression forces are transmitted by the nucleus pulposus, it can distend the annulus by slightly changing the angle between the collagen fiber bundles (Fig. 9–3).

The Nucleus Pulposus. The white, glistening, amorphous substance of the nucleus pulposus consists predominantly of semisolid matrix with some collagen fibers embedded without any specific orientation. Matrix and fibers are produced by the sparse cells found in the nucleus. The cells resemble chondrocytes. The nucleus pulposus has a capacity for absorbing water which it looses when compressed. Its extent can be demonstrated radiographically (Fig. 9–4).

Nutrition and Degenerative Changes. Apart from the most superficial layers of the annulus fibrosus, the intervertebral disk in adult life is avascular. Its nutrition relies on diffusion across the hyaline cartilage from the spongy bone of the vertebra. During the growth period, however, radial

vascular channels are present in the hyaline cartilage. Degenerative changes begin in the intervertebral disk during the third decade. These changes are due to the mechanical stresses imposed on the disk and are most marked and common in the last two lumbar disks. The changes consist of thinning of the hyaline cartilage plate, dehydration, and loss of pliability in the nucleus pulposus with accompanying cell death and fragmentation of fibers in the annulus fibrosus. The latter phenomenon is particularly marked posteriorly where the annulus is thinner. These factors contribute to reduction in the height of the disk and predispose to rupture of the annulus with consequent herniation of the disk into the vertebral canal or intervertebral foramina (see also Chap. 10).

Joints of the Vertebral Arch

Consecutive vertebral arches articulate with one another via their articular prosesses (Fig. 9–1). The joints are synovial, and a capsule encloses the facets of a pair of mating superior and inferior articular processes. Since the intervertebral disk permits movement in any direction, the types of motion possible between a pair of vertebrae are determined by the synovial joints of the arch. The vertebral arch joints are of the plane or ellipsoid variety. The vertebral arch is more mobile than the vertebral body, and this fact is consistent with the synovial nature of vertebral arch joints and with the presence of a symphysis between vertebral bodies.

Ligaments

The ligaments which reinforce the intervertebral symphysis are tough and inelastic, while the ligaments associated with the vertebral arch contain many elastic fibers and are stretchable.

Ligaments Associated with the Intervertebral Disk. Between the skull and the sacrum the **anterior** and **posterior longitudinal ligaments** run uninterruptedly on respective surfaces of the vertebral bodies (Fig. 9–1). The ligaments resist anterior and posterior displacement of vertebrae on one another. Both ligaments are firmly attached to each intervertebral disk but allow some blood vessels to pass deep to them over the vertebral bodies.

Ligaments Associated with the Vertebral Arch. Ligaments run between laminae and spinous

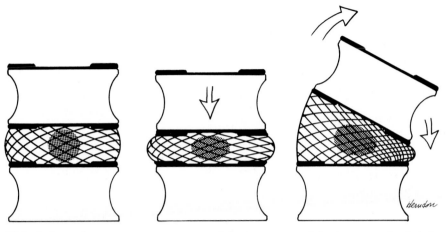

FIG. 9-3. Schematic representation of the structure of the intervertebral disk. The crisscross arrangement of collagen fiber bundles in the annulus fibrosus permits rotation between the vertebrae and also allows for bulging when the nucleus pulposus is compressed.

FIG. 9-4. A discogram. A radioopaque, water-soluble substance is injected into the center of the intervertebral disk and it outlines the extent of the nucleus pulposus which, in this case, is normal. (Courtesy of Dr. Rosalind H. Troupin)

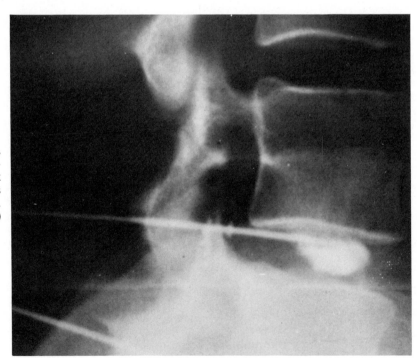

and transverse processes of consecutive vertebrae (Fig. 9–1). There are no ligaments between pedicles where the intervertebral foramen is located. During flexion of the spine the ligaments become stretched and limit the movement.

The **ligamentum flavum** connects the laminae of adjacent vertebrae and is rich in elastic fibers. The rather thin **interspinous ligaments** attach along the superior and inferior edges of spinous processes, while the **supraspinous ligament** is a strong fibrous cord and connects the tips of spinous processes. The latter ligament is liable to tear in flexion injury. The **intertransverse ligaments** are functionally insignificant.

REGIONAL SPECIALIZATION IN THE VERTEBRAL COLUMN

While the basic structure of vertebrae and intervertebral joints is the same throughout the spine, specializations exist in all five regions (Fig. 9–5). The seven cervical vertebrae provide freedom of movement for the head; the 12 thoracic vertebrae articulate with the ribs; the bodies of the 5 lumbar vertebrae are larger than those in other regions; the 5 sacral vertebrae have fused into a single bone, and coccygeal vertebrae have become vestigial. In each region, the vertebrae are held together in curvatures of differing radius with alternating forward convexity and concavity. Exaggeration of a normal thoracic curve is known as **kyphosis** and an exaggerated lumbar curve is a **lordosis.** These Greek words mean convexity and concavity, and were originally used to describe the curves as seen by the examiner standing behind the patient. The normal curves impart an undulating lateral profile to the whole column which greatly increases its springiness. The freedom of movement is greater in anteriorly convex regions of the spine.

Cervical Spine

The first two cervical vertebrae are specially adapted for the free movement of the head but joints between the remaining cervical vertebrae also subserve this function.

Atlantooccipital and Atlantoaxial Joints. The first cervical vertebra is the bearer of the "globe" and is known as the **atlas** (Fig. 9–6). The atlas is the most slender vertebra, consisting of an anterior and posterior bony arch, and it lacks a body. The skull rests with its occipital condyles on a pair of articular facets situated at the junction of the two

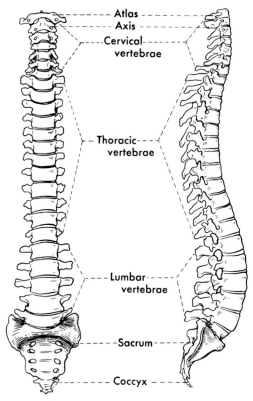

FIG. 9-5. The anatomic regions of the vertebral column seen from the anterior and lateral aspects. (Hollinshead WH: Textbook of Anatomy, 3rd ed. Hagerstown, Harper & Row, 1974)

arches. The second cervical vertebra is called the **axis** because it provides the axis upon which the atlas, bearing the head, can rotate. However, only its toothlike (odontoid) process, the **dens,** which projects upward from its body, subserves this function. The first intervertebral disk is encountered between the axis and the third cervical vertebra and provides for the stabilization of the axis.

The joints responsible for the greatest range of head movements are all synovial. These include a pair of atlantooccipital joints and three atlantoaxial joints. The concave ellipsoid, superior articular facets of the atlas (Fig. 9–6) permit nodding or flexion and extension of the head and some lateral bending. The inferior articular facets of the atlas are plane and they match the corresponding facets of the axis, permitting free sliding at the lateral atlantoaxial joints during head rotation (Figs. 9–6, 9–7). The median atlantoaxial joint functions as a pivot. It is located between the anterior arch of the atlas and the dens (Figs. 9–6, 9–8A).

The stability of these mobile joints is secured through a number of strong ligaments. The most important of these is the **transverse ligament of the atlas** (Fig. 9–6). It retains the dens in position, preventing impingement on the spinal cord. However, when rheumatoid arthritis affects this joint, the ligament may become eroded and may rupture, leading to a fatal outcome even in minor whiplash injuries (Fig. 9–8). Normally, the ligament is so strong that when subjected to trauma, as in judicial hanging or in other cases of violent trauma (automobile accidents), it will often not give way, rather, the bone will fracture (hangman's fracture).

C3–C7 Spine. Movements in the lower cervical spine extend the range obtained between the skull and the first two cervical vertebrae. Flexion reverses the cervical forward convexity of the spine, and at its extreme places the chin on the chest. While the intervertebral disks secure stability during flexion, the vertebral arches and spinous processes spread apart. A sickle-shaped elastic membrane replaces the supraspinous ligaments in this region and helps to support the head in the flexed position. The membrane is the **ligamentum nuchae.** Flexion, extension, and lateral bending require free sliding of the **articular facets** at the synovial joints of the vertebral arches. These joints are visible in a lateral x-ray of the cervical spine (Fig. 9–9). The facets of these joints are placed in the coronal plane (Fig. 9–10) thus providing freedom for these movements and also permitting but a small degree of rotation between consecutive vertebrae.

In adult life, small cavities appear in the posterolateral parts of the cervical intervertebral disks. The cavities have been mistaken for synovial joints (joints of Luschka). They are absent at birth and most likely represent degenerative changes in the disks.

The **vertebral foramen** of all cervical vertebrae is large in comparison with their body (Fig. 9–10). It provides room for the spinal cord which is of the greatest diameter in this region. On the other hand, the **intervertebral foramina** are relatively small in the cervical region. Flexion tends to open up the foramina while extension, lateral bending, and rotation tend to crowd these spaces. Symptoms due to nerve root compression will be exaggerated by these movements. This may be appreciated by studying the radiologic anatomy of the cervical spine (Fig. 9–10), particularly in the oblique projection.

The **transverse process** of all cervical vertebrae, including the atlas and axis, is perforated (Figs.

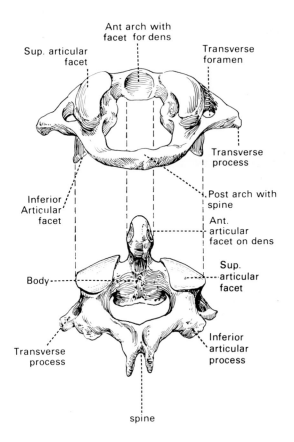

Ant arch with facet for dens
Sup. articular facet
Transverse foramen
Transverse process
Inferior Articular facet
Post arch with spine
Ant. articular facet on dens
Body
Sup. articular facet
Inferior articular process
Transverse process
spine

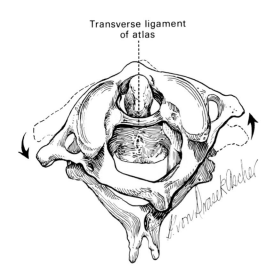

Transverse ligament of atlas

FIG. 9-6. The atlas and axis vertebrae. The atlas pivots around the dens carrying the head with it.

9–6, 9–10). The foramina transmit the vertebral artery with its sympathetic nerve plexus and the vertebral veins. The vertebral artery is the main source of blood supply to the hind brain as well as to the cervical spinal cord and cervical spine. The intimate relationship of these vessels renders them susceptible to compression by abnormalities of the cervical spine, superimposing an additional element on nerve root and spinal cord compression that is special to this region.

Thoracic Spine

The rib cage is supported on the thoracic spine, and thoracic vertebrae bear facets for articulation with the ribs (Fig. 9–11). The thoracic spine is concave anteriorly. Its flexion, extension, and lateral bending are limited by the rib cage but most of the rotation possible along the vertebral column below C2 is obtained in this region. **Costal cartilages** join the ribs anteriorly to the **sternum** and

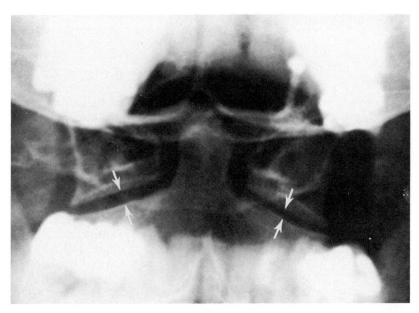

FIG. 9–7. The dens of the axis projecting above the two lateral atlanto-axial joints **(arrows),** the plane articular surfaces of which permit gliding as the atlas, bearing the head, pivots around the dens. This anteroposterior x-ray is taken through the open mouth, and the tip of the dens can be seen to be on level with the hard palate. (Courtesy of Dr. Rosalind H. Troupin)

FIG. 9–8. Lateral x-rays of the cervical spine of a patient suffering from rheumatoid arthritis. **(A)** The head is ex- ▶ tended and the anterior arch of the atlas **(stemmed arrow)** is closely apposed to the dens **(arrowhead).** The hardly perceptible radiolucency separating them represents the articular cartilage of the median atlantoaxial joint. **(B)** In flexion the dens moves away from the anterior arch of the atlas, indicating that the transverse ligament, which normally retains it in position, has been eroded away. (Courtesy of Dr. Rosalind H. Troupin)

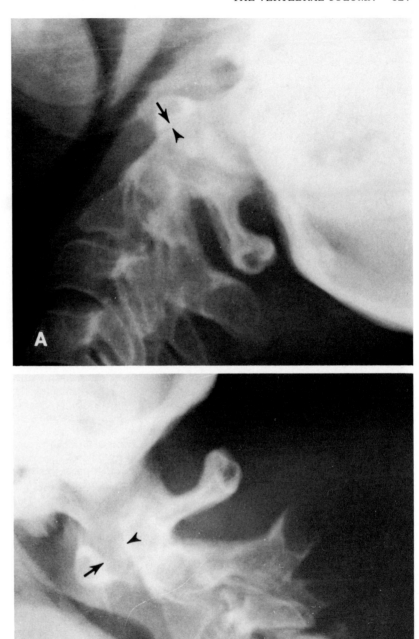

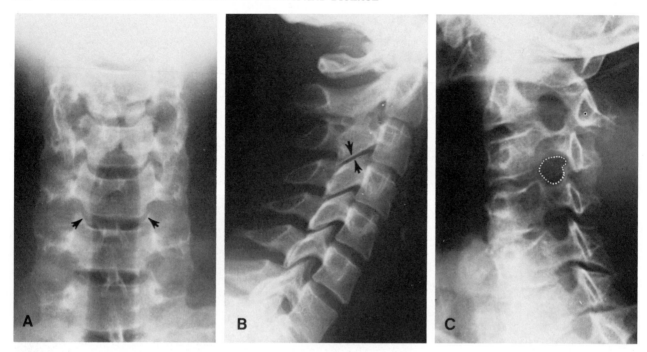

FIG. 9-9. Radiologic anatomy of the cervical spine. **(A)** In the anteroposterior view the most superior vertebra is C3; C1 and C2 are obscured by the jaw. The lateral lip of the superior surface of the vertebral body projects upward **(arrows).** The so-called joints of Luschka are situated here, replacing the posterolateral part of the intervertebral disk. The central radiolucent shadow is the trachea which tapers into the larynx superiorly. **(B)** In the left lateral projection all cervical spinous processes are visible, the vertebral bodies and disks are well outlined, and the joint space is clearly seen between superior and inferior articular processes **(arrows). (C)** A right oblique projection demonstrates the intervertebral foramina to best advantage (one of them outlined). The foramina are bounded by a pedicle above and below, anteriorly by the disk and by part of the vertebral body above and below the disk. The posterior boundary of the foramen is formed by the articular processes and the joint capsule. The circular or C-shaped profile in the vertebral bodies anteriorly is the outline of the transverse process on the right side. (Courtesy of Dr. Rosalind H. Troupin)

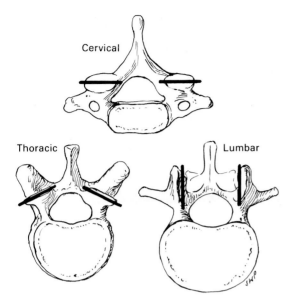

Cervical

Thoracic

Lumbar

FIG. 9-10. Superior view of a cervical, thoracic, and lumbar vertebra illustrating the major differences between vertebrae of these three regions (see text). Solid lines have been placed across the articular surfaces of the vertebral arch joints in order to illustrate the different planes in which the facets of these joints lie. Only in the thoracic region does the positioning of these facets permit an appreciable amount of rotation between consecutive vertebrae.

furnish the plasticity to the rib cage necessary during vertebral rotation and in the movements of respiration.

Forces that support and move the ribs are transmitted to the vertebrae and provide a series of splints to the thoracic spine. Due to their bilateral symmetry, these forces contribute to the lateral stability of the thoracic vertebral column.

Costovertebral and Costotransverse Joints. Each typical rib abuts with its head against an intervertebral disk, and a synovial joint joins it to the bodies of the vertebrae above and below (Fig. 9-11). This costovertebral joint is enclosed in a capsule reinforced by ligaments. **Costotransverse ligaments** secure the neck of the rib to the transverse process of the two vertebrae. At the costotransverse joint, the lower transverse process articulates with the tubercle of the rib, which bears the same number as that vertebra. Slight movements at these joints will result in greatly amplified excursions of the rib shaft and will be transmitted to the sternum. These movements increase the anteroposterior and lateral diameters of

the thoracic cage during inspiration. In deep inspiration, the thoracic spine extends, thus facilitating the separation of the ribs. Abnormalities of the thoracic spine which interfere with rib movements and with the symmetry of the rib cage may seriously impair cardiovascular–respiratory function.

Thoracic Rotation. The facets of synovial joints on the thoracic vertebral arches are positioned along the arc of a circle whose center is in the vertebral body (Fig. 9-10). The mechanism is ideally suited for rotation of vertebrae on one another around this imaginary center. Rotation is the characteristic motion of a thoracic vertebra.

Lumbar Spine

Lumbar vertebral bodies are large in comparison with other vertebrae and in comparison with their own vertebral canal. The intervertebral foramina are spacious. The characteristic radiologic features of the lumbar spine are illustrated in Figure 9-12.

The lumbar spine is convex ventrally and possesses a relatively wide range of movement. However, the effective range of flexing the trunk is greatly augmented by movement at the hips. The planes of articular facets on the vertebral arch face in a sagittal plane (Fig. 9-10). They slide effectively on one another in flexion, extension, and lateral bending but there is hardly any freedom for rotation.

Shearing stresses imposed on the last intervertebral disk are the greatest along the entire column. This is due to weight transmission and to the presence of the **lumbosacral angle** created by the change in spinal curvatures and by the angulation of the superior surface of S1 (Fig. 9-13A). The facets of the vertebral arch joints at the lumbosacral joint take a great share in supporting the lumbar spine on the sacrum as these facets have changed from the sagittal to a transverse orientation. The bone of the vertebral arch of L5 that intervenes between superior and inferior articular processes plays a key role in this mechanism (Fig. 9-12C). When this **pars interarticularis** is disrupted (spondylolysis), the fifth lumbar vertebra and the rest of the spine with it slip forward on the sacrum (Fig. 9-13B). The condition is known as **spondylolisthesis.** Defects of the pars interarticularis and spondylolisthesis may occur at other vertebrae but are most common between L5 and S1. In addition to nerve root compression in the intervertebral foramen, the cauda equina also may come to danger.

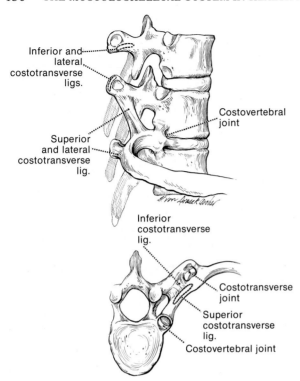

Inferior and lateral costotransverse ligs.

Costovertebral joint

Superior and lateral costotransverse lig.

Inferior costotransverse lig.

Costotransverse joint

Superior costotransverse lig.

Costovertebral joint

FIG. 9–11. The thoracic spine and costovertebral and costotransverse joints with their associated ligaments.

The Sacrum

The sacrum is formed by the complete fusion of all elements of five vertebrae. The rami of sacral spinal nerves emerge from the sacral canal through foramina on the anterior and posterior aspects of the triangular bone. The sacrum is wedged in between the two hip bones and the weight of the body is transmitted to these bones via the **sacroiliac joints.** Although the joints are synovial, the irregular, interlocking surfaces and the strong **sacroiliac** and **iliolumbar ligaments** permit little movement, converting the sacrum and the two hip bones into the rigidly constructed pelvis.

DEVELOPMENT OF THE VERTEBRAL COLUMN

The vertebrae are preformed in hyaline cartilage which develops from the segmental **sclerotomes.** Ossification centers soon define the **centrum** and two halves of the vertebral arch. At this stage of development, the vertebral arches are also known as neural arches. From the centrum develops most of the vertebral body. At birth, vertebrae consist of these three pieces of bone united by hyaline cartilage (Fig. 9–14). Initially, enlargement of vertebrae depends on over-all growth of the cartilage but after the appearance of **secondary ossification centers** around the age of puberty, growth proceeds mainly at the epiphyses. A **ring-shaped epiphysis** is present along the superior and inferior surfaces of vertebral bodies (Fig. 9–14E), and secondary ossification centers appear also at the tips of spinous and transverse processes (Fig. 9–14D).

Congenital Malformations

In order to understand congenital malformations of the spine, it is necessary to state the developmental sequence in slightly greater detail.

The development of the centrum is associated with the **notochord,** whereas the neural arches are influenced by the spinal cord. Cells migrate bilaterally from each of the somites (see Fig. 12–1), and by uniting around the notochord, segmental sclerotomes are established (Fig. 9–15A). Soon a fissure splits each sclerotome (Fig. 9–15B), and the caudal half of one sclerotome fuses with the cranial half of the next (Fig. 9–15C). Thus, each centrum is actually derived from four mesodermal elements with the notochord running through its center and also through the sclerotomal fissure which defines the position of the future intervertebral disk. From this sclerotomal primordium, cells of the vertebral arches migrate dorsally around the spinal cord and their extensions establish also the future vertebral processes. In addition, all vertebrae possess a **costal element** which grows ventrally from the sclerotome in the region of the future intervertebral disk. Chondrification and ossification occur in these anlagen.

Malformations of the Centrum. Some of the cells of the nucleus pulposus are derived from the notochord but the notochordal canal is obliterated in the vertebrae. Notochordal rests in sacral vertebrae may develop into a *malignant chordoma.* Persistence of the notochordal canal together with nonunion of right and left sclerotomes is responsible for *cleft* or *butterfly vertebra* (Fig. 9–16).

Although normally only a single ossification center can be identified for each centrum, failure of the right or left half of the center to appear results in **hemivertebra.** The other half of the vertebra remains cartilaginous and usually becomes compressed, predisposing to lateral curvatures of the spine.

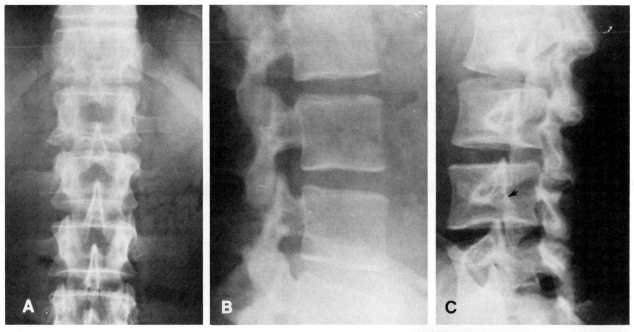

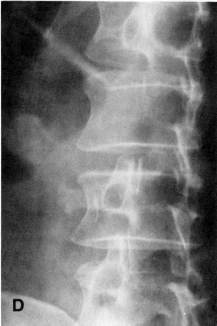

FIG. 9-12. Radiologic anatomy of the lumbar spine. **(A)** In the antero-posterior view clearly identifiable are 1) the vertebral body, 2) the space occupied by the intervertebral disk, 3) the roots of the pedicles, 4) transverse and spinous processes, 5) the superior margin of the laminae, 6) superior and inferior articular processes with the joint space between their facets (refer to Fig. 9–2). **(B)** In the lumbar region the lateral projection gives a good view of the intervertebral foramina and of the structures that form their boundaries. **(C)** The oblique projection in the lumbar region provides a good view of the superior and inferior articular processes and of the bridge of bone that unites their bases which is known as the *pars interarticularis*. Though somewhat fanciful, it helps orientation to recognize the outline of a Scotty dog over the posterior half of the vertebra. The dog's head is the root of the pedicle, its large eye the base of the transverse process, its ear the superior articular process, and front legs the inferior articular process. The neck of the dog **(arrow)** is the pars interarticularis. **(D)** An oblique view of the lumbar spine of the same patient shown in Figure 9–2D. The Scotty dog is missing in one of the vertebrae. (Courtesy of Dr. Rosalind H. Troupin)

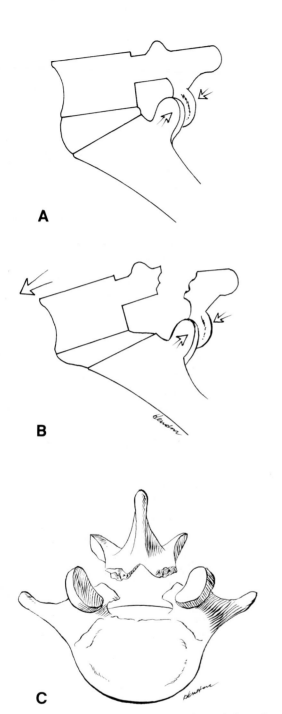

FIG. 9-13. **(A)** The lumbosacral angle and the role of the articular processes in supporting the vertebral column on the sacrum. **(B)** Disruption of the pars interarticularis (spondylolysis) leads to spondylolisthesis. **(C)** Superior view of L5 with pars interarticularis defect.

Vertebral Fusion. The centrum of the atlas fuses with the centrum of the axis and is represented by the dens. In the sacral region such intervertebral fusion unites all five vertebrae. The fifth lumbar vertebra is not uncommonly sacralized (Fig. 9-16). In other regions *block vertebrae* are produced by the same process.

Supernumerary Ribs. Only in the thoracic region does the costal element become a separate bone. In cervical and lumbar vertebrae it is incorporated into the transverse process, while in the sacrum costal elements fuse in the lateral masses of the bone. Thus, supernumerary ribs in cervical and lumbar regions may be readily explained. They may give rise to symptoms due to compression of nerves and blood vessels.

Malformation of the Vertebral Arch. The most common congenital anomalies of the spine affect the vertebral arch. Defects in midline union exist in different degrees. The simplest is **spina bifida occulta** which is asymptomatic. More serious degrees of nonunion are associated with meningeal and spinal cord abnormalities which are most commonly seen in the lumbosacral region (Fig. 9-17). The swelling may or may not be covered by skin and is known as a **meningocele** when it contains cerebrospinal fluid. In a **meningomyelocele** nerves of the cauda equina or the spinal cord itself are present. When the central canal of the spinal cord is also distended, or when the cord is laid open due to nonunion of the neural folds, the condition is known as **myelocele.** The latter is invariably associated with serious neurologic abnormalities and other malformations.

Rarely, the cartilage persists between ossification centers of the arch and the centrum (Fig. 9-14). Such defects of the **neurocentral junction** are situated in the posterolateral part of the vertebral body because the ossification center of the arch contributes to formation of the vertebral body.

No developmental explanation can be offered for defects of the **pars interarticularis** (Figs. 9-12C, 9-13). The ossification center of a developing arch is uninterrupted across the bases of the articular processes, and the defect is not present at birth.

Development of the Curvatures

The fetal spine is curved like a C and is concave ventrally. This primary curvature persists in the thoracic and sacral regions. After birth, the sec-

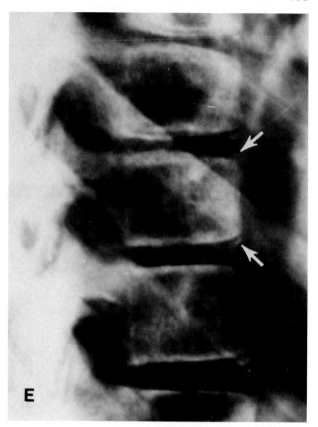

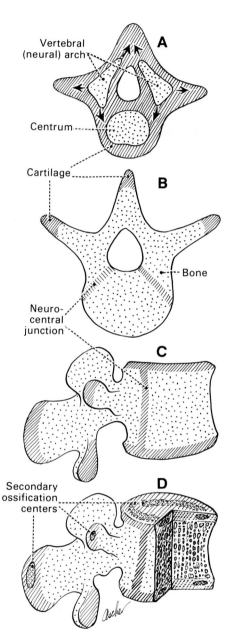

FIG. 9-14. Development of a vertebra. **(A)** Ossification center for the centrum and neural arch at the time of birth. **(B and C)** Before puberty. **(D)** Secondary ossification centers. **(E)** Lateral x-ray of the lumbar spine at the age of 13. The ring epiphysis is visible anteriorly at the superior and inferior margins of vertebrae **(arrows)**. **(E.** Courtesy of Dr. Rosalind H. Troupin)

ondary curves appear which are convex anteriorly. Development of the cervical curvature is associated with the ability of the infant to raise its head, while the lumbar curve appears when the child begins to walk. Normally, there are no lateral curvatures in the spine.

Abnormal curves may develop in the vertebral column during the growth period, or as a consequence of disease in the vertebrae and intervertebral joints. Curves may also result from interference with the normal function of the spinal musculature. Pathologic curvatures will be dealt with after the muscles that move the vertebral column have been discussed.

MUSCLES OF THE VERTEBRAL COLUMN

The range and type of movement possible in each region of the spine is determined by the vertebral arch joints but the control and strength of the movements depend on muscles. Muscles are also essential for the stability of the spine. The muscles

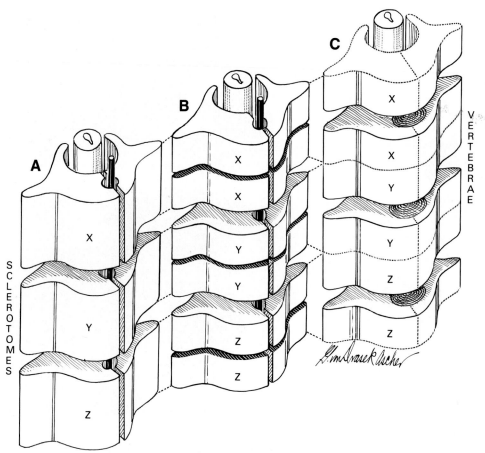

FIG. 9-15. The sclerotomal origin of vertebrae. The notochord is represented as a black rod and the spinal cord as a white cylinder. For explanation, see text.

fall into two groups: extensors and flexors. Both groups are also capable of rotating and laterally bending the column.

Extensors

The extensors of the spine are placed posterior to the laminae and transverse processes and span the entire back between the sacrum and the occiput. This large muscle bulk is composed of numerous individual muscles which are collectively known as the **erector spinae** (Fig. 9–18). The muscle is not responsible for holding the spine erect during standing, but, as its name inplies, restores it to the erect position. In addition to producing extension, it controls flexion of the spine by "paying out rope" against gravity. The contraction of the muscle is just as powerful, and may be palpated both during bending over to tie a shoe lace and during straightening up from the bent position.

The erector spinae contains all the myotomal cells that migrated dorsal to the spinal cord. Although some of these cells have fused into muscles that span several vertebrae, the deepest muscles of the erector spinae have retained a truly segmental arrangement. However, even the longer muscles conform to a segmental pattern in their innervation. **The erector spinae is the only muscle in the body supplied by dorsal rami of spinal nerves.** Segmental spasm and pain will be induced in the muscle when a single nerve root is irritated. Conversely, segments of the muscle may go into spasm to guard against movement when a painful lesion is present.

In the cervical region parts of the erector spinae are specialized for head movements, but the names of individual muscles in any region of the spine are beyond the scope of this book. It is relevant, however, to note that most of the muscles originate and insert by multiple tendinous slips. The various muscles ascend and descend in diagonal lines from spinous processes to transverse processes, or from transverse processes to ribs, from ilium or sacrum to spines or ribs, and *vice versa*. They cross each other in different layers establishing a system of guy ropes or trusses (Fig. 9–18). Clearly, such an arrangement is ideal for providing lateral stability to the vertebral column. When this mechanism is defective on one side, a pathologic lateral curvature or scoliosis will result.

The subdivision of this muscle mass by innumerable connective tissue planes, and the multiple attachments of tendons over small areas of periosteum on vertebral processes may suggest why pain

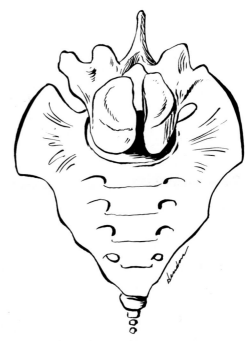

FIG. 9–16. Cleft fifth lumbar vertebra, the transverse process of which has fused with the sacrum on the left side, thus sharing the fate of the sacral transverse processes.

or spasm is so common in the extensor musculature of the spine, and why it is so difficult to offer specific anatomic explanation for it.

A strong fascia envelops the entire erector spinae in the lumbar region (Fig. 9–19). It is known as the **thoracolumbar** or **lumbodorsal fascia,** and numerous muscle fibers of the erector spinae take origin from it. The anterior layer of this fascia is anchored to the transverse processes, and anterior and posterior layers meet along the lateral edge of the erector spinae, where muscles of the anterior abdominal wall arise from it. The fascia is much thinner in the cervical and thoracic regions. Two flat sheets of muscle are superficial to the fascia in the back. These are the trapezius superiorly and the latissimus dorsi inferiorly. They conceal the erector spinae in the back. Both muscles serve the upper limb and do not belong to spinal extensors.

Flexors

Flexor musculature is virtually confined to the cervical and lumbar regions of the spine, reflecting the fact that these are the most mobile regions of the vertebral column. Gravity plays a major part in

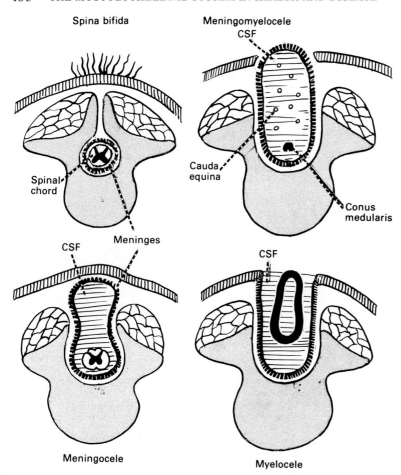

FIG. 9-17. Congenital anomalies of the vertebral arch. For explanation see text.

flexion, and therefore the flexor muscles of the spine are best demonstrated when they are made to work against gravity, as during raising the head or the trunk from the supine position.

Anatomically, the **prevertebral musculature** is the flexor counterpart of the erector spinae. The muscles which are in close apposition to the vertebral column anteriorly are ineffectual as a flexor unit because of their poor mechanical advantage. These prevertebral flexors retain their original function only in the cervical region where they are chiefly represented by the **longus colli** and the **scalene muscles** (Fig. 9–20). In the thoracic region this muscle group has disappeared while in front of the lumbar spine it is chiefly represented by the **psoas major** (Fig. 9–19). The psoas muscle no longer functions as a flexor of the spine (Fig. 9–21). The distal attachment of the psoas has migrated to the lower limb, and when it contracts it flexes the entire trunk on the lower limb at the hip. It cannot produce flexion at intervertebral joints.

More powerful are the muscles which flex the spine indirectly. They are placed more anteriorly and operate at a better advantage than the prevertebral muscles. The **sternomastoid muscles** attach superiorly to the skull and inferiorly to the manubrium and clavicles (Fig. 9–20). They not only draw the head forward but flex the cervical spine. This composite movement anticipates food being placed into the mouth.

The flexors of the lumbar spine are the anterior abdominal wall muscles (Fig. 9–22). The two **rectus abdominis** muscles are attached to the rib cage and to the pubis. They are assisted by the **external** and **internal obliques.** These muscles approximate the rib cage to the pelvis. The muscles are put to work during sit ups, especially when the hips and knees are kept flexed. With extended hips, sit ups mainly exercise the psoas.

The prevertebral and the anterior abdominal wall muscles are derived from ventral extensions of the myotomes and they are all supplied segmentally by the ventral rami of spinal nerves. The sternomastoid muscles are an exception; they are supplied from cervical spinal cord segments via the spinal accessory nerve whose relationship to spinal nerves is not clearly understood.

Lateral Bending

Unilateral contraction of spinal flexors and/or extensors will produce lateral bending. The rotation element which some of these muscles produce has to be cancelled out by appropriate antagonists. A muscle which functions purely in lateral bending of the lumbar spine is the **quadratus lumborum** (Fig. 9–21).

Rotation

Rotation is possible in the cervical and thoracic regions, but for practical purposes it is nonexistent

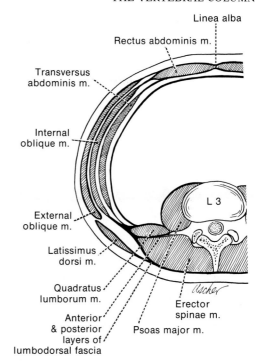

FIG. 9–19. A schematic transverse section across the trunk at the level of L3 to show the arrangement of the main muscle groups and fascial layers.

in the lumbar spine. When the head is turned fully to one side, 70 percent of the movement occurs at the **atlantoaxial** and **atlantooccipital joints** and rotation between the remaining cervical vertebrae accounts for only 30 percent of the movement.

The sternomastoid is the most powerful rotator, but a combination of muscles is called into action. Although parts of the erector spinae running between the transverse process of one vertebra and the spinous process of the vertebra above do exert a rotatory action (Fig. 9–18), the most powerful rotators of the thoracic spine are the abdominal flank muscles, namely the external and internal obliques (Fig. 9–22). These muscles run obliquely in opposite directions between the pelvis and the thoracic cage. The right external oblique acts in union with the left internal oblique and together they rotate the costal margin toward the left side.

ABNORMAL SPINAL CURVATURES

Pathologic exaggeration of the thoracic curvature is known as **kyphosis** and may be due to congenital

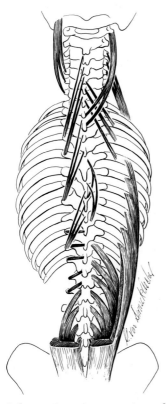

FIG. 9–18. Schematic representation of some of the individual components of the erector spinae to give an impression of the composition of this multilayered muscle whose individual units crisscross each other in different planes. (For description see text.)

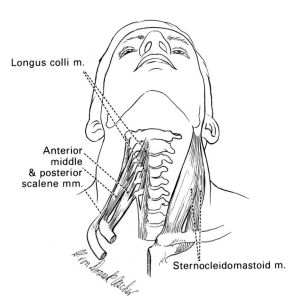

FIG. 9-20. Flexor muscles of the cervical spine.

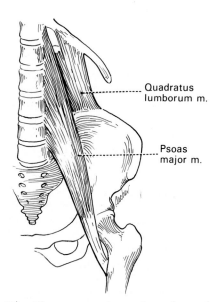

FIG. 9-21. The psoas major and quadratus lumborum muscles.

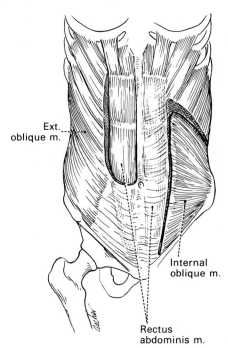

FIG. 9-22. Anterior abdominal wall muscles. On the right side the upper portion of the aponeurosis of the external oblique has been cut open to expose the rectus abdominis. On the left, the inferolateral part of the external oblique has been removed to expose the internal oblique. See also Figure 9–19.

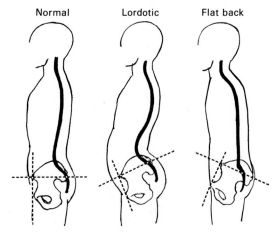

FIG. 9-23. Variations of posture. Tilting the pelvis is associated with changes in the spinal curvatures. In the normal, the line drawn across the anterior and posterior superior iliac spines lies horizontal while the pubic tubercle and the anterior superior iliac spine lie in the same vertical plane. Forward tilting of the pelvis produces lordosis, and its backward tilt flattens the normal lumbar curve.

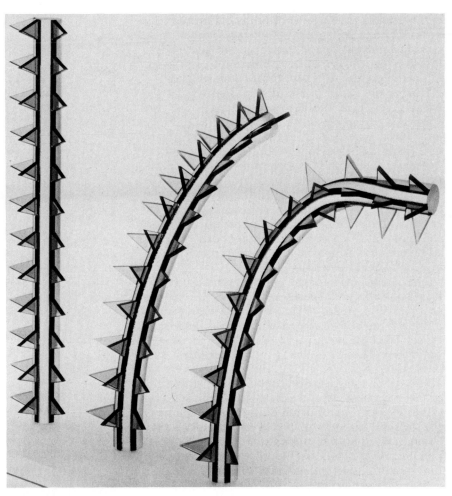

FIG. 9-24. Three models built to illustrate the composite deformity in scoliosis. Plexiglass columns have been inlayed with three black lines into which are fixed spines to correspond to the transverse and spinous processes of vertebrae. One of the columns is straight, the second is bent in one plane, mimicking the thoracic spinal curvature. If, without any twisting or rotation, the third bent column is bent once more in a plane at right angles to the plane of the primary curvature, the black lines and the spines will be caused to spiral around the column, demonstrating the obligatory, concomitant rotation. It is this second curve which accounts for the composite deformity of scoliosis. (Model constructed by Dr. WD Rubin) (Photography by Roy Hayashi)

hemivertebra or, more commonly, to growth abnormalities or collapse of a vertebral body or disk. If such abnormalities are localized, the acute angulation deformity is called a **gibbus.** However, in the majority of cases the kyphosis is generalized.

During the rapid phase of spinal growth in the preadolescent and adolescent age group, the ring epiphysis of vertebral bodies may suffer damage anteriorly, where it is less protected. The result will be wedge-shaped vertebrae because growth proceeds posteriorly at a normal pace while anteriorly it is retarded. The condition must be watched for since the deformity can be prevented by wearing an appropriate brace during the growth phase. In the older age group the most common cause of kyphosis is osteoporosis of the spine which is frequently complicated by the collapse of vertebral bodies.

The exaggeration of the normal lumbar convexity is spoken of as **lordosis.** Lordosis usually represents an adjustment of the spine in an attempt to maintain the body's center of mass over the feet. It is seen in obese people and in the later months of pregnancy. Lordosis, as a rule, develops secondarily to a thoracic kyphosis, and is an invariable sequela to hip flexion contracture, tightening, or over activity of the soleus musculature (see Chap. 19). **Any factor producing a change in one of the spinal curvatures requires compensatory changes in the other curves to maintain balance.** The degree of tilting of the pelvis even in normal individuals causes recognizable variations in posture which are reflected in the spinal curvatures (Fig. 9–23).

Lateral curves (curvatures in the coronal plane) are always abnormal curves. It is a mechanical principle that one cannot bend a column in one plane without a concomitant rotation (Fig. 9–24).

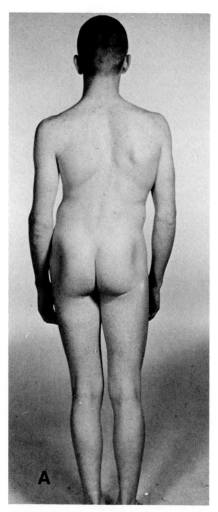

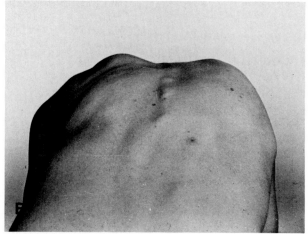

FIG. 9–25. **(A)** A scoliotic curve of the thoracic spine is evident; the curve is convex to the right. A secondary curve of the lumbar spine is also present which is convex to the left. The pelvis and gluteal folds appear symmetrical; the right shoulder is higher than the left and the gap between the arm and flank is greater on the right than on the left side. An imaginary plumb line dropped from the occiput aligns with T1 but not with the natal cleft. **(B)** When the patient bends forward the lateral curves of the spine remain visible but the asymmetry of the contour of the rib cage becomes exaggerated. The rib hump on the right obscures the scapula from view at this angle, while on the left the scapula is still visible, the curve of the rib cage being much lower than on the right.

Hence, a **lateral bending deformity of the spine must be accompanied by rotation, and this complex deformity is termed scoliosis.**

The cause may be congenital abnormality of the vertebrae such as a hemivertebra, block vertebra, or vertebral bar. Scoliosis is more frequently acquired due to a variety of abnormalities. For instance, a short leg or hip adduction contracture (Chap. 19) produces scoliosis because the pelvis must dip to that side in order for both feet to remain on the ground. Sciolosis may also be due to unilateral muscle spasm provoked by pressure on a nerve caused by a prolapsed intervertebral disk. Unilateral muscle paralysis due, for example, to poliomyelitis is still a frequent cause of scoliosis. In each case the imbalance of forces acting on the spine is responsible for the scoliosis. The most common type of scoliosis, however, is idiopathic; that is, the cause or causes cannot be determined. Idiopathic scoliosis is usually associated with rapid growth and is most prevalent in the preadolescent and the adolescent age. It can, however, occur in the very young infant or in the younger child, usually five to seven years of age. Once scoliosis has started, it will usually progress during the growth period. The degree of deterioration of the curve cannot be predicted and, therefore, once diagnosed it must be followed closely in order to prevent a serious deformity. The deformities include structural changes not only in the vertebrae but also in the ribs associated with vertebral rotation (Fig. 9–24). Severe scoliosis will alter respiratory function by diminishing the capacity of the thorax and shifting the mediastinum. It will also compromise the height of the individual.

The abnormality is best picked up by observing the disrobed patient from the back (Fig. 9–25A). As the patient bends to 90°, even a slight scoliosis can be picked up by the asymmetry of the height of the rib cage. The *rib hump* (Fig. 9–25B) is due to the displacement of the ribs by the rotation element of the scoliosis. Physical examination should include testing of the strength of the trunk musculature in extension and lateral bending. However, the physician is largely dependent on x-ray evaluation (Fig. 9–26) to determine the cause and to follow the progress of the condition.

While scoliosis is most frequently identified in the thoracic region, it may also occur at the thoracolumbar junction and in the lumbar spine. Such curves are more difficult to diagnose clinically but can be identified by careful examination of the disrobed patient. Special attention must be paid to asymmetry of the pelvis, failure of the ex-

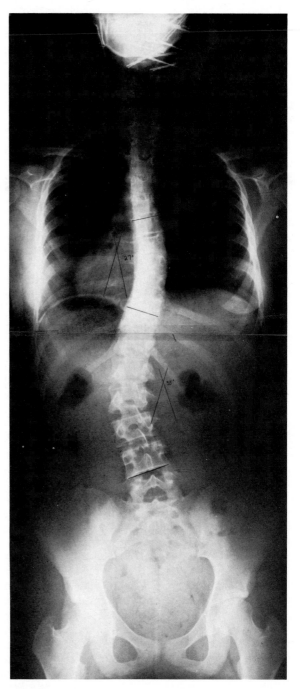

FIG. 9–26. Composite radiograph of a patient with idiopathic scoliosis. In addition to the primary curve in the thoracic spine there is a secondary compensatory curve in the lumbar region. On close examination the rotatory element of the deformity may be appreciated from the changes in the alignment of the spinous processes and of the bases of the pedicles from vertebra to vertebra.

ternal occipital protuberance and the first thoracic vertebra to line up with the natal crease along a plumb line, and to asymmetry of the erector spinae musculature in the lumbar region.

CLINICAL EVALUATION OF THE VERTEBRAL COLUMN

Because the vertebral column is so intimately associated with the spinal cord and spinal nerves, physical examination of the spine integrates evaluation of structural elements with the assessment of spinal nerves. In practice, these two components of the examination are inseparable, but in this book they have to be considered independently. This section is concerned with detecting structural deformities and testing the ranges of movement and the strength of the spinal musculature. The evaluation of certain segments of the cord and the testing of spinal nerves is deferred to Chapter 12, because it requires knowledge of the contents of the vertebral canal (Chap. 10) and the distribution of spinal nerves (Chaps. 11 and 12).

Diseases and disorders of the vertebral column manifest themselves principally with the symptoms and signs which are described below.

Symptoms

Pain. Back pain occurs in most people at one time or another. It is the principal complaint that brings patients with vertebral disorders to the doctor. It must be remembered, however, that many diseases and disorders in other organ systems may also produce back pain. It is also important to understand that approximately one half of the patients with back pain show no clear-cut physical or radiologic signs to permit an accurate diagnosis. To disguise ignorance, such patients are often said to have postural back pain, though this cannot be accepted as a disgnosis.

Back pain may vary from a mild ache to a severe lancinating type of pain. If the back pain is truly vertebral in origin, it will be aggravated by motion. Pain is usually felt several segments distal to the actual site of the lesion. This is most commonly noted in low back disease, when the patient frequently refers to pain in the buttocks and thigh.

Inability to Perform. Disability may result from pain and/or restricted motion. Determination of the character, periodicity, precise location, and radiation of pain, as well as what relieves or aggra-

vates it, is helpful in establishing a diagnosis and is an integral part of the examination.

Physical Signs

Signs of vertebral column disorders include deformity, loss of motion, tenderness on palpation and percussion, weakness, and signs of neurologic involvement of the spinal cord or spinal nerve roots. The latter are dealt with in Chapter 12.

Inspection. Posture, gait, ease and smoothness of motion should be observed as the patient enters, and also as he or she disrobes for the examination. The entire back, including shoulders and hips must be exposed. The patient is inspected from the front, back, and side views, paying attention to:

1. General posture (Fig. 9–23) and shape of the chest.
2. Soft tissue contours, localized swellings, scars, sinuses, hairy or discolored patches on the skin.
3. Symmetry in height of the shoulders and of the iliac crests (the latter confirmed by palpation); symmetry in the prominence of the scapulae, ribs, and the flanks (Fig. 9–25).
4. Cervical, thoracic, and lumbar curvatures in the back and side views.
5. Vertical alignment of the spine, using a tape measure as a plumbline, if necessary, held up to the occiput.

A deepening of the median furrow in the lumbar region is suggestive of increased lordosis. In addition to the secondary causes of lordosis, spondylolisthesis must be suspected. Thoracic scoliotic curves are best confirmed by looking for the rib hump as the patient bends forward.

Palpation and Percussion. For palpation and percussion to be informative in the clinical assessment of the spine the anatomy of palpable bony points and vertebral levels must be reviewed. The importance of this will be reinforced in Chapters 10 and 12.

PALPABLE BONY POINTS. Bony points of the vertebral column available for palpation are essentially limited to the tips of the spinous processes. In addition, the transverse processes of the atlas can be felt in the gap between the mastoid process and the angle of the jaw. The atlas has no true spinous process. Slight passive extension of the head or resting it in the supine position relieves tension in the ligamentum nuchae and provides access to the spinous process of C2–C6. The spine of C7 is the *first* prominent spinous process designating the vertebra as the *vertebra prominens,* often undeservedly, because the spine of T1 may protrude as much or more as C7. Slightly lateral to the cervical spines, ill-defined bony masses can be discerned which represent the articular processes. These may be tender when the cervical spine is affected by arthritis.

In the midthoracic region, the spinous processes overlap the body of the vertebra below, but pain over the spinous process is related to its own vertebra. In the lumbar region the spinous processes are at the level of their own bodies. The posterior surface of the sacrum, with its rudimentary spinous process, is quite superficial. The coccyx and the anterior aspect of the sacrum are best palpated by a finger inserted into the patient's rectum.

VERTEBRAL LEVELS. Counting vertebrae is accomplished with the aid of some landmarks. The anterior arch of the atlas is on level with the hard palate. Cervical and upper thoracic vertebrae can be counted with reference to the prominent processes of C7 and T1. Lower thoracic and upper lumbar spines can be identified by locating the 12th rib. The inferior angle of the scapula is usually opposite the spine of T7, and L4 vertebra is on level with the superior border of the iliac crest.

CLINICAL EVALUATION. The cervical spine is best palpated while the patient is lying comfortably supine. In this position the cervical paravertebral muscles should also be felt for tenderness and localized spasm. The sternomastoids and lymph nodes of the neck should also be palpated by sliding the hands forward.

For palpating the spinous processes below C6, the patient has to be sitting or lying prone. The latter position is advantageous in the lumbar region because it relaxes the erector spinae. Spasm in this muscle is most readily detected in the prone position. Muscle spasm is frequently unilateral and may present as a firm and tender mass. If the muscle spasm is not relaxed in this position, irritation of a nerve root should be suspected. Tenderness between spinous processes is suggestive of ligamentous tear incurred in a flexion injury.

Percussion of the spinous process is best done with the patient sitting or standing. The cervical and lumbar regions have to be flexed slightly. As emphasized previously, pain elicited by percussion is indicative of pathology within the percussed vertebra.

Estimation of Range of Movement. It is not possible clinically to measure movement between individual vertebrae, nor is it feasible to measure movement in any one region of the spine in actual degrees, although this may be done radiographically. Examination is usually limited to comparison of movements in opposite directions and to visual estimates of the range. The manner in which the movement is carried out should be smooth, with comparable ease of recovery of the erect stance. The examiner should note whether the movement is limited by pain or reflex. All movements should be performed actively by the patient.

CERVICAL SPINE.

1. Full flexion of the cervical spine and of the atlantooccipital joints should put the chin on the chest with the mouth closed (Fig. 9–27A).
2. Full extension of the same joints catches the examiner's finger between the occiput and C7, but does not trap it (Fig. 9–27B).
3. As the examiner steadies the shoulders, keeping them horizontal, each ear is approximated toward the shoulder, demonstrating the range of lateral bending. The total range between left and right side is somewhat less than 90°.
4. Rotation of the head and neck to the right and left brings the chin level with the shoulders (Fig. 9–27C) as the examiner steadies the shoulders.
5. Combined extension and rotation to one side compresses the cervical intervertebral foramina maximally and exaggerates cervical nerve root pain (Chap. 12).

It must be remembered that the range of cervical motion varies from individual to individual.

THORACOLUMBAR SPINE. Flexion, extension, and lateral bending occur mainly in the lumbar region while rotation of the trunk takes place predominantly in the thoracic spine. Limitation of flexion, extension, and rotation can be camouflaged by movement at the hip joint and this must be excluded by stabilizing the pelvis. If there is pain, flexion is the last movement to be tested.

1. Extension. Even in the erect, neutral position, the normal lumbar curvature holds the lumbosacral angle in extension. If the L5-S1 joint is damaged or diseased, further extension produces pain. The range of extension is only about 15–30° if movement at the hips is not allowed to

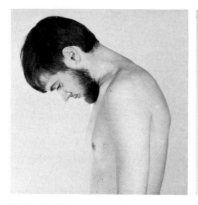 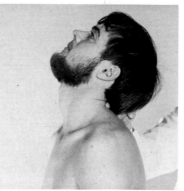 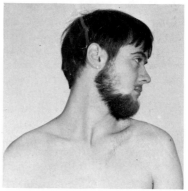

FIG. 9–27. Flexion (**A**), extension (**B**), and rotation (**C**) of the cervical spine and head. For description see text.

contribute. Extension exaggerates the normal lordotic curvature.

2. Lateral bending can be measured by asking the patient to slide the hand down the side of the thigh as far as possible. Normally, the patient can reach the head of the fibula, without flexing the hip or knee. The distance from the fingertips to the fibula is a reliable measure of the range of the lateral bend.

    If the patient complains of pain on the concave side while bending laterally, nerve root compression should be suspected. Pain on the convex side is usually related to muscle and tendon abnormalities. The etiology for both may be degenerative joint disease of the vertebral arch joints, or degeneration of the intervertebral disks (Chaps. 10 and 12).

3. Rotation. Pelvic rotation at the hips must be excluded. Therefore, the examiner standing behind the patient stabilizes the pelvis by placing a hand on the iliac crest, while the patient twists the trunk looking back at the examiner. Alternatively, the patient may be seated while the trunk is rotated. The range of movement is assessed by the change in the position of the shoulders.

4. Flexion. The patient should be asked to bend forward as far as possible with the knees extended. Normally, there should be no asymmetry in the erector spinae muscles during this process and this should be confirmed by palpating the muscle as the patient bends down. The range of motion is best recorded by placing a tape measure between T1 and a fixed point on the sacrum in the upright position, and recording the increase in the distance between these two points as full flexion is attained. This measurement is preferable to the distance between the fingertips and the floor because the contribution by hip flexion is excluded.

Estimation of Muscle Strength. The erector spinae is tested as a group, with the patient in the prone position. The patient is asked to raise the head and shoulders from the examining table. The examiner may apply resistance to the head or shoulders, testing the strength of the muscles in the cervical and thoracic regions. Contraction of the lumbar part of the muscle can also be observed during the same maneuver, or alternatively the patient may be asked to elevate the legs, hips, and the pelvis from the table. This is only possible if the hip extensors are intact. The movement achieved is minimal, but the contraction is visible and palpable.

Weakness of the erector spinae is rarely associated with pathology except in the paralytic conditions. More commonly back symptoms are related to weakness of the flexor muscles, particularly the rectus abdominis and the flank muscles. No back evaluation is complete without having the patient attempt sit ups, keeping the knees in the flexed position. Inability to do sit ups in this position signifies marked weakness of the abdominal musculature. The umbilicus should be observed during the exercise. If there is segmental weakness, the umbilicus will shift away from the direction of weakness, whereas if the weakness is generalized the umbilicus will maintain its position. The two recti may be compared by placing the hands over them while the patient is performing the sit ups.

SUGGESTED READING

Coventry, M. B. Anatomy of the intervertebral disk. Clin. Orthop. 67:9, 1969
A well-illustrated article on the normal anatomy and pathology of degenerating intervertebral disks.
Hollinshead, W. H. Anatomy for Surgeons, Vol. 3, 2nd ed. New York, Harper & Row, 1969
Chapter 2 gives a scholarly comprehensive presentation of

anatomy with extensive bibliography. An excellent source for reference.

MacConnaill, M. A., and Basmajian, J. V. Muscles and Movements. Baltimore, Williams & Wilkins, 1968
Chapter 8 deals briefly in an interesting manner with the muscles and movements of the vertebral column.

Morris, J. M. Biomechanics of the spine. Arch. Surg. *107*:418, 1973
The mechanics of vertebral movement and the various compression forces operating on the spine are illustrated with interesting examples.

Olsen, G. A., and Hamilton, A. The lateral stability of the spine. Clin. Orthop. *65*:143, 1969
An interesting account of how the spinal musculature functioning as guy ropes and trusses lends lateral stability to the spine and how failure of this mechanism leads to scoliosis.

Parke, W. W. Development of the spine. *In* Rothman, R. H., and Simeone, F. A. (eds): The Spine. Philadelphia, W. B. Saunders, 1975
A brief description of development, well illustrated with anatomical specimens and x-rays.

Ruge, D., and Wiltse, L. L. (eds): Spinal Disorders, Diagnosis and Treatment. Philadelphia, Lea & Febiger, 1977.
A multiauthor volume which, in addition to dealing with normal structure, development, deformities, congenital anomalies, tumors, infections, trauma and other disorders that affect the vertebral column, discusses diagnosis, the problem of pain, as well as operative and nonoperative management of the various disorders.

Schmorl, G., and Junghanns, H. The Human Spine in Health and Disease, 2nd ed. New York, Grune & Stratton, 1971
A classic monograph dealing with all aspects of normal and pathological anatomy as well as clinical manifestations of various disorders.

10
The Vertebral Canal and Its Contents

CORNELIUS ROSSE

The vertebral canal contains the spinal cord invested in its meninges. The roots of 32 pairs of spinal nerves issue from the cord and traverse the canal exiting through the intervertebral foramina. The vertebral canal also contains blood vessels which contribute to the supply of the spinal cord, the vertebrae, and the intervertebral joints. It is important to understand the anatomy of the vertebral canal, because function will be seriously impaired even by relatively minor lesions which compromise available space within the inexpansible canal, or within its portals of exit, the intervertebral foramina. The resulting functional loss may be complex and may manifest itself in structures anatomically removed from the spine. A diagnosis of the causative lesions will only be possible if the anatomy of the vertebral canal and of its contents is fully understood.

THE VERTEBRAL CANAL

The vertebral canal is formed by the serial superimposition of the vertebral foramina. It commences at the **foramen magnum** and terminates at the **sacral hiatus** just above the coccyx. The vertebral bodies and intervertebral disks make up the anterior wall of the canal over which the posterior longitudinal ligament is draped. Posteriorly, the laminae and ligamenta flava roof over the canal. Laterally, nerves and blood vessels leave and enter the canal through the intervertebral foramina which are separated from one another by the pedicles (see Fig. 9–1). The foramina are bounded anteriorly by vertebral body and disk and posteriorly by the articular processes and the capsule of the synovial joints (see Figs. 9–1, 9–9C, 9–12B).

THE MENINGES

The spinal cord is suspended in the vertebral canal within a triple envelope of meninges made up of the **pia, arachnoid,** and **dura mater** (Fig. 10–1). The pia is closely applied to the spinal cord, spinal nerve roots, and rootlets. Blood vessels arborize in it.

Between the dorsal and ventral row of nerve rootlets the pia extends laterally in the form of a septum which attaches at regular intervals to the arachnoid and dura. This membranous extension of the pia is the **ligamentum denticulatum,** and it suspends the cord in the subarachnoid space.

The space between pia and arachnoid, called the **subarachnoid space,** is filled by cerebrospinal fluid (CSF) which protects the cord like a water jacket. The space communicates freely with the intracranial subarachnoid space. Outermost is the dura, anchored to bone at the foramen magnum and via a narrow fibrous band, the **filum terminale,** to the coccyx. The dura is also attached in places to the posterior longitudinal ligament. Between dura and arachnoid, the potential **subdural space** contains only a film of fluid (lymph) but the **epidural space** is filled with fat in which a rich plexus of veins (vertebral venous plexus) is embedded.

The dural or thecal sac sends sleevelike projections into the intervertebral foramina (Figs. 10–1, 10–7) where the dura blends with the epineurium of the spinal nerves and with connective tissue in the foramina. The latter anchor the dural sleeves which can thus protect the nerve roots from being stretched during movements of the spine.

The dural sac and the subarachnoid space terminate in the vertebral canal at the level of S2 or S3. The sac can be punctured by a needle inserted between the lumbar spinous processes into the

147

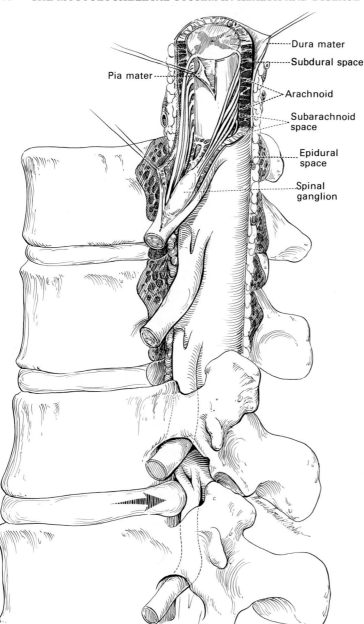

Dura mater

Subdural space

Pia mater

Arachnoid

Subarachnoid space

Epidural space

Spinal ganglion

FIG. 10–1. The contents of the vertebral canal. The spinal cord is illustrated with its meninges and associated spaces. Note the rootlets of spinal nerves as they form dorsal and ventral roots per segment. A fusiform ganglion is present on the dorsal root. A dural sleeve invests the roots and the ganglion as far as the intervertebral foramen. The subarachnoid space is interlaced by delicate strands of the arachnoid and is filled by CSF. The disk between L1 and L2 vertebrae is prolapsed and compresses the roots of L2 nerve.

median gap that exists between the ligamenta flava. Such a **lumbar puncture** is performed for measuring intrathecal pressure, for sampling the cerebrospinal fluid, or for delivering drugs or radiologic contrast media into the subarachnoid space (Fig. 10–7).

A rise in intrathoracic and intraabdominal pressure is freely transmitted into the vertebral canal via the free communication of the vertebral venous plexus with veins of the thoracic and abdominal cavity. Intracranial pressure will also be increased via the jugular veins. Forceful expiration against a closed glottis (Valsalva maneuver) as occurs during straining or coughing causes a rise in CSF pressure and may induce or exaggerate pain due to lesions that increase tension in the vertebral canal. Similarly, temporary compression of the jugular veins leads to increase in intracranial pressure which is transmitted to CSF in the spinal subarachnoid space (Queckenstedt maneuver) if there is no obstruction in the foramen magnum or in the vertebral canal.

THE SPINAL CORD

The spinal cord is the continuation of the medulla oblongata. The diameter of the cord is small compared to the diameter of the vertebral canal. Its circumference is enlarged in two regions from which the upper and lower limbs are supplied. These are the **cervical** and **lumbar enlargements.** At its distal end, the cord tapers to the **conus medullaris** and continues as the nonneural **filum terminale** with which the dura mater blends.

The division of the cord into symmetrical right and left halves is suggested on its surface by two longitudinal grooves, the **anterior median sulcus** and **posterior median fissure.** There are no signs of segmentation on the surface of the cord. The dorsal and ventral rootlets of spinal nerves emerge along uninterrupted longitudinal rows on the posterolateral and anterolateral surfaces and are subsequently gathered on each side into a single dorsal and ventral root per segment (Fig. 10–1).

The spinal cord is shorter than either the vertebral canal or the dural sac. In the adult, its lower end is most commonly found at the lower level of the first lumbar vertebra, while in the newborn it may reach to L3. However, by two months of age it attains its adult level. This results from a faster rate of growth of the vertebral column than of the cord. Consequently, the segments of the spinal cord do not lie opposite the corresponding verte-

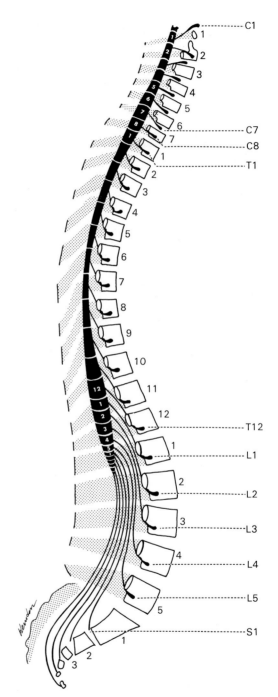

FIG. 10-2. A schematic representation of the relationship of spinal cord segments and spinal nerves to the vertebrae. (Based on Haymaker W, Woodhall B: Peripheral Nerve Injuries. Philadelphia, WB Saunders, 1967)

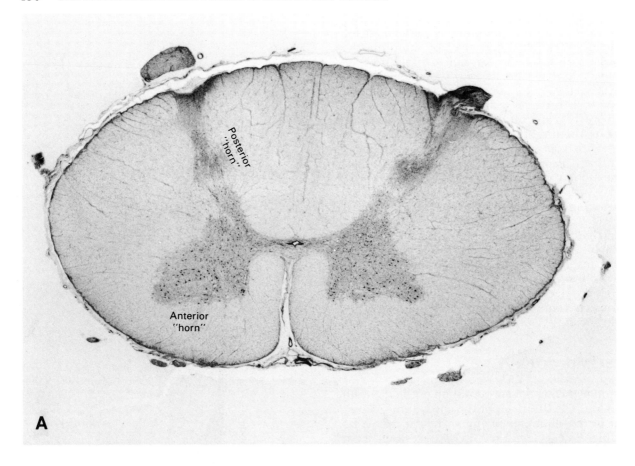

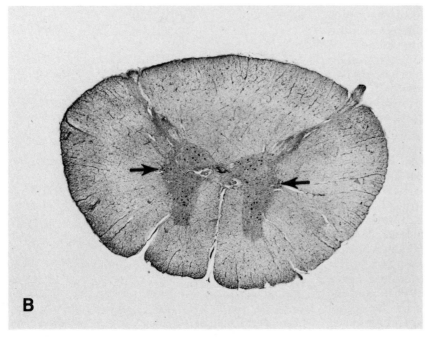

FIG. 10-3. Photomicrographs of transverse sections of the spinal cord stained with cresyl violet. (× 10) **(A)** Cervical enlargement. **(B)** Midthoracic region. The lateral horn is indicated by arrows. Compare the size of the anterior columns of grey matter in **A** and **B.** At this magnification the neurons are visible as black dots. (Everett NB: Functional Neuroanatomy, 6th ed. Philadelphia, Lea & Febiger, 1971)

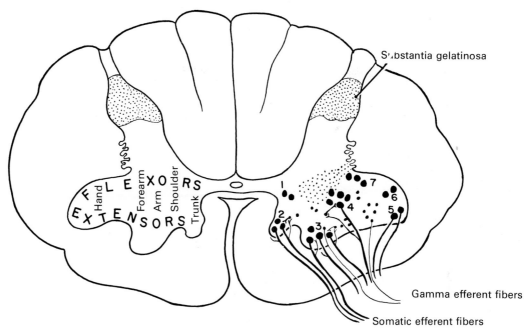

FIG. 10-4. A diagram of the groups of motor neurons in the anterior grey column of the cervical enlargement. On the left is shown the general location of anterior horn cells that send motor axons to specific muscle groups of the upper limbs. Individual motor nuclei are designated by numbers on the right. Neurons and axons of gamma efferents are smaller than those of alpha efferents. (Truex RC, Carpenter MB: Strong and Elwyn's Human Neuroanatomy, 5th ed. Baltimore, Williams & Wilkins, 1964)

brae (Fig. 10–2). This is an important point to appreciate in cases of cord compression associated with spinal lesions and injuries.

As a general rule, the tip of the spine of a cervical vertebra corresponds to the level of the succeeding cord segment (C6 spine opposite C7 segment); the difference is two segments in the upper thoracic region and three segments in the lower thoracic region with reference to the tips of the spinous processes (tip of T10 spine opposite L1 segment). Lumbar and sacral segments are telescoped in the canal of T11 and T12 and L1 vertebrae. T12 spine is opposite S1 segment.

Internal Structure

The **central canal,** barely visible to the naked eye, runs down along the length of the spinal cord as the distal continuation of the ventricles of the brain (Fig. 10–3). Around this canal are aggregated in more or less well defined groups all neurons of the spinal cord, while more peripherally the substance of the cord is made up exclusively of nerve fibers. Therefore, on a transverse section, **white matter**

representing the myelinated fibers surrounds the central core of **grey matter,** which contains the neurons.

The grouping of neurons is such that in cross-sectional profile the grey matter is roughly H-shaped, presenting two anterior and two posterior *horns,* which correspond to the **anterior** and **posterior columns** of grey matter. Somatic motor neurons giving rise to both alpha and gamma efferents are located in the anterior grey column, and some degree of functional localization has been demonstrated among the groups (Fig. 10–4). The anterior horn in the cervical and lumbar enlargements is augmented laterally by groups of neurons concerned with the supply of the limbs (Fig. 10–3A). Neurons of the posterior grey column receive and relay incoming impulses. In segments T2-L1 an additional group of neurons forms the **lateral column** of grey matter (lateral horn or intermediolateral cell column, Fig. 10–3B). These are preganglionic sympathetic neurons and they furnish the sympathetic nerve supply to the entire body, including the limbs. A similar cell column in segments S2-S4 contains preganglionic parasym-

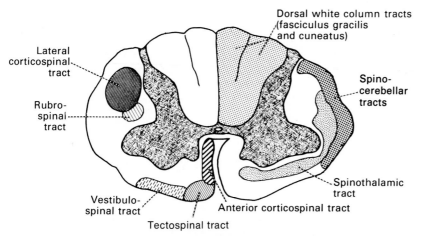

FIG. 10-5. A simplified diagram of the main tracts in the white matter in the spinal cord. The ascending tracts are shown on the right side of the figure and the descending tracts on the left. (Adapted from Warnick R, Williams PL (eds): Gray's Anatomy, 35th ed. Philadelphia, WB Saunders, 1973)

pathetic neurons which, as far as it is known, are concerned exclusively with the innervation of viscera.

The white matter of the cord contains ascending and descending nerve fiber tracts, the more important of which are identified in Figure 10-5. Most of these have been discussed in Chapter 4.

THE NERVE ROOTS

The ventral and dorsal **roots** of spinal nerves gathered from their respective **rootlets** proceed independently toward their respective intervertebral foramina traversing the subarachnoid space within the dural sac and dural sleeves. The **spinal nerve** is formed by the union of the dorsal and ventral roots in the intervertebral foramen (Figs. 10-1, 12-2).

In spite of the malalignment of the segments and vertebrae, the spinal nerves themselves emerge through the intervertebral foramen above or below their corresponding vertebrae. C1 to C7 spinal nerves leave the vertebral canal above the pedicles of the corresponding vertebrae, but since there are only seven cervical vertebrae, C8 passes below the pedicle of C7. From T1 distally, the spinal nerves leave the vertebral canal by passing below the pedicle of their respective vertebrae (Fig. 10-2). The intradural course of the nerve roots is oblique and increases greatly from cervical to sacral segments. Below L1 vertebra, the bundle of nerve roots resembles a horse's tail as the roots pass toward their respective intervertebral foramina. These roots are collectively called the **cauda equina** (Fig. 10-6).

The **spinal ganglion** is a fusiform enlargement on the dorsal root just proximal to the point of union with the ventral root (Figs. 10-1, 12-2). In the ganglion are located the cell bodies of all sensory nerve fibers contained in a spinal nerve. The ganglia are situated in the intervertebral foramina. Those of sacral roots are within the sacral canal. In all presacral regions, the first division of the spinal nerve takes place in the intervertebral foramen. The resulting branches are the **dorsal and ventral rami** (see Fig. 12-2).

Sacral spinal nerves divide in the sacral canal, and ventral and dorsal rami emerge through the anterior and posterior sacral foramina. In presacral regions the dorsal rami pass posteriorly, skirting the articular processes, while the ventral rami proceed laterally to supply the body wall and the limbs.

In cervical intervertebral foramina the spinal nerve is directly related anteriorly to the intervertebral disk, but in the thoracic and lumbar regions the disk is not in contact with the nerve (Fig. 10-1). The nerves hook around the inferior border of the pedicles and are related anteriorly to the vertebral body. In the lumbar vertebral canal, the nerve roots enclosed in their dural sleeves cross the disk proximal to the pedicle below which they exit (Fig.

10–1). Therefore, herniation of cervical intervertebral disks into the intervertebral foramina directly compresses the exiting nerve (Fig. 10–7A), while disk protrusion in the lumbar region stretches the nerve roots that cross the disk in the vertebral canal (Figs. 10–1, 10–7B,C). Because cervical nerves pass above, and lumbar nerves below their own pedicles, in both regions the nerve roots affected by a disk bear the number of the vertebra placed just inferior to the disk. For instance, a disk lesion between C4 and C5 vertebrae will affect C5 nerve, and a disk protrusion between L1 and L2 vertebrae will stretch the roots of L2.

Space occupying lesions within the canal, or irregularities in its walls (e.g., intervertebral disk prolapse) may be demonstrated radiographically by instilling radiopaque contrast material into the subarachnoid space. Such **myelograms** are shown in Figure 10–7.

INTERVERTEBRAL DISK SYNDROME

Degeneration of intervertebral disks is a common cause of back pain and disability. The degeneration may or may not be complicated by prolapse or herniation of the disk. In most cases the disk herniates posterolaterally, compressing the spinal nerve or its roots in the intervertebral foramen. A large prolapse may compress the spinal cord. The clinical syndrome is described briefly because it illustrates the diagnostic importance of understanding anatomic relationships within the vertebral canal.

Etiology. Physical, biochemical, and histologic changes occur in intervertebral disks with aging (see p. 122). Beyond the third decade the disks have a reduced ability for imbibing water, their collagen content increases while proteoglycans diminish. The regularity of the collagen fiber architecture in the annulus becomes deranged, and signs of cavitation and desiccation appear in the nucleus pulposus. However, these universal changes do not invariably manifest themselves in disease, though inevitably they predispose to it.

The etiology of intervertebral disk degeneration and prolapse is unknown. Heredity, trauma, and poor nutrition of the disk resulting from reduced mobility of the spine may all play a role.

Pathogenesis. As the disk degenerates it narrows and thereby disturbs the mechanics of the back. The vertebral arch joints settle and have to bear an

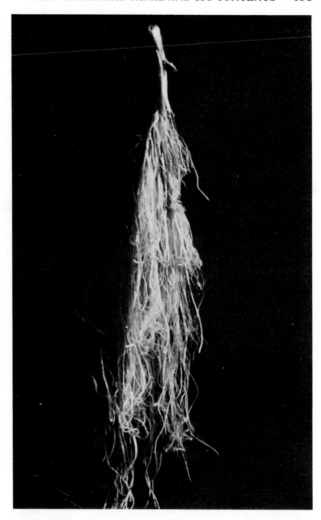

FIG. 10–6. The human cauda equina. The specimen was prepared by John Hunter. (Courtesy of the Hunterian Museum, Royal College of Surgeons, London)

increased amount of weight, requiring adaptive changes in the capsule and ligaments. All these changes may be associated with back pain. Once the disk undergoes degenerative changes, it is subject to prolapse. When an intervertebral disk prolapses, part of the nucleus pulposus, annulus fibrosus, and the hyaline cartilage plate protrude beyond their normal confines. These tissues may herniate in any direction, and they stretch and tear other tissues barring their way. This, in itself, generates pain because the posterior longitudinal ligament and the annulus fibrosus itself are innervated. However, the prolapse attains particular clinical significance when the displacement is pos-

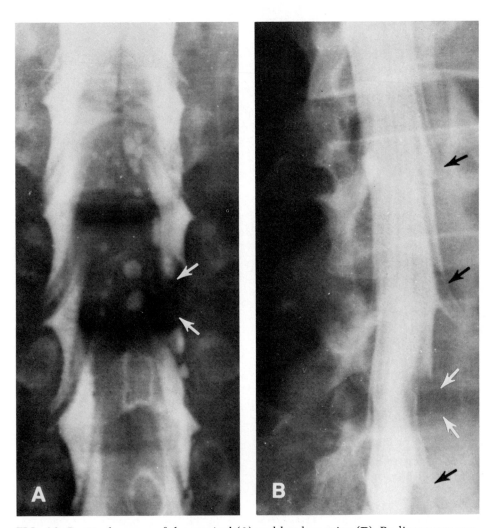

FIG. 10-7. Myelograms of the cervical **(A)** and lumbar spine **(B).** Radioopaque contrast medium has been injected into the subarachnoid space via a lumbar puncture. The table was then tilted allowing the contrast medium to flow to the area of diagnostic interest before x-rays were taken. **(A)** Contrast medium fills the subarachnoid space on each side of the cervical spinal cord (which is radiolucent) and some drops of the medium are superimposed over the cord. The dorsal and ventral roots are discernible as radiolucent strands as they pass toward the intervertebral foramina within the lateral extensions of the subarachnoid space in the dural sleeves. The regularity of the scalloped pattern along the lateral edge of the thecal sac is distorted by a radiolucent lesion **(arrows)** situated between C4-C5 vertebrae. The patient, a 19-year-old college student, injured his neck rupturing C4-C5 disk during wrestling. In addition to neck pain, he had symptoms and signs in his upper limb attributable to compression of C5 nerve. **(B)** A slightly oblique view of the lumbar spine in a 35-year-old male. The thecal sac is filled by contrast medium in which the spinal nerve roots of the cauda equina can be discerned. L3, L4, and S1 dural sleeves are clearly identifiable **(black arrows),** but the sleeve around L5 is obliterated by a radiolucent lesion **(white arrows)** which represents herniation of L5-S1 disk. The patient experienced severe back pain on straightening up from a bent position and had a positive straight-leg-raising sign on the left. (Courtesy of Dr. Rosalind H. Troupin)

terior or posterolateral and impinges upon the spinal cord, cauda equina, or as it happens most frequently, on the nerve roots.

Incidence.   Prolapse occurs most frequently in the lumbar region, less so in the cervical spine, and rarely in the thoracic spine. It may occur at any age, but the incidence is maximal in the 30 to 50 age group. There is a slightly higher incidence in the male than in the female.

Clinical Picture.   The dominant symptom is pain, the onset of which can often be related to some minor trauma. A jarring or twisting strain sustained in the neck or lower back is followed by agonizing pain, precipitated, often a few hours or days later, by twisting, bending, or coughing. The neck or the lower back become stiff, and pain severely limits movement, but usually not in all directions. Some time later the pain may radiate into the arm or leg depending on the location of the lesions. The pain is aggravated by coughing, sneezing, or straining. Tingling and numbness may develop in dermatomal regions of the affected limb (see Chap. 12). Such acute attacks may subside with rest but will recur intermittently unless the lesion is allowed to heal completely or is removed.

During an acute attack examination reveals that spinal motion is limited, the patient's movements are hesitant and guarded, and the affected region of the spine is splinted by muscle spasm. The cervical spine is usually held in some degree of lateral flexion, whereas in the lumbar spine the normal curvature is obliterated, and this flattening of the back is associated with scoliosis or some lateral bend (listing). There is visible and palpable spasm in the erector spinae.

Localized tenderness may be detected over the erector spinae, and in an acute attack pressure over the vertebral spines adjacent to the damaged disk may also be painful. There is no limitation of joint movement in the limbs (except in the straight-leg-raising test), nor is there any tenderness even if pain radiates into the limb.

There are valuable clinical maneuvers which test increased intrathecal pressure and tension of the nerve roots. Intrathecal pressure may be increased by the Valsalva maneuver or by compression of the jugular veins for 10 sec. or so. Exaggeration of symptoms by either test is indicative of increased tension in an intrathecal structure. Compression of the cervical spine by pressing down on the head exaggerates the pain due to nerve root compression in cervical intervertebral

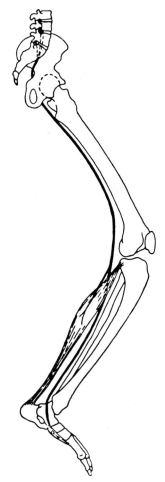

FIG. 10-8.   The course of the sciatic nerve, explaining why the straight-leg-raising test increases the tension in the nerve roots of the sacral plexus. The nerve is anchored at the vertebral column and below the knee joint. It is put on tension when the hip is flexed while the knee is kept extended. The tension is further increased by dorsiflexion of the foot. (Cram RH: J Bone Joint Surg. 35-B:192, 1953)

foramina, whereas traction applied to the head tends to relieve the cervical symptoms.

The dural sleeves anchored in the intervertebral foramina may be stretched by asking the patient to raise the head and shoulders from the supine position, and then flex the head, pressing the chin or the chest with the help of his own arms or with those of the examiner. This maneuver pulls the thecal sac upward in the vertebral canal and exaggerates the pain due to a taut nerve root.

For testing disk herniation in the lumbar spine, the most useful diagnostic maneuver is the

straight-leg-raising test. Figure 10–8 illustrates the anatomic mechanism by which tension is transmitted to spinal nerves L4, L5, and S1 through pulling indirectly on the sciatic nerve.

While the patient is lying supine, the leg on the affected side is raised passively by the examiner, keeping the knee fully extended. The range of hip flexion will be limited by pain felt in the back which may radiate into the leg. The smaller the angle of hip flexion obtained, the more tension there is on the affected nerve root. If the leg is lowered below the point where pain was experienced, passive dorsiflexion of the foot will elicit the pain again, because this movement also pulls on the sciatic nerve.

In cases of severe nerve entrapment, raising the opposite leg may also be painful because the thecal sac is being pulled over toward the side of the raised leg. However, the pain in this case is experienced on the side of the leg which is resting on the table; that is, on the side of the disk herniation.

If it is suspected that the patient is malingering, the straight-leg-raising test should be repeated actively. While the patient is trying to raise the leg on the side of the suspected lesion, the examiner supports the opposite heel in the cup of his hand just above the table. If the patient is really trying, the heel of the sound leg will press down firmly into the examiner's palm.

Herniation of the disks between L1 and L5 vertebrae may be tested by increasing the tension in L2-L4 spinal nerve roots. This can be activated by stretching the femoral nerve which enters the thigh over the anterior aspect of the hip. The maneuver is the mirror image of the sciatic nerve stretch. The hip is passively extended while the patient is lying prone or on his side.

A dermatomal pattern of pain distribution is characteristic for each intervertebral disk lesion. Muscle weakness and atrophy also conform to the segmental pattern of spinal nerve distribution in the limbs. These patterns are explained in Chapter 12 which also deals with their clinical evaluation. A neurologic examination that includes testing of cutaneous sensation in dermatomes, muscle strength, and atrophy, as well as deep tendon reflexes is mandatory in all cases where nerve root or spinal cord involvement is suspected.

The cervical spinal cord may be compressed by a large disk prolapse. Such lesions may interfere with the blood supply of the cord, or may compress some of the descending and ascending tracts, particularly in the anterior white columns. The neurologic picture may be complex. It may include weakness and incoordination in the legs, wide-based, jerky gait and paresthesias.

Confirmatory Investigations. Plain x-rays of the spine are usually uninformative unless advanced disk degeneration has narrowed the intervertebral spaces. Myelography (Fig. 10–7) is carried out only if special indications call for it. The cerebrospinal fluid is usually normal, although there may be some increase in protein.

Management. Rest is prescribed in the acute stage in order to allow the inflammatory reaction accompanying the prolapse to subside. In cervical lesions a suitably fitted soft collar immobilizes and supports the neck. For lumbar lesions bed rest for up to two weeks on a firm mattress is the treatment of choice. Analgesics and muscle relaxants are also helpful. As pain subsides, gentle, graded muscle exercises must be instituted. An exercise program is the cornerstone of management which is designed to improve nutrition of the avascular disk and to increase the efficiency of spine flexors. The long range aim of the program is to improve standing and sitting posture and to decrease lumbar lordosis. If the patient fails to respond to these measures, surgical excision of the prolapsed disk is required.

VASCULATURE AND INNERVATION

The clinical importance of blood vessels associated with the vertebral canal is two fold: 1) They provide for the nutrition of neural tissues and the vertebrae. 2) They furnish the route of access for bacteria and infective and neoplastic emboli to the cancellous bone of vertebrae. In addition to the arteries and venous plexuses, this section also deals with the sensory nerves which supply the intervertebral joints and their ligaments, the meninges, epidural tissues, bone, and the periosteum. These nerves have already been mentioned in connection with the intervertebral disk syndrome.

Arteries

Two major groups of arteries enter the vertebral canal: 1) **anterior** and **posterior spinal arteries** which descend on the surface of the spinal cord from the posterior cranial fossa through the foramen magnum, 2) **spinal branches** of the segmental arteries, or their equivalents, which enter the canal through each intervertebral foramen.

Blood Supply of the Spinal Cord. The anterior spinal artery lies in the anterior median sulcus, and its central branches supply two-thirds of the cross-sectional area of the cord. Since no arterial anastomosis takes place in the substance of the cord, compression of a segment of the anterior spinal artery has serious consequences. The smaller, posterior spinal arteries run bilaterally along the attachments of the dorsal rootlets to the cord. All these longitudinal arterial channels are reinforced segmentally by **radicular branches,** which reach the cord along the dorsal and ventral roots. The radicular arteries are given off by the spinal branch of the segmental artery (Fig. 10–9) in each intervertebral foramen. In fact, the blood supply of the lower two-thirds of the cord depends entirely on this segmental input. In the lower cervical and upper thoracic regions several of the radicular arteries may be quite large. The largest radicular artery *(arteria radicularis magna)* is unilateral and, though variable in position, is found most often at L1 (Figs. 10–9, 10–10). It ascends, feeding into the anterior spinal artery, and supplies the lower part of the cord.

Blood Supply of the Vertebrae. In the T2-L5 regions, spinal branches arise from the segmental intercostal or lumbar arteries (Figs. 10–9, 10–10). In the cervical and sacral regions these segmental vessels have fused into vertical arterial channels (vertebral, deep cervical, and lateral sacral arteries) which dispatch spinal branches segmentally into the vertebral canal. The segmental spinal arteries entering the intervertebral foramen supply the dura and epidural tissues, give off the radicular arteries, and also a branch that penetrates the posterior aspect of the vertebral bodies. This branch supplies the spongy bone and its marrow, as well as the peripheral layers of the annulus fibrosus. No arterial branches enter the intervertebral disk, the metabolic turnover of which depends on diffusion to and from the vertebral body across the hyaline cartilage plate. The blood supply of the vertebral body is supplemented by branches of the segmental artery, which enter the bone on its anterior aspect (Fig. 10–9).

The Vertebral Venous Plexuses

Venous blood from the vertebrae and from the spinal cord is collected into irregular sinuses in the

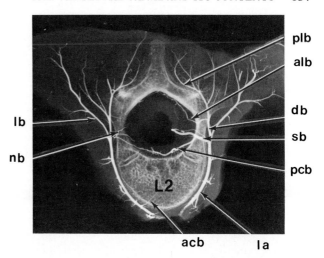

FIG. 10–9. Radiograph of an anatomic specimen in which the arteries in the lumbar region have been injected with a radioopaque substance. The segmental artery (in this instance a pair of lumbar arteries, 1a) divides in front of the transverse process into lateral (1b) and dorsal (db) branches. From the point of division or from the dorsal branch, the spinal branches (sb) enter the vertebral canal through the intervertebral foramen. One of these on the right side is the **arteria radicularis magna** (sb). Visible are also smaller radicular arteries (nb) and the anastomosing branches on the posterior aspect of the vertebral body (pcb). Small branches enter the vertebra anteriorly from the lumbar artery (acb). The dorsal branch distributes to the vertebral canal (alb) and to bone and soft tissues of the back (plb). (Parke WW, chap 2 in Rothman RH, Simeone FA (eds): The Spine. Philadelphia, WB Saunders, 1975)

epidural space, which form cross-connected, ladderlike venous channels, a pair of which runs along the posterior aspect of the vertebral bodies, and another pair is apposed to the laminae. The largest tributaries of this **internal vertebral venous plexus** are the **basivertebral veins,** which issue from a large foramen on the posterior aspect of each vertebral body. Each basivertebral vein empties into a cross connection between the two anterior vertical venous channels.

Through the intervertebral foramina the internal vertebral venous plexus connects with the **external vertebral venous plexus,** which is smaller but resembles in its arrangement the internal plexus. The plexuses drain into the caval and azygos systems via their connections with the intercostal and lumbar veins. They also communicate freely with veins of the pelvis and in the neck with the deep cervical and jugular veins.

The spacious, thin-walled irregular sinuses of

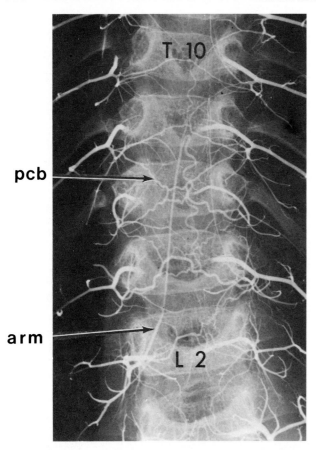

FIG. 10-10. An anatomic preparation of the lower thoracic and upper lumbar regions of the spine in a 6-year-old child. On this x-ray the injected spinal branches of the segmental arteries are visualized. Note the interlocking anastomotic pattern in the vertebral canal over the posterior aspect of the vertebral bodies (pcb), and especially the straight ascending *arteria reticularis magna* (arm), arising in this specimen from L2 on the right side. (Parke WW, chap. 2, in Rothman RH, Simeone FA (eds): The Spine. Philadelphia, WB Saunders, 1975)

traabdominal pressure, which is freely transmitted via the valveless connections of the vertebral veins (see p. 149). A notable exception to the lack of valves are the small radicular veins, in which small valves prevent venous congestion of the spinal cord when the internal vertebral venous plexus becomes engorged.

Because of the unimpeded, copious, to and fro flow of blood in the vertebral venous plexuses, septic and neoplastic emboli from pelvic, abdominal, and other organs readily sequester to venous sinusoids in the bone marrow of the vertebrae, or even up into the cranial cavity. Neoplasms of the

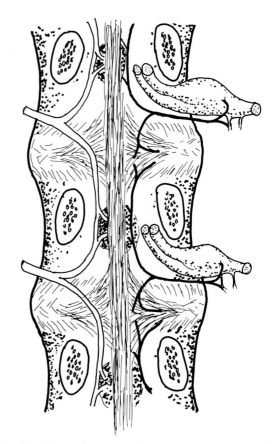

FIG. 10-11. A drawing of the posterior aspect of the vertebral bodies with the pedicles cut and removed. The posterior longitudinal ligament is shown in the center and on the right the origin, course, and distribution of the sinuvertebral nerves **(black).** Periosteal and meningeal branches have been omitted. The left side shows the distribution of spinal arteries to the vertebrae **(white).** (Parke WW, in Rothman RH, Simeone FA (eds): The Spine. Philadelphia, WB Saunders, 1975)

the internal vertebral plexus can accommodate considerable volumes of blood, and provide an alternative route for venous return to the caval and azygos systems in cases of venous obstruction in the body cavities or in the neck. Blood can flow freely up or down in the plexuses because they are devoid of valves. The distended veins function in the vertebral canal as a water jacket around the thecal sac, and the fluctuations of venous pressure are transmitted to the CSF. This fluctuation is brought about by changes in intrathoracic and in-prostate, lung, breast, thyroid, and kidney metastasize to the vertebrae via these venous channels.

Innervation of the Spine

A recurrent meningeal branch is given off by each spinal nerve as soon as it is formed in the intervertebral foramen. This branch, known also as the **sinuvertebral nerve** reenters the vertebral canal (Fig. 10–11), and carries with it sensory as well as sympathetic fibers. Each nerve divides into ascending and descending branches and supplies the periosteum, the posterior longitudinal ligament, and the outer laminae of the annulus fibrous over at least two adjacent vertebrae. No nerve fibers enter the deeper layers of the annulus nor the nucleus pulposus. Due to the overlapping territories of distribution, pain induced by a herniating disk is mediated by more than one sinuvertebral nerve. The sinuvertebral nerves are sensory also to the meninges and to the walls of the vertebral venous plexuses.

Proprioceptive and pain sensation from the vertebral arch joints are mediated by branches of the dorsal ramus of each spinal nerve (see Fig. 12–2) as the ramus courses dorsally around the articular processes. Thus in case of a prolapsed disk there may be three different sources of pain: 1) ruptured annulus, torn posterior longitudinal ligament and periosteum, innervated by sinuvertebral nerves of at least two segments; 2) compression of the spinal nerve or its roots; 3) both vertebral arch joints, innervated by dorsal rami, may become painful because of their disturbed mechanics.

SUGGESTED READING

Armstrong, J. R. Lumbar Disc Lesions, 3rd ed. Baltimore, Williams & Wilkins, 1965
A comprehensive monograph which treats normal structure and function quite extensively. The pathogenesis, clinical picture and treatment of disk disease are instructively described.

Batson, O. V. The function of the vertebral veins and their role in the spread of metastases. Am. J. Surg. *112*:138, 1940
A classical study of the vertebral venous plexus.

Everett, N. B. Functional Neuroanatomy, 6th ed. Philadelphia, Lea & Febiger, 1971
Chapter 4 presents a clear description of the anatomy of the spinal cord.

Parke, W. W. Applied anatomy of the spine. In Rothman, R. H., and Simeone, F. A. (eds): The Spine, Philadelphia, W. B. Saunders, 1975
A well-written, well-illustrated, concise account, paying special attention to vasculature and nerve supply.

Pedersen, H. E., Blunck, C. F. J., and Gardner, E. The anatomy of lumbosacral posterior rami and meningeal branches of spinal nerves (sinu-vertebral nerves). J. Bone Joint Surg. [A] *38*:377, 1956
A detailed anatomical study of the innervation of structures in the vertebral canal and of the vertebral arch joints.

Rothman, R. J., and Simeone, F. A. Lumbar disc disease. In Rothman, R. H. and Simeone, F. A., (eds): The Spine. Philadelphia, W. B. Saunders, 1975, p. 443
This paper deals with the pathogenesis, clinical picture, differential diagnosis and treatment of intervertebral disk lesions.

Simeone, F. A., and Rothman, R. H. Cervical disc disease. In Rothman, R. H. and Simeone, F. A., (eds): The Spine, Philadelphia, W. B. Saunders, 1975, p. 387
This paper deals with the pathogenesis, clinical picture, differential diagnosis and treatment of intervertebral disk lesions.

11
Basic Structural Plan and Functional Adaptations in the Limbs

CORNELIUS ROSSE

The upper and lower limbs are distinguished by some striking morphologic and functional differences, yet both pairs of limbs are built essentially on the same basic plan. The understanding of this plan simplifies the learning of limb anatomy and provides the key for the appreciation of anatomic adaptations that subserve the functions unique to each limb. The upper limb of man has evolved to explore as large a space as possible in which the hand can be positioned as a sensory and effector organ capable of performing innumerable complex, manipulative tasks. In comparison, freedom of movement is restricted in the lower limbs. Their robust construction ideally serves the support of the erect trunk while giving resilience and power to the bipedal pattern of locomotion. When the normal anatomy of limbs becomes deranged, treatment has to aim for restoring these respective functions.

SKELETON AND JOINTS

The bones of the limbs constitute the appendicular skeleton. The **pectoral** and **pelvic girdles** unite the free parts of the limbs to the axial skeleton. Each girdle consists of three bony elements which are differently modified in the two limbs. In the pectoral girdle bony fusion unites the coracoid to the scapula, but only ligaments append the coracoid to the clavicle (Fig. 11–1A). All three bones of the pelvic girdle have fused into a single bone; the **ilium, ischium,** and **pubis** constitute the **hip bone (os coxae)** (Fig. 11–2A). In both girdles, the area of bony union presents a socket which receives the head of the humerus or femur. Both joints are synovial of the ball and socket variety.

The pectoral girdle articulates with the axial skeleton only at the medial end of the clavicle (Fig. 11–1B). This **sternoclavicular joint** allows a free range of movement for the clavicle, greatly enhancing the mobility of the scapula which can slide freely around the rib cage. There is no direct connection with the vertebral column. By contrast, the articulation of the pelvic girdle with the sacrum is massive. The **sacroiliac joints** securely unite the pelvic girdle to the spine and the girdle is further strengthened by a symphysis between the pubes (Fig. 11–2B). The direct connection between the corresponding bones of the pectoral girdle is represented by a functionally relatively unimportant interclavicular ligament. The length and free mobility of the clavicle are the chief factors responsible for extending the operational sphere of the upper limb above the head.

The proximal segment of the free portion of the limb is built around a single bone represented by the **humerus** or **femur,** while there are two bones in the intermediate segment of each limb. In the intermediate segment, the respective **preaxial bones** are the **radius** and **tibia,** and the respective **postaxial bones** are the **ulna** and **fibula** (Fig. 11–3A). The hinge joint between proximal and intermediate segments involves all three bones at the elbow, whereas at the knee, in man, the postaxial bone has receded from the articulation (Fig. 11–4A).

The lower limb has rotated and extended during its development (Figs. 11–3B,C; 11–4A) which resulted in important adaptations to bearing weight:

161

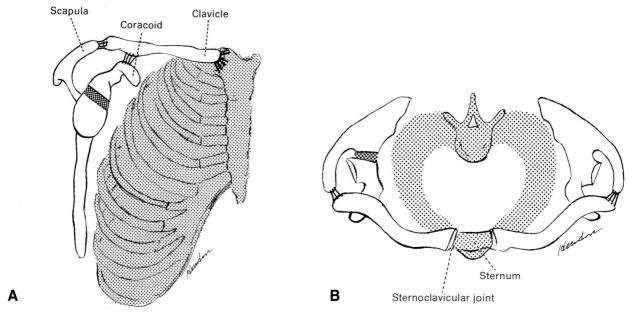

FIG. 11-1. Schematic representation of the bones of the pectoral girdle, shown in white, and their relation to the axial skeleton (stippled). **(A)** The coracoid is united by cartilage to the scapula in the glenoid fossa. This union is ossified by birth. Ligaments secure the clavicle to the other two bones of the girdle. **(B)** Direct connection between the pectoral girdle and the axial skeleton is restricted to the insubstantial sternoclavicular joints.

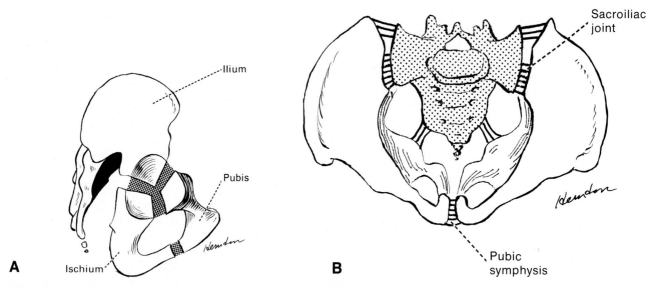

FIG. 11-2. Schematic representation of the bones of the pelvic girdle. **(A)** Ilium, ischium, and pubis are united to one another by cartilage in the acetabulum. The cartilage ossifies at puberty. **(B)** The pelvic girdle is united to the axial skeleton by the robust sacroiliac joints, and the two hip bones are fixed to one another by the pubic symphysis.

FIG. 11-3. Development of the limbs. **(A)** The axis of the limb buds is defined by the single bone primordium in the proximal segment (stippled). Cranial to this axis is the preaxial border of the limb and caudal to it is the postaxial border. In the intermediate segment of each limb the preaxial bone is shown black and the postaxial bone white. **(B)** Frontal view of the same stage of development. **(C)** Before the limbs are extended the position of preaxial and postaxial bones is symmetrical in the upper and lower limbs. Figure 11-4A shows the outcome of extension and also medial rotation in the lower limb. (Based on O'Rahilly R, Gardner E: Anat Embryol 148:1, 1975)

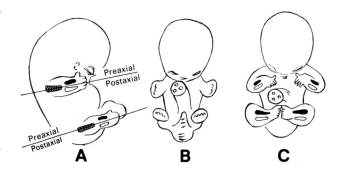

1. The limbs have been brought in line with the long axis of the body.
2. The preaxial border of the limb has turned medially.
3. The extensor surface of the limb has turned anteriorly.

Therefore, the plantar surfaces of the feet have been brought in contact with the ground. The upper limb of man can assume a similar position, but in order to place the palm of the hand on the ground, the radius has to cross over the ulna, placing the distal end of the preaxial bone medially (Fig. 11-4B). The developmental rotation of the lower limb achieves this position without crossing the tibia over the fibula and these bones cannot move in relation to one another. Their fixed relationship stabilizes the ankle joint. The movements of the radius in relation to the ulna in pronation and supination are unique to the upper limb. They provide an additional dimension for hand movements which is essential for a fully functional hand.

Both the hand and the foot are built on a primitive **pentadactylar** pattern, but the human foot has become more highly specialized than the hand. The **carpal** and **tarsal** bones contain the homologues of the primitive pentadactylar limb, but different elements have become fused in car-

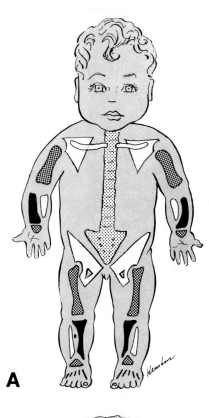

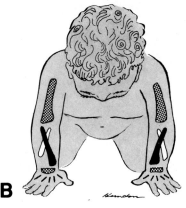

FIG. 11-4. **(A)** Extension and medial rotation of the lower limb has placed the preaxial border and preaxial bone medially while in the upper limb the preaxial border became lateral. **(B)** Placing the preaxial border medially in the upper limb requires crossing of the two bones in the intermediate segment (pronation).

pus and tarsus. At the wrist the postaxial bone has withdrawn from the articulation with the carpus, whereas at the ankle both bones articulate with the tarsus (Fig. 11–4A). However, forces from the carpus or tarsus are transmitted to the preaxial bone (radius or tibia) at the wrist and at the ankle joints. Movement is supplemented at the wrist by abduction and adduction while the ankle developed into a uniaxial joint, shaped like a mortice. The **metacarpals** and **metatarsals** as well as the **phalanges** are clearly equivalent. In the foot these elements are held together to form a segmented lever lending power and spring to the foot, while in the human hand the digits possess much greater freedom, particularly the thumb. The joints and musculature of the thumb impart a versatility to the human hand which is quite unmatched in any other vertebrate.

MUSCULATURE AND INNERVATION

The basic pattern of musculature and innervation is already evident in the limb buds of 8–11 mm human embryos. The limb buds arise ventrolateral to the somites from unsegmented body wall. The axial region of limb bud mesenchyme forms the blastemata of skeletal elements and the musculature of the limbs develops *in situ* from surrounding mesenchyme. The central skeletal axis and preaxial and postaxial borders of the limb already foretell a division into two compartments: a ventrally placed **flexor compartment** and a dorsally placed **extensor compartment.**

Segmental spinal nerves growing out of the spinal cord contact the differentiating muscle anlagen and areas of developing skin. The limbs are innervated only by ventral rami of spinal nerves because the limb buds emerge from that part of the body wall which is served by the ventral and not the dorsal rami. The upper limb bud is invaded by the **ventral rami** of C5-T1 spinal nerves and the lower limb bud by ventral rami of L2-S3 spinal nerves. At the root of the limb bud each ventral ramus splits into an **anterior** and **posterior division** (Fig. 11–5). Nerves formed by the union of anterior divisions will proceed to the flexor compartment and make contact with flexor muscle primordia and with areas of skin on the flexor surface of the limb. The posterior divisions proceed in like manner to the extensor compartment.

The rearrangement of nerve fibers of the ventral rami constitutes at the root of the limb bud the **brachial** and **lumbosacral plexuses,** from which

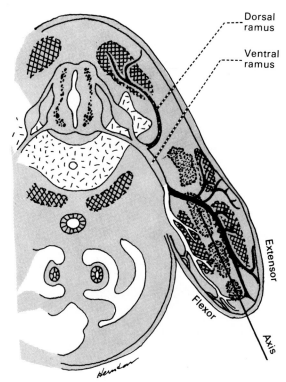

FIG. 11-5. A schematic representation of a transverse section of an embryo to illustrate the basic innervation plan of the limb bud. Flexor and extensor compartments are demarcated by the limb bud axis defined by the bone primordia. The ventral ramus of the spinal nerve bifurcates into an anterior division (white), distributed to the flexor compartment, and a posterior division (black) which supplies the musculature and skin of the extensor compartment.

issue the major named nerves of the upper and lower limbs, respectively. The plexuses provide intermingling of nerve fibers derived from different segments. One ventral ramus may contribute to several named nerves. There is, however, no mixing between fibers of anterior and posterior divisions nor between flexor and extensor nerves.

The major nerves derived from posterior divisions in the brachial plexus are the **axillary** and **radial nerves** (Fig. 11–6). The anterior divisions of the plexus are rearranged to form three major nerves: the **musculocutaneous, median,** and the **ulnar nerves** (Fig. 11–8). In the lumbosacral plexus likewise two major nerves are formed by posterior divisions: the **femoral** and **common peroneal** (Fig. 11–7); anterior divisions are distributed along three major nerves; **obturator, medial** and **lateral plantar nerves** (Fig. 11–9). The latter

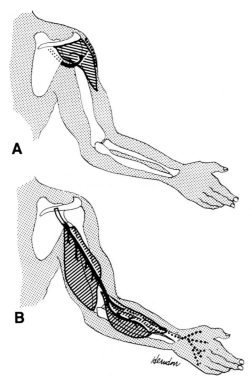

FIG. 11-6. Distribution of the major nerves derived from the posterior divisions of the brachial plexus. **(A)** The axillary nerve supplies a powerful abductor of the shoulder (deltoid) derived from the extensor compartment and the overlying skin. **(B)** The radial nerve supplies all the muscles in the extensor compartment of the arm and forearm, as well as much of the overlying skin.

compartment to the front. The primitive arrangement is retained in the upper limb.

It is not understood how nerve fibers derived from specific segments establish contact with specific groups of muscle masses and skin areas. The segmental pattern of nerve supply to the skin and musculature of the limbs is described in Chapter 12.

Some of the muscles formed in the limb bud migrate proximally and gain attachment to the axial skeleton. They produce limb movements relative to the trunk and include such muscles as the latissimus dorsi. The musculature of the limb girdles is supplied by minor branches of the plexuses. This nerve supply will be retained even in those muscles which gain attachment to the vertebral

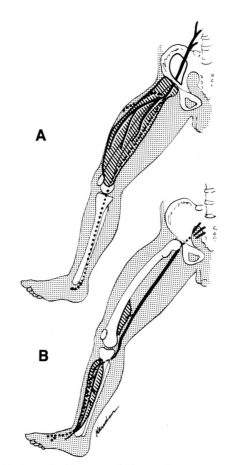

FIG. 11-7. Distribution of the major nerves derived from the posterior divisions of lumbosacral plexus. **(A)** The femoral nerve supplies the extensor muscles of the knee (quadriceps) and a large area of skin. **(B)** The common peroneal nerve is distributed to extensors of the ankle and toes and to the overlying skin.

two are terminal branches of the **tibial nerve** and in the foot correspond to the median and ulnar nerves of the hand. This striking similarity between the major branches of the brachial and lumbosacral plexuses is apparently confounded by the fact that connective tissue binds the common peroneal and tibial nerves into a large nerve trunk known as the sciatic nerve. The sciatic nerve from a functional point of view, however, is not an entity.

Adductor muscles are derived from the flexor compartment of a limb and abductors from the extensor compartment. They are innervated respectively by nerves derived from anterior and posterior divisions of the plexuses.

The discussion of skeletal homologues in upper and lower limbs should make it comprehensible that the developmental rotation of the lower limb places its flexor compartment, which was originally anterior, to the back and brings the extensor

FIG. 11-8. The three main nerves derived from the anterior divisions of the brachial plexus. **(A)** The musculocutaneous nerve supplies the flexors of the elbow and an area of skin on the preaxial border of the forearm. **(B)** The median nerve supplies the flexors of the wrist and digits situated mainly in the preaxial two-thirds of the flexor compartment, and it is the chief sensory nerve of the palmar surface of the hand. **(C)** The ulnar nerve supplies the remaining flexors in the postaxial portion of the forearm, most of the small muscles in the hand, and the skin on the postaxial digits.

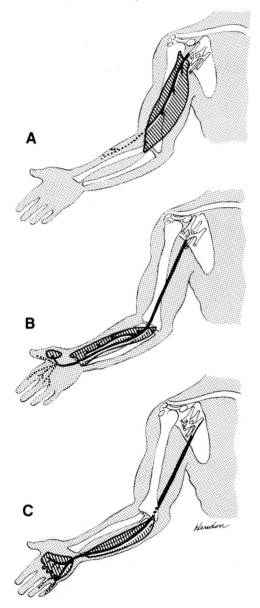

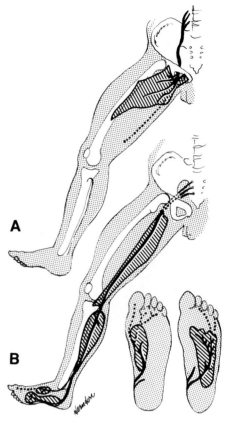

FIG. 11-9. The three main nerves derived from the anterior divisions of the lumbosacral plexus. **(A)** The obturator nerve supplies the adductors of the thigh, which are derived from the flexor compartment, and the overlying skin. **(B)** The other two nerves are represented by the tibial nerve as far down as the ankle. The tibial nerve supplies the flexor muscles of the ankle and the toes in preaxial and postaxial halves of the flexor compartment. In the foot the medial and lateral plantar nerves separate and their muscular and cutaneous distribution resembles those of the median and ulnar nerves, respectively.

column and move their site of origin some distance from the girdle skeleton.

BLOOD SUPPLY

The main arteries and veins of upper and lower limbs are similar, although their precise development is more complex in the lower limb.

Arteries

There is a single major arterial trunk along the proximal segment of each limb and two arteries in the intermediate segment, and in the hand and foot superficial and deep anastomotic arcades or arches give rise to arteries that supply the digits (Fig. 11–10). Because of the presence of the arches, adequate arterial blood will reach the extremities even if one of the proximal arteries is occluded. Anastomoses exist also around the major joints. A deep branch is given off in the proximal and intermediate segments for the supply of the more deeply seated muscles and the bones. At the root of each limb branches of the main artery establish an anastomosis with arteries of the trunk securing a potential, alternative arterial route to the limb which becomes important when the main artery is occluded.

The main artery in the upper limb is the **brachial** and in the lower limb the **femoral artery.** The brachial artery is the continuation of the **axillary artery,** while the femoral is the continuation of the **external iliac artery.** Below the elbow, the brachial artery divides into **radial** and **ulnar arteries,** while the femoral artery below the knee gives rise to the **anterior** and **posterior tibial arteries.** In the hand and foot, the arterial arcades are the **superficial** and **deep palmar** or **plantar arches** and the arteries springing from them are the **metacarpal** or **metatarsal arteries,** which terminate in the digital branches. The deep branches for the supply of arm and thigh musculature are called the **profunda brachii** and **profunda femoris arteries.** The deep branch in the forearm is the **interosseous artery** which divides into anterior and posterior branches for the supply of flexor and extensor musculature; the deep branch in the leg is the **peroneal artery.** Although these arteries of the upper and lower limbs are not exact developmental homologues, there is a striking similarity in their distribution.

Veins

Pressure from the palm of the hand and sole of the foot divert most of the venous blood to the dorsal aspects of the extremities. From the venous plexuses on the dorsum of the hand and foot, a superficial vein runs along each of the postaxial and preaxial borders of the limbs. The preaxial vein in the arm is the **cephalic vein** and in the leg the **long saphenous vein;** the postaxial veins are the **basilic** in the arm and the **short saphenous** in the

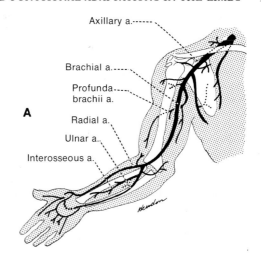

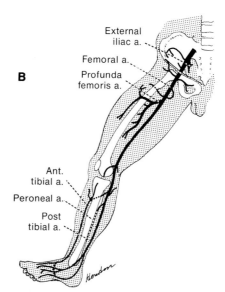

FIG. 11–10. The basic plan of arterial supply in the upper (**A**) and lower (**B**) limbs.

leg. In addition, **deep veins** accompany the arteries in each limb which are usually known as **venae comitantes** of the respective arteries. The two venae comitantes of the brachial artery become the **axillary vein** which receives the two superficial veins of the upper limb. A large **femoral vein** accompanies the femoral artery. Behind the knee, the **short saphenous,** and at the groin, the **long saphenous vein** empty into it.

Both upper and lower limb veins are interrupted

by venous valves which prevent retrograde flow favored by gravity. Centripetal flow in the veins is due to contractions of the limb musculature.

LYMPHATICS

The lymph drains from rich capillary plexuses of the hands and feet into lymphatic vessels that run predominantly along the superficial veins. A lymph node interrupts the flow at the elbow and behind the knee. Lymph from deep structures is conveyed proximally in lymphatics that run along the arteries. All the lymph from the upper limb passes through groups of lymph nodes situated in the axilla while lymph from the lower limbs is filtered by inguinal lymph nodes situated in the groin. Inflammation of the nodes gives rise to pain

and tenderness. This must be borne in mind in differential diagnosis of painful conditions at the respective joints. Lymph nodes become secondarily involved in septic and neoplastic diseases of their territory of drainage.

SUGGESTED READING

O'Rahilly R, Gardner E The timing and sequence of events in the developing of the limbs in the human embryo. Anat. Embryol. *148*:1, 1975.
An interesting account of the morphogenesis of human limb buds based on original observations. Extensive review of the literature.

Warwick R, Williams PL Gray's Anatomy, 35th British ed. Philadelphia, W. B. Saunders, 1973.
The section on The Appendicular Skeleton (p. 315) concisely reviews the phylogeny of limb development and presents interesting functional comparisons.

12
Segmental Innervation

CORNELIUS ROSSE

All vertebrates are built on a basic segmental anatomic pattern. Although this segmentation is less evident in man than in more primitive vertebrates, its existence may readily be appreciated during embryonic development. Between the 21st and 31st days of human embryonic development, the paraxial mesoderm condenses into segments or **somites** (Fig. 12–1A). Later development of somites produces **sclerotomes, dermatomes,** and **myotomes** (Fig. 12–1B). The sclerotomes are destined to become the axial skeleton, the dermatomes the integument, and the myotomes skeletal muscle. At an early stage the spinal nerve corresponding to each somite makes contact with its differentiating subdivisions. This relation remains throughout life. In essence there is a nerve, muscle, bone, an artery, and a vein for each segment. The orderly segmental arrangement is clearly retained in the trunk but is obscure in the limbs. Nevertheless, the innervation of the limbs is also segmental.

The appreciation of segmental distribution of nerves to muscle, skin, and even to viscera is not only helpful for grasping the basic anatomic structure, but is of considerable clinical importance. It is essential to understand the segmental pattern of innervation for the following reasons:

1. It forms the basis of the functional interrelation between the central nervous system and the musculoskeletal system.
2. Lesions of the spinal cord and its nerve roots often manifest themselves by affecting the musculoskeletal system in a segmental fashion.
3. Pain referred from viscera may affect the cutaneous and neuromuscular segments which are innervated from the same cord segments as the viscera.

This chapter deals with the distribution of spinal nerves to skeletal muscle and skin. The cranial nerves and their territory of distribution are omitted. The last section of the chapter presents the clinical evaluation of spinal nerves. Usually, this evaluation forms an integral part of the physical examination of the spine (Chap. 9).

ANATOMY OF A SPINAL NERVE

The formation of spinal nerves from dorsal and ventral roots was discussed in Chapter 10, and their intrathecal course was also described. The spinal nerve divides as it emerges from the intervertebral foramen yielding a ventral (anterior primary) ramus and a dorsal (posterior primary) ramus (Fig. 12–2).

Each **dorsal ramus** supplies a vertebral arch joint, a segment of the erector spinae, and a strip of skin on the back. None of the dorsal rami contribute nerves to the limbs.

The **ventral rami** are larger, and they supply the limbs (bones, joints, skin, and muscles), the prevertebral muscles, and the ventrolateral portion of the neck and the trunk. Ventral rami of thoracic nerves retain a truly segmental arrangement similar to that of the dorsal rami, but in the cervical, lumbar, and sacral regions ventral rami form plexuses. The **cervical plexus** (C1-C4) supplies all muscles of the neck anterior to the vertebrae as well as the skin of the neck anterolaterally and on the posterolateral aspect of the head. Ventral rami of C5-T1 are distributed to the upper limbs via the **brachial plexus,** and those of L2-S3 proceed through the **lumbosacral plexus** to the lower limb. Ventral rami supplying the limbs do not innervate structures in the trunk. All the layers of the body wall are supplied by ventral rami of T2-L1, including the skin down to the groin.

Composition of Spinal Nerves

Spinal nerves are composed predominantly of somatic efferent and somatic afferent nerve fibers.

169

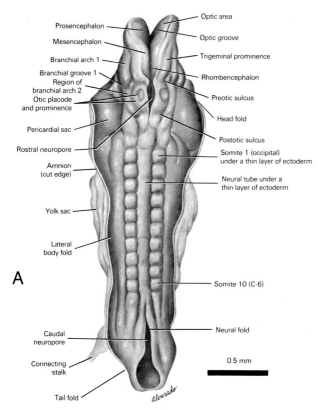

A

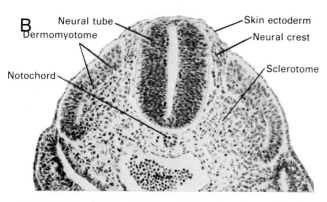

B

FIG. 12-1. Differentiation of the segmental paraxial mesoderm. (**A**) Dorsal view of an embryo in which 10 somites are identifiable. Altogether, 4 somites develop in the occipital region, 8 in the cervical, 12 in the thoracic, 5 each in the lumbar and sacral regions, and as many as 10 coccygeal somites may appear. By the time the caudal somites form, more rostral somites have differentiated. (**B**) Transverse section of an embryo similar to that in **A**. The cells of the somite in this segment have separated into the dermomyotome and sclerotome. (**A** from Gasser RF: Atlas of Human Embryos. Hagerstown, Harper & Row, 1975; **B** from FitzGerald MJT: Human Embryology, Hagerstown, Harper & Row, 1978) Both embryos are from the Carnegie Collection.

Somatic efferents are the axons of neurons in the anterior grey column contributed to the spinal nerve via its ventral root. They innervate skeletal muscle. **Somatic afferents** convey from the skin and deep structures impulses concerned with pain, temperature, touch, pressure, vibration, and position sense to the spinal cord. Their cell bodies are in the spinal ganglia. Each spinal nerve contains, in addition, **visceral efferent** and **visceral afferent** nerve fibers which may belong either to the sympathetic or parasympathetic divisions of the autonomic nervous system. **Parasympathetic** nerves are confined to the sacral segments of the cord and are concerned exclusively with the innervation of viscera. **Sympathetic** nerves, on the other hand, supply besides viscera the smooth muscle of blood vessels throughout the body, as well as all the sweat glands. Both these facts are of diagnostic importance in the musculoskeletal system.

All preganglionic **sympathetic efferents** originate in the intermediolateral cell column of T1-L2 segments (see Fig. 10–3), and the ventral roots of these segments only contain such fibers. They leave T1-L2 spinal nerves (via so-called white rami communicantes) and distribute themselves up and down the sympathetic chain (see Fig. 13–17). After relaying in one of the ganglia of the chain, postganglionic fibers rejoin each spinal nerve (via so-called grey rami communicantes) and reach their destination along its dorsal and ventral rami. Other fibers leave the chain for the viscera (medial or splanchnic branches). **Visceral afferents** enter the ganglia of the sympathetic chain, join the spinal nerve, and reach the spinal ganglia where their cell body is located among the ganglion cells of somatic afferents. The central processes of all spinal ganglion cells pass via the dorsal root to the posterior grey column of the spinal cord, where they either relay, cross to the contralateral side, or ascend in the white matter of the cord. Although it is of somewhat academic interest, pain sensation from the arteries and veins of the limbs may be mediated by *visceral* rather than somatic afferents.

Myotomes, Dermatomes, Sclerotomes

The mass of skeletal muscle innervated by the dorsal and ventral rami of a single spinal nerve is often spoken of as a **myotome**. A myotome includes portions of several muscles, and many muscles contain portions of more than one myotome. This concept is clinically useful, but the myotome thus defined should not be confused with the portion of the somites designated by the same name. All evidence is against migration of myotomal cells of the

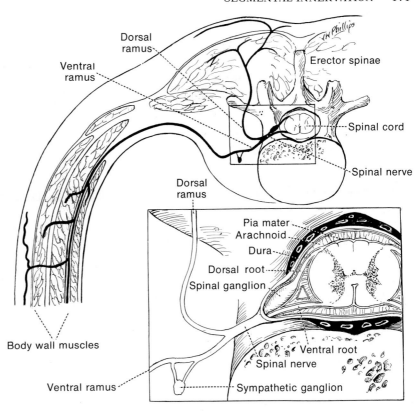

FIG. 12-2. Origin, division, and course of a typical spinal nerve.

somites into the limb buds (Chap. 11), yet all muscles in the limbs incorporate portions of myotomes according to the definition based on spinal nerve distribution. The same pertains to the dermatome. The dermatomal portion of a somite is not necessarily synonymous with the area of skin supplied by the dorsal and ventral rami of a single spinal nerve. Such an area of skin is defined as a **dermatome.** The cell bodies of these sensory nerve fibers are located in a single spinal ganglion.

It has been proposed that **sclerotomes** also exist in the sense that areas of bone and periosteum can be defined which are innervated by individual spinal nerves. Such a definition of a sclerotome is not identical with the embryonic sclerotome. There is no evidence that the skeleton of the limbs is derived from the embryonic, paraxial sclerotomes, yet their periosteum is also segmentally innervated.

SEGMENTAL INNERVATION OF MUSCLES

The segmental arrangement of myotomes in the

trunk clearly emerges from the distribution of spinal nerves T1-L1. Their dorsal rami supply the thoracic and lumbar portions of the erector spinae segmentally and their ventral rami innervate the intercostal muscles, abdominal flank muscles, and the rectus abdominis in a strictly segmental fashion.

The columns of motor neurons concerned with the supply of individual muscles in the limbs have been identified experimentally, as well as by correlating paralysis of individual muscles with the patchy distribution of motor neuron death in cases of poliomyelitis. Such cell columns in the anterior horns are constant and, depending on the muscle, may span 2–4 segments. However, the majority of motor neurons responsible for the contraction of the muscle are contained in just one or two of these segments. Thus, from a functional point of view, some segments in the motor neuron column of each muscle are more important than others. The cell columns that innervate muscles sharing the same action at a particular joint are found in the same segments of the spinal cord. Therefore, muscle groups operating as prime movers at a particular joint may be viewed as a segmentally innervated

TABLE 12–1. Segmental Innervation of the Upper Limb Musculature*

Joints/Prime Movers	Cord Segments				
	C5	C6	C7	C8	T1
Shoulder					
Abductors	X	x			
Extensors	X	X	X	x	
Lateral Rotators	X	x			
Adductors		X	X	x	
Flexors	x	X	X	x	
Medial Rotators	x	X	X	x	
Elbow					
Flexors	X	x			
Extensors		x	X	X	
Forearm					
Supinators	x	X			
Pronators		x	X	X	x
Wrist					
Flexors		X	X	x	x
Extensors		X	X	x	
Fingers					
Flexors		X	X	x	
Extensors		X	X	x	
Intrinsic Hand Muscles				x	X

*The cord segments principally concerned with various movements are indicated by boldface capital **X**s. Movements are so grouped as to make the existence of *joint centers* more readily appreciable.

functional unit. The innervation of prime movers for different joints of the upper and lower limbs is shown in Tables 12–1 and 12–2.

From the overview of these tables, a few general features emerge which are helpful in understanding the basic arrangement:

1. Muscles with a common primary action on a joint share at least two adjacent segments of the spinal cord.
2. The segments of the cord which supply the antagonists of the muscle group either overlap or run in numerical sequence with the cord segments for that group. For instance, elbow flexors are supplied by C5 and C6, while the chief supply of the extensors is from C7 and C8.
3. In general, the segments which innervate the muscles of a joint that is more distal in the limb lie *en bloc* more distal in the cord.

The segments concerned with the chief supply of muscles of a joint might be thought of as a *joint center* in the spinal cord. With the aid of Figure 12–3, it is an easy matter to commit to memory which movements are innervated by which segments and *vice versa*. Knowing the principal action of a muscle, it is possible also to deduce its segmen-

tal innervation. This knowledge is useful clinically, and provides a sound basis for being aware of the spinal segments evaluated when testing muscle strength or eliciting deep tendon reflexes.

Deep Tendon Reflexes

The stretch reflex as the physiologic basis of tendon jerks was discussed in Chapter 4. The clinically most useful tendon reflexes are the biceps, triceps, and brachioradialis tendon jerks in the upper limb and the knee and ankle jerks in the lower limb. The biceps jerk tests spinal cord segment C5, the biceps being a flexor of the elbow, while the triceps is an elbow extensor and its jerk gives information about segments C7 and C8. The brachioradialis jerk involves chiefly C6 segment. In eliciting a knee jerk, the tendon of the extensor muscle (quadriceps) is tapped, testing segments L3 and L4, while the ankle jerk tests S1 and S2, because the muscles subjected to momentary stretch are the plantar flexors of the ankle. It has to be remembered, however, that in addition to the appropriate

TABLE 12–2. Segmental Innervation of the Lower Limb Musculature*

Joints/Prime Movers	Cord Segments						
	L2	L3	L4	L5	S1	S2	S3
Hip							
Flexors	X	X	x				
Adductors	X	X	x				
Medial Rotators	X	X	x	x	x	x	
Extensors			x	X	X	x	
Abductors			x	X	X	x	
Lateral Rotators				X	X	x	
Knee							
Extensors	x	X	X				
Flexors			x	X	X	x	x
Ankle							
Extensors (dorsiflexors)			X	X	x		
Flexors (plantarflexors)				x	X	X	
Pretalar-Subtalar Joint							
Invertors			X	X	x		
Evertors			X	X	x		
Toes							
Extensors			X	X	x		
Flexors				X	X	x	
Intrinsic Foot Muscles						X	x

*The cord segments principally concerned with various movements are indicated by boldface capital **X**s. Movements are so grouped as to make the existence of *joint centers* more readily appreciable.

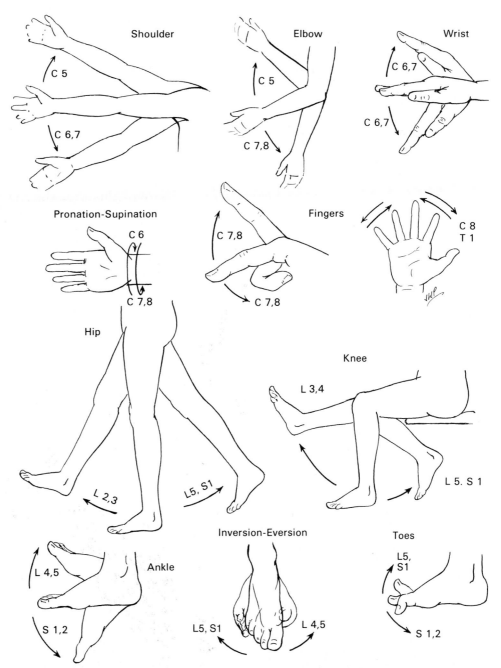

FIG. 12–3. Segmental innervation of the muscle groups producing movement in the limbs. Only segments principally responsible for the innervation of a movement are shown. These are the segments of greatest practical usefulness. For a more complete account refer to Tables 12–1 and 12–2. (Based on Last RJ: Anatomy. London, Churchill, 1972)

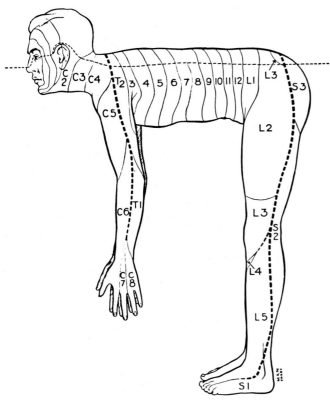

FIG. 12-4. Segmental innervation of the skin: dermatomal map according to Foerster. The body is shown in the quadruped position to emphasize the regular distribution of dermatomes. The interrupted vertical lines in the limbs represent the dorsal axial lines along which dermatomes migrated to the extremities of the limbs, and along which the neighboring dermatomes belong to noncontiguous segments. Although the ventral axial lines cannot be seen in this position, it can be appreciated that the skin covering the preaxial border of the limbs between ventral and dorsal axial lines is innervated by the more proximal segments of the limb plexus, while the skin covering the postaxial border is innervated by the distal segments. In the case of the upper limb, skin has been borrowed from trunk dermatomes proximally and distally. The interrupted line along the back marks the boundary between the distribution territory of dorsal and ventral rami. (Haymaker W, Woodhall B: Peripheral Nerve Injuries, 2nd ed. Philadelphia, WB Saunders, 1953)

spinal cord segments, all anatomic components of the stretch reflex must be intact (see Fig. 4–8).

The sensitivity of deep tendon reflexes is modulated by suprasegmental input to the spinal motor neuron pool. Exaggerated or abnormally brisk tendon jerks are indicative of upper motor

neuron lesions, which remove suprasegmental influence from the spinal reflex centers (Chaps. 4 and 27).

SEGMENTAL INNERVATION OF THE SKIN

Like the myotomes, dermatomes of the trunk are arranged in regular bands from T2 to L1 (Figs. 12–4, 12–5). T2 is at the sternal angle, T10 at the level of the umbilicus and L1 in the region of the groin. There is considerable overlap between neighboring dermatomes of the trunk, and no anesthesia can be demonstrated clinically in a dermatome if its spinal nerve is the only one blocked. This is not the case in the limbs. Limb dermatomes cover larger areas of skin, and although there is overlap between neighboring dermatomes, compression or anesthetic block of a single spinal nerve that feeds into one of the plexuses does produce hypoesthesia or even anesthesia over part of the appropriate dermatome.

Each of the two dermatomal maps currently in use represents the synthesis of a large number of isolated clinical observations. The map of Foerster (Fig. 12–4) is based largely on patients in whom specific dorsal roots have been surgically divided. Keegan and Garrett's map (Fig. 12–5) is constructed largely from cases of nerve compression by herniating intervertebral disks in the cervical and lumbosacral regions, verified in most instances by surgery.

In Foerster's map the dermatomes represented in the limbs are completely missing in the trunk, while according to Keegan and Garrett, both C5 and T1 appear anteriorly on the trunk, and none of the segments is missing posteriorly. Lately, Keegan and Garrett's map has gained wider clinical acceptance. The developmental explanation put forward by these authors postulates that sensory branches of limb nerves grew down the developing limb bud along its dorsal surface and wound themselves around both the preaxial and postaxial borders to the ventral surface, meeting along a line called the **axial line** (Fig. 12–6A). Therefore, neighboring dermatomes across this line are noncontiguous with respect to number, and overlap across the axial line is minimal. In Foerster's map both ventral and dorsal axial lines exist. He postulated that during development the central dermatome of each limb bud became drawn out in its entirety to cover the most distal

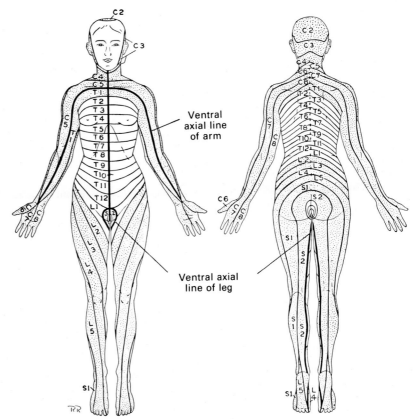

FIG. 12-5. Segmental innervation of the skin: dermatomal map according to Keegan and Garrett. Axial lines exist only on the ventral surface of the limb, which in the lower limbs are posterior in consequence of the developmental rotation of the limb. (Keegan JG, Garrett FV: Anat Rec 102:409, 1948)

segment of each limb, leaving behind discontiguous dermatomes in contact with one another across dorsal and ventral axial lines (Fig. 12–6B). Whichever explanation is correct, the existence of ventral axial lines is universally accepted. Ventral axial lines are clinically useful because testing cutaneous sensation across these lines is the least complicated by dermatomal overlap.

Superficial Reflexes

Stimulation of the skin by stroking or scratching in certain dermatomal areas provokes reflex muscle contraction. These so-called superficial reflexes depend on the integrity of the appropriate sensory and motor peripheral nerves and spinal cord segments, as well as on intact suprasegmental input to the spinal reflex centers. Unlike deep tendon re-

flexes, superficial reflexes are abolished by upper motor neuron lesions. The most useful superficial reflexes are the abdominal, cremasteric, plantar, and anal reflexes.

Scratching the skin some distance away from the umbilicus in any one quadrant of the anterior abdominal wall causes contraction of the underlying abdominal muscles. The umbilicus will be drawn toward the side of the contraction.

The **abdominal reflex** in the upper quadrant depends on segments T7-T9, and in the lower quadrants on segments T10-T12.

The **cremasteric reflex** tests L1-L2 segments and is elicited in males by stroking the medial side of the thigh. This provokes reflex contraction of the cremaster muscle causing prompt and visible elevation of the testis.

The **plantar reflex** is elicited by scratching the

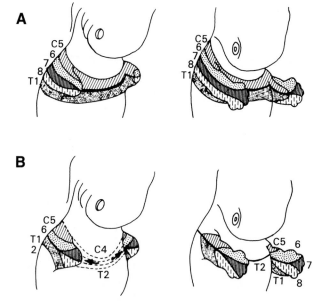

FIG. 12–6. Development and explanation of the dermatomes in the upper limb. (**A**) According to Keegan and Garrett. (**B**) According to Foerster. (**A** from Bowdon REM, Abdullah S, Gooding MR: In Brain Lord, Wilkinson M (eds): Cervical Spondylosis. Philadelphia, WB Saunders, 1967) Each is shown at two successive stages of development.

sole along its lateral aspect from heel to toes (dermatomes L5,S1) which provokes plantar flexion of the toes. Segments L5,S1 and S2 are chiefly involved. In upper motor neuron lesions the great toe will extend while the other toes are flexed (Babinski's sign).

The **anal reflex** is elicited by scratching the skin in the perianal region (dermatome S3). A visible contraction of the external anal sphincter causes puckering of the anus. Segments S2,S3 and S4 are involved.

CLINICAL EVALUATION OF SPINAL NERVES

The evaluation of spinal nerves and cord segments forms an integral part of the examination of the vertebral column. Having dealt with the anatomy of the vertebral canal (Chap. 10) and with the functions associated with spinal cord segments, a screening neurologic examination can be described meaningfully which must be performed as a continuation of the physical examination presented in Chapter 9.

Pain in dermatomal or myotomal areas suggests irritation of spinal nerves. It may also be referred from viscera via autonomic afferents which terminate in the same spinal cord segment. Anesthesia or paresthesia of dermatomal distribution and muscle wasting and weakness that involve functional muscle groups and joints are likely to be due to pathology of cord segments or spinal nerves and must be distinguished from lesions of peripheral nerves.

Myotomes of the limbs should be tested by evaluating the strength of prime movers at the various joints and by eliciting appropriate reflexes. Dermatomes are evaluated by pricks of a safety pin or by firmly scratching the skin with the pin drawing it across dermatomal boundaries. In the limbs this should be done across axial lines. In addition, the degree of vasodilation and sweating should be compared with adjacent areas. The skin becomes flushed and dry when it is deprived of its sympathetic nerve supply. In addition, the clinical maneuvers which increase the tension or compression of specific spinal nerves are of great diagnostic importance (pp. 155, 156).

The neurologic examination may be performed proceeding from segment to segment testing myotomes and dermatomes, or, as it is more commonly done, by first evaluating the strengths of prime movers at joints of the upper and lower limbs, then eliciting all the reflexes, and finally testing the dermatomes. Below are summarized the chief physical signs which are helpful in distinguishing the compression or interruption of neighboring spinal nerves.

C5. Decreased power of shoulder abduction and elbow flexion; the biceps reflex is absent or grossly diminished even if C6 is intact; sensory changes over the deltoid and lateral aspect of the arm.

C6. Decreased power of supination; wrist flexion and extension; the brachioradialis reflex is abolished; sensory changes over the lateral aspect of the forearm, including the thumb.

C7. Decreased power of elbow extension, pronation, finger flexion and extension; decreased or abolished triceps reflex; sensory changes most pronounced over palmar and dorsal surface of middle finger.

C8. Similar distribution of muscle weakness as with a C7 lesion but intrinsic muscles of the hand are also affected. This is assessed by testing the power of spreading the fingers (Chap. 15). There is no specific reflex; the triceps reflex may be diminished. Sensory changes affect the little finger and the medial side of the forearm.

T1. Intrinsic muscles of the hand are severely affected; more proximal muscles are spared and all reflexes are normal; sensory changes along the medial aspect of the arm.

T2-T12. Isolated spinal nerve lesions are difficult to detect; distribution of pain, tenderness, muscle spasm, and careful evaluation of sensory changes are the chief factors in the diagnosis. Lesions of upper thoracic nerves may abolish the sympathetic input to the upper limb and head and neck. Abdominal reflexes will be absent usually only if more than one of T6-T12 spinal nerves are blocked or interrupted.

L1-L2. Absent cremasteric reflex; sensory changes over the groin.

L2-L3. Weakness in hip flexors and adductors; some weakness of the quadriceps (knee extension) but only minimal, if any, detectable change in the knee jerk; sensory changes over the anterior aspect of the thigh.

L4. Weakness of knee extension, ankle dorsiflexion and inversion; the knee jerk is greatly diminished or absent; sensory changes over the medial side of the leg and great toe. (Foerster's original data include the great toe in L4 dermatome. Later, charts constructed from these data erroneously assigned the great toe to L5 dermatome, and this error has been perpetuated in many subsequent reproductions of the chart.)

L5. Numerous muscle groups are affected, but weakness of toe extensors (particularly that of the great toe) distinguishes this lesion from L4. Furthermore, both knee and ankle jerks are normal. Sensory changes involve the dorsum of the foot.

S1. Plantar flexors of the ankle (calf muscles), evertors of the foot, long flexors and extensors of the

toes are affected. The most useful test is the strength of the evertors (peronei). The ankle jerk is absent or greatly diminished. Sensory changes involve the lateral side of the dorsum and sole of the foot.

S2-S3. Paralysis of intrinsic foot muscles presents with deformities of the toes and the arches of the foot (Chap. 18). Innervation of the bladder may be affected; the ankle jerk may be diminished. Sensory change with an S2 lesion involves the back of the leg and the thigh.

Lesions involving part or the whole of spinal cord segments are complicated by damage to ascending and descending tracts. Their description is beyond the scope of this chapter. For such clinical syndromes one of the references should be consulted.

SUGGESTED READING

Bowden, R. E. M., Abdullah, S., and Gooding, M. R. Anatomy of the cervical spine, membranes, spinal cord, nerve roots and brachial plexus. In Brain, W. R., and Wilkinson, M. (eds.): Cervical Spondylosis. Philadelphia, W. B. Saunders, 1967.
In addition to describing the anatomy, the segments directly concerned with the supply of various movements of the upper limb are tabulated.

Foerster, O. The dermatomes in man. Brain 56:1, 1933.
Many interesting cases are presented in whom dorsal roots have been cut and areas of remaining sensitivity have been outlined. These and many other cases form the basis of Foerster's dermatomal map.

Haymaker, W., and Woodhall B. Peripheral Nerve Injuries, 2nd ed. Philadelphia, W. B. Saunders, 1953.
The first two chapters deal with the composition of spinal nerves and their segmental distribution to skin and muscles. The segmental innervation of all muscles of upper and lower limbs is presented in a handy tabular form. The book is profusely illustrated with clinical cases.

Hoppenfeld, S. Physical Examination of the Spine and Extremities. New York, Appleton-Century-Crofts, 1976.
The methods of eliciting various reflexes and other diagnostic maneuvers are clearly described and well-illustrated. Chapters 4 and 9 deal with the physical examination of the spine, including a screening neurologic evaluation.

Hoppenfeld, S. Orthopedic Neurology. Philadelphia, J. B. Lippincott, 1977.
A diagnostic guide to neurologic levels. Well-written and well-illustrated.

Inman, V. T., and Saunders, J. B. deC. M. Referred pain from skeletal structures. J. Nerv. Ment. Dis. 660, 1944.
The clinical significance of sclerotomes is discussed.

Keegan, J. J., and Garrett, F. D. The segmental distribution of the cutaneous nerves in the limbs of man. Anat. Rec. *102*:409, 1948.
The original report of numerous cases of intervertebral disk prolapse with resultant changes in cutaneous sensitivity. The authors comprehensively review the earlier literature and pre-

sent a hypothesis for explaining developmentally their own dermatomal map.

Last, R. J. Innervation of the limbs. J. Bone Joint Surg., [B] *31*:452, 1949.
An illuminating presentation of the basic plan for the innervation of musculature and skin in the limbs. Some of the segmental values given for some movements have been modified by more recent studies.

Ruge, D. Neurologic evaluation. In Ruge, D., and Wiltse, L. L. (eds): Spinal Disorders. Philadelphia, Lea & Febiger, 1977, p. 53.

An informative, brief account of the clinical syndromes associated with spinal nerve compression and with segmental damage to the spinal cord.

Sharrard, W. J. W. The distribution of the permanent paralysis in the lower limb in polyomyelitis. J. Bone Joint Surg. [B] *37*:540, 1955.
The columns of motor neurons in the ventral horn are reconstructed, based on cases of poliomyelitis. Segmental values of innervation for lower limb muscles are based largely on this study.

13
The Shoulder Region and the Brachial Plexus

CORNELIUS ROSSE

Placing the hand in positions required for function relies on movements also at the shoulder and elbow. Combinations of shoulder and elbow movements position the hand within a space somewhat larger than a hemisphere whose diameter is essentially the span of the upper limbs. This is possible only when there is free mobility at all joints, adequate muscle power and muscle control, and freedom from pain. **Appreciation of functional interdependence of the various parts of the upper limb is essential.**

The diagnosis of disorders and their localization to individual structures are only possible with the knowledge of functional anatomy. Anatomy and physical examination are considered together in this chapter to emphasize the functional importance of various structures.

THE PECTORAL AND SHOULDER REGIONS

The **clavicle** and the **scapula** are associated with a number of muscles which attach the upper limb to the trunk. In addition to providing movement of the bones, the muscles are important in uniting the scapula and clavicle to the axial skeleton. By definition, this mechanism can be regarded as a *joint* and is described as the *scapulothoracic joint*.

Movements between the scapula and clavicle take place at the **acromioclavicular joint**, and the clavicle, in turn, articulates with the manubrium at the **sternoclavicular joint**. In all movements of the shoulder, the scapulothoracic, sternoclavicular, and acromioclavicular joints work together with the **glenohumeral joint** in a synchronized rhythm (Fig. 13–1).

Bony Landmarks

Verification of the normal or abnormal positions of the clavicle, scapula, and humerus in relation to one another is based on palpation of the bones. Palpation of bony landmarks is the key to the examination of the shoulder region. Figure 13–2 illustrates the relationship of the bones to one another around the shoulder joint.

Clavicle. The entire clavicle may be palpated from its medial expanded end to the flat, lateral, or acromial end. In its medial two thirds the bone is convex anteriorly as it arches over the brachial plexus, while in its lateral third a concavity is directed forward. Fractures due to indirect violence usually occur along the middle third. This is due not only to the change in curvature, but to the fact that a pair of ligaments anchor the medial and lateral thirds of the clavicle (Fig. 13–1). The ligaments are not palpable because they are attached to the inferior surface of the bone. Two **coracoclavicular (conoid** and **trapezoid) ligaments** fix the lateral third, while the medial third is bound to the first rib by the **costoclavicular ligament** which consists of two laminae. Both pairs of ligaments slant posteriorly as they approach the clavicle, and therefore when the clavicle is elevated, putting the ligaments on a stretch, the clavicle automatically rotates posteriorly. The movement is easily appreciated by placing the hand on the clavicle during abduction of the arm.

The clavicle may become dislocated or subluxed at either end. In **acromioclavicular separation,** the weight of the arm pulls the scapula down leaving the lateral end of the clavicle abnormally prominent. The capsule of the joint (acromioclavicular ligament) is usually torn and so may be the conoid

179

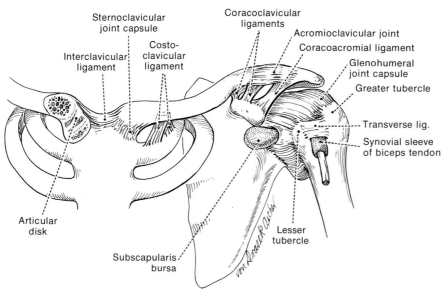

FIG. 13-1. The sternoclavicular, acromioclavicular, and glenohumeral joints with associated ligaments seen from the front.

and trapezoid ligaments, in cases where the distracting force is large.

Dislocation at the sternoclavicular joint is restrained chiefly by the articular capsule and by an **articular disk** of fibrocartilage (Fig. 13–1). The articular capsule of the joint is the key structure in supporting the weight of the entire upper limb. It is reinforced by **anterior** and **posterior ligaments** and by an **interclavicular ligament.** The chief concern in posterior dislocation of the clavicle is compression of the trachea.

Scapula. Unlike the clavicle, the scapula is largely covered by muscles. It is a flat, triangular bone which lies with its anterior surface against the thoracic cage. Of its three borders and three angles, only the **medial** (or vertebral) **border** and the **inferior angle** are readily palpable. The lateral angle presents the **glenoid cavity** (or fossa) and two processes—the acromion and coracoid.

Anteriorly, the **acromion** meets the clavicle at the acromioclavicular joint, which is medial to the tip of the acromion (Fig. 13–2). On the lateral aspect of the tip of the shoulder, the acromion is subcutaneous and readily palpable between the attachments of the trapezius and the deltoid (Fig. 13–3). The subcutaneous bone continues posteriorly into the **spine of the scapula** which can be traced to the vertebral border. The base of the scapular spine is opposite the spinous process of

T3 while the inferior angle of the bone is on level with T7.

The tip of the **coracoid** is palpable 2.5 cm below the depth of the concavity of the clavicle (Fig. 13–3). It is felt as a definite, blunt tubercle, placed more laterally than one intuitively anticipates. It is quite sensitive to pressure. The beaklike process arches over the major neurovascular structures of the axilla, and its base is situated more superomedially. During abduction of the arm, the coracoid process can be felt moving away from the palpating finger. During the same movement, maximum excursion is shown by the inferior angle of the scapula which slides forward, around the chest wall.

Fractures of the scapula are best assessed clinically by compressing the bone between the coracoid process and inferior angle. Pain with or without crepitus is a positive sign.

The **coracoacromial ligament** (Fig. 13–1) spans the gap between the coracoid and acromion completing a strong osseoligamentous arch over the glenoid cavity and the head of the humerus (Fig. 13–2). The ligament cannot be palpated. It represents vestigial portions of the girdle musculature and it can be resected without loss of function. The ligament provides reinforcement to the glenohumeral joint.

Proximal End of the Humerus. Palpable portions

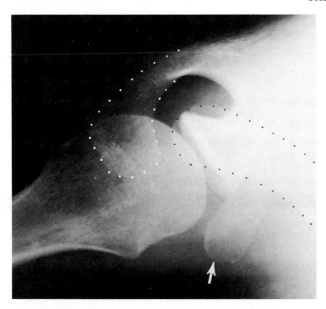

FIG. 13–2. A transaxillary x-ray of the shoulder. The x-ray film is placed above the acromion and the x-rays travel through the axilla. The acromion **(white dots)** overhangs the humeral head and is separated from the lateral end of the clavicle **(black dots)** by a radiolucent gap which is occupied chiefly by articular cartilage, and an articular disk, in the acromioclavicular joint. The clavicle is superimposed over the glenoid, the shallow fossa of which is separated from the humeral head by radiolucent articular cartilage. The beaklike coracoid projects forward, its tip **(arrow)** being level with the lesser tubercle. The coracoacromial ligament (invisible) bridges the gap between the coracoid and acromion. (Courtesy of Dr. Rosalind H. Troupin)

on the proximal end of the humerus include the head covered with articular cartilage, the greater and lesser tubercles, and the intertubercular sulcus. The **head of the humerus** is accessible only in the axilla with the arm abducted. The **greater tubercle** is felt through the deltoid just below the acromion, and 2.5 cm anterior to it is the **intertubercular groove** or sulcus which separates it from the **lesser tubercle** (Fig. 13–3).

The tendon of the long head of the biceps is retained in the groove by the **transverse humeral ligament** (Fig. 13–1). Inflammation of the synovial sheath around the tendon causes pain and tenderness. The tendon may snap in and out of the groove if the ligament is degenerated or torn.

The normal position of the humeral head can be confirmed with reference of the lesser tubercle, to the coracoid and the tip of the acromion. The three points mark the angles of a regular triangle (Fig.

13–3). The humerus may dislocate anteriorly or posteriorly; either case resulting in obvious deformity. The normal relationship of the three bony points will, of course, become distorted (Fig. 13–4), and the humeral head will be palpable in the abnormal position. The normal relationship of the three bony points will not be altered, however, if the **surgical neck** of the humerus is fractured (Fig. 13–4). Continuity of the proximal end of the bone with the distal end is tested by feeling for movement at the proximal end when the humerus is rotated passively at the elbow. If the humeral neck fracture is impacted, this test will not detect the fracture.

Movements

The shoulder girdle can be elevated, depressed, protracted, retracted, and rotated. These are the movements which extend the functional range obtained at the shoulder joint. However, it is both instructive and clinically important to analyze these movements independent of glenohumeral motion. The scapula and clavicle move together in all these movements.

In the normal limb, the limits to all scapular movements are imposed by the clavicle. The sternal end of the clavicle moves in a direction opposite to that of its lateral end, like two ends of a lever move around a fulcrum. This relation no longer exists if 1) the clavicle is fractured, 2) the coracoclavicular or costoclavicular ligaments are torn, or

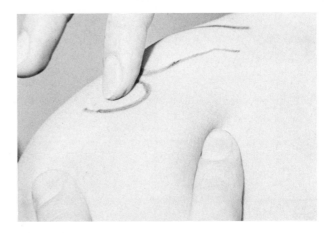

FIG. 13–3. The relationship of the acromion, lesser tubercle, and coracoid process. The index finger of one hand is on the tip of the acromion, that of the other hand on the coracoid, and the middle finger of the same hand on the lesser tubercle. The three bony points outline a regular triangle. This relationship is disturbed when the humerus is dislocated.

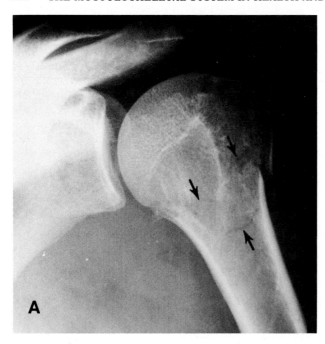

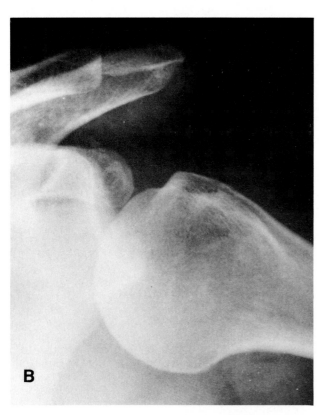

FIG. 13-4. (A) Fracture of the surgical neck of the humerus. The points where the fracture line interrupts the cortex on the medial and lateral aspect of the neck are clearly seen. The fracture has been caught in two profiles between these two points because of its obliquity and is visible as an irregular streak of radiolucency (**arrows**). Note that a normal relationship is retained between the humeral head, glenoid, and acromion. (**B**) Dislocation of the humerus. Only physical examination or a transaxillary projection (Fig. 13–2) can resolve whether the dislocation is anterior or posterior. Note that the relationship of the glenoid and the humerus is distorted, and the latter is widely separated from the acromion. (Courtesy of Dr. Rosalind H. Troupin)

3) the acromioclavicular joint is dislocated. Other clinically important abnormalities of the shoulder girdle arise from deranged function of the acromioclavicular and sternoclavicular joints, and from muscle paralysis.

Elevation. The scapula and clavicle become elevated in full arm abduction. The movement can be performed independently, however, during shrugging of the shoulders. The muscles concerned are the levator scapulae, the rhomboids, and the upper portion of the trapezius (Fig. 13–5).

The **levator scapulae** arises from the transverse processes of upper cervical vertebrae and the **rhomboids** from the spinous processes of the same or lower vertebrae. The muscles insert in continuity into the medial border of the scapula, the levator having the greatest advantage for scapular elevation. All these muscles are innervated by a branch of the brachial plexus (dorsal scapular nerve, C5), though the levator also receives some fibers directly from cervical ventral rami above the brachial plexus. The muscles are concealed by the trapezius and, consequently, their contraction is not easy to demonstrate.

The **trapezius** is the most superficial muscle in the back and plays an important role in elevation and retraction of the shoulder as well as in scapular rotation. Each muscle is a large triangle with the base attached to all thoracic spinous processes, the ligamentum nuchae and the skull (Fig. 13–5). Only the upper fibers that insert along the scapular spine, acromion, and into the lateral third of the clavicle are capable of elevating the shoulder girdle. The muscle is readily demonstrated by testing the power of shoulder elevation or better by opposing abduction of the arms. When the muscles contract, lack of symmetry of the upper fibers along the contour of the neck is the best indication of

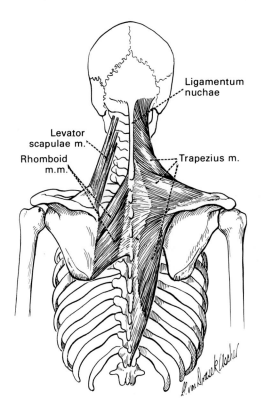

FIG. 13–5. Muscles of the pectoral girdle capable of elevating and retracting the pectoral girdle. The trapezius has other actions as well. Posterior view.

weakness or paralysis. The trapezius is innervated by the *spinal* accessory nerve and by ventral rami of C2,C3, and C4. It does not receive any fibers from the brachial plexus and the reasons for this have not been explained. The strength of the elevators of the shoulder can be assessed by opposing the patient's attempts at shrugging the shoulder.

Depression. Only during climbing and during walking on crutches is active depression of the pectoral girdle called for. In the back, the lower fibers of the **trapezius** (Fig. 13–5) and the **latissimus dorsi** (Fig. 13–6, via its attachment to the humerus) are the muscles concerned. Anteriorly, the **pectoralis minor** and the lower portion of the **pectoralis major** (Fig. 13–7, via the humerus) assist in the movement. The small **subclavius** depresses and rotates the clavicle but is probably more important in shunting the clavicle toward the manubrium in violent movements of the arm (throwing, hitting out).

Protraction. The shoulder is thrust forward by the serratus anterior (Fig. 13–8) and pectoralis minor (Fig. 13–6). The movement commonly accompanies shoulder flexion as in reaching forward, throwing, and stabbing. Sliding of the scapula around the rib cage is governed by the serratus anterior. The lateral end of the clavicle moves passively with the scapula.

Even at rest, the **serratus anterior** is responsible for retaining the scapula in apposition with the chest wall. It is a complex, fan-shaped muscle which arises by fleshy digitations from the anterolateral aspect of the upper eight to ten ribs and converges on the anterior lip of the medial border of the scapula (Fig. 13–8). The muscle hugs the rib cage (forming the medial wall of the axilla) before it inserts into the scapula. Mainly, its upper half is responsible for protraction. The lower (and, therefore, the larger) four to five digitations insert into a relatively small area on the anterior surface of the inferior angle (Fig. 13–8). Exerting force at this point, they are an important agent in scapular rotation. The muscle is supplied segmentally (C5,C6,C7) by a branch of the brachial plexus (long thoracic nerve).

In muscular subjects its serrated edge is readily seen in the axilla. It is best tested by demonstrating its ability to keep the scapula in apposition with the chest wall. When it is weak or paralyzed, *winging of the scapula* will occur when the subject pushes against an immovable object in front of him (Fig. 13–9). The test is the more sensitive, the less the force applied. It is chiefly the serratus anterior which does not allow the scapula to be pushed away from the trunk during push ups when the body weight is supported on the arms.

Retraction. The **rhomboids** and the horizontal fibers of the **trapezius** brace the shoulders back (Fig. 13–5).

Rotation. Scapular and clavicular rotation form such an integral part of arm abduction that the movement will be described in that context.

THE SHOULDER JOINT

The humerus articulates with the pectoral girdle at the glenohumeral, or shoulder, joint. Being the most mobile joint in the body, stability is sacrificed for mobility. This functional requisite is reflected in the anatomy of the joint.

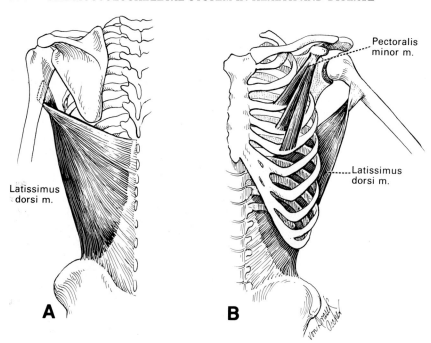

FIG. 13-6. Some of the muscles capable of depressing the pectoral girdle. The latissimus dorsi acts on the girdle via the shoulder joint. **(A)** Posterior view. **(B)** Anterior view.

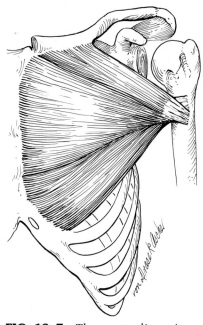

FIG. 13-7. The pectoralis major.

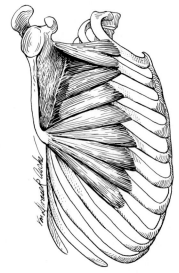

FIG. 13-8. The serratus anterior

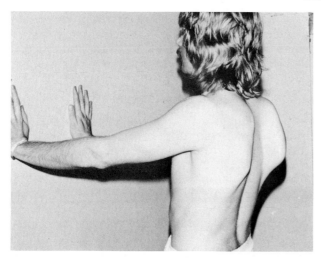

FIG. 13-9. Winging of the scapula due to paralysis of the serratus anterior. The patient is pushing against the wall. (Courtesy of Dr. David M. Chaplin)

Anatomy of the Joint

The shoulder is a **polyaxial synovial joint** in which the **ball-and-socket**-shaped articular surfaces make movement possible in any direction.

Articular Surfaces. The humeral head is larger than the glenoid cavity (Fig. 13–2) even though the latter is slightly enlarged and deepened by a rim of fibrocartilage, the **glenoidal labrum** (Fig. 13–10). Hyaline articular cartilage covers the bony surfaces. Since neither the ball nor the socket represent segments of a perfect sphere, only limited areas of the mating surfaces are in contact in any position, permitting the humeral head to slide and/or spin freely on the glenoid (Chap. 5). The close-packed position is obtained in abduction and lateral rotation when the congruity between ball and socket is maximal, the ligaments are rendered taut and humerus and scapula are transformed into a single rigid unit.

The Fibrous Capsule and Ligaments. The loose sleeve of the fibrous capsule puts no restraints on joint movement except in the close-packed position. The capsule is attached just peripheral to the glenoidal labrum, and on the humerus it follows the articular margin except inferiorly where it extends to the surgical neck enclosing the epiphyseal line of the humeral head within the joint cavity (Fig. 13–10). The ligamentous reinforcements of the capsule (glenohumeral ligaments) are inconse-

quential except for the **coracohumeral ligament** which supports much of the weight of the pendent arm. The tendons of the so-called rotator cuff strengthen the capsule superiorly by fusing with it, but inferiorly the capsule hangs loose.

The Synovial Membrane. The capsule is lined by synovial membrane. A sleeve of synovial membrane invests the tendon of the long head of the biceps (Figs. 13–1, 13–10). The tendon is intra-articular from its attachment to the upper lip of the glenoid fossa and labrum to the transverse ligament in the intertubercular groove. The synovial membrane of the joint is continuous with that of the subscapularis bursa which always communicates with the joint (Fig. 13–1).

Nerve Supply. The capsule is supplied by sensory nerves and the synovial membrane predominantly by sympathetic vasomotor nerves. Both types are

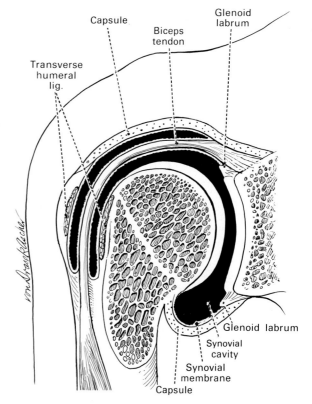

FIG. 13-10. The glenohumeral joint. Schematic representation of a coronal section to show the relationship of the glenoid cavity, the labrum, capsule, and biceps tendon.

derived from articular branches of the nerves that supply the prime movers of the joint. Most important are the axillary and suprascapular nerves.

Movements

Practically all movements in which the humerus swings or slides on the glenoid fossa are accompanied by scapulothoracic and sternoclavicular movements. Scapular and clavicular movements become more pronounced as the humeral swing increases and may continue after the close-packed position has been obtained at the shoulder joint. For the understanding of shoulder mechanisms and also in clinical evaluation of this region, glenohumeral movements are more profitably analyzed by considering the joints in succession rather than simultaneously. The shoulder joint may be abducted and adducted, flexed and extended, and laterally and medially rotated. An uninterrupted succession of these movements produces circumduction.

Abduction. The total range of abduction is 180°, and at its maximum the medial surface of the arm

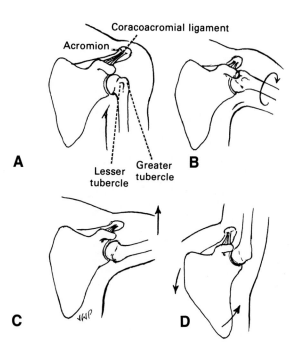

FIG. 13–11. Conjunct rotation of the humerus laterally places a large area of articular surface above the glenoid cavity (**B** and **C**), extending the range of glenohumeral abduction from around 90° to 120°. An additional 60° of movement is attained by scapular rotation (**D**). (Based on Last RJ: Anatomy, 5th ed. London, Churchill, 1973)

can touch the ear. The harmony between glenohumeral and scapulothoracic movement is particularly well illustrated during abduction of the arm. For every 15° of movement, 10° occur at the glenohumeral joint and 5° at the scapulothoracic joint. From a clinical point of view, abduction is the most useful movement to test. A significant anatomic defect of the shoulder may be ruled out if the arm can be abducted through 180° without pain and under perfect control.

When abduction is analyzed on the skeleton, it is easy to appreciate that moving the humerus from a pendent position until the humeral and glenoid articular surfaces come edge to edge superiorly, 90° of abduction can be obtained (Fig. 13–11). This range can be increased to 120° by rotating the humerus laterally, so that the large area of the humeral head now facing downward comes to lie superiorly. The remaining 60° of abduction are accounted for by scapular and clavicular movement.

The fixed point of the scapula is at the acromioclavicular joint, and at 120° of abduction, close-packed position of the glenohumeral joint was secured. Therefore, humerus and scapula will be moved as one unit by the abduction force in relation to the fixed point at the acromioclavicular joint. This force is provided by rotator muscles of the scapula which increase the angle between the superior border of the scapula and the clavicle. This angulation generates tension in the coracoclavicular ligaments and, therefore, the clavicle will be elevated and rotated mainly via forces acting on the scapula.

It was emphasized at the outset that movement occurs simultaneously at all joints almost from the start of abduction. However, it is possible to restrain scapular and clavicular movements by grasping the scapula firmly by its inferior angle. Glenohumeral movement can then be assessed independently.

The **rotation element** of humeral abduction needs clarification. The humerus *rotates laterally* during abduction. In the majority of individuals (though not in all), voluntary medial rotation of the humerus restricts glenohumeral abduction. Contrary to common opinion, the cause of lateral rotation is not impingement of the greater tubercle on the acromion. In all instances, the tubercle slides under the acromion. Its passage is facilitated by a large bursa (subacromial-subdeltoid bursa) and the tubercle never *bumps* (Fig. 13–12B,C). The rotatory element in abduction is an inevitable outcome of the geometric properties of the articulating surfaces. In the loose-packed position of the joint, the point of contact between humerus and glenoid slides along a succession of arcs on an ovoid surface. The rotation will occur *passively* (consequential movement or **conjunct rotation**) as a result of abduction force without the assistance of lateral rotators. The point in question was introduced in Chapter 5 (see Fig. 5–12) and is instructively demonstrated by an interesting exercise.

Press the palm of the hand against the thigh and, henceforth, keep the hand in this position. Now flex the arm to the horizontal and then swing it out laterally (i.e., extend it). When the hand is returned to the thigh, the palm of the hand faces forward. Repeating the same cycle all over, starting from this position, will place the back of the hand against the thigh. The humerus has clearly rotated laterally as a consequence of flexion, extension, and adduction without any *active* rotation. It can be made to rotate medially in a like manner by performing the exercise in the reversed sequence.

The Force of Abduction. The prime movers of glenohumeral abduction are the **supraspinatus** and the **deltoid** (Fig. 13–13). The large size of the deltoid and the prominent acromion, from which the deltoid largely arises, are features characteristic of the shoulder of man. The deltoid provides the power of abduction while the supraspinatus is particularly important in initiating abduction and stabilizing the humeral head in its shallow socket. The supraspinatus is assisted in the latter task by the other short scapular muscles: **subscapularis**, **infraspinatus**, and **teres minor** (Fig. 13–14). These four muscles converge upon the greater and lesser tubercles, and before reaching them their tendons fuse with the capsule of the shoulder joint and with each other, forming in effect a cuff around the superior aspect of the joint. The integrity of this mechanism, known as the **rotator cuff** is essential for abduction and plays an important stabilizing

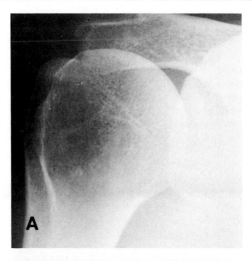

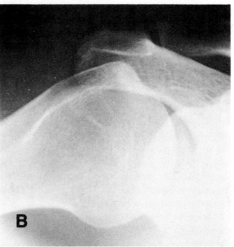

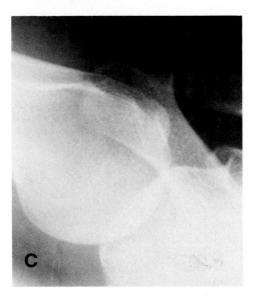

FIG. 13–12. Sequential x-rays taken during abduction of the humerus to show that the greater tubercle slides under the acromion and impingement of the tubercle on the acromion plays no part in bringing about lateral rotation of the humerus. **(A)** Neutral position. **(B)** At approximately 90° abduction the greater tubercle passed well beyond the lateral margin of the acromion. **(C)** At about 120° the acromion shelters a large part of the proximal end of the humerus. Scapular rotation has already taken place. (Courtesy of Dr. Rosalind H. Troupin)

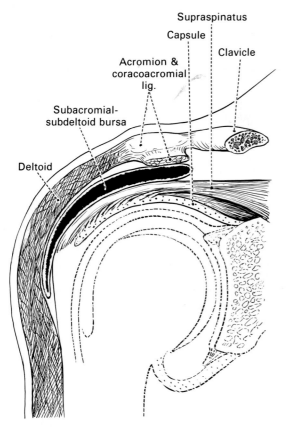

Supraspinatus

Capsule

Clavicle

Acromion &
coracoacromial
lig.

Subacromial-
subdeltoid bursa

Deltoid

FIG. 13-13. Coronal section of the shoulder joint shown schematically to illustrate the position of the deltoid and supraspinatus in relation to the subacromial bursa and the shoulder joint capsule. For orientation refer to Figure 13-10.

role in all the movements of the humerus. Although the term *rotator cuff* is widely used, not all the muscles contributing to it are rotators of the humerus. Notably, the supraspinatus, most frequently involved in rotator cuff lesions, is purely an abductor. *Tendinous cuff* is a preferable term.

The triangular, bulky mass of the **deltoid** is composed of three parts. Anterior and posterior fibers which arise from clavicle and scapular spine, respectively, are parallel and are more suited for flexing and extending the joint than abducting it. The central portion of the muscle takes origin by shorter fibers from the acromion and these fibers insert into tendinous septa within the muscle from which in turn new fibers originate. This multipennate arrangement lends power to the muscle and it is this central portion which is active in abduction. All three parts of the muscle insert into a rough tuberosity half way down the shaft of the humerus.

Thus, the general direction of all muscle fibers is vertical.

Although activity is evident in the muscle from the beginning of abduction, it can only exert abduction power if the humeral head is stabilized. If it is not, the deltoid simply elevates the humerus in the pendent position without any abduction. The deltoid is innervated by the **axillary nerve,** (C5, C6). The nerve reaches the muscle by passing along the inferior aspect of the joint capsule as it leaves the axilla and then skirts around the surgical neck of the humerus. It is susceptible to injury in shoulder dislocation, in humeral neck fracture, and when injections are delivered into the deltoid. When the deltoid is wasted, the point of the shoulder becomes prominent. The power of the muscle is best tested by opposing abduction at about 45°. Once the arm is raised above the head, the deltoid largely relaxes.

The **supraspinatus** is active throughout abduction. The muscle is said to be the *workhorse of abduction*. It fills the supraspinous fossa where its hard muscle belly may be palpated during abduction through the trapezius (Fig. 13-14B). The muscle is ideally placed for initiating abduction by spurt action, and its contraction is necessary for the deltoid to obtain a purchase (Fig. 13-13). The supraspinatus is innervated chiefly by C5 through a branch of the brachial plexus (suprascapular nerve).

Force Couples and Rotator Cuff Defects. Both supraspinatus and deltoid exert an upward force on the humeral head, which has to be counterbalanced if the humerus is to remain stabilized on the glenoid fossa. The weight of the arm provides such a counterforce, and the contractions of subscapularis and teres minor due to the obliquity of their fibers exert a force on the humeral head which has a downward component (Fig. 13-14). Normal shoulder abduction depends on the operation of these force couples. One vector is provided by the prime movers of abduction and the other by the weight of the arm plus the short scapular muscles.

Consideration of the force couples explains why tears or paralysis in rotator cuff musculature (not only of the supraspinatus) seriously impair shoulder abduction. In cases of acute tears the limiting factor will be pain. Muscle paralysis is assessed by feeling for contraction over the respective muscle bellies.

In typical cases of supraspinatus tendon tear or paralysis, abduction cannot be initiated actively, but will proceed normally through deltoid action if the limb is moved passively into 20–30° abduction. The patient may achieve this much abduction by automatically leaning toward the affected side and letting the arm hang. Some patients may abduct the arm in the presence of rotator cuff lesions, and may support it above the head without difficulty. However, in either case, the patient will be unable to support the arm at 90° of abduction because one of the members of the force couple is missing.

Scapular rotation, the final element of arm abduction, is also achieved through force couples, that is forces pulling tangentially on prominences of the scapula to bring about its rotation. The upper part of the **trapezius** and the lower half of the **serratus anterior** turn the scapula like a wing-nut, the wings being the acromion and the inferior angle of the scapula. The portion of the trapezius which attaches to the base of the scapular spine also aids this action (Fig. 13–15).

Adduction. The powerful axillary fold muscles adduct the arm. Anteriorly, the pectoralis major (Fig. 13–7) and posteriorly the latissimus dorsi (Fig. 13–6) and teres major are the prime movers. A functionally insignificant muscle, the coracobrachialis, which originates from the coracoid and inserts into the humeral shaft, is also a prime adductor and represents the only counterpart in the upper limb of the massive adductor musculature of the lower limb.

Adduction is limited by contact between the arm and the rib cage, but the movement may be continued in front of the chest. Protraction of the pectoral girdle contributes significantly to the latter phase of the movement. Powerful adductor movements are required in climbing. The adductor muscles may also be called into action as accessory muscles of respiration when a breathless individual leans on the arms. The points of insertion being now stabilized, these attachments function as points of origin and the chest wall will be lifted by contraction of adductor musculature.

The **pectoralis major** (Fig. 13–7) is a large fan-shaped muscle that covers the front of the rib cage from clavicle to the sixth or seventh rib. From such a wide area of origin, the fibers converge and twist

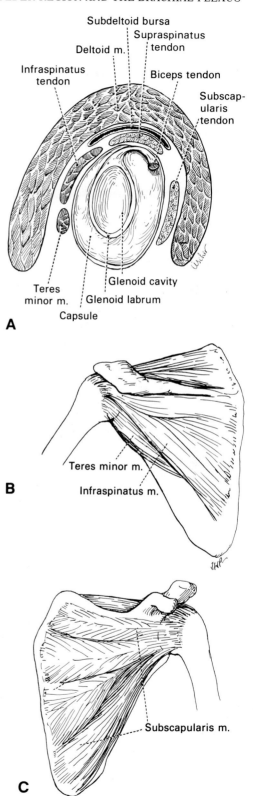

FIG. 13–14. Muscles and tendons of the rotator cuff sheltered by the deltoid. **(A)** Lateral view of the socket of the shoulder joint after the humerus with its muscles has been removed. **(B)** The posterior and **(C)** the anterior aspects of the rotator cuff muscles.

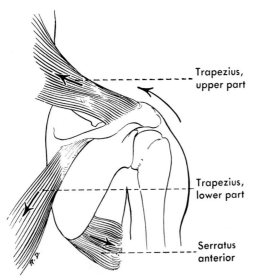

FIG. 13–15. The muscles which rotate the scapula upward during abduction of the arm. (From Hollinshead WH: Anatomy for Surgeons, vol. 3, 2nd ed. New York, Hoeber, 1969)

upon themselves in the axillary fold before inserting into the lateral lip of the intertubercular sulcus as a ribbonlike tendon. The fibers most active in adduction arise from the manubrium and sternum. The clavicular fibers, on the other hand, are prime movers in flexion, and the costal fibers extend the flexed humerus (the latter also depress the shoulder). Both muscles will spring into prominence if the hands are pressed together in the position of prayer, some distance in front of the body. The pectoralis major is supplied segmentally by C5-T1 through two branches of the brachial plexus (lateral and medial pectoral nerves). The central portion concerned chiefly with adduction receives C7 and C8.

The **latissimus dorsi** (Fig. 13–6) has migrated further from the upper limb bud than any other upper limb muscle. The muscle is superficial to the erector spinae and covers the lower half of the back. From a very extensive origin, the thin muscular sheet converges toward the posterior axillary fold where it twists around the teres major, similar to the twist of the pectoralis major upon itself. Together with the teres major, the latissimus dorsi inserts into the medial lip of the intertubercular groove. The muscle is supplied by the thoracodorsal branch (C6,C7,C8) of the brachial plexus.

The **teres major** arises from the posterior aspect of the inferior angle of the scapula and it is supplied by yet another branch of the brachial plexus (lower subscapular nerve, C6,C7). Both teres major and latissimus dorsi can be demonstrated in the posterior axillary folds when the arm is adducted against resistance which is the method for testing their strength clinically. Clearly, both muscles are well situated also for shoulder extension. It is a peculiarity of the teres major that activity cannot be recorded in it during active adduction or extension, but only when these movements are resisted or during involuntary movements like swinging the arms during walking.

Flexion-Extension. Although the scapula is placed obliquely, for most purposes it is adequate to measure flexion and extension in the sagittal rather than in an oblique plane. The prime movers have already been described. The flexors are the clavicular portion of the pectoralis major and clavicular fibers of the deltoid. The extensors are the latissimus dorsi, teres major, and posterior fibers of the deltoid.

Rotation. Lateral rotation may be tested by swinging the forearm laterally when it is flexed in the horizontal position. A simple way of assessing medial rotation is to ask the patient to place his hand between his two scapulae. These movements may also be checked in the supine position (Fig. 13–16).

Muscles which attach anterior to the vertical axis of the humerus will medially rotate the humerus; those that attach posterior to the axis will laterally rotate it. Prime movers in medial rotation are the subscapularis, pectoralis major, latissimus dorsi, teres major, and clavicular fibers of the deltoid. Prime movers of lateral rotation are the infraspinatus, teres minor, and posterior fibers of deltoid.

Factors of Stability

Unlike at the hip, bony contours of the shoulder joint do not contribute anything to stability. Of the capsular ligaments only the coracohumeral ligament plays a significant role in supporting the weight of the arm. **Stability is effected mainly by muscle action.** The chief muscular stabilizers are the rotator cuff muscles (Figs. 13–13, 13–14). The coracoacromial arch, consisting of the acromion, coracoacromial ligament, and coracoid process (Fig. 13–1), the rotator cuff, and the biceps tendon

(Figs. 13–10, 13–14) are structures which reinforce the joint on its upper aspect. They have no counterparts inferiorly; hence, dislocation usually occurs in this direction. In the majority of cases, the head of the dislocated humerus rests in the axilla just below the coracoid (anterior or subcoracoid dislocation) (Fig. 13–4B), where it may be palpated. Compression of the brachial plexus, the axillary artery, and particularly, the axillary nerve must be looked for in these cases. The muscles which run in relation to the inferior aspect of the joint (triceps, short head of biceps, coracobrachialis) play no active role in stabilizing the joint.

THE AXILLA

The axilla is a space through which the blood and lymph vessels and the nerves pass as they course between the thorax, the neck, and the upper limb. It is a pyramid-shaped space and is bordered medially by the serratus anterior covering the thoracic cage, posteriorly by the subscapularis covering the scapula, anteriorly by the deep surfaces of the pectoral muscles and clavicle, and laterally by the arm. The base or floor consists of the axillary fascia. Its more important contents are the axillary artery and vein, lymph nodes, and the brachial plexus with its branches. These structures are embedded in fat.

The **axillary artery** is the continuation of the subclavian artery and itself becomes the brachial artery, which is the main artery of the upper limb. The artery is surrounded by the cords of the brachial plexus and the major nerves arising from this plexus. The branches of the axillary artery supply the muscles and joints of the shoulder and pectoral regions. They establish a free anastomosis around the scapula between the branches of the subclavian and brachial arteries **(circumscapular anastomosis),** so that occlusion of the artery in the axilla does not interfere seriously with the blood supply of the upper limb.

Lymph nodes of the axilla receive and filter the lymph from the upper limb and from the anterior and posterior aspects of the trunk as far distal as the umbilicus and iliac crest. Lymph from the breasts drains predominantly to the axillary nodes and also to the parasternal nodes inside the rib cage.

Examination of the axilla should include palpation of the axillary artery and the axillary lymph

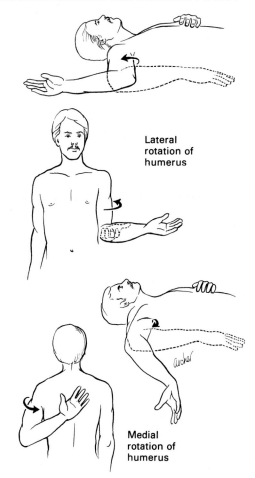

FIG. 13–16. Methods of testing lateral and medial rotation of the humerus in the erect and supine patient.

nodes. The latter, particularly if enlarged or inflamed, may be palpated against the ribs deep in the axilla, while the artery is best felt by compressing it against the humerus.

CLINICAL EVALUATION OF THE SHOULDER REGION

The region of the shoulder is a complex area, in which complaints may arise from arthritis or injury in three different joints (sternoclavicular, acromioclavicular, and glenohumeral) as well as from neuromuscular dysfunction, degeneration in tendons and ligaments, or from inflammation of muscles, fasciae, bursae, and synovial sheaths. An end stage phenomenon resulting from a variety of these inflammatory processes is known as the **frozen shoulder** in which adhesions, deformities, and contractures materially restrict all movements of the shoulder and any attempt at movement is aggravated by pain. In addition, complaints may be due to compression of related nerves and blood vessels or due to pain referred to the shoulder from the cervical spine or from the thorax and abdomen. In childhood, septic arthritis may affect the glenohumeral joint, while in the adult degenerative changes commonly involve a number of structures individually or in combination. Major and minor injuries and the sequelae are common causes of pain and disability in this region. Meticulous, systematic evaluation of the patient is essential because complaints in the shoulder region are especially prone to misinterpretation.

Evaluation of the brachial plexus and its branches is usually included in the physical examination of the shoulder, but in this book will be deferred until the anatomy of the plexus and the distribution of its branches have been presented.

Symptoms

Pain, swelling, clicking, and limitation of movement are the usual complaints.

Pain from the acromioclavicular and sternoclavicular joints is usually localized to the joints themselves, but may radiate from the latter to the anterior chest wall. Pain from the glenohumeral joint is felt over the tip of the shoulder and characteristically radiates in most cases as far down the arm as the insertion of the deltoid. Problems with the rotator cuff, subacromial-subdeltoid bursa, and the biceps tendon have a pain distribution similar to that of the glenohumeral joint itself. Pain from nerve or nerve root compression conforms to the area of distribution of the structure involved, and may radiate into the neck. Pain from the thoracic or abdominal surface of the diaphragm is referred mainly to dermatome C4 (see Fig. 12–4) and is usually associated with thoracic or abdominal symptoms and signs. If physical examination of the shoulder does not identify any structural lesion, a general survey and examination of other parts of the body is called for.

Clicking is usually associated with specific movements and may be due to recurrent dislocation of the humerus, subluxation of the sternoclavicular or acromioclavicular joints, or displacement of the biceps tendon from its groove.

In acute cases, **limitation of movement** may be due to pain or to injury or paralysis of various structures which have to be identified by examination.

Physical Examination

Inspection. Both shoulders, pectoral regions, and upper limbs have to be bare of clothing, including shoulder straps. Comparison of the two sides is the key to detecting abnormalities.

The patient is inspected in the standing or sitting position from the front, side, and then from back views as well as from above the shoulder, paying attention in each view to

1. Symmetry of bony prominences including the clavicle (medial end, body, lateral end), spine and inferior angle of the scapula, curvature of the vertebral column.
2. Symmetry of soft tissue contours including the neck, back, shoulder, pectoral region.
3. Localized swellings, scars, discoloration of skin.
4. Muscle bulk, noting especially trapezius, supraspinous and infraspinous fossae, deltoid, pectoralis major, biceps.
5. Muscle fasciculation.

An abnormally prominent tip of the shoulder may be due to atrophy of the deltoid, dislocation of the humerus, or acromioclavicular separation. Spinal curvatures displace the scapula and distort the symmetry of the level of the shoulders. The scapula may be congenitally high on one side.

Palpation. All bones, joints, and potential sites of common pathology should be palpated systematically. Standing behind the patient, the examiner should place one hand on each shoulder and commence palpation medially. As palpation proceeds laterally, attention should be paid to areas of tenderness, increased skin temperature, swellings, bony irregularities, and consistency of the muscles. A typical sequence for the palpation is as follows:

1. Jugular notch, interclavicular ligament, insertion of the sternomastoids, sternoclavicular joint.
2. Convex and concave curves of the clavicle.
3. Acromioclavicular joint and acromion.
4. The greater tubercle, just lateral and inferior to the tip of the shoulder. This small area is of great diagnostic importance and should be palpated with precision.

Lateral rotation of the arm produces palpable movement of the tubercle, verifying that the palpating hand is on the humerus. This movement also makes the intertubercular groove more accessible as palpation proceeds anteriorly. Tenderness may be due to tear or degeneration in the supraspinatus tendon or in other tendons of the cuff, as well as to inflammation in the subacromial-subdeltoid bursa or to pathology in the biceps tendon and its synovial sheath.

In lateral rotation, the biceps tendon should be palpated down to the fleshy belly. Then the arm should be passively extended, which rotates the superior surface of the greater tubercle anteriorly, exposing it for palpation just anterior to the acromion. In this position, the insertion of the rotator cuff muscles is better palpable. Tenderness due to inflammation of the bursa usually extends more inferiorly and laterally, and it is not specifically localized over the intertubercular groove. Furthermore, when the bursa is involved, the patient usually resists all attempts to move the joint.

5. With the arm hanging and laterally rotated the lesser tubercle is palpable anterior to the groove, and on level with it medially is the tip of the coracoid process.

6. Returning to the acromion, the spine of the scapula should be palated along its edges (feeling for tenderness in the insertion of the trapezius) and then along the vertebral border of the scapula (feeling the insertion of the levator scapulae and rhomboids).

7. The following muscles should be palpated: the superolateral edge of the trapezius in the neck, supraclavicular and infraclavicular fossae; posterior, middle, and anterior parts of the deltoid; pectoralis major, biceps, including its short head running in the axilla to the coracoid process.

8. In the axilla, the head of the humerus, the axillary artery, the chest wall, lymph nodes.

9. In the supraclavicular fossa, nerve trunks of the brachial plexus, lymph nodes.

Range of Motion. Passive range of movement must be tested if the active range is found to be limited. The most important movement to evaluate is abduction. If no abnormality was detected by palpation and if the patient performs 180° of abduction smoothly without any pain or effort, other movements need not be tested. If there is limitation of abduction, the cause and site of the limitation must be determined by evaluating separately glenohumeral, scapulothoracic, and sternoclavicular movements. These movements have been described adequately along with other move-

ments of the shoulder in the preceding sections. Testing of **muscle strength,** the next item in the physical exam, has likewise been described along with the anatomy of individual muscles.

THE BRACHIAL PLEXUS

The brachial plexus is an ordered network of large nerves through which the sensory and motor nerve supply is distributed to all structures that constitute the upper limb. The brachial plexus is formed by the ventral rami of C5-T1 spinal nerves, and it conforms to the general plan of a limb plexus already discussed in Chapters 11 and 12. Understanding of the plexus is essential for comprehension of normal and disordered neuromuscular and sensory functions in the upper limb.

Types of Nerve Fibers

The brachial plexus is composed predominantly of somatic nerve fibers, both efferent and afferent, but nerves from the sympathetic component of the autonomic nervous system also join the brachial plexus and are distributed to the limb with its branches (Chap. 10).

Somatic Efferent Fibers. Motor fibers for skeletal muscle of the upper limbs arise in anterior horn cells of segments C5-T1. Groups of these motor neurons constitute the lateral portions of the anterior horns in these segments (Fig. 10–4). They serve all the motor units in upper limb musculature.

Somatic Afferent Fibers. Exteroceptive (pain, temperature, pressure, touch) and proprioceptive (joint and position sense, muscle spindle) impulses are conveyed from the limb by afferent fibers whose cell bodies are located in spinal ganglia C5-T1.

Sympathetic Nerve Fibers. Presynaptic sympathetic nerve fibers for the upper limb originate in the lateral horn neurons of upper thoracic segments (T2-T5), pass along the sympathetic chain, and relay in cervical and thoracic sympathetic ganglia (Fig. 13–17). Postsynaptic fibers reach the brachial plexus via grey rami communicantes associated mainly with C8 and T1 spinal nerves. The sympathetic nerves are distributed with the branches of the brachial plexus to smooth muscle of the blood vessels and hair follicles and to sweat glands.

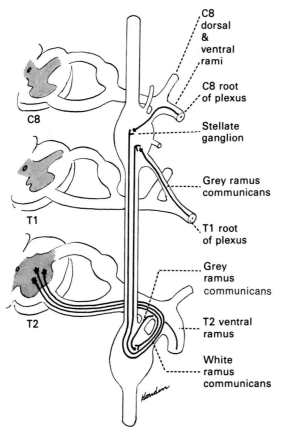

C8
dorsal
&
ventral
rami

C8 root
of plexus

C8

Stellate
ganglion

T1

Grey ramus
communicans

T1 root
of plexus

Grey
ramus
communicans

T2

T2 ventral
ramus

White
ramus
communicans

FIG. 13–17. Origin and course of the sympathetic nerve fibers which are distributed to the upper limb via the brachial plexus.

Formation and Component Parts

The basic plan of the plexus is shown in Figure 13–18. The ventral rami of C5-T1 spinal nerves are known as the **roots** of the brachial plexus. Before splitting into divisions, the roots unite to form three **trunks.** C5 and C6 form the **upper trunk,** C7 continues alone as the **middle trunk,** and C8 and T1 unite into the **lower trunk.** The regrouping of nerve fibers destined for the flexor and extensor compartments takes place at this level. Each trunk splits into an **anterior** and a **posterior division.** The respective sets of divisions unite to form the **cords** of the plexus. All the posterior divisions merge in the **posterior cord** and, therefore, in it are gathered all nerves (C5-T1) for the extensor compartment. It lies posterior to the axillary artery. The axillary artery splits the **anterior cord** into two; the two halves being known as the **lateral** and **medial cords.** The lateral cord gathers the anterior divi-

sion of the upper and middle trunks (C5,C6, and C7) and the medial cord is made up by the continuation of the anterior division of the lower trunk (C8,T1). The two cords together supply the flexor compartment.

The spinal cord segments that contribute to the plexus are suprisingly constant and so is the organizational plan of the plexus. Rarely, there may be a substantial input from C4, in which case the plexus is said to be *prefixed.* When T2 contributes significantly, the plexus is *postfixed.* Both instances result in appropriate shifts in the apportionment of different segments to the cords and main branches. Although connective tissue which defines the usual anatomic subdivisions of the plexus may not separate them according to the plan described, the normal subdivisions are usually demonstrable by splitting connective tissue planes in the plexus.

Branches

The main nerves of the upper limb (see Chap. 11) are terminal branches of the cords. In addition, a number of small branches are given off from the roots, trunks, and cords for the supply of pectoral girdle musculature and to the skin along the medial aspect of the limb.

Main Terminal Branches (Figs. 13–18, 11–8, 11–10). The testing of the main nerves will be discussed after the musculature and joints of the free limb have been studied. It is useful, however, to attach from the outset a broad functional designation to each of these nerves.

The **posterior cord** terminates in two main nerves: the radial and axillary.

1. The **radial nerve** (C5-T1) supplies the extensor musculature of the elbow, wrist, and digits. It is sensory to the skin on the extensor surface of the arm, forearm, and hand. *The radial nerve is the nerve of extension.*
2. The **axillary nerve** (C5,C6) *supplies the chief abductor of the shoulder,* the deltoid, and the skin overlying it. It is also sensory to the shoulder joint.

The two **anterior cords** terminate in three major nerves. Both **lateral and medial cords** contribute to the formation of the median nerve; the musculocutaneous nerve originates from lateral cord and the ulnar nerve from the medial cord.

1. The **musculocutaneous nerve** (C5,C6) is *the chief nerve of elbow flexion.* It also supplies skin on the preaxial border of the forearm.

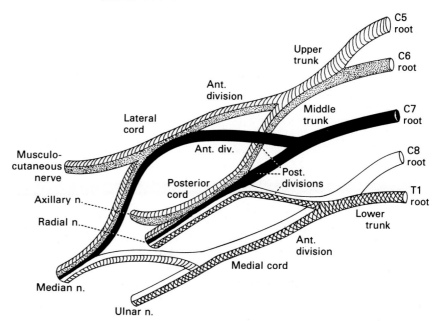

FIG. 13-18. The basic plan of the brachial plexus and its major terminal branches. Each root of the plexus is identified by a different pattern of shading to illustrate the manner of its distribution as it proceeds through the plexus.

2. The **median nerve** (C6,C7,C8,T1) is *the chief nerve of sensation in the hand* because it supplies the pulp of the digits commonly used for feeling. It is also the *chief nerve for pronation* and for flexion of the wrist and of the digits. It supplies the bulk of the muscles in the flexor compartment of the forearm, and in the hand most of the muscles of the thumb.

3. The **ulnar nerve** (C8, T1, C7) is the *chief nerve of the intrinsic muscles of the hand.* It also supplies some forearm muscles in the flexor compartment, and skin over the postaxial half of the hand. The nerve receives a contribution from the anterior division of C7, sometimes as a delicate slip in the plexus, other times lower down as a communicating branch from the median nerve.

Small Branches of the Plexus (Fig. 13–19). Brachial plexus injuries can be localized more precisely by testing the smaller branches which originate from different parts of the plexus. The testing of all the muscles these branches supply has been discussed with the movements of the pectoral girdle.

From C5 root the **dorsal scapular nerve** proceeds posteriorly to the rhomboids and levator scapulae. C5, C6 and C7 roots give origin to the **long thoracic**

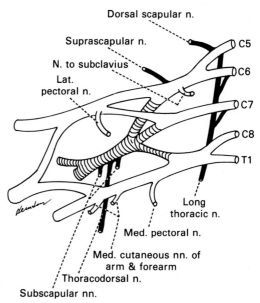

FIG. 13-19. Smaller branches of the brachial plexus from roots, trunks, and cords. The posterior divisions and cord are shaded.

nerve which descends posterior to the roots and continues in the axilla on the surface of the serratus anterior which it supplies.

Two branches arise from the upper trunk; the other trunks have none. The **suprascapular nerve** (C5,C6) heads for the supraspinatus, passing through the notch in the upper border of the scapula, supplies the muscle, and continues to the infraspinatus. It is also sensory to the shoulder and acromioclavicular joint. The second small branch of the upper trunk supplies the subclavius muscle which is concealed by the clavicle and cannot be tested.

In addition to their terminal branches, one nerve is given off by the lateral cord and three by each medial and posterior cord. The **lateral pectoral nerve** (C5,C6,C7) is the branch of the lateral cord (hence its name) and together with the **medial pectoral nerve** (C8, T1), given off by the medial cord, they supply the pectoralis major and minor. The remaining two branches of the medial cord are cutaneous: the **medial cutaneous nerves** of the arm and forearm. On the posterior cord the thoracodorsal nerve originates between two subscapular nerves. The **thoracodorsal nerve** (C6,C7,C8) supplies the latissimus dorsi, and the two **subscapular nerves** (C5,C6) supply the subscapularis and teres major (the teres minor is supplied by the axillary nerve).

Anatomic Relations, Compression Syndromes, and Injuries

The roots and trunks of the brachial plexus are in the neck, the divisions are behind the clavicle, the cords and major nerves are in the axilla grouped around the axillary artery. Clearly, branches of the roots and trunks are above the clavicle and those of the cords inferior to it. In the neck, the plexus may be palpated posterior to the sternomastoid and feels like a bunch of tense cords. The cords of the plexus, however, are not discernible in the axilla.

The roots of the plexus emerge between the scalene muscles. The prevertebral fascia continues with them laterally and encloses the entire plexus in a fascial sleeve. The axillary artery is also within the sleeve but the axillary vein lies outside and more anterior. During movements of the arm the fascial sleeve facilitates sliding of the brachial plexus in the axilla. It will also confine local anesthetic injected around the plexus.

Compression Syndromes. The brachial plexus is subject to compression in three areas: 1) between the scalene muscles, over the first thoracic rib, by a cervical rib or its fibrous vestige, 2) behind a deformed clavicle, 3) underneath the coracoid process and pectoralis minor.

Arterial compression is usually part of the syndrome in all three instances. Consequently, the pulse at the wrist is weaker, or may disappear on the affected side. The vein may also be compressed by the coracoid or the clavicle, resulting in swelling and edema of the hand and arm. Pain and paresthesia (tingling, numbness) have the distribution of the affected nerves as do muscle weakness and atrophy.

Most commonly T1 root is compressed either by a rib or by increased tone in the scaleni (**scalene syndrome** or **thoracic outlet syndrome**). The symptoms and signs are exaggerated by extension of the arm and retraction of the shoulder. Irritation of the sympathetic fibers in the affected roots may result in vasoconstriction leading to painful ischemic changes in the hand (Raynaud's disease) and may lead to gangrene. Hyperextension of the arm at 45° abduction will reproduce the syndrome of clavicular or coracoid compression of the neurovascular structures. The radial pulse may be obliterated by this manuever in many normal individuals who have no symptoms or signs.

Injuries. In addition to compression (described above) the brachial plexus may be injured by penetrating wounds or by traction on the upper limb. Penetrating injuries are localized, and may occur anywhere in the plexus, while traction injuries usually affect the roots of the plexus. The latter are more common and more serious.

Traction force may be applied to the plexus in two ways: 1) by increasing the angle between the neck and the shoulder and 2) through the abducted arm.

When the body is forcefully thrown and lands with the shoulder against the ground, neck and shoulder will be forced apart and the upper roots of the plexus (C5,C6) become evulsed. The same type of injury may result from pulling on the fetal head during delivery. On the other hand, when the arm is wrenched or when it catches the weight of the body falling from a height, the lower roots (C8,T1) will suffer damage. C5-C6 lesions will leave the patient with a greatly disabled shoulder, but a reasonably functional hand, whereas damage to C8-T1 will produce the reverse picture.

The prognosis is influenced by the actual site of the tear. This may be fairly precisely located by knowledge of anatomic distribution of sensory and motor components of the affected roots and of the branching pattern of spinal nerves. With the aid of Chapters 11 and 12 and this chapter, it should be possible to construct the clinical picture which results from the interruption of individual roots, trunks, or cords of the plexus. Some of the references listed will be helpful in such an endeavor. This diagnostic exercise has to be performed in the reverse in clinical practice where the lesion has to be identified from the clinical picture.

SUGGESTED READING

Adams, J. C. Outline of Orthopedics, 6th ed. Baltimore, Williams & Wilkins, 1968.
Chapter 5 gives a concise, clear description of important disorders of the shoulder and discusses their diagnosis and treatment.

Aids to the Investigation of Peripheral Nerve Injuries. Medical Research Council War Memorandum No. 7, 2nd ed. London, Her Majesty's Stationary Office, 1943.
A brief pictorial guide to the testing of nerves and muscles.

Bateman, J. E. The Shoulder and Neck. Philadelphia, W. B. Saunders, 1972.
A comprehensive monograph dealing with the normal and surgical anatomy, evolution, embryology, congenital anomalies of the shoulder as well as with the diagnosis and treatment of many abnormalities. Extensive bibliography with each chapter and good illustrations of basic concepts and clinical cases.

Haymaker, W., and Woodhall, B. Peripheral Nerve Injuries, 2nd ed. Philadelphia, W. B. Saunders, 1967.
Many examples of nerve injury are illustrated and discussed.

Hollinshead, W. H. Anatomy for Surgeons, Vol. 3, The Back and Limbs, 2nd ed. New York, Harper & Row, 1969.
Chapters 3 and 4 give a scholarly account of the shoulder region and brachial plexus including variations and such important abnormalities as brachial plexus lesions. Extensive bibliography.

Hoppenfeld, S. Physical Examination of the Spine and Extremities. New York, Appleton-Century-Crofts, 1976.
Chapter 1 is probably the best description of the physical examination of the shoulder in the literature. The diagnostic tests are simple and well-illustrated.

Inman, V. T., Saunders, J. B. deC. and Abbott, L. C. Observations on the function of the shoulder joint. J. Bone. Joint Surg. [A] 26:1, 1944.
A classical experimental study which deals with the shoulder from a comparative anatomical and dynamic point of view. The function of individual muscles is analyzed during movements of the shoulder.

Lucas, D. B. Biomechanics of the shoulder joint. Arch. Surg. 107:425, 1973.
A brief article dealing with the concept of force couples.

MacConnaill, M. A., and Basmajian, J. V. Muscles and Movements. Baltimore, Williams & Wilkins, 1969.
Chapter 10 gives an interesting analysis of movements of the shoulder and of the muscles concerned. Description of conjunct rotation of the humerus in the present chapter is based on this book.

Stanwood, J. E., and Kraft, G. H. Diagnosis and management of brachial plexus injuries. Arch. Phys. Med. Rehab. 52:52, 1971.
A concise description of brachial plexus injuries and their prognosis. A very practical and useful article.

14

The Arm, Forearm, and Wrist

CORNELIUS ROSSE

In the previous chapter, the topographic and functional anatomy of the shoulder region was discussed with reference to movements possible at the shoulder. The anatomy of the arm, forearm, and wrist will be treated in the same way, and physical examination will be presented together with the anatomy.

The large muscles which flex and extend the elbow occupy the flexor and extensor compartments of the arm. The respective compartments of the forearm house the flexor and extensor musculature of the wrist and digits. The latter are regarded as the extrinsic muscles of the hand. Although the hand can also be abducted and adducted, specific muscles do not exist for these movements in the forearm. Abduction and adduction of the hand is performed by combined action of wrist flexors and extensors on the radial or ulnar side of the limb. Both flexor and extensor compartments of the forearm contain muscles that move the forearm bones in relation to one another. These are the pronators and supinators. Disease or structural defects in any part of the upper limb will affect hand function, and in the last analysis the evaluation of functional anatomy of the upper limb has to be based on the hand.

THE SKELETON OF THE FREE LIMB INCLUDING THE HAND

The bones and joints of the hand, forearm, and arm are frequently injured. The diagnosis often has to be made on physical signs, as x-rays may be negative. It is essential that the student and the clinician should be familiar with the anatomy of the bones not only on the skeleton, but also in the living limb and on x-rays.

Humerus

The cylindrical shaft of the humerus is palpable through the muscles from the surgical neck of the bone to the elbow. The shaft is most accessible medially, between the flexor and extensor muscles. The palpable features of the proximal end have already been described in Chapter 13. The lower end is expanded but flattened, and its sharp edges project laterally and medially as the **supracondylar ridges** (Fig. 14–1). Both are palpable. Each ridge terminates in a bony prominence, the **medial** and **lateral epicondyles.** The condyle or articular portion of the lower end is between them and is out of reach. It will be described with the elbow joint.

Above the epicondyles, a fibrous membrane projects from each supracondylar ridge and augments the bony surfaces for muscle attachments. These are the **intermuscular septa** (Fig. 14–7). Together with the humerus, the septa separate the flexor and extensor compartments.

Radius and Ulna

In the resting position of the arm and also during the performance of most common tasks, the radius is crossed over the ulna, and the forearm is pronated. The parallel or supinated position of the bones is the *anatomic position* but not the natural position of the limb.

Both radius and ulna have an expanded and a narrow end, joined by a shaft. The narrow end of each bone is its *head*. The head of the radius is at the elbow while the head of the ulna is at the wrist. Both heads are palpable. The **head of the radius** is just distal to the lateral epicondyle. It can be felt rotating during pronation and supination, and it is visible when the elbow is extended. The radial

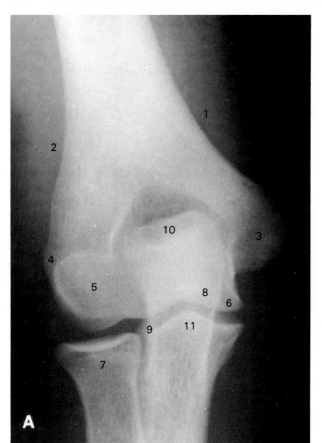
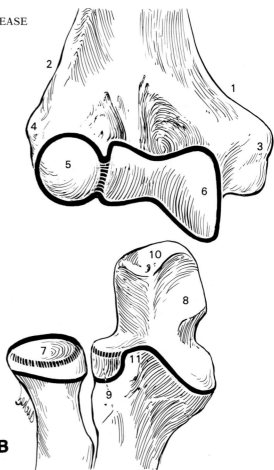

FIG. 14-1. An x-ray of the right elbow joint **(A)** compared with a schematic drawing of the bones **(B).** On the drawing the articular facets are accentuated by heavy lines. (1) medial, (2) lateral supracondylar ridges, (3) medial, (4) lateral epicondyles, (5) capitulum, (6) trochlea, (7) head of the radius, (8) trochlear notch of the ulna, (9) radial notch of the ulna, (10) olecranon process, (11) coranoid process. (**A** courtesy of Dr. Rosalind H. Troupin)

head is covered on its upper surface and around its periphery by articular cartilage (Fig. 14–1B) and will be studied later. In the pronated forearm the **head of the ulna** is visible as a smooth prominence on the back of the wrist in line with the little finger. In the supinated hand it is no longer visible but may be grasped between finger and thumb if the tendons around the wrist are relaxed.

The **styloid process** of the ulna projects toward the carpal bones beyond the head (Figs. 14–2, 14–3A). It is fixed to the posterior edge of the head of the ulna. The inferior surface of the head is covered with hyaline cartilage and faces toward the wrist joint but does not directly articulate with the carpal bones (Fig. 14–3A). The styloid process of the radius is more blunt and also projects toward the carpus from the expanded inferior end of the bone.

Its tip is at a slightly lower level than that of the ulnar styloid (Figs. 14–2, 14–3A).

The **expanded end** of the radius articulates with the carpal bones and the expanded end of the ulna with the humerus. On the dorsal aspect of the wrist the radius feels superficial but only its styloid process and its **dorsal tubercle** are truly subcutaneous. The tubercle is in line with the index finger. The flexor tendons make the anterior surface of the radius inaccessible at the wrist.

The proximal end of the ulna terminates in two stout processes which grasp the trochlea of the humerus (Fig. 14–1). Of these, only the **olecranon process** is palpable behind the elbow. It is subcutaneous and a bursa separates it from the skin. The **coronoid process** is buried in muscles in the depth of the cubital fossa.

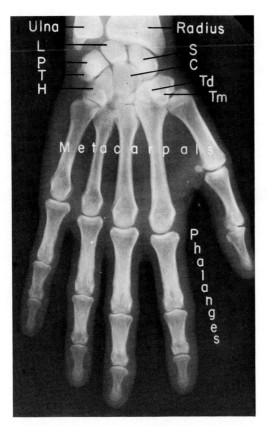

FIG. 14–2. An x-ray of the right hand. Note that the relative positions of the radius and ulna are reversed when compared with that in Figure 14–1 because the hand was x-rayed in the palm down or prone position. *Proximal row of carpal bones:* S = scaphoid; L= lunate; T = triquetrum; P = pisiform. *Distal row:* Tm = trapezium; Td = trapezoid; C = capitate; H = hamate. Note that the pisiform is superimposed on the triquetrum, the head of the ulna is separated by a wide radiolucent gap from the carpal bones, which is occupied by an articular disk.

The shaft of the ulna is subcutaneous from olecranon to styloid process, but only the distal third of the radial shaft is directly palpable; more proximally it is covered in muscles.

Radius and ulna articulate with one another at both ends. The joints are the proximal and distal **radioulnar joints.** The head of the radius is received by the radial notch of the ulna (Fig. 14–1), while the head of the ulna is accommodated by the ulnar notch of the radius (Fig. 14–3A). The **interosseous membrane** stretches between the shafts of the two bones and provides additional area for muscle attachment.

The Hand

The Carpus. The proximal segment of the skeleton of the hand consists of eight irregular bones which are collectively known as the carpus. These bones are equally divided between a proximal and a distal row (Fig. 14–2). In the proximal row, the **scaphoid, lunate,** and **triquetrum** articulate with the radius at the **radiocarpal** or **wrist joint;** the fourth bone, the **pisiform,** articulates only with the triquetrum. **Trapezium, trapezoid, capitate,** and **hamate** form the distal row. They articulate with the proximal row at the **midcarpal joint** and with the metacarpal bones at the **carpometacarpal joints.** Members of each row articulate with each neighboring bone (intercarpal joints). Clearly, the carpus is a pliable region and its movements amplify those that occur at the radiocarpal joint.

The **dorsal aspect of the carpus** is convex because the bones are united to form the carpal arch. The scaphoid and the lunate can be precisely palpated on the dorsum of the wrist. They are the most frequently affected bones in traumatic injuries. The scaphoid is palpable just distal to the styloid process of the radius in a depression called the *anatomic snuffbox.* The lunate is easily felt during flexion and extension of the wrist just distal to the dorsal tubercle of the radius. Most of the other carpal bones, though palpable, cannot be separately identified, and they are of lesser clinical importance.

The scaphoid is the largest carpal bone (Fig. 14–3). It is dumbell-shaped, and except for its narrower waist it is covered by articular cartilage. Blood vessels have access to it only over the nonarticular waist. During a fall on the outstretched hand, this is the area where the bone fractures (Fig. 14–3B), and this is the reason for the ischemic necrosis that often follows.

The semilunar-shaped lunate is perched with its concavity on the *head* of the capitate. Due to a fall on the outstretched hand, the bone may slip from this position and it usually dislocates in a palmar direction into the carpal tunnel.

The **palmar aspect of the carpus** presents a gutter because the bones are narrower on their palmar aspect than on the dorsal (Fig. 14–4). The gutter is deepened by bony prominences at its edges. Only these prominences are palpable in the palm. On the radial side the tubercle of the scaphoid and the tubercle of the trapezium, and on the ulnar side the pisiform and the hook of the hamate protrude into the palm. All four points are palpable in the living hand. A strong ligament, the **flexor retinaculum,**

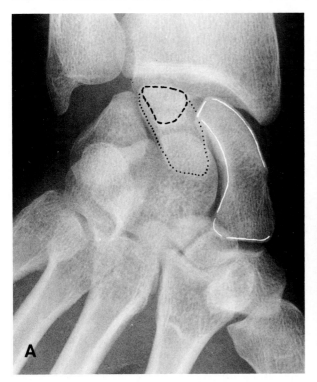 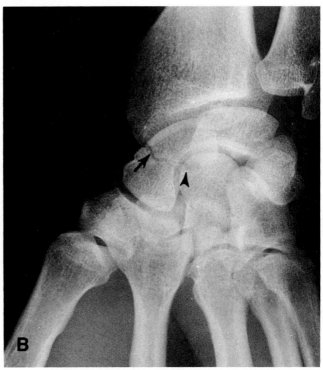

FIG. 14–3. X-rays of a left (**A**) and of a right (**B**) wrist taken in abduction to give a complete view of the scaphoid. In **A** which is normal, the surfaces of the scaphoid covered by articular cartilage are indicated by white lines. The profile of the lunate facing toward the dorsum of the wrist is identified by a black interrupted line, and black dots outline the rest of the bone perched on top of the capitate. **B** was taken 14 days after the patient fell on his outstretched hand and sprained his wrist. A fracture of the scaphoid is identified at the waist of the bone by an arrow, and its extension into the surface which articulates with the capitate is marked by an arrowhead. (Courtesy of Dr. Rosalind H. Troupin)

attaches to these four bony prominences and converts the gutter into the **carpal tunnel.** Its contents shall be studied later.

The position of the carpal bones is more proximal than commonly appreciated. The level of the radiocarpal joint is about 2 cm above the distal skin crease of the wrist (Fig. 14–19), and the plane of the carpometacarpal joints is level with the proximal border of the outstretched thumb.

The Metacarpals and Phalanges. The intermediate segment of the skeleton of the hand is represented by the metacarpals and the distal segment by the phalanges (Fig. 14–2). They are miniature long bones. Their proximal expanded end is their base and the distal end is the head. The metacarpal bone of the thumb is separated from the other four and together with its carpal bone (trapezium) it has rotated into a plane at right

angles to the others. These features and the mobility of its carpometacarpal joint enable the thumb to oppose with any of the fingers. The joints of the hand will be discussed in Chapter 15.

THE ELBOW JOINT

The Anatomy of the Joint

The elbow joint is a compound synovial joint in which the radius and ulna articulate with the humerus (Fig. 14–1). The joint cavity is continuous with that of the proximal radioulnar joint, and the two joints are enclosed by a single capsule (Fig. 14–5). Both joints are uniaxial; the elbow functions basically as a hinge permitting flexion and extension of the forearm while the proximal radioulnar joint is a pivot which permits rotation of the radius

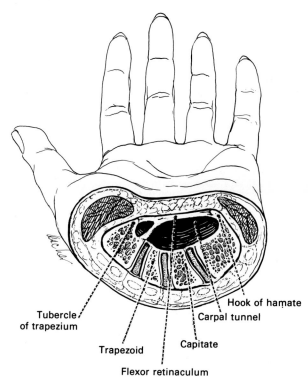

Tubercle of trapezium

Carpal tunnel

Hook of hamate

Trapezoid

Capitate

Flexor retinaculum

FIG. 14-4. Schematic representation of a section cut across the distal row of carpal bones to show their anterior concavity. The flexor retinaculum converts this bony gutter into the carpal tunnel.

during pronation and supination. The latter movements are possible in any position of elbow flexion or extension.

The integrity of the proximal radioulnar joint is essential for elbow flexion and extension. Ligaments hold the head of the radius in close apposition to the radial notch of the ulna converting the distal articular surface into two condyles, while the proximal condyles in the elbow joint are represented by the capitulum and the trochlea of the humerus.

Articular Surfaces. The two humeral condyles are covered by uninterrupted articular cartilage, but the continuity of the inferior articular surface is interrupted by the proximal radioulnar joint (Figs. 14–1, 14–5). The lateral condyles are the **capitulum of the humerus** and the **head of the radius** (humeroradial joint), and the medial condyles are the **trochlea of the humerus** and the **trochlear notch of the ulna** (humeroulnar joint). Only if a joint is subluxed and abnormal movements take place does a lateral condylar surface come in contact with the medial condylar sur-

face of the other bone. In normal movements, lateral condylar surfaces remain in contact with one another and the same is true for the medial condylar surfaces.

The slightly concave superior surface of the radial head slides on the spheroidal capitulum during elbow flexion, and spins on it during pronation and supination. Both the trochlea and the trochlear notch are divided into unequal medial and lateral facets (Fig. 14–1B). The trochlea is shaped like an hourglass lying on its side, the medial half of which projects further inferiorly than the lateral half. The trochlear notch occupies the upper surface of the coronoid process and the anterior surface of the olecranon process. A smooth ridge on the trochlear notch corresponds to the groove on the trochlea. The coronoid articular surface is level with the plateau of the radial head but the articular surface on the olecranon reaches upward behind the trochlea which is grasped by the two ulnar processes (Figs. 14–1, 14–6).

Maximum congruity between the trochlea and trochlear notch is obtained when the elbow is fully extended. This is the close-packed position of the joint in which its stabilizing ligaments become taut. In all positions between full extension and full flexion some abduction and adduction can be elicited passively in the joint due to the fact that the articular surfaces on the medial condyles are not congruent. This incongruity also permits some movement of the ulna during active pronation and supination.

Because the articular surfaces on the medial condyles make angles greater than 90° with the shafts of the respective bones, the forearm makes an angle of 150–160° with the shaft of the humerus if the elbow is extended with the hand in the supinated (anatomic) position. This is the **carrying angle.** The carrying angle disappears when the forearm is pronated. The same is the case when the elbow is flexed, due to the fact that the less angulated lateral facets of the trochlea and trochlear notch have been brought into contact. This movement places the supinated hand over the shoulder or in front of the face. Fractures of the humeral shaft which are allowed to unite with the distal fragment rotated will distort this relationship, and the patient may experience difficulty performing such essential movements as placing food into the mouth.

Capsule and Ligaments. The capsule of the elbow joint is thin anteriorly and posteriorly, but collateral ligaments reinforce the joint on each side (Fig. 14–5). Anteriorly, the capsule's attachment to the

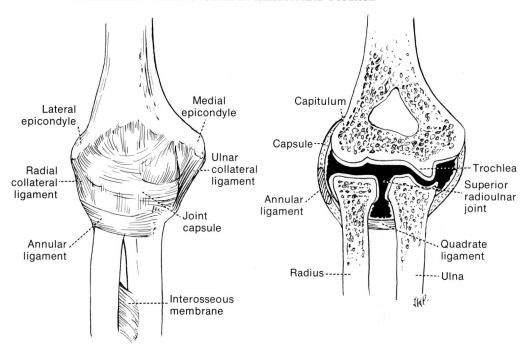

FIG. 14-5. The elbow joint. On the left the joint capsule is shown with its associated ligaments. The coronal section of the joint on the right shows the relation of the superior radioulnar joint to the elbow joint.

humerus encloses the coronoid and radial fossae situated above the two condyles and posteriorly the attachment is to the upper margin of the olecranon fossa. Both epicondyles are outside the capsule. The epiphyseal line for the distal epiphysis is intraarticular but that of the medial epicondyle is not. Inferiorly, the capsule attaches to the articular margins on the coronoid and olecranon processes but over the radius it blends with the ligaments which retain the radius and ulna in articulation at the proximal radioulnar joint. These ligaments are the **annular** and **quadrate ligaments** (Fig. 14–5). The annular ligament is a strong, nearly complete fibrous circle which attaches to the margins of the radial notch and encircles the head of the radius. The quadrate ligament runs between the inferior edge of the radial notch and the neck of the radius. It represents the inferior part of the joint capsule that bridges the gap between the two bones (Fig. 14–5).

The **medial** or **ulnar collateral ligament** is a triangular fibrous band that spans the space between medial epicondyle, coronoid process, and the subcutaneous edge of the olecranon. The **lateral** or **radial collateral ligament** fans out from the lateral epicondyle and blends with the annular ligament.

The **nerve supply** of the capsule is derived chiefly from the nerves that innervate the prime movers of the joint. Anteriorly the musculocutaneous nerve and posteriorly the radial nerve supply the joint capsule and the synovial membrane.

The Synovial Membrane. The capsule is lined by synovial membrane which is attached to the articular margins. It encloses a synovial cavity common to the humeroulnar, humeroradial, and radioulnar joints. The membrane doubles back on itself at the lines of capsular attachment and is draped over the fat pads which occupy the coronoid, radial, and olecranon fossae. The fat pads are compressed by the radius and ulna and function to spread the synovial fluid when they are allowed to expand. They also retain the synovial membrane in contact with the articular cartilage of the condyles where they are free from contact with the apposing articular surface.

Movements

The elbow can be flexed and extended. The prime movers of flexion and extension occupy the flexor and extensor compartments of the arm and only they will be discussed in this section. Those muscles of the forearm which originate from the humerus and cross the joint can also produce movement at the elbow but they become important in flexion and extension only when the chief prime movers are paralyzed. Normally, three muscles are concerned with flexing the elbow and three with extending it. The flexors are the brachialis, biceps brachii, and brachioradialis (Fig. 14–7), the extensors are the medial (or deep), lateral, and long heads of the triceps (Fig. 14–8). In both movements gravity plays an important part and must be taken into account when the muscles are being tested.

Flexors. The **brachialis** is the most important flexor of the elbow (Fig. 14–7). Flexion is the only action this large muscle is capable of, and it partakes in this act whether the movement is performed slowly or rapidly, whether the forearm is pronated or supinated, whether a load is being lifted or only the force of gravity acting on the forearm has to be overcome. It is the servile muscle among elbow flexors, and it has been aptly named the workhorse of elbow flexion. The muscle is often insufficiently appreciated because the superficial bulk of the biceps obscures it.

The brachialis arises from the anterior surface of the lower half of the humeral shaft and from the two intermuscular septa. The muscle fibers converge on a short tendon deep in the cubital fossa which inserts into the coronoid process of the ulna. The muscle is ideally placed for fast or spurt action (see Fig. 4–1), but it gives power to elbow flexion under all circumstances. By its isometric contraction it maintains the flexed position, especially when resistence or weight is applied to the forearm. When the flexed forearm is extended by the force of gravity, it is the brachialis that controls elbow extension by gradual relaxation while the triceps is quiescent. "It picks up the drink and puts down the empty glass" (R. J. Last). The hardened belly of the brachialis may be palpated on either side of the biceps and its tendon when flexion is opposed.

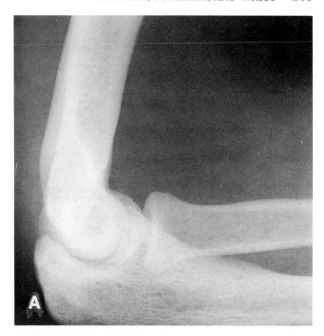

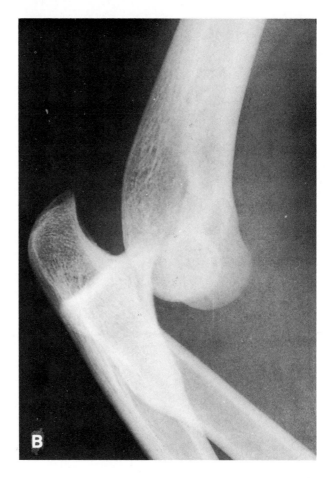

FIG. 14–6. Lateral x-rays of the elbow joint. **(A)** Normal anatomy. The plateau of the radial head abuts against the capitulum; the trochlea is grasped by the olecranon and coronoid processes. **(B)** Posterior dislocation of the ulna and radius. The normal relationship of these two bones to one another is retained. (Courtesy of Dr. Rosalind H. Troupin)

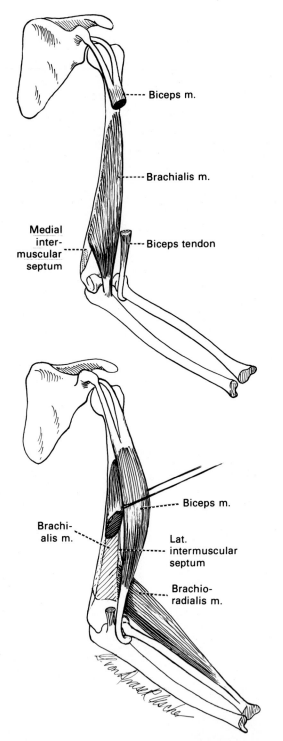

Biceps m.

Brachialis m.

Medial inter-muscular septum

Biceps tendon

Biceps m.

Brachi-alis m.

Lat. intermuscular septum

Brachio-radialis m.

FIG. 14-7. Flexors of the elbow. The upper drawing shows the brachialis, the bulk of the biceps having been resected. The lower drawing illustrates the biceps and the brachioradialis.

The chief segmental nerve supply from C5 to C6 reaches the muscle via the **musculocutaneous nerve.** Apparently paradoxically, a minor branch of the radial nerve (C7) also supplies the brachialis. This anomaly is probably due to the fact that in the embryonic limb the lateral portion of the muscle may have been in the extensor compartment.

The chief function of the **biceps** (Fig. 14–7) is to supinate the pronated forearm. This will be apparent from its mode of insertion. However, it is also a powerful prime mover when the supine or semi-prone forearm is flexed. The biceps remains quiescent during flexion if full pronation is maintained. It functions chiefly as a reserve muscle of elbow flexion, being called into action when power is required. The biceps arises by two heads; the short head from the coracoid process together with the coracobrachialis, and the long head via a long tendon from the supraglenoid tubercle inside the shoulder joint. The two muscle bellies fuse on the surface of the brachialis, and above the elbow the muscle terminates in a tendon which crosses the elbow joint and inserts into the tuberosity of the radius. In the supinated position, the tuberosity faces toward the ulna but in pronation it is rotated posteriorly. The tendon, attached to the posterior lip of the tuberosity, is wrapped around the radial neck in pronation (with a bursa intervening between tendon and bone). It is clear, therefore, that contraction of the biceps will first reverse rotation of the radius (i.e., supinate) before the muscle will act as an elbow flexor. From the proximal end of the tendon a fibrous band, the **bicipital aponeurosis** crosses medially over the forearm muscles that originate from the medial epicondyle (Fig. 14–10). The aponeurosis fuses with the deep fascia of the forearm. This attachment subserves only elbow flexion.

Like the brachialis, the biceps is innervated by C5 and C6 via the **musculocutaneous nerve.** The biceps tendon is used for eliciting the biceps reflex, which tests spinal cord segments C5 and C6, but chiefly C5, and both afferent and efferent limbs of the reflex arc that involve the musculocutaneous nerve and the brachial plexus.

In addition to providing power to supination and elbow flexion, the biceps also contributes to glenohumeral flexion via its short head and to glenohumeral abduction via its long head.

The **brachioradialis** (Fig. 14–7) can flex the elbow joint but functionally belongs to a different class of muscles than the brachialis and biceps brachii. It is the typical example of a shunt muscle (see Fig. 4–1).

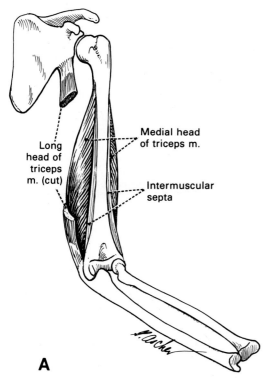

cle is also active when weight is lifted in the semi-prone position. When flexion is restrained in this position by an examiner the muscle will be thrown into prominence. Contrary to previous teaching, the brachioradialis has been shown to be inactive during pronation and supination. The brachioradialis is innervated by the **radial nerve** (C5,C6,C7). It is used clinically for eliciting a tendon reflex which tests the same cord segments as the biceps tendon reflex, but chiefly C6. The reflex however assesses different pathways through the brachial plexus and peripheral nerves than those tested by the biceps reflex.

Extensors (Fig. 14–8). The functional counterpart of the brachialis is the so-called **medial head of the triceps.** The muscle is misnamed; the head lies deep, not medial, and is the mirror image of the brachialis in the extensor compartment of the arm. It originates from the humerus and intermuscular septa below the radial groove, and the other two heads of the triceps are superficial to it. The **lateral head** originates from a narrow area on the humerus above the radial groove. The **long head** lies medially and arises from the infraglenoid tubercle of the scapula just outside the shoulder joint. Lateral and long heads merge half way down

FIG. 14–8. The triceps muscle seen from the front (**A**) and from the back (**B**).

The brachioradialis originates from the proximal part of the lateral supracondylar ridge and from the lateral intermuscular septum and inserts into the lower end of the radius just proximal to the styloid process. In contrast to the brachialis and biceps, the brachioradialis originates close to the joint and inserts far away from it. Its pull on the radius will be greater *along* the shaft of the radius than *across* it (the reverse of the dominant direction of pull exerted by the biceps or by the brachialis), and in any position it will tend to pull the radius toward the humerus. On the other hand, once a certain degree of flexion is obtained, the biceps and brachialis will tend to pull the radius and ulna away from the humerus. Due to the spurt action of these muscles, any point on the forearm will move on a curved path, and a centripetal force directed toward the axis of movement is required if the point is not to fly off at a tangent to the curved path. This centripetal force at the elbow is provided by the brachioradialis which is called into action when the movement is rapid, be it flexion or extension. During slow movement at the elbow, the brachioradialis is quiescent. The mus-

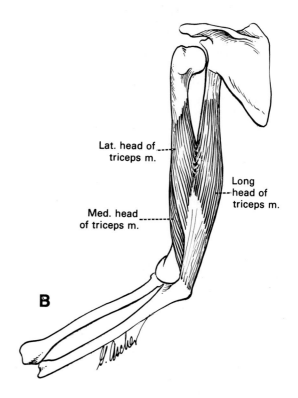

the arm, giving rise to a tendon that remains superficial to the fleshy medial head and lower down is joined by some of its fibers. The three heads insert via a stout tendon into the upper surface of the olecranon.

The three heads participate in elbow extension in an unequal manner. The medial head is always active, the long head is quiescent during active extension, and the lateral head shows minimal activity. However, when resistance has to be overcome, the lateral and long heads are recruited. In this respect they resemble the two heads of the biceps. For instance, all parts of the triceps are active during push-ups or when a heavy object is being pushed with the arms. The triceps is called into action as a synergist when the semiflexed forearm is forcefully supinated. It cancels out the flexor action of the biceps. The muscle is quiet, however, when the forearm is extended by the force of gravity.

Two small muscles are considered parts of the triceps: the **articularis cubiti** and the **anconeus.** The former is deep to the medial head and is inserted into the capsule of the elbow joint, preventing it from being caught by the olecranon. The anconeus is an extension of the triceps and inserts into the lateral surface of the olecranon and posterior aspect of the annular ligament. Some of its fibers arise from the lateral epicondyle.

The triceps is supplied by several branches of the **radial nerve** (C6,C7,C8). The level at which the branches arise is of clinical importance in cases of radial nerve injury. The medial head receives two branches; one given off in the axilla which descends with the ulnar nerve (ulnar collateral nerve); the other originates in the radial groove. The branch to the long head also originates high, before the nerve enters the radial groove, while the lateral head receives its branch in the radial groove. Clinically, the triceps tendon reflex is used for testing cord segments C7 and C8. The peripheral afferent and efferent pathways involve the radial nerve and respective parts of the brachial plexus.

ANATOMIC RELATIONS IN THE ARM AND CUBITAL FOSSA

The Arm

The general anatomic plan of the arm is simple (Fig. 14–9). The large flexor and extensor muscles occupy the anterior and posterior compartments.

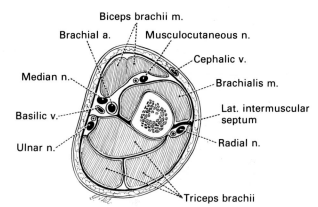

FIG. 14–9. A transverse section across the lower third of the arm.

Between them on the medial side, the **brachial artery** approaches the elbow accompanied by the **median** and **ulnar nerves,** neither of which give off any branches in the arm. They are nerves of the forearm and hand. After leaving the axilla, the musculocutaneous and radial nerves make their way through the flexor and extensor muscles, and distribute their branches as they pass in a lateral direction toward the elbow. The **musculocutaneous nerve** passes between the biceps and brachialis, supplies both, as well as the coracobrachialis (which is a vestigial adductor on the medial side in the upper half of the arm). The **radial nerve** passes between the deep and superficial heads of the triceps in the middle third of the arm and reaches the lateral intermuscular septum above the elbow. In the radial groove it is much closer to the bone than the musculocutaneous nerve, hence, more vulnerable in humeral fractures. The radial nerve lies on the most proximal fibers of the medial head of the triceps as they arise from the radial groove, and the nerve is covered by the lateral and long heads. It may be rolled against the bone in this position. The **profunda brachii artery** accompanies the nerve. This branch of the brachial artery is the chief source of arterial blood for the arm musculature. When the radial nerve reaches the lateral edge of the humerus, it pierces the lateral intermuscular septum and continues inferiorly in the anterior compartment, lying between the brachialis and brachioradialis. It is here that it gives its branches to these muscles and to the elbow. It also supplies the extensor carpi radialis longus, which originates on the lateral supracondylar ridge just below the brachioradialis. In front of the lateral epicondyle the

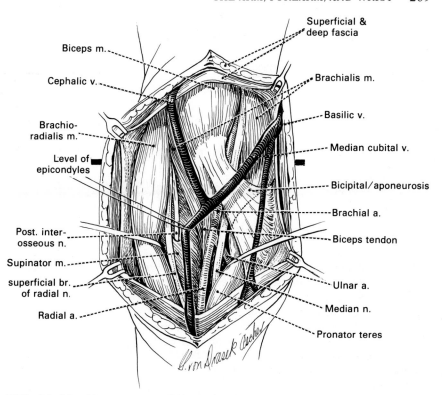

FIG. 14-10. The contents of the cubital fossa exposed by pulling the brachioradialis and pronator teres to the side. The level of the epicondyles, shown in the intact arm by a skin crease, is indicated by a black bar.

nerve divides into a superficial and a deep branch. The **superficial branch** retains the name of its parent in the forearm but supplies no muscles. It will be distributed to skin on the dorsum of the hand. More important is the **deep branch,** called the **posterior interosseous nerve** which supplies all extensor muscles in the forearm (except the extensor carpi radialis longus).

When the musculocutaneous nerve emerges on the lateral side of the biceps above the elbow, it has spent all its motor fibers. Hence, it assumes the name of **lateral cutaneous nerve of the forearm** and is distributed to skin on the preaxial border of the limb below the elbow.

The median nerve keeps company with the brachial artery but the ulnar nerve leaves it about the middle of the arm. The nerve pierces the medial intermuscular septum and descends in the extensor compartment. The ulnar nerve reaches the posterior aspect of the elbow where is passes between the olecranon and the medial epicondyle. Here it may be readily palpated because it is subcutaneous.

The Cubital Fossa

The biceps and brachialis lead into an intermuscular space as they pass to their insertions in front of the elbow. The triangular space is the cubital fossa, the apex of which points inferiorly (Fig. 14–10). The greater part of the floor of the fossa is formed by the brachialis and supinator muscles, the lateral boundary by the brachioradialis, and medially the fossa is limited by the pronator teres, a muscle that originates on the medial epicondyle. The cubital fossa is important anatomically and clinically because with the exception of the ulnar nerve, it contains all the major nerves and vessels that supply the forearm and hand.

The **brachial artery** enters the fossa along the medial side of the biceps tendon, and the vessel divides into the **ulnar** and **radial arteries** deep in the fossa, on level with the radial tuberosity. The **median nerve** accompanies the brachial artery into the fossa, lying just medial to it, and will cross the ulnar artery superficially, close to the origin of the vessel. Just above this point several motor branches are given off by the nerve to muscles which arise from the medial epicondyle; just distal to this point the **anterior interosseous nerve** branches off which supplies the more deeply seated muscles in the forearm. Both the brachial artery and the median nerve are held down in the cubital fossa by the bicipital aponeurosis which crosses superficial to them and to the pronator teres.

The **radial nerve** divides into superficial and deep terminal branches at the lateral corner of the cubital fossa, being sheltered by the brachioradialis. The superficial branch descends in the lateral boundary of the fossa underneath that muscle but the deep division **(posterior interosseous nerve)** turns posteriorly and exits from the fossa.

The posterior interosseous nerve is accompanied by the **posterior interosseous artery,** and the anterior interosseous nerve by the **anterior interosseous artery.** They originate by a common stem from the ulnar artery. Other branches of the ulnar and radial arteries ascend through the fossa and establish a **circumarticular** (trochlear) **anastomosis** with more proximal branches of the brachial and profunda brachii arteries.

The fossa is roofed over by the bicipital aponeurosis and the deep, investing fascia of the forearm. Embedded in the superficial fascia passes the **cephalic vein** on the lateral side and the **basilic vein** on the medial side. The two veins are interconnected by the **median cubital vein.**

During venipuncture and other manipulations around the elbow, it is useful to bear in mind the relationship of nerves and vessels to one another across a line that joins the two epicondyles (Fig. 14–10). The line is marked by a skin crease and represents the base of the triangular fossa. Proceeding from the lateral to medial epicondyle, the order of structures is as follows: 1) superficial to the brachioradialis over the lateral epicondyle is the cephalic vein, and deep to the muscle is the radial nerve, 2) in the center is the biceps tendon, 3) medial to the tendon the brachial artery with the median nerve on its medial side, 4) the bicipital aponeurosis separates the artery and nerve from the median cubital vein, and 5) the basilic vein is superficial to the pronator teres over the medial epicondyle.

SUPINATION AND PRONATION

The movements of supination and pronation are unique to the forearm. They are made possible by two synovial joints that unite the radius and ulna at their proximal and distal ends. These are the radioulnar joints. The essence of the movements is rotation of the radius. While the head and neck of the radius spin around a fixed axis, the distal end of the bone describes an arc of about 180° around the head of the ulna, carrying the hand with it. When radius and ulna are crossed, the back of the hand looks forward or toward the ceiling if the elbow is flexed. This is the position of **pronation.** In **supination** the two bones are parallel and the palm looks forward or, with elbow flexion, toward the ceiling.

The distal end of the axis is not fixed. The hand can be supinated and pronated with the ulna lying on the table. The finger tips will move along arcs, the largest of which is described by the thumb, while the little finger has practically no excursion. Objects grasped by the index finger and thumb can thus be manipulated in a large volume of space with great precision. When the forearm is free, supination and pronation will carry the thumb and little finger along arcs of identical radius. In this instance, the palm of the hand and the middle finger move the least. Thus, a twisting force can be exerted on an object such as a doorknob or a screwdriver.

Slight movements of the head of the ulna are synchronized with excursions made by the distal end of the radius. The movements are an exaggeration of the slight play permitted by the incongruity between the medial condyles in the elbow joint.

The **range of pronation** and supination should be measured from the midprone position. This should be done with the elbow flexed. The normal range is 90° in either direction. When the forearm is extended, the range of supination and pronation is considerably augmented by humeral rotation. In this position, the latter movement can mask, or compensate for, a reduced range of supination or pronation.

The Radioulnar Joints

Both proximal and distal radioulnar joints are pivot joints. At both joints the radius is the moving bone. The disk-shaped radial head is covered by articular cartilage not only on its upper surface but around its entire circumference, where the radius articulates with the radial notch of the ulna and the inner aspect of the annular ligament (Figs. 14–1B, 14–5). Only three quarters of the circumference of the ulnar head is covered by articular cartilage upon which the concave ulnar notch of the radius slides (Fig. 14–3A). The chief structure responsible for the integrity of the proximal joint is

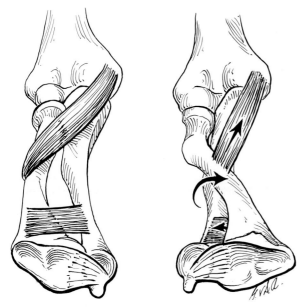

FIG. 14-11. Pronation. Contraction of the pronator teres (upper muscle) and pronator quadratus (lower muscle) swing the radius across the ulna. The articular disk between the ulnar styloid process and ulnar notch of the radius guides this movement. The annular ligament, which stabilizes the radial head, is not shown. (Adapted from MacConnaill MA, Basmajian JV: Muscles and Movements, Baltimore, Williams & Wilkins 1969)

the annular ligament, while at the distal end a triangular **articular disk** retains the two bones in apposition and, at the same time, permits the radius to move (Fig. 14-11).

The annular ligament and articular disk beautifully illustrate how different types of movements correlate with different anatomic arrangements in joints. The annular ligament has already been studied, and it is easy to appreciate how the radial head, stabilized by the capitulum superiorly, can spin in the articular ring constructed by the ligament and the radial notch. The triangular fibrocartilaginous disk attaches with its apex to the root of the ulnar styloid process and with its base to the radius along the inferior edge of the ulnar notch (Fig. 14-11). These attachments secure the two bones but also permit movement. The disk, twisting at its apex, moves with the radius while its upper surface slides on the inferior aspect of the ulnar head that is covered by articular cartilage. Inferiorly, the disk faces into the wrist joint. The articular disk separates the synovial cavities of the radiocarpal and the distal radioulnar joints. However, occasionally the disk may be perforated. As noted before, the proximal joint always shares a common cavity with the elbow joint.

Muscles of Pronation and Supination

The movements are accomplished by two pairs of muscles: the **pronator teres** and **pronator quadratus** represent one pair, and the **supinator** and **biceps** the other.

Pronators (Fig. 14-11). Both pronators are in the anterior compartment of the forearm. Work is not equally divided between them. The pronator quadratus is always active while the pronator teres is recruited during swift or powerful pronation.

The **pronator quadratus** is the deepest muscle in the forearm. Its parallel fibers run, like a broad band, over the anterior surfaces of the radius and ulna, reaching about a hand's breadth above the wrist. The ulnar attachment represents the origin. The fibers are at their greatest length when the radius and ulna are uncrossed. The anterior interosseous nerve supplies the muscle (C8).

The **pronator teres** is one of the superficial muscles of the forearm and it delimits the cubital fossa medially. Its main origin is from the medial epicondyle. The muscle crosses the forearm obliquely and inserts into the point of greatest convexity on the radial shaft. At its insertion, the muscle is covered by the brachioradialis. Consideration of the mechanical advantages these attachments offer will explain why the muscle is well suited for quick and powerful pronation (spurt action). The pull of the muscle generates a significant force vector along the shaft of the radius which ensures good contact between the capitulum and the radial head when pronation is performed rapidly (shunt action). The muscle is supplied by the first branch of the median nerve given off in the cubital fossa (C6,C7). Of the two pronators only the pronator teres can be demonstrated by opposing pronation.

Injury to the median nerve above the elbow results in a complete loss of active pronation.

Supinators. The muscle which is always active in supination is the supinator. The biceps lends power and speed to the movement. The biceps is inactive when the extended forearm is supinated, but participates in the movement when the elbow is flexed.

The **supinator** is deeply placed in the extensor compartment of the forearm (Fig. 14-14). It wraps itself around the upper third of the radius. The muscle originates from the posterior aspect of the lateral epicondyle, the radial collateral ligament of the elbow joint, and the lateral surface of the ulna below the radial notch. The ulnar fibers encircle the neck of the radius and are deep to those that originate on the epicondyle. The muscle inserts into the radius over a wide area between the neck and the point of insertion of the pronator teres. The fibers are at maximum length when the forearm is pronated, and their contraction restores the radius into a position parallel with the ulna. The posterior interosseous nerve and vessels pass between the deep and superficial parts of the muscle. The nerve supplies the supinator before it enters it (C5,C6).

The origin and insertion of the **biceps** have already been examined (Fig. 14–7). The biceps exerts its powerful supinator action due to the fact that its tendon of insertion wraps around the neck of the radius in the pronated position. Both biceps and supinator generate forces that spin the head of the radius, but each muscle also pulls the radial head toward the capitulum to stabilize it during the movement.

The demonstration and testing of the biceps has been discussed with elbow flexion. The biceps can also be tested by opposing supination of the forearm. The supinator is difficult to demonstrate. It is noteworthy that the two muscles with supinator action are innervated by two different nerves—the posterior interosseous and musculocutaneous nerves.

ANATOMIC RELATIONS IN THE FOREARM

The anatomy of the forearm is more complex than that of the arm. Its anterior and posterior compartments are separated not by one but by two bones with the **interosseous membrane** stretching between them. In addition to housing the prime movers of the wrist, these compartments accommodate the supinators and pronators already discussed and the muscles that flex and extend the digits. The power of hand movements is largely generated by muscle bellies confined to the forearm. These muscles exert their action on the hand via long tendons. No muscle belly crosses the wrist. The wrist and carpus are surrounded anteriorly and posteriorly by tendons that are retained in position by fascial bands known as retinacula. These represent reinforcements in the deep fascial sleeve of the forearm (antebrachial fascia) and their function is to prevent bow stringing of the tendons when the muscles contract. The tendons that negotiate the wrist include also those of the wrist prime movers. Wrist flexors and extensors insert into the carpal bones and the bases of the metacarpal bones, thereby they exert action on

the carpometacarpal, intercarpal, and radiocarpal joints. The tendons serve as landmarks for locating the nerves and vessels around the wrist as they enter the hand.

The **posterior interosseous nerve,** derived from the radial, is the only nerve in the extensor compartment. It proceeds toward the wrist on the interosseous membrane, buried deeply among the extensor muscles. The **anterior interosseous nerve,** derived from the median, has a similar course in the flexor compartment. This compartment contains also the three large nerves that are destined primarily for the hand, having spent their motor branches to forearm muscles in the region of the elbow. The nerves are the **radial, median,** and **ulnar** nerves.

All nerves in the forearm are accompanied by arteries. The **anterior** and **posterior interosseous arteries** and the **median artery** are relatively small. All three are derived from the ulnar artery in the cubital fossa, and they terminate at the wrist by forming an anastomosis around the carpal bones. The large arteries in the forearm are the **radial** and **ulnar arteries.** They feed into the hand.

The Grouping of Muscles

The functional groups have been identified above. These are:

1. Prime movers of the wrist
2. Supinators and pronators
3. Prime movers of the digits (or extrinsic muscles of the hand)

In the latter group, it is useful to consider muscles of the thumb separately from those of the fingers.

Anatomically, muscles of the anterior and posterior compartments are divided into **superficial** and **deep groups.** In each compartment, the superficial group consists of muscles that originate from the epicondyles and the supracondylar ridges, while the deep muscles arise from the respective surfaces of the radius and ulna and the interosseous membrane. Once the muscles of each functional group are identified, they can be placed logically among deep or superficial muscles of the respective compartments (Figs. 14–12 to 14–14).

Prime Movers of the Wrist. The flexor and extensor muscles of the carpus send their tendons along the radial and ulnar margins of the wrist. Hence, they are named **flexor carpi radialis, flexor carpi ulnaris, extensor carpi radialis (longus** and **brevis),**

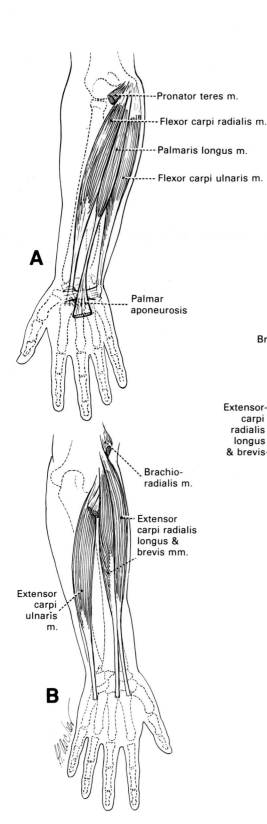

FIG. 14–12. Flexor and extensor muscles of the wrist in the anterior (**A**) and posterior (**B**) compartments of the forearm. **C** is a transverse section at the junction of the upper and middle thirds of the forearm.

Pronator teres m.

Flexor carpi radialis m.

Palmaris longus m.

Flexor carpi ulnaris m.

Palmar aponeurosis

Brachio-radialis m.

Extensor carpi radialis longus & brevis mm.

Extensor carpi ulnaris m.

Pronator teres m.

Brachioradialis m.

Flexor carpi radialis m.

Palmaris longus

Flexor carpi ulnaris

Extensor carpi radialis longus & brevis

Supinator

Extensor carpi ulnaris m.

and **extensor carpi ulnaris** (Fig. 14–12). All these muscles are superficial. They are tested by opposing flexion or extension of the wrist, when their respective tendons will stand out or become palpable. The innervation of the muscles follows the anticipated pattern: the median nerve supplies the flexor carpi radialis, the ulnar nerve the flexor carpi ulnaris, the radial nerve the extensor carpi radialis longus, and the posterior interosseous nerve the extensor carpi radialis brevis and extensor carpi ulnaris. The spinal cord segments distributed to both flexor and extensor muscles are C7 and C8, with some representation of C6 on the radial side.

Supinators and Pronators. The muscles were discussed on page 211 (Figs. 14–7, 14–11, 14–14).

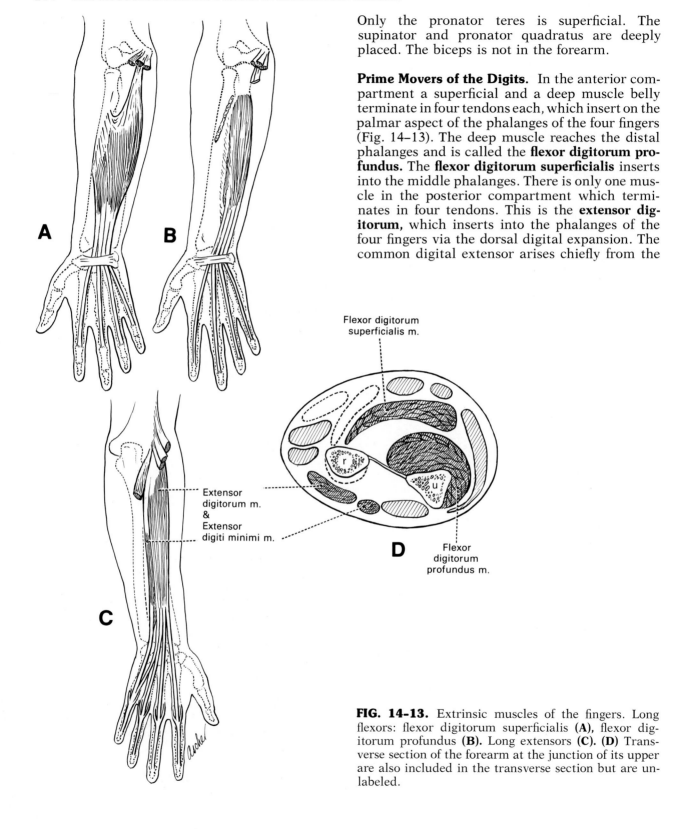

Only the pronator teres is superficial. The supinator and pronator quadratus are deeply placed. The biceps is not in the forearm.

Prime Movers of the Digits. In the anterior compartment a superficial and a deep muscle belly terminate in four tendons each, which insert on the palmar aspect of the phalanges of the four fingers (Fig. 14–13). The deep muscle reaches the distal phalanges and is called the **flexor digitorum profundus.** The **flexor digitorum superficialis** inserts into the middle phalanges. There is only one muscle in the posterior compartment which terminates in four tendons. This is the **extensor digitorum,** which inserts into the phalanges of the four fingers via the dorsal digital expansion. The common digital extensor arises chiefly from the

FIG. 14–13. Extrinsic muscles of the fingers. Long flexors: flexor digitorum superficialis **(A),** flexor digitorum profundus **(B).** Long extensors **(C). (D)** Transverse section of the forearm at the junction of its upper are also included in the transverse section but are unlabeled.

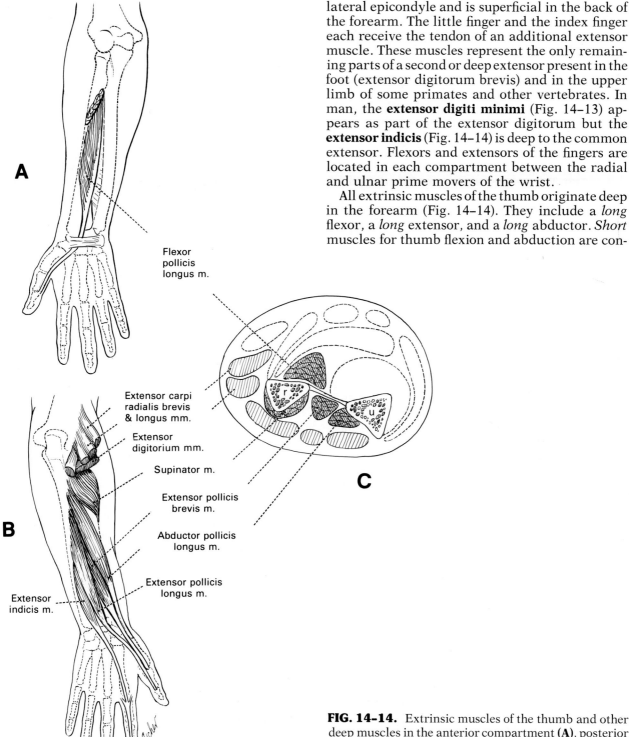

lateral epicondyle and is superficial in the back of the forearm. The little finger and the index finger each receive the tendon of an additional extensor muscle. These muscles represent the only remaining parts of a second or deep extensor present in the foot (extensor digitorum brevis) and in the upper limb of some primates and other vertebrates. In man, the **extensor digiti minimi** (Fig. 14–13) appears as part of the extensor digitorum but the **extensor indicis** (Fig. 14–14) is deep to the common extensor. Flexors and extensors of the fingers are located in each compartment between the radial and ulnar prime movers of the wrist.

All extrinsic muscles of the thumb originate deep in the forearm (Fig. 14–14). They include a *long* flexor, a *long* extensor, and a *long* abductor. *Short* muscles for thumb flexion and abduction are con-

A

Flexor
pollicis
longus m.

Extensor carpi
radialis brevis
& longus mm.

Extensor
digitorium mm.

Supinator m.

Extensor pollicis
brevis m.

Abductor pollicis
longus m.

Extensor pollicis
longus m.

Extensor
indicis m.

B

C

FIG. 14–14. Extrinsic muscles of the thumb and other deep muscles in the anterior compartment (**A**), posterior compartment (**B**), and in a transverse section cut at the (**C**). The transverse section also shows muscles identified in Figs. 14–12, 14–13, but they are unlabeled.

fined to the hand, but the *short* extensor originates in the forearm. In comparison with other primates, the extrinsic muscles of man's thumb are particularly well developed and have attained independence from other extrinsic muscles of the fingers. Close to the wrist, the tendons of the pollex (thumb) emerge between the flexors or extensors of the fingers and the radial prime movers of the wrist. Least accessible is the **flexor pollicis longus.** But on the dorsum of the wrist the tendons of the extrinsic muscles of the thumb are prominent. The tendon of the **extensor pollicis longus** skirts around the radial tubercle and then forms the ulnar boundary of the anatomic snuffbox. The **extensor pollicis brevis** and the **abductor pollicis longus** together form the radial boundary of this fossa. All three cross the tendons of extensor carpi radialis longus and brevis superficially (Fig. 14–18).

The **palmaris longus** is a vestigial member of the superficial flexor group (Fig. 14–12). In many species the muscle acts on the claws. When present in man the slender, superficial tendon of the muscle descends midway between the two styloid processes and terminates in the palmar aponeurosis.

All the extensor muscles are supplied by the posterior interosseous nerve. The anterior interosseous nerve supplies the deep flexors but the ulnar nerve innervates the ulnar half (little and ring fingers) of the flexor digitorum profundus. The superficial flexors each receive a branch from the median nerve. The segmental innervation of all extrinsic muscles of the digits is from C7 and C8, with the latter dominating in both groups. Flexor muscles receive a contribution also from T1.

Arteries and Nerves

Figures 14–15 and 14–16 summarize the relationship of nerves and arteries to the muscles.

Distal to the cubital fossa, the **radial** and **ulnar arteries** diverge toward each side of the forearm and descend to the two styloid processes (Fig. 14–15). They run between the deep and superficial muscles. The radial artery is sheltered by the brachioradialis and the ulnar artery by the flexor carpi ulnaris, but near the elbow the ulnar artery is crossed by all the muscles that originate on the medial epicondyle. The radial artery becomes superficial along the medial side of the brachioradialis tendon about half way down the forearm and may be palpated here against the radius. The ulnar artery only surfaces in the vicinity of the wrist where it is palpable against the ulna on the radial side of the flexor carpi ulnaris tendon.

At the wrist the ulnar artery enters the hand passing superficial to the flexor retinaculum along the lateral side of the pisiform bone. The radial artery, on the other hand, turns posteriorly below the styloid process, passes deep to the tendons of the extensor pollicis brevis and abductor longus, crosses the scaphoid in the snuffbox, and enters the hand between the first two metacarpal bones. Before it changes its direction, it sends a superficial palmar branch into the hand through the muscles of the thenar eminence.

In the forearm, the **radial** and **ulnar nerves** follow the same course as the respective arteries (Fig. 14–15). They retain the same relative position to the arteries as they had at the elbow: the radial nerve is lateral to the artery, and the ulnar nerve is medial to the ulnar artery. The ulnar nerve enters the hand with the artery. The radial nerve, however, deviates posteriorly sooner than its artery. The nerve descends along the back of the lower third of the forearm and lies superficial to all tendons as it crosses the wrist. A dorsal branch is given off by the ulnar nerve a hand's breadth above the wrist which behaves like the radial nerve. It passes posteriorly and descends to the back of the hand in the superficial fascia.

The **median nerve** crosses the ulnar artery in the cubital fossa and descends along the midline of the forearm between the flexor digitorum superficialis and flexor digitorum profundus (Fig. 14–15). The nerve is held to the deep surface of the superficial flexor by connective tissue (Fig. 14–16). The median artery, a small branch of the anterior interosseous artery, accompanies the median nerve. At the wrist, it becomes superficial between the tendons of the flexor digitorum superficialis and flexor carpi radialis. The prominent tendon of the palmaris longus, when present, is a good guide to the nerve. The median nerve enters the hand through the carpal tunnel. Before doing so, a small palmar cutaneous branch originates from it which passes superficially to skin over the thenar eminence.

The anterior and posterior **interosseous nerves** and **arteries** are buried among the deep muscles of the respective compartments (Fig. 14–16).

STRUCTURES AROUND THE WRIST

The Retinacula

On the dorsal and palmar surface of the wrist, the flexor and extensor retinacula retain the tendons in place. Both retinacula represent reinforcements in

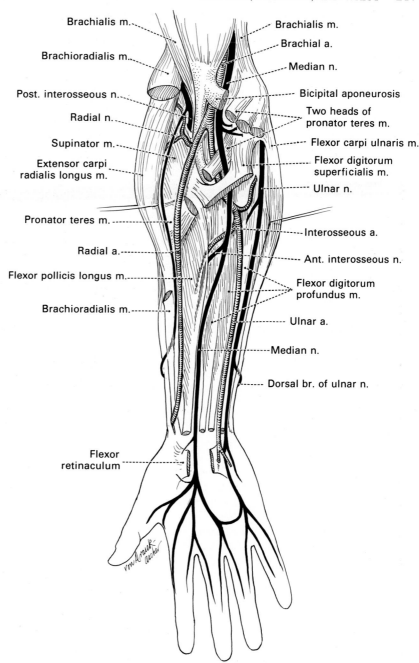

Brachialis m.

Brachioradialis m.

Post. interosseous n.

Radial n.

Supinator m.

Extensor carpi
radialis longus m.

Pronator teres m.

Radial a.

Flexor pollicis longus m.

Brachioradialis m.

Flexor
retinaculum

Brachialis m.

Brachial a.

Median n.

Bicipital aponeurosis

Two heads of
pronator teres m.

Flexor carpi ulnaris m.

Flexor digitorum
superficialis m.

Ulnar n.

Interosseous a.

Ant. interosseous n.

Flexor digitorum
profundus m.

Ulnar a.

Median n.

Dorsal br. of ulnar n.

FIG. 14-15. Nerves and arteries in the anterior compartment of the forearm.

the deep fascia that invests the upper limb. The flexor retinaculum is distal to the radiocarpal joint and is attached only to carpal bones. The extensor retinaculum, on the other hand, crosses the wrist joint and the distal radioulnar joint. Its bony attachments are to the radius and to the carpal bones on the ulnar edge of the hand.

The **flexor retinaculum** roofs over the the carpal tunnel (Fig. 14–4). Its bony attachments have already been examined (p. 201). It is deep in the palm of the hand and both thenar and hypothenar muscles arise from its anterior surface. The tendons it retains in the carpal tunnel are those of the flexor digitorum superficialis and profundus and flexor

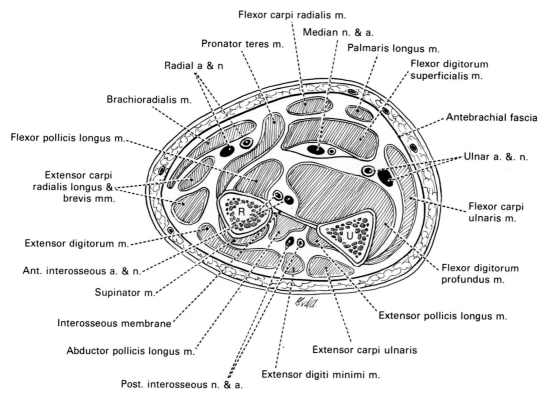

FIG. 14-16. Transverse section at the junction of the middle and upper thirds of the forearm drawn to show the relationship of nerves and arteries to the muscles. R = radius; U = ulnar.

pollicis longus (Fig. 14–17). The flexor carpi radialis tendon occupies a separate compartment in the groove of the trapezium. The median nerve passes through the tunnel on the palmar surface of the flexor digitorum superficialis tendons, and it is immediately deep to the retinaculum.

The **extensor retinaculum** is a ribbonlike band, thinner, broader, and longer than its flexor counterpart (Fig. 14–18). Its attachments are such that the retinaculum does not restrict radial movement during pronation and supination, nor does it become slack in pronation. From its attachment to the anterior border of the radius above the styloid process, the retinaculum slopes downward to blend with deep fascia and periosteum over the pisiform and triquetral bones. Fibrous septa bind it down to bony prominences on the dorsal aspect of the radius which prevent side-to-side displacement of the extensor tendons. All tendons in the back of the wrist pass deep to it, but the radial artery and the branches of the radial and ulnar nerves are superficial to it.

Synovial Sheaths

Flexor and extensor tendons are invested by synovial sheaths as they pass underneath the retinacula. The general arrangement of synovial sheaths around tendons is illustrated in Figure 14–17. The anatomic location of these sheaths has clinical importance. Inflammation due to irritation or infection (tenosynovitis) will distend the sheaths and pressure will have to be released surgically otherwise the tendons will die due to ischemia. Because of the slow turnover of collagen, tendon rupture may not occur for several weeks, but the median nerve will suffer damage in the carpal tunnel in a very short time.

In the carpal tunnel, all eight flexor tendons of the fingers share a common sheath *(ulnar bursa)*, as do the four tendons of the extensor digitorum on the back of the wrist (Figs. 14–17, 14–18, 14–19). Other tendons are enveloped by individual synovial sheaths. However, communications may exist between them underneath the retinacula. None of

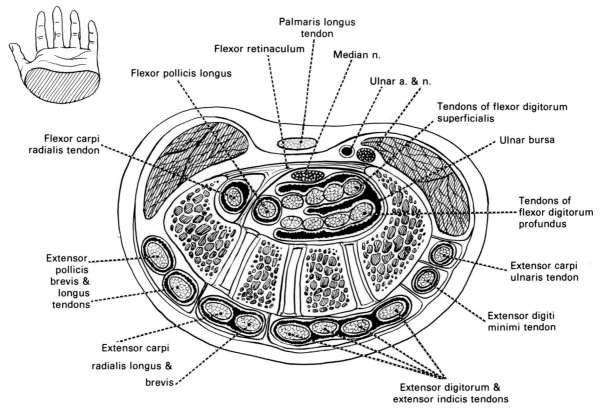

FIG. 14-17. Transverse section of the wrist across the carpal tunnel. Synovial membrane is indicated as a ruffled white line. Synovial fluid within synovial sheaths is shown in black, and, for the purpose of clarity, its quantity is exaggerated.

the synovial sheaths extends into the fingers on the dorsal aspect, but in the palm the common flexor sheath extends into the little finger and the sheath of the flexor pollicis longus covers the tendon to the terminal phalanx of the thumb (Fig. 14–19). The flexor tendons are invested in synovial sheaths also in the remaining three digits. Only rarely does one other of these sheaths retain continuity with the ulnar bursa that occupies the carpal tunnel. Such a possibility, however, has to be kept in mind with penetrating wounds of all fingers, not only of the little finger and thumb.

Apart from these communications, both flexor and extensor sheaths end blindly proximal and distal to the retinacula. Distension of the common flexor sheath may present as a tender swelling in the palm of the hand or proximal to the skin crease of the wrist. Painful irritation of the synovial sheath is common at the point where the tendons of the extensor pollicis brevis and abductor longus

cross over those of the extensor carpi radialis longus and brevis (Fig. 14–18).

Location of Tendons, Nerves, and Arteries

Direct and indirect trauma commonly involves structures around the wrist. An accurate knowledge of anatomy in this area is essential for diagnosis.

Tendons. In learning the order of tendons around the wrist, it is best to proceed on anterior and posterior aspects from the radial styloid process to that of the ulna. On the anterior aspect, the tendons of the flexor carpi radialis, palmaris longus, and flexor carpi ulnaris are the important landmarks. On the dorsum, the boundaries of the snuffbox are helpful in physical examination.

Anteriorly, the only tendons which do not pass through the carpal tunnel are those of the palmaris

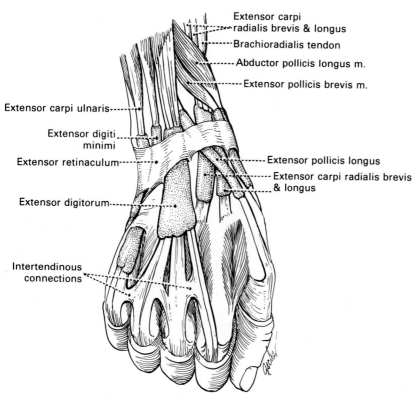

FIG. 14–18. The extensor retinaculum with the tendons and their synovial sheaths on the dorsum of the wrist.

longus and the flexor carpi ulnaris. The former ends in the palmar aponeurosis and the latter inserts into the pisiform. Its true insertion is into the hamate and the fifth metacarpal bone via the pisohamate and pisometacarpal ligaments. Therefore, the pisiform may be regarded as a sesamoid bone in the tendon of the flexor carpi ulnaris.

Nerves and Arteries. The **median nerve** enters the carpal tunnel at the distal skin crease of the wrist. Above this line it lies just deep to the prominent tendon of the palmaris longus (See Fig. 15–6). If that muscle is absent, the nerve can be located on the medial side of the flexor carpi radialis. It is superficial to the tendon of the flexor pollicis longus.

The palmar cutaneous branch of the radial artery enters the palm parallel with the median nerve but remains superficial to the retinaculum. In lacerations, the small vessel may bleed profusely.

The **ulnar nerve** is located adjacent to the lateral side of the tendon of the flexor carpi ulnaris. Here it may be rolled against the head of the ulna. The

ulnar artery is medial to the nerve. Both structures remain superficial to the retinaculum. The course of the **radial artery** has already been traced as have the dorsal cutaneous branches of the ulnar and radial nerves (p. 216).

THE JOINTS OF THE WRIST AND CARPUS

The types of movements possible at the wrist are determined by the radiocarpal or wrist joint. The range of motion, however, is a summation of movement obtained at the radiocarpal, midcarpal, intercarpal, and carpometacarpal joints. It will be evident from the anatomy of the radiocarpal joint that the wrist may be flexed, extended, abducted, and adducted. True rotation is not possible. The combination of all movements produces circumduction. Functional rotation of the hand is amply provided for by the radioulnar joints (pronation and supination).

The **range of movement** can be tested by placing

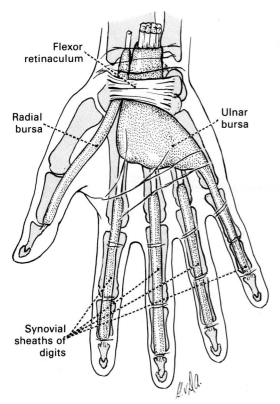

FIG. 14–19. Synovial sheaths of the flexor tendons in the carpal tunnel and the hand. Note the proximal extent of the radial and ulnar bursae in relation to skin creases of the wrist, the upper limit of the retinaculum, and the joint line of the wrist joint. Note also the relationship of the digital synovial sheaths to skin creases of the palm and to the joints.

the hands together in the position of prayer (extension) and then reversing the position by putting the backs of the hands together (flexion). The range of abduction (radial deviation) and adduction (ulnar deviation) may be measured by placing the supine hand on a piece of paper and drawing a line along the little finger in full abduction and adduction while keeping the forearm fixed. Wrist abduction is much more limited than adduction. There is considerable variation in the range of all movements from individual to individual. The progress of a disease or healing process can, however, be monitored in any patient by making such measurements from time to time.

Anatomy of the Joints

The Radiocarpal Joint. The wrist joint is a biaxial, synovial joint of the ellipsoid variety. The proximal, concave **articular surface** is shallow, and consists of the triangular articular disk and the distal surface of the radius. The scaphoid, lunate, and triquetral bones are held together by intercarpal interosseous ligaments and present a continuous, convex articular surface (Fig. 14–20). Because the transverse diameter of the surfaces is much longer than the anteroposterior diameter, rotation of the carpus as a whole is not possible in the socket.

It is usually not appreciated that the ulnar styloid process is covered by articular cartilage on its tip and along its lateral side. The process articulates with a **meniscus** which is distinct from the articular disk and usually separates the pisotriquetral joint from the wrist joint (Fig. 14–20). Ossification may occur in the meniscus.

The stability of the joint depends on its capsular ligaments and the tendons that surround the wrist. The so-called collateral ligaments are ill defined on both the radial and ulnar side of the joint. More important are the *palmar radiocarpal* and *radioulnar* ligaments which are positioned to absorb hyperextension force at the wrist, sustained for instance during falling on the outstretched hand.

The synovial cavity of the wrist joint does not

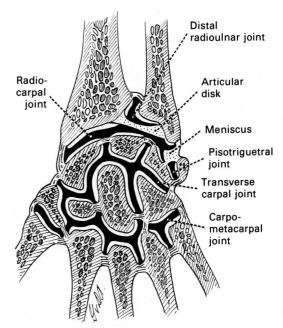

FIG. 14–20. The joints of the wrist and carpus. (Adapted from Lewis OJ, Hamshere RJ, Bucknill TM: J Anat 106:539, 1970, after Warwick R, Williams PL (eds): Gray's Anatomy, 35th ed. Philadelphia, WB Saunders, 1973)

communicate with the more distal joints of the carpus, but it sends an extension toward the ulnar styloid above the meniscus. The meniscus or the disk may be perforated, in which case the pisotriquetral or the distal radioulnar joints will communicate with the wrist joint.

The Midcarpal Joint. The complex joint between the proximal and distal rows of carpal bones is the midcarpal joint (Fig. 14–20). It contributes especially to the range of wrist flexion. In abduction and adduction, the sinuous outline of the joint locks the distal and proximal rows of carpal bones together and ensures that the hand moves as a whole.

The joint cavity is continuous with that of the intercarpal and carpometacarpal joints. There are two exceptions: the carpometacarpal joint of the thumb and the pisotriquetral joint which are separate. Capsular ligaments are attached to the palmar and dorsal surfaces of all bones in continuity with the capsule of the wrist joint. The bones are further secured by interosseous ligaments that run between their nonarticular deep surfaces.

Muscles and Movements

Flexor and extensor muscles of the carpus have already been studied. They all cross both the radiocarpal and midcarpal joints. The radial flexors and extensors acting together produce abduction, while the ulnar flexors and extensors together adduct the hand.

The second important function of the prime movers of the wrist is to stabilize that joint while other muscles act on the fingers. When the fingers are flexed, flexion of the wrist is prevented by contraction of the extensores carpi radialis and ulnaris. Their contraction is readily verified. Similarly, when the fingers are extended without extending the wrist, contraction of the flexor carpi radialis and ulnaris becomes palpable. The prime movers of the wrist are also called into action to increase the mechanical advantage of the finger muscles in order to ensure maximum power of grip. This is **synergistic action.** The importance of the synergistic action becomes evident when one compares the power of grip with the wrist flexed and extended. The tendons of the extensor digitorum are not long enough to allow maximum flexion of the fingers and of the wrist at the same time. In fact, the range of wrist flexion is limited by tension in the extensor digitorum, and more flexion is possible at the wrist when the fingers are extended than when they are flexed. Conversely, when complete finger flexion is required for a powerful grip, the wrist is automatically extended.

CLINICAL EVALUATION

Diseases and injuries in the arm, elbow, forearm, and wrist may seriously compromise hand function. In some injuries an accurate and prompt anatomic diagnosis is essential in order to prevent permanent disability in the hand. In addition to trauma, joint disease and inflammation of bursae and tendon sheaths may cause pain and loss of function. Of the bones of the upper limb the humerus is most often involved in osteomyelitis in the young, and it is also the most frequent site of primary neoplasms or metastases.

The bones of the upper limb may break due to direct or indirect violence. A fall on the outstretched hand may sprain ligaments of the wrist, elbow, and shoulder, but it may also fracture or dislocate some of the bones through which the major component of the force is transmitted. The more common injuries are fracture of the scaphoid (Fig. 14–3B), dislocation of the lunate, fracture of the distal end of the radius (Colles' fracture) or intraarticular fracture of its head, dislocation of the elbow (Figs. 14–6A, 14–21) and supracondylar fracture of the humerus (Fig. 14–21). The same force may dislocate the shoulder or break the clavicle. The brachial artery and median and ulnar nerves are particularly liable to compression or laceration with supracondylar fractures and elbow dislocation. The radial nerve may be injured in the radial groove by diaphyseal fractures of the humerus. A dislocated lunate and a Colles' fracture may be complicated by carpal tunnel syndrome.

Symptoms

Pain, limitation of movement, deformity, and loss of function are the chief complaints which must be pursued as outlined in Chapter 7. Fracture should be suspected at the wrist or elbow following even minor sprains, especially if the pain persists. Fractures may reveal themselves for the first time radiologically only 8–10 days after the injury when sufficient absorption of bone along the fracture line has taken place (Fig. 14–3B).

Whether or not the injured limb is enclosed in a cast or dressing, it is important to be vigilant about the development of pain in the forearm or hand

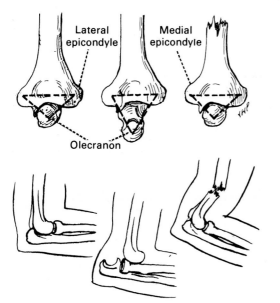

FIG. 14–21. Relation of the olecranon and medial and lateral epicondyles to one another in the normal joint, in posterior dislocation, and in supracondylar fracture of the humerus.

which follows injury around the elbow. If the pain is caused by ischemia of the forearm muscles due to interference with their blood supply (compartment syndrome), necrosis of the muscles and subsequent contracture (Volkmann's ischemic contracture) can only be prevented if treatment is instituted as an emergency measure.

Muscle atrophy, tingling, and numbness in the hand may be due to more proximal compression of the nerves not only in acute injury but during the reduction of fractures and dislocations. Gradual and chronic compression may be caused by fascial bands around the elbow, increased pressure in the carpal tunnel, callus of a healing fracture, or by stretching of the ulnar nerve at the elbow deformed by a fracture that healed a long time ago.

Physical Examination

Because of the continuity of structures between the forearm and hand, physical examination of the two segments of the upper limb is logically performed in continuity. In fact, many structures present in the forearm can only be tested in the hand. These include the extrinsic muscles of the hand and, to some extent, the three major nerves. So clinical evaluation of the hand, dealt with in the next chapter, will be a summary of much of the func-

tional anatomy discussed in these preceding pages. This section is concerned chiefly with those aspects of the physical examination which do not directly implicate the hand.

Inspection. Both upper limbs should be bared, including the shoulders. Comparison of the two sides is the basis for detecting most abnormalities.

Many fractures and dislocations produce obvious and characteristic deformity as well as generalized or localized swelling due to bleeding and edema. In nontraumatic cases, examination should include comparison of the carrying angles, muscle bulk and soft tissue contours in the arm and forearm, inspection for generalized swelling of the joint regions as well as a search for localized swellings and signs of inflammation.

An increase in the carrying angle (cubitus valgus) is usually the result of retarded growth of the lateral humeral condyle due to injury (e.g., supracondylar fracture) during childhood. A varus deformity reverses the normal carrying angle (gunstock deformity) and is due to similar causes on the medial side. Both predispose to degenerative joint disease of the elbow. Cubitus valgus, in addition, may cause neuritis of the ulnar nerve.

Varus and valgus deformity at the wrist are likewise usually due to growth disturbances at the distal epiphysis.

A swollen or distended elbow joint obliterates the hollows on either side of the olecranon, and if the joint is also painful, the forearm will be flexed to about 45° in the midprone position. The wrist, similarly affected, will be held slightly extended. Localized swellings around the elbow may be due to a distended olecranon bursa (student's elbow), rheumatoid nodules, or gouty tophi. A so-called ganglion is a common cystic swelling on the back of the wrist due, it is thought, to mucoid degeneration of synovial membrane of the tendon sheaths.

Palpation. Preceding sections of this chapter were oriented toward physical examination and the location and accessibility of palpable structures were described in detail. Here they will be enumerated in a sequence logically followed in the assessment of a patient. In addition to normal anatomy, potential sites of pathology should be palpated, and attention should be paid to areas of tenderness, and to the size, shape, consistency, and temperature of any swellings and masses encountered. Feeling with the back of the fingers, skin temperature and moisture should be compared over corresponding areas of the limbs. The following structures should be palpated:

1. In the arm
   a. the shaft of the humerus
   b. the biceps, brachials and the triceps
2. Around the elbow
   a. lateral and medial supracondylar ridges leading to the respective epicondyles. Tendinitis or microscopic tears in the common tendon of origin of the extensor muscles causes tenderness localized over the anterior aspect of the lateral epicondyle. The condition is known as **tennis elbow.** The pain is aggravated by stretching the muscles by wrist flexion.
   b. the olecranon process. In the extended elbow, the tip of the olecranon is more or less level with the two epicondyles but when the elbow is flexed these three bony points outline an equilateral triangle (Fig. 14–21). The triangle remains undisturbed in supracondylar fractures but is distorted by dislocation of the elbow.
   c. the head of the radius immediately distal to the lateral epicondyle. Rotation of the head should be verified during pronation and supination. It will be missing when the radius is pulled out of the sling of the annular ligament, a frequent injury in children who were suddenly pulled by the hand.
   d. the joint capsule in the regions of the medial and lateral collateral ligaments
   e. the ulnar nerve behind the medial epicondyle
3. In the forearm
   a. the shaft of the ulna and radius
   b. flexor muscles originating on the medial epicondyle, and extensor muscles on the lateral epicondyle and supracondylar ridge.
4. In the cubital fossa
   a. biceps tendon
   b. brachial artery pulse just medial to the tendon
5. Around the wrist
   a. styloid process of the radius and ulna and the head of the ulna
   b. the extensor tendons in their synovial sheaths under the extensor retinaculum between the two styloid processes across the back of the wrist.
   Frictional tenosynovitis is a common cause of tenderness, especially where the abductor pollicis longus and extensor pollicis brevis cross the tendon of the wrist extensors just proximal to the radial styloid process (Fig. 14–18).
   c. the joint line on the dorsum of the wrist between the two styloid processes

   d. the lunate bone distal to the dorsal tubercle of the radius, and the scaphoid in the anatomic snuffbox
   e. the flexor tendons in their synovial sheaths between the two styloid processes
   f. in the palm of the hand, the pisiform bone and the hook of the hamate on the ulnar side, and on the radial side of the tubercle of the scaphoid, palpable through the thenar muscles
   g. the flexor retinaculum between these bony points
   h. the pulse of the radial and ulnar arteries

Range of Motion and Muscle Strength. Passive range of movement must be tested when the active range is limited. Full flexion of the elbow (150°) brings in contact the brachioradialis with the biceps. The ranges of pronation, supination, wrist flexion-extension, abductor, and adductor have been described with the anatomy of the joints, and these movements have to be tested. The method of testing groups and individual muscles has been described with their anatomy. Testing of the extrinsic muscles of the hand will be discussed in the next chapter which deals with the hand.

Joint Stability. Collateral ligaments of the elbow are tested by applying force in a lateral or medial direction to the wrist grasped by one hand of the examiner while the other hand stabilizes the humerus above the extended elbow. No movement is possible if the ligaments are intact. A similar maneuver at the wrist is less informative about the ligaments because of the normal range of abduction and adduction. The functionally most important ligaments are the palmar, radiocarpal, and radioulnar ligaments which are difficult to test.

SUGGESTED READING

Basmajian JV, Latif A: Integrated actions and functions of the chief flexors of the elbow. A detailed electromyographic analysis. J Bone Joint Surg [A] 39: 1106, 1957
Much of the discussion of the muscles of the elbow are based on this paper and other publications of Basmajian
Hollinshead WH: Anatomy for Surgeons, Vol 3, The Back and Limbs, 2nd ed. New York, Harper & Row, 1969
Chapters 5 and 6 present a detailed, well-illustrated account of the anatomy of the arm, elbow, forearm and wrist with clinical correlations and extensive bibliography
Hoppenfeld S: Physical Examination of the Spine and Extremities. New York, Appleton-Century-Crofts, 1976
Chapters 2 and 3 describe the comprehensive physical examination of the region. Extensively illustrated

Iversen LD, Clawson DK: Manual of Acute Orthopedic Therapeutics. Boston, Little, Brown, 1977
Though the book is primarily oriented toward management of orthopedic cases, Chapters 11, 12 and 13 discuss, in a concise format, injuries of the arm, elbow, forearm and wrist

Kauer JMG: The interdependence of carpal articulation chains. Acta Anat (Basel) *88*: 481, 1974.
The paper deals with the functional anatomy of the wrist and analyzes components of wrist movement

Lewis OJ, Hamshere RJ, Bucknill TM: The anatomy of the wrist joint. J Anat *106*:539, 1970
A scholarly paper dealing with the phylogeny, developmental and gross anatomy of the human wrist joint

Spinner M: Injuries to the Major Branches of Peripheral Nerves of the Forearm. Philadelphia, WB Saunders, 1972
Good correlation of anatomy, diagnosis and treatment

The following are selected articles relevant to clinical anatomy:

Bacron RW, Kurzke JF: Colles' fracture: a study of two thousand cases from the New York State Women's Compensation Board. J Bone Joint Surg [A] *35*: 643, 1953

Conwell HE: Injuries to the elbow. Clin Symp *21*: 35, 1969

Mital MA, Patel UH: Fractures and dislocations about the distal forearm, wrist and hand. Am J Surg *124*: 660, 1972

15
The Hand

CORNELIUS ROSSE

Anatomically, the hand of man is a relatively primitive structure. It is less specialized than the foot or the hand of several other primates. Yet the attainments of our civilization in science, technology, and art must largely be attributed to the infinite variety of purposeful actions the human hand is capable of. The versatility of the manipulative and prehensile functions of the hand is a reflection of the complexity of man's cerebral cortex and not of functional adaptations within the hand. The movements comprise flexion, extension, abduction, adduction of all digits, and opposition of the thumb. While testing of the individual movements of the digits is a requisite in clinical evaluation of the hand, the assessment of hand function must recognize the manner in which these movements are combined in using the hand for power grip and precision grip.

The hand is a sensory organ as well as a manipulative tool. In the manipulation of the environment, the hand relies on sensation for the gathering of information and for the execution of tasks that require precision grip. Precision and power are integrated by the interplay of the extrinsic and intrinsic muscle groups as they operate the adaptable skeletal framework of the hand.

SKELETAL FRAMEWORK AND JOINTS

The carpus and metacarpus are a deformable unit whose plasticity is essential for normal hand function. The carpus and its joints have been described and identified already (see Chap. 14, Fig. 14–2). The carpometacarpal joints are important in grasping because they permit the formation of the transverse metacarpal arch. The carpometacarpal joint of the thumb is specially adapted for the free range of movement which distinguishes this digit.

The metacarpophalangeal joints of the fingers permit abduction and adduction in addition to flexion and extension. The laxity of the ligaments and disparity of the articular surfaces at these joints allows for a considerable passive range of movement in all positions of these joints, except in full flexion. Together with the transverse metacarpal arch, the passive movements at the metacarpophalangeal joints enhance the plasticity of the hand and facilitate its adaptability to the shape and size of the object being grasped. Movement at the interphalangeal joints is restricted to flexion and extension.

The Transverse Metacarpal Arch

When the wrist and fingers are extended, the palm of the hand is flat and the heads of the metacarpal bones lie in one plane. Flexion of the wrist causes cupping of the palm and the metacarpal heads come to lie along an arc. This is a reflection of the *carpal arch* (see Fig. 14–4) with which the metacarpals articulate.

In the extended position the fingers are of different lengths and are spread apart. Flexion of the fingers brings them together, and their tips contact the palm along a straight line. The knuckles, which represent the metacarpal heads, form an arc in this position. The curvature of the arc becomes exaggerated as the power of the grip is increased. The arc described by the metacarpal heads in the clenched or cupped hand is the *transverse metacarpal arch*. The mobility of the fourth and fifth metacarpal bones is largely responsible for changes in the arch.

The transverse metacarpal arch permits the tips of the fingers to meet and work together in any position of flexion. The arch provides an important mechanism for the effectiveness of both power grip and precision grip. It is clinically important to take note of the fact that due to the metacarpal arch, each finger when flexed individually contacts the ball of the thumb and points toward the tuberosity of the scaphoid. Fractures of the metacarpals should be immobilized using this relationship as a guide, otherwise, the fracture will unite with the distal fragment rotated and the resulting finger deformity will interfere seriously with hand function. Furthermore, in the treatment of hand injuries the position chosen for immobilization must maintain the metacarpal arch. Scar formation and fibrosis in the flat position will prevent reformation of the arch and will compromise hand function.

Joints

The Carpometacarpal Joint of the Thumb. The thumb is unique among the digits because it can be opposed to each finger and because it can be moved very freely. These characteristics are due to the independence of the first metacarpal bone from the others, and to the saddle-shaped articular surfaces between the trapezium and the metacarpal.

The trapezium is set in the carpus in such a manner that the long axis of its sellar articular surface makes an angle of nearly 90° with the palm. This determines the orientation of the first metacarpal and the neutral or resting position for describing thumb movements (Fig. 15–1). The joint is biaxial (Fig. 5–9) but the curvatures of the articular surface on the metacarpal are greater than on the trapezium, and, therefore, the joint is very loose in all positions except in full abduction and adduction. Joint stability in these positions is essential for hand function. In precision grip the thumb metacarpal is abducted and the joint is stabilized, while in power grip, the joint becomes stable in the adducted position. In both positions, the thumb is opposed as well. The taut capsular ligaments on the dorsal and lateral aspects of the joint are the chief factors of stability in abduction and adduction. In the neutral position, the capsule is very loose, and free passive movements are permitted.

It is inherent in the nature of the incongruous articular surfaces that when the thumb moves in an ulnar direction, the metacarpal bone rotates medially along its long axis. This results in the opposition of the pulp of the thumb against the palm or against the pulp of any of the fingers. A special muscle exists for bringing about this movement actively; this is the opponens pollicis. However, rotation of the metacarpal is inevitable and even if the opponens is paralyzed, the thumb will swing into opposition when the flexor muscle pulls the metacarpal in an ulnar direction (conse-

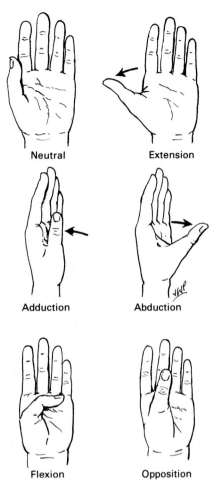

FIG. 15–1. Movements of the thumb.

quential movement). The carpometacarpal joint of the thumb is chiefly responsible for opposition, abduction, adduction, and circumduction of this digit. It contributes also to flexion and extension but these movements occur mainly at the more distal joints.

The Metacarpophalangeal (MCP) Joints. The condyloid articular surface on the metacarpal heads extends further on the palmar aspect than dorsally and is also wider in the palm than on the knuckles (Fig. 15–2). The shallow, ovoid facet of the proximal phalanx is much smaller than the metacarpal head, and when the ligaments are lax, accessory movements are freely elicited at the joint which include rotation. Active movements consist of

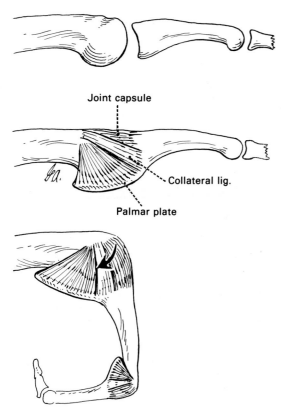

FIG. 15-2. The metacarpophalangeal and interphalangeal joints.

flexion, extension, abduction, adduction, and circumduction. The joint line is palpable on the knuckles, but in the palm it is about 2 cm proximal to the free edge of the finger web.

On the palmar aspect the **capsule** has thickened into a stiff, fibrocartilaginous plate called the **palmar ligament** or **palmar plate** (Fig. 15-2). The plate is grooved by the flexor tendons as they cross the joint, and its deep surface articulates with the metacarpal head. The palmar plates are firmly attached to the base of the phalanx and always move with it. A much thinner portion of the capsule attaches the proximal edge of the palmar plate to the metacarpal. The thin portion of the capsule may become torn and when a dislocated joint is reduced, the palmar plate may become caught between the metacarpal head and the phalanx.

Three types of ligaments attach to the palmar plate. These are the collateral ligaments, the deep transverse metacarpal ligaments, and the fibrous digital sheaths.

The oblique, cordlike portion of the **collateral**

ligament is attached dorsally to the metacarpal head and distally to the base of the proximal phalanx (Fig. 15-2). However, a fan-shaped portion of the collateral ligament blends with the palmar plate. The collateral ligaments are lax in extension, and deviation and passive rotation of the fingers is possible. As the phalanx is flexed, the cordlike ligament is drawn over the broader portion of the metacarpal head and becomes increasingly tight. Due to this tension, the fingers cannot be spread apart (actively or passively) in the fully flexed position (90°) and no accessory movements can be elicited. **If an injured ligament is allowed to heal with the joint in extension, it will be too short to permit flexion and the fingers will become stiff in the extended position.** Therefore, an injured hand should be immobilized with the MCP joints in approximately 90° flexion.

The **deep transverse metacarpal ligaments** are in the depth of the finger webs and run between the edges of the neighboring palmar plates of the four fingers (Fig. 15-3). These connections restrict independent flexion of the middle and ring fingers, and prevent separation of the metacarpal heads. However, they permit the required mobility of these bones during changes of the transverse metacarpal arch. The deep transverse metacarpal ligament is not to be confused with the superficial transverse metacarpal ligament which is part of the palmar aponeurosis (Fig. 15-22).

The third ligamentous structure attached to the palmar plate is the **fibrous digital sheath** (Fig. 15-3) which forms a retention sling for the long flexor tendons. Dorsally, the thin capsule of the metacarpophalangeal joint is protected by the dorsal digital expansion (Fig. 15-10).

Two **sesamoid bones** articulate with the palmar aspect of the head of the first metacarpal (see Fig. 14-2) and, rarely, such bones may be present also at other metacarpals.

The Interphalangeal (IP) Joints. The pulley-shaped articular surfaces of the distal (DIP) and proximal (PIP) interphalangeal joints function as pure hinge joints. Only flexion and extension are possible. The structure of the joints and the arrangement of the ligaments, including the palmar plates, is similar to that of the metacarpophalangeal (MCP) joint (Fig. 15-2), but there is no equivalent, of course, for the transverse metacarpal ligament. The palmar plates of the IP joints are important factors in preventing hyperextension of the joints.

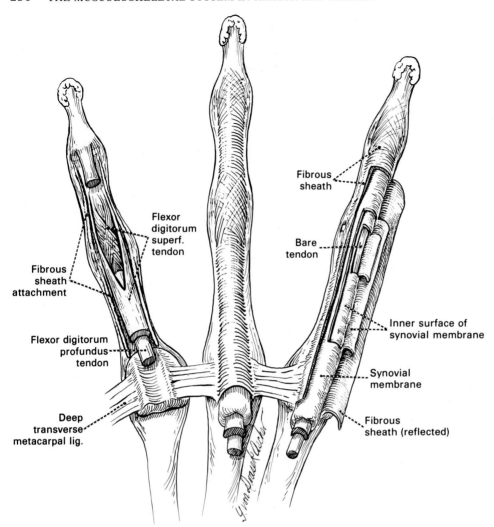

FIG. 15–3. The arrangement of flexor tendons, synovial membrane, and fibrous flexor sheaths in the fingers.

MUSCLES OF THE HAND

In the palm and on the dorsum of the hand, the extrinsic muscles are represented only by tendons. The muscle bellies of the intrinsic hand muscles are confined to the palm and their tendons proceed to the digits. The latter muscles are principally responsible for abduction, adduction, and opposition of the digits. Although flexion and extension are primarily the function of the extrinsic muscles, intrinsic muscles play an important role also in these movements. The only movement not influenced by intrinsic muscle action is flexion of the IP joints. Without intrinsic muscles, the hand is re-duced to functioning as a simple hook, whereas the intact intrinsic muscles enable the hand to perform as the most versatile tool, combining power and precision.

The Flexor Tendons

After the tendons of the flexor digitorum superficialis and profundus emerge from the carpal tunnel, they proceed in pairs toward the MCP joints where they enter another osseofibrous tunnel formed by the fibrous digital sheaths. Between these two tunnels in the palm of the hand they are covered by the palmar aponeurosis. Within the

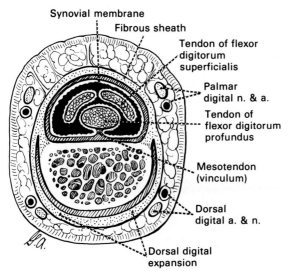

FIG. 15-4. A transverse section across the proximal phalanx of a finger to show the arrangement of flexor tendons and their synovial membrane within the fibrous flexor sheaths.

fibrous digital sheaths, the tendon of the flexor digitorum superficialis inserts into the middle phalanx and the profundus into the distal phalanx.

The **fibrous digital sheaths** are sheaths of dense fibrous tissue that span over the tendons from the metacarpal head to the base of the distal phalanx. The sheaths attach on each side of the tendons to the phalanges and the palmar plates of the MCP and IP joints (Fig. 15–3). They are thinner and more pliable over the joints. The tunnels are lined by synovial membrane which reflects onto the tendons (Fig. 15–4). These are the **digital synovial tendon sheaths** and their relationship to the synovial sheaths found in the carpal tunnel has been discussed already (see Fig. 14–19).

Within the fibrous digital sheath, the tendon of the flexor digitorum superficialis splits over the proximal phalanx, Each half passes dorsal to the tendon of the flexor digitorum profundus and attaches along the middle phalanx (Fig. 15–3). The latter then proceeds to the base of the distal phalanx. The tendons receive their blood supply via delicate mesotendons called **vincula** (Fig. 15–4). Only one tendon occupies the osseofibrous tunnel in the thumb, that of the flexor pollicis longus.

Testing of the Flexor Tendons. It is evident from the attachment of the tendons that the distal phalanx is flexed by the flexor digitorum profundus only. The integrity of the muscle and tendon

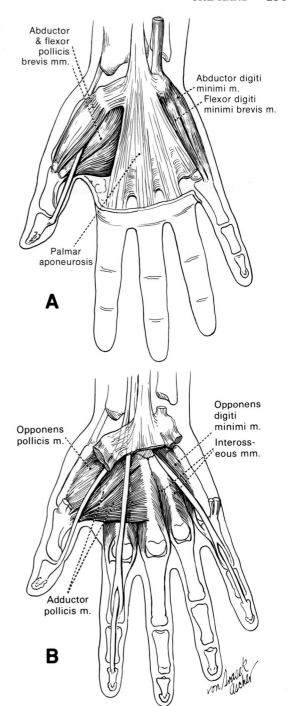

FIG. 15-5. The thenar and hypothenar muscles. In **A** only the superficial fascia of the palm has been reflected. In **B** the dissection has been carried further by removing the palmar aponeurosis as well as the flexor tendons of the middle and ring fingers. In addition, the two superficial muscles in both thenar and hypothenar eminences have been resected.

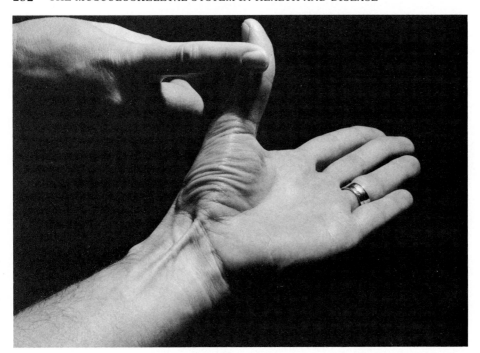

FIG. 15-6. Contraction of the abductor pollicis brevis plicates the skin of the thenar eminence and reflexly invokes the contraction of the palmaris longus, throwing its tendon into prominence. The latter muscle contracts to stabilize the palmar aponeurosis from which the short abductor arises. The test, as demonstrated, verifies the integrity of the median nerve, both in the proximal forearm and at the wrist.

can be tested by holding all joints of a finger in extension, releasing the DIP joint, and then asking the patient to flex the tip of the finger.

Both the superficial and the deep flexor tendons produce flexion at the PIP and MCP joints. The flexor digitorum superficialis can, however, be tested in the middle, ring, and little fingers independent of the profundus by the following maneuver. Holding all fingers in extension at all joints immobilizes the flexor digitorum profundus. If the finger to be tested is freed, and the patient is requested to flex it, flexion will occur at the PIP and MCP joints due to contraction of the flexor digitorum superficialis. Under these conditions, the profundus cannot flex the finger at either interphalangeal joint because its individual tendons cannot be operated separately by its muscle belly. This is demonstrated in the normal hand by the inability to flex the DIP joint of a finger when the other fingers are immobilized in extension.

Testing the profundus tendon in the index and middle finger demonstrates integrity of the anterior interosseous branch of the median nerve (C8,T1) and testing the tendon in the little and ring fingers provides the same information for the ulnar nerve (C8,T1) in the forearm. The flexor digitorum superficialis is innervated by the median nerve in the forearm (C7 and C8). The flexor pollicis longus (anterior interosseous nerve, C8 and T1) inserts into the distal phalanx of the thumb and is tested the same way as the flexor digitorum profundus. When a finger remains in extension in the resting hand, it is an indication that a flexor tendon of the finger is interrupted.

Intrinsic Muscles of the Hand

The intrinsic muscles of the hand may be divided into three groups: 1) the muscles of the thumb (thenar muscles), 2) the muscles of the little finger (hypothenar muscles), and 3) the interosseous and lumbrical muscles. Both thenar and hypothenar muscles produce a fleshy eminence on the radial and ulnar side of the palm, respectively (Fig. 15-5A). The interosseous muscles are the deepest structures in the palm, filling the spaces between the metacarpal bones (Fig. 15-5B). They are deep to the flexor tendons while the lumbricals are asso-

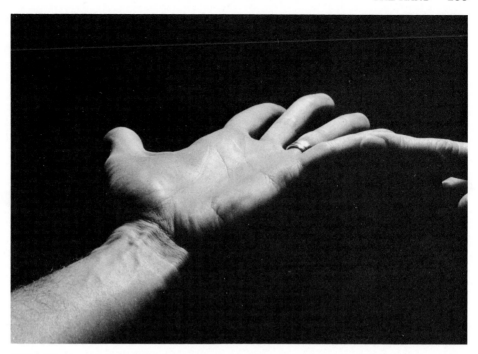

FIG. 15–7. Contraction of the abductor digiti minimi plicates the skin of the hypothenar eminence and reflexly invokes the contraction of the flexor carpi ulnaris to stabilize the pisiform bone from which the abductor muscle originates. The test, as demonstrated, verifies the integrity of the ulnar nerve in the proximal forearm and at the wrist.

ciated with the tendons of the flexor digitorum profundus.

Muscles of the Thumb. The thenar eminence is produced by three muscles. The **abductor pollicis brevis** and **flexor pollicis brevis** are superficial (Fig. 15–5A), deep to them is the **opponens pollicis** (Fig. 15–5B). A fourth muscle called the **adductor pollicis,** the largest, does not contribute to the eminence because it is more deeply placed. The principal actions of these muscles are proclaimed by their names. However, it should be borne in mind that they can and do contribute actively to thumb movements other than their names imply.

The three muscles of the thenar eminence originate from the flexor retinaculum and the trapezium. Some superficial fibers of the **abductor** originate from the palmar aponeurosis and from the deep fascia that covers the thenar eminence. These two areas of origin are helpful in testing the contraction of this muscle which, of all hand muscles, is the most informative in the evaluation of the median nerve. During abduction of the thumb, the tendon of the palmaris longus reflexly springs into prominence as the muscle tightens the aponeurosis, and the skin over the eminence becomes plicated (Fig. 15–6). The abductor inserts into the base of the proximal phalanx on the radial side and the short flexor on the ulnar side of the same bone. A sesamoid bone is present in each tendon of insertion (Fig. 14–2).

The tendon of the flexor pollicis longus apparently separates a small portion of the flexor pollicis brevis from the more bulky superficial part of the muscle. The deep head lies in the plane of the adductor pollicis and has much in common with it. The opponens pollicis inserts into the shaft of the first metacarpal (Fig. 15–5B).

The **adductor pollicis** is a fan-shaped muscle. Its proximal fibers constitute the oblique head and arise from the bases of the first three metacarpals. The distal fibers originate on the shaft of the third metacarpal and represent the transverse head. Both heads converge on the sesamoid bone on the ulnar side of the MCP joint and insert into the base of the proximal phalanx. Thus, of the four thenar muscles only the opponens attaches to the metacarpal shaft while the remaining three insert via sesamoid bones into the base of the proximal phalanx. However, all these muscles can move the carpometacarpal joint, the most important joint of the thumb.

The **innervation pattern** of thenar muscles is important in the diagnosis of nerve injuries sustained around the wrist or in the hands. The rule usually stated assigns the adductor to the ulnar nerve and the other three muscles to the median nerve. However, this holds true only for a proportion of cases. Most constant is the innervation of the adductor by the deep branch of the ulnar nerve (97%), and the abductor pollicis brevis by the median nerve (95%). The deep head of the flexor brevis is usually supplied by the ulnar nerve and the superficial part by the median. The opponens is innervated in 80 percent of cases by both the median and ulnar nerves and only in the remaining 20 percent is it supplied entirely by the median nerve. Rarely, it is supplied completely by the ulnar nerve. The segmental supply to thumb muscles is overwhelmingly from T1 with some input from C8, as it is to all intrinsic hand muscles.

Muscles of the Little Finger. The hypothenar eminence, like the thenar eminence, consists of three muscles. These are the **abductor digiti minimi, flexor digiti minimi brevis,** and **opponens digiti minimi.** Their arrangement and mode of insertion mirror those of the thenar muscles (Fig. 15–5). There is no named adductor for the fifth digit; its adduction is obtained by one of the interossei. All muscles are innervated by the deep branch of the ulnar nerve (C8,T1).

Testing of the abductor digiti minimi is particularly informative in evaluation of the ulnar nerve. The muscle arises from the pisiform bone, and when it contracts the pisiform has to be stabilized at the pisotriquetral joint. As soon as abduction of the little finger is initiated, the tendon of the flexor carpi ulnaris reflexly springs into prominence in a manner analogous to that of the palmaris longus during testing of the abductor pollicis brevis (Fig. 15–7). These two tests demonstrate that the ulnar or median nerves are intact not only in the hand, but also in the proximal forearm.

The **palmaris brevis** is a thin muscle sheet located in the superficial fascia over the hypothenar eminence. It has no counterpart on the thenar side, but it tethers the skin like some fibers of the abductor pollicis brevis over the thenar eminence. The palmaris brevis is the only muscle supplied by the superficial division of the ulnar nerve.

The Interosseous Muscles. The muscles are so named because they fill the spaces between the metacarpal bones. They are divided into two groups; the palmar and dorsal interossei. Both groups are located in the palm of the hand, where they form the deepest muscle layer (Fig. 15–8).

The **dorsal interossei** are larger and they are visible also on the back of the hand. Each dorsal interosseous originates by two heads from adjacent sides of two metacarpal bones and inserts into the proximal phalanx and dorsal digital expansion. The tendons leave the palm by passing dorsal to the deep transverse metacarpal ligament, but their line of pull is such that they flex the MCP joint (Fig. 15–10, 15–11). There are four dorsal interossei; the tendons of two insert into the middle finger (one on each side), one into the radial side of the index finger (this is the first dorsal interosseous), and one into the ulnar side of the ring finger. This pattern of insertion can be reasoned from one of the actions exerted by the dorsal interossei at the MCP joint. They *abduct* or spread all fingers away from the imaginary axis of the middle finger. Clearly, no dorsal interossei are associated with the thumb or the little finger as these possess their own abductors.

There are only three **palmar interossei** (Fig. 15–8). Each originates from one metacarpal bone anterior to the attachment of the dorsal interosseous. The tendon leaves the palm passing dorsal to the deep transverse metacarpal ligament and inserts into the dorsal digital expansion (Fig. 15–10). Acting together with the dorsal interossei, they too flex the MCP joint. The palmar interossei *adduct* the fingers at the MCP joint toward the imaginary axis of the middle finger. The palmar interosseous of the index passes the MCP joint on the ulnar side and those of the ring and little finger on the radial side. The middle finger has none, and only sometimes is a vestigial palmar interosseous associated with the thumb. Thus, one palmar or dorsal interosseous tendon joins the dorsal digital expansion on each side in each finger (Fig. 15–10) except in the fifth, which has none on the ulnar side.

The interossei are responsible for three distinct types of finger movements: 1) flexion of the MCP joint, 2) abduction-adduction of the MCP joint, and 3) by virtue of their insertion into the dorsal digital expansion, they extend the PIP and DIP joints.

All interossei are innervated by the deep branch of the ulnar nerve (C8,T1). The most readily palpable muscle in the group is the **first dorsal interosseous** which becomes hard and prominent when the

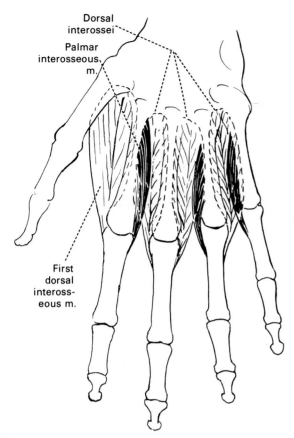

FIG. 15–8. Palmar and dorsal interosseous muscles.

The Extensor Tendons and the Dorsal Digital Expansion

After the extensor tendons of the digits emerge from underneath the extensor retinacula they fan out along the back of the hand toward the digits. **Intertendinous connections** join the four tendons of the extensor digitorum to one another just proximal to the MCP joints (see Fig. 14–18). This explains why independent extension of the middle and ring fingers is difficult and unnatural. The index and little fingers enjoy much greater independence in extension because each is served by an additional extensor (extensor indicis and extensor digiti minimi) which are not bound to the extensor digitorum. The thumb has its own two extensors, the extensor pollicis longus and brevis.

Cutting any one of the extensor digitorum tendons proximal to the intertendinous connections results in little or no loss in finger extension, but if the tendon of the middle or ring finger is cut distal to the connections, extension of the MCP joint will no longer be possible.

The insertion of the extensor tendons of the thumb is relatively simple; the extensor pollicis brevis attaches to the base of the proximal phalanx and the long extensor to the distal phalanx. (Sometimes the extensor brevis continues to the distal phalanx and is capable of extending it even with the tendon of the extensor pollicis longus cut.) Aponeurotic expansions from the tendons of the

index is abducted against resistance or when it is pinched hard against the thumb (Fig. 15–9). However, it is not the best muscle to use for ulnar nerve tests, because rarely it may be innervated by the median nerve. The power of abduction and adduction in the other fingers gives more reliable indication of ulnar nerve integrity in the hand.

The Lumbricals. Four slender muscles arise from the tendons of the flexor digitorum profundus in the palm of the hand. They are the lumbricals. Their tendons pass along the palmar surface of the deep transverse metacarpal ligaments on the radial side of the fingers and join the dorsal digital expansion (Figs. 15–10, 15–11). Via this insertion they extend the interphalangeal joints. Due to the manner in which they pass the PIP joint, they prevent its hyperextension by the extensor digitorum. As a rule, the radial two lumbricals are innervated by the median nerve and the other two by the deep branch of the ulnar nerve.

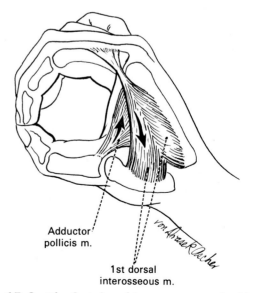

FIG. 15–9. The first dorsal interosseous and adductor pollicis contract during precision grip.

abductor pollicis brevis and adductor pollicis contribute some transverse fibers to the long extensor tendon. The insertion of the extensor tendons of the fingers is much more complex. The tendons form an aponeurotic expansion over the MCP joints and phalanges, which is reinforced by the tendons of the interossei and lumbricals and by some intrinsic bands of connective tissue. This triangular structure is properly called the **dorsal digital expansion** but is also known as the **extensor hood** or the **extensor aponeurosis**.

The Dorsal Digital Expansion. The ribbonlike tendon of the extensor digitorum trifurcates over the proximal phalanx (Fig. 15–10). The **central slip** inserts into the base of the middle phalanx and the two **lateral bands** pass on either side of the PIP joint, fuse with each other beyond it, and insert into the base of the distal phalanx. The trifurcate tendon is held centered over the finger by transverse fibers in the expansion (transverse retinacular ligaments).

On each side the **tendon of an interosseous muscle** comingles with the lateral band of the extensor digitorum and becomes an integral part of it (Figs. 15–10, 15–11). The fusion occurs over the middle phalanx. Proximal to this point, the interosseous tendon fans out into an aponeurosis, some fibers of which fuse with the central slip of the extensor digitorum, while others arch over it and blend with the interosseous aponeurosis on the other side of the finger. On the radial side, the tendon of a lumbrical joins the expansion in the region of the PIP joint, just distal to the interosseous tendon.

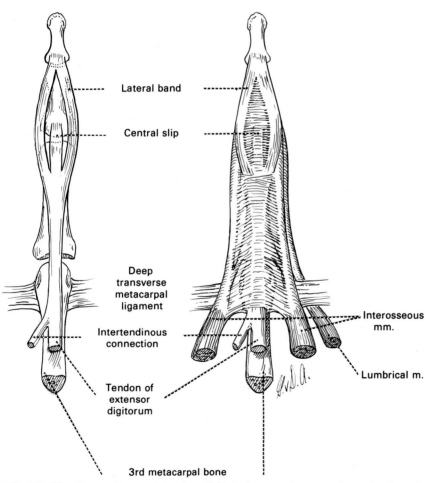

FIG. 15–10. Components of the dorsal digital expansion seen from the dorsal aspect.

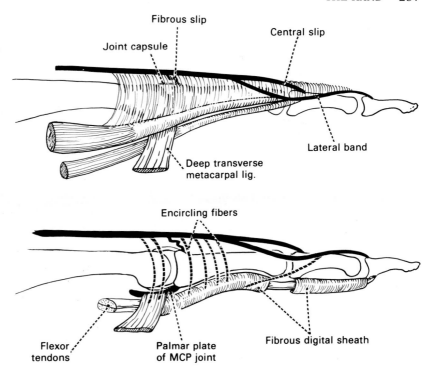

Fibrous slip

Joint capsule

Central slip

Lateral band

Deep transverse metacarpal lig.

Encircling fibers

Flexor tendons

Palmar plate of MCP joint

Fibrous digital sheath

FIG. 15–11. The dorsal digital expansion seen from the side and some of its components illustrated schematically.

Each trifurcate extensor digitorum tendon transmits, therefore, forces generated by two interossei and a lumbrical and by its own muscle belly. These forces extend the proximal and distal interphalangeal joints. Extension of the MCP joint is also mediated via the dorsal digital expansion. The extensor digitorum tendon sends a fibrous slip from its deep surface into the capsule of the MCP joint, which inserts into the base of the proximal phalanx via the capsule (Fig. 15–11). This structure, however, plays little or no role in MCP extension because it remains lax during all phases of the movement and is tight only in hyperextension. A series of fibers derived from the dorsal digital expansion encircle the MCP joint and the proximal phalanx and fuse on the palmar aspect of the finger with the deep transverse metacarpal ligament and with the fibrous digital sheaths (Fig. 15–11). These fibers, and not the fibrous slip, transmit the pull of the extensor digitorum to the proximal phalanx and bring about extension of the MCP joint.

Several other components have been described in the dorsal digital expansion (e.g., retinacular ligaments) whose functional importance remains controversial except when they limit movement due to their scarring or contracture. The normal function and the disorders of the extensor mechanism in the fingers can be explained by understanding the interplay of the major components described above.

Integration of Finger Movements by the Dorsal Digital Expansion. The MCP joint may be flexed or extended whatever the position of the interphalangeal joints. On the other hand, movement at the PIP and DIP joints is always synchronized. The middle phalanx cannot be extended without extending the distal phalanx also, and the same is true in reverse. This is because the muscles that exert force through the central slip of the expansion also exert force along the lateral bands. The mechanism requires that the lengths of these tendons be precisely balanced.

During flexion of the interphalangeal joints, the two lateral bands of the dorsal digital expansion bowstring in a palmar direction because flexion shifts their point of distal attachment in this direction (Fig. 15–12). The bands slide onto the wider palmar aspect of the head of the proximal phalanx which prevents their slackening. When the PIP

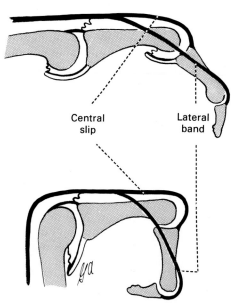

FIG. 15-12. Integration of movement at the interphalangeal joints by components of the dorsal digital expansion. For explanation see text. (Adapted from Harris C, Rutledge GL Jr: J Bone Joint Surg 54-A:713, 1972)

Central slip

Lateral band

joint is flexed completely, the distal phalanx cannot be extended because the central slip of the expansion has been put under tension passively and, therefore, fixes the entire extensor hood. In the reverse of the movement, the middle phalanx will come into extension first as the central slip of the expansion extends the PIP joint. Then the lateral bands approximate each other on the dorsum of the finger as the pull is transmitted along them. The lumbricals may play a role in integrating flexor and extensor mechanisms as they are attached to both flexor and extensor tendons. Some fibrous bands in the digital expansion (oblique retinacular ligaments) which run between the lateral bands and the fibrous flexor sheaths (Fig. 15-11) may have a similar function.

Finger Deformities Due to Disrupted Extensor Mechanisms. A brief review of some common finger injuries is instructive because it emphasizes the functional importance of various structures.

When the extensor tendon is evulsed from the distal phalanx, with or without a chip of bone, or when the lateral bands are ruptured or cut, a flexion deformity results at the DIP joint (*baseball* or *mallet finger*, Fig. 15-13). The torn ligament or the fracture may heal if the finger is immobilized with the DIP joint in extension. The deformity will not be completely corrected, however, if the healed ligament is longer than the normal structure.

If the central slip of the digital expansion is ruptured, minimal deformity results as long as the transverse fibers of the expansion remain intact. If they are also torn, a deformity is produced at the PIP joint, which the English speaking orthopaedic community calls the *"boutonnière" deformity* while the French call it the "button hole." In this case, all extensor force will be transmitted to the distal phalanx by the intact lateral bands, producing hyperextension of the DIP joint. The PIP joint buckles into flexion and protrudes through the breech in the extensor hood. The two lateral bands will now run on the palmar aspect of the PIP joint and will exaggerate flexion. Correction of the deformity must aim at reattachment of the central slip and must not interfere with the lateral bands.

Hyperextension of the PIP joint with associated flexion of the DIP joint is known as the *swan neck* deformity. Some young people can produce it voluntarily. Hyperextension at the PIP joint allows the lateral bands to bowstring on the dorsal aspect of the middle phalanx which gives them sufficient slackness to permit the flexor digitorum profundus to flex the DIP joint. When due to trauma or disease, the cause is evulsion or rupture of the palmar plate of PIP joint. The deformity is commonly seen in rheumatoid arthritis (see Fig. 22–5).

The dorsal digital expansion and the extensor tendons are often severely involved in inflammatory changes associated with rheumatoid arthritis. In this case, the extensor tendons usually slip in an ulnar direction from their central position at the MCP joints. Flexion of the fingers displaces the tendons further. Extension at these joints becomes impossible but the tendon may snap back into a more central position whence extension will proceed.

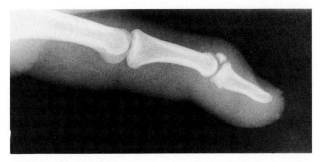

FIG. 15-13. Evulsion of the attachment of the lateral bands of the dorsal digital expansion from the distal phalanx with a chip of bone (baseball or mallet finger). (Courtesy of Dr. Rosalind H. Troupin)

Swelling or nodule formation in the flexor tendons or in their synovial sheaths or a narrowing of the fibrous digital sheaths may produce a *trigger finger* (Fig. 15–14). During flexion, the swelling may be pulled out of the osseofascial tunnel of the finger into the palm of the hand. Its reentry into the tunnel during extension will be retarded, but when the resistance is overcome by extension force, the finger will snap into extension (sometimes audibly). This is painful and commonly occurs in traumatic or degenerative conditions.

MOVEMENTS OF THE HAND

Movements of the Hand as a Whole

Individual digits can be tested separately and the range of each movement can be recorded in degrees but the movements which transform the hand into the functional unit it is cannot be measured in this way. These movements are complex biomechanical operations involving all joints at the same time. Most important of these are the movements concerned with prehension which involve grasping an object. Although they are complex, the movements can be broken down into two basic acts: power grip and precision grip. The thumb and the radial two fingers are chiefly (but not exclusively) concerned with precision grip, while the ulnar half of the hand contributes greatly to power grip. It is a requirement in both types of grip that the object be held securely and, therefore, joint stability is an important factor in hand function.

In **power grip** the fingers form one jaw of a clamp, the other jaw of which is the palm. The thumb is wrapped around the dorsum of the clenched fingers and serves as a buttress. It is powerfully adducted. If precision needs to be combined with power, it is the thumb that supplies precision as it shifts its point of contact to the side of the index finger and comes to direct the object that is grasped. These movements may be observed when a rope, hammer, steering wheel, or handle of a pitcher are held in the hand. During these movements, the wrist is stabilized in the neutral position.

Precision grip employs the pulp of the thumb, index, and middle fingers, that is, the sensory surface of the digits (Fig. 15–9). The wrist is stabilized in extension, the position most advantageous for the action of extrinsic hand muscles. The carpometacarpal joint of the thumb becomes stable in abduction and opposition. The ulnar half of the

hand may retain power grip over an object while the thumb and radial fingers manipulate it with precision. These basic movements can be combined in a constantly changing chain of actions.

Movements of the hand as a whole will be impaired by anatomic defects and pain in the hand. To diagnose such defects it is necessary that individual movements are thoroughly understood. The anatomy and clinical testing of the various digital movements is the subject of the next sections.

A second major cause of functional impairment

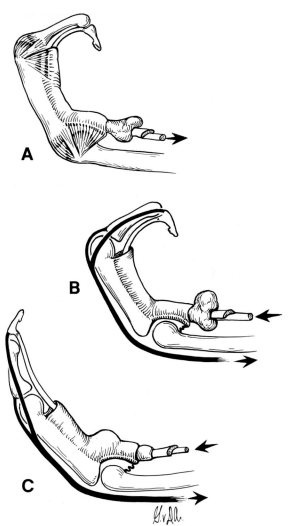

FIG. 15-14. Trigger finger. **(A)** Flexion displaces a swelling in the synovial sheath of the flexor tendon from the fibrous flexor sheath into the palm. **(B)** Extension is limited by the resistance the swelling encounters in reentering the narrow osseofibrous tunnel. **(C)** When this resistance is overcome by extensor force, the finger snaps into extension.

of the hand is interference with its central control. In cerebral palsy and other diseases of the central nervous system, the complicated hand movements suffer the greatest loss, and during recovery they are the last to return. Reference is made to these conditions in Chapter 27.

Movements of the Digits

Although anatomists of antiquity had a fair knowledge of the actions of specific hand muscles, much research was done in recent times to provide an understanding of the interplay of various muscle groups during movements of the digits.

Finger Movements. In the position of rest, all muscles are relaxed and the fingers are held partially flexed due to what has been called the viscoelastic properties of the flexor digitorum profundus. In natural or habitual movements of the hand, the four fingers tend to move together, and under these circumstances only the prime movers contract; their antagonists remain quiescent. When only one finger is moved, most commonly the index or little finger, the others have to be immobilized and then there is activity in both prime movers and antagonists.

Opening and closing the hand is the function of the extrinsic muscles. The intrinsic muscles modify these basic movements. They do not participate in closing the hand fully, but come into play when different movements are required at different joints. The interossei and lumbricals are responsible for producing the combined position of metacarpophalangeal flexion and interphalangeal extension. This posture is an important component of numerous activities such as writing, drawing, cutting with a knife and fork, or holding a spoon. The interossei also produce controlled abduction and adduction of the fingers. These movements are components of such complex activities as playing musical instruments or using a typewriter. In the extended hand, uncontrolled abduction of the fingers can result from the pull of the extensor digitorum tendons as they fan out from the wrist. Likewise, uncontrolled adduction of the fingers occurs during flexion.

The sole extensor of the MCP joints is the extensor digitorum. This muscle is active in interphalangeal extension, whatever the position of MCP joints. The interossei and lumbricals, in addition to contributing to interphalangeal extension as prime movers, render the action of the extensor

digitorum at the DIP joint more efficient because they prevent hyperextension at the PIP joint. This joint would tend to hyperextend due to the attachment of the central slip of the digital expansion to the base of the middle phalanx. Hyperextension is prevented as the interossei and lumbricals pull the extensor hood in a palmar direction on each side of the finger.

Thumb Movements. The importance of thumb movements in hand function has already been emphasized. The natural movement of the thumb is opposition. The opponens pollicis controls this movement when the thumb is gently opposed to the index and middle fingers. However, when the thumb approaches the ring and little finger, the latter begin to move reflexly toward the thumb from the inception of thumb movement. Thus, thenar and hypothenar muscles contract in unison.

When firm opposition is required, not only the opponens pollicis, but the abductor and flexor pollicis brevis, as well as the adductor pollicis, become active. Interestingly, the hypothenar muscles are recruited during firm opposition, even when this movement is performed against the radial two fingers. The thenar and hypothenar muscles acting together exaggerate the transverse metacarpal arch. These muscle groups are ideally positioned for this purpose as they diverge from their attachment to the flexor retinaculum toward the MCP joints of the first and fifth digits.

INNERVATION AND BLOOD SUPPLY OF THE HAND

It is important to understand the over-all plan of innervation and blood supply in the hand before proceeding to the description of significant details.

The **median nerve** is the chief nerve of sensation in the hand because it supplies the palmar surfaces of the digits most commonly employed for feeling and for precision grip. In addition, it is motor to the thenar eminence musculature. The **ulnar nerve** is the chief motor nerve of the intrinsic muscles of the hand, and it is sensory only to the ulnar one and a half fingers. The **radial nerve** supplies no muscle in the hand and its sensory distribution is confined to the dorsum. Division of either the median or ulnar nerves seriously impairs hand function, whereas interruption of the superficial branch of the radial nerve above the wrist is barely perceptible. In the diagnosis of nerve injuries, motor, sensory, and

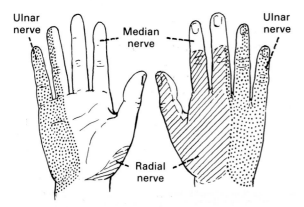

FIG. 15–15. The typical sensory distribution of the median, ulnar, and radial nerves in the hand. The considerable overlap between these areas is not indicated.

sympathetic components of the nerves must be taken into account. The three nerves also share the supply of the joints of the hand.

The motor distribution of the median nerve is essentially confined to the thenar muscles and all other muscles are supplied by the ulnar nerve. The ulnar nerve frequently encroaches on the motor territory of the median nerve but the reverse is hardly ever the case. There is considerable overlap in the cutaneous distribution of the three nerves both on the palmar and dorsal aspects of the hand. This is due to communicating branches as well as to some variation in the true anatomic distribution pattern. The typical sensory distribution of the three nerves, shown in Figure 15–15, contrasts with the skin areas whose supply is always derived only from one nerve (Fig. 15–16). Clearly, the latter are the most valuable in discriminatory testing.

Blood is delivered to the hand by the **radial** and **ulnar arteries.** Two anastomotic arcades connect these two vessels in the palm of the hand; the **superficial** and **deep palmar arches** (Fig. 15–17). The arches ensure that occlusion of one artery does not impair blood supply to the hand. If blood is squeezed out of the cutaneous capillary bed by powerfully clenching the fist, and either the radial or the ulnar artery is compressed above the wrist, when the hand is opened, the skin becomes pink due to filling of the peripheral vascular bed. However, if both arteries are compressed simultaneously, the hand will remain blanched when opened. The patency of one or other vessel can be readily assessed by this test.

The **metacarpal** and **digital arteries** run in the palm and only smaller branches reach the dorsum of the hand. The large venous channels, on the other hand, are on the dorsum, and the veins that accompany the main arteries are relatively small.

The Median Nerve

In the carpal tunnel, the median nerve lies between the flexor retinaculum and the tendons of the flexor digitorum superficialis which are wrapped in their synovial sheath, the ulnar bursa (Fig. 15–18). As soon as the nerve emerges at the distal border of the retinaculum it breaks up into branches. The **branches** are 1) a muscular branch (sometimes called recurrent branch) to the thenar eminence, 2) palmar ditigal nerves for the thumb, and 3) palmar digital nerves for the index and middle finger and for the radial half of the ring finger.

At their origin, the branches are embedded in loose connective tissue on the deep surface of the palmar aponeurosis. The digital nerves of the fingers continue in this layer and are accompanied by the common digital arteries, branches of the superficial palmar arch. The muscular and digital

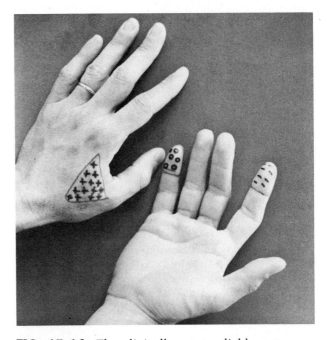

FIG. 15–16. The clinically most reliable cutaneous areas for testing the radial (crosses), ulnar (circles), and median nerves (dashes) in the hand. In these areas there is the least likelihood of overlapping innervation from the neighboring nerves. (Courtesy of Dr. Frederick A. Matsen III)

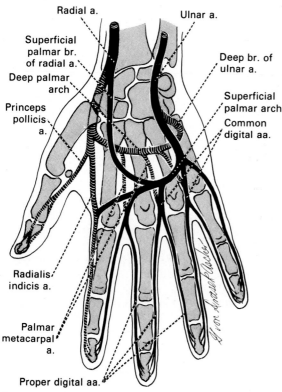

FIG. 15–17. The arterial supply of the hand.

The branching pattern of the **palmar digital nerves of the fingers** is shown in Figure 15–18. The first two lumbricals are supplied by these nerves in the palm. The common digital nerves divide into proper digital branches before entering the finger web, and then they are distributed to the skin of the fingers in a similar way as the nerves of the thumb. The palmar digital nerves supply the digital arteries with sympathetic vasomotor fibers, and the sweat glands of the skin with sudomotor fibers.

Carpal Tunnel Syndrome. The median nerve is liable to compression in the carpal tunnel. The syndrome provides an instructive demonstration of the distribution of the median nerve, and only by knowing its anatomy is it possible to distinguish this condition from other syndromes that cause paresthesias and muscle atrophy in the hand.

The condition is more common in women and often there is no identifiable cause. The syndrome may be precipitated by arthritis of the wrist or

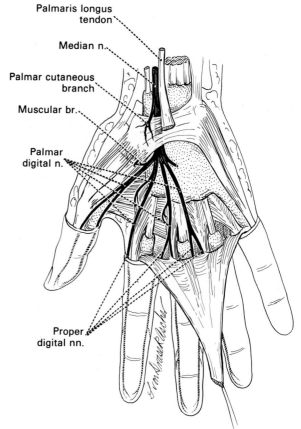

FIG. 15–18. The median nerve in the hand. The palmar aponeurosis has been reflected.

branches to the thumb turn laterally and enter the fascial envelope which encloses the thenar eminence.

Before the median nerve enters the carpal tunnel, it sends a **palmar cutaneous branch** over the anterior surface of the retinaculum which remains in the superficial fascia and is distributed to skin over the thenar eminence and the center of the palm.

The **muscular branch** turns anteriorly and curves around the free edge of the flexor retinaculum. It is the first or most lateral branch of the median nerve in the palm. It crosses the surface of the flexor pollicis brevis before penetrating it. The superficial portion of that muscle as well as the abductor pollicis brevis and opponens are supplied by the nerve. The ulnar nerve sometimes contributes to the innervation of these muscles. The muscle most consistently supplied by the median nerve is the abductor pollicis brevis.

The two **palmar digital nerves of the thumb** may originate by a common stem. They supply the palmar surface of the digit and the dorsum of the distal phalanx.

intercarpal joints (e.g., rheumatoid arthritis), dislocation of the lunate, distension or swelling of the synovial sheaths (tenosynovitis, rheumatoid arthritis), a tumor (ganglion), or by diseases in which there is generalized swelling (myxedema, toxemia of pregnancy) or overgrowth of bone (acromegaly). Initially, irritation of the nerve causes tingling in the sensory distribution area of the nerve, and twitching of the thenar muscles may be experienced. These symptoms can be reproduced by pressure over the flexor retinaculum. With nerve paralysis the thenar muscles atrophy and there is anesthesia in the sensory distribution area of the median nerve. Movements of the fingers are, of course, unaffected, and even those of the thumb are not seriously impaired. Flexion is accomplished by the flexor pollicis longus (anterior interosseous nerve) and by the deep head of the flexor pollicis brevis (ulnar nerve). Though the opponens pollicis is lost, opposition is obtained by the pull of the flexor muscles, and abduction is provided by the abductor pollicis longus (posterior interosseous nerve). Fine, coordinated movements of the hand may suffer due to the sensory loss.

Symptoms and signs of the compression syndrome are relieved by division of the flexor retinaculum at the wrist. In long standing cases, nerve regeneration may not take place.

Median Nerve Injuries. When the median nerve is cut at the wrist, the clinical picture is identical with that of complete compression in the carpal tunnel. In both conditions, there will be, in addition, vasodilation and lack of sweating in the cutaneous distribution area. As pointed out before, the best muscle to test in this case is the abductor pollicis brevis (Fig. 15–6). In spite of the fact that the thumb possesses another abductor, the test, if properly performed, provides unambiguous information about the status of the abductor pollicis brevis.

If the nerve is cut in the forearm above the level of the innervation of the long flexor muscles, the resulting hand disability and deformity will be much more severe. In addition to the sensory and motor loss described for the carpal tunnel syndrome, flexion will not be possible at all in the thumb, index, and middle fingers except at the MCP joints. The latter can be flexed by the interossei. The ulnar half of the flexor digitorum profundus will be unimpaired and flexion of the ring and little fingers will not be seriously affected by paralysis of the flexor digitorum superficialis. The position of the hand has been likened to that assumed in the act of dispensing blessing, and the deformity is therefore known as the *benediction attitude.*

The Ulnar Nerve

The ulnar nerve enters the hand on the lateral side of the pisiform bone with the ulnar artery. Both structures are in front of the flexor retinaculum but are beneath a fascial band which is a mere reinforcement in the deep fascia that invests the forearm and hand (Fig. 15–19). This band is sometimes identified as the *palmar carpal ligament* or the *superficial lamina of the flexor retinaculum.* A triangular space deep to this ligament is bounded, in addition, by the pisiform and the flexor retinaculum proper. The space is known as the *canal of Guyon.* The nerve may suffer compression underneath the ligament.

The ulnar nerve divides into a superficial and a deep branch at the level of the pisiform (Figs. 15–19, 15–20). The superficial branch contains motor fibers only for the palmaris brevis, otherwise it is cutaneous. The deep branch supplies all the hypothenar muscles, all the interossei, the ulnar two lumbricals, and the adductor pollicis. In addition, it usually innervates the deep head of the flexor pollicis brevis and more rarely the opponens pollicis.

The **superficial division** (Fig. 15–19) passes over the hypothenar eminence where it divides into digital nerves that serve the palmar surface of the little finger and the ulnar half of the ring finger. The **deep division** of the nerve heads toward the depth of the palm with the deep branch of the artery. They pass between the abductor digiti minimi and flexor digiti minimi brevis. At the root of the hook of the hamate, a fibrous arch from which these muscles arise protects the nerve but sometimes it may compress it (Fig. 15–20). The nerve dispenses its branches to the hypothenar muscles and then runs across the surface of the interossei lying deep to the flexor tendons. Its course follows the deep palmar arch and is close to the bases of the metacarpals.

In addition to the branches described, a **palmar cutaneous branch** arises from the ulnar nerve above the wrist, which shares the supply of the skin in the palm with a similar branch of the median nerve. The **dorsal branch** of the ulnar nerve originates also above the wrist, winds its way around to the dorsum of the hand and breaks up into dorsal digital nerves which supply the ulnar one and a half or two and a half fingers (Fig. 15–15). The other

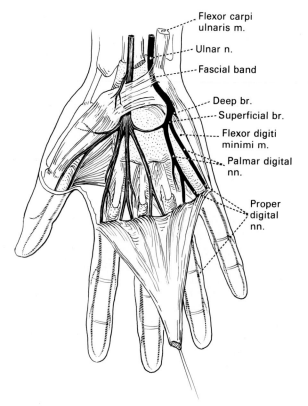

FIG. 15–19. The ulnar nerve at the wrist and its superficial branches in the hand. A frequent communicating branch with the median nerve is illustrated. The palmar aponeurosis has been reflected.

digits are supplied by dorsal digital branches of the radial nerve.

Like the median nerve, all branches of the ulnar and radial nerves also contribute sympathetic branches to blood vessels and sweat glands.

Compression and Injuries. Unlike the median nerve, compression or injury of the ulnar nerve near the wrist leads to a worse deformity than division of the nerve in the region of the elbow. The major loss in each case is the intrinsic musculature of the hand. The deformity is the result of the muscle imbalance created at the MCP and interphalangeal joints. The imbalance is less severe when not only the interossei but the ulnar half of the flexor digitorum profundus is also deprived of its nerve supply by a proximal ulnar nerve lesion.

When the ulnar nerve is damaged in the region of the wrist, the innervation of the ulnar half of the flexor digitorum profundus remains unaffected but the hypothenar muscles, interossei, ulnar two

lumbricals, and the adductor pollicis are paralyzed. Because of the loss of the interossei, the MCP joints will be hyperextended due to overpull by the extensor digitorum. Also, because of the lacking interosseous action, the interphalangeal joints will be flexed due chiefly to overpull by the flexor digitorum profundus. Interphalangeal flexion will be less pronounced in the index and middle fingers because their intact lumbricals provide for some balance. Muscle imbalance at the thumb leads to abduction of this digit. The transverse metacarpal arch will become flat. The characteristic, composite deformity is known as the *ulnar claw hand*. Sensation will be lost in the distribution area of the nerve distal to the lesion.

The ulnar nerve may be injured directly at the wrist or it may be compressed by the fascial band

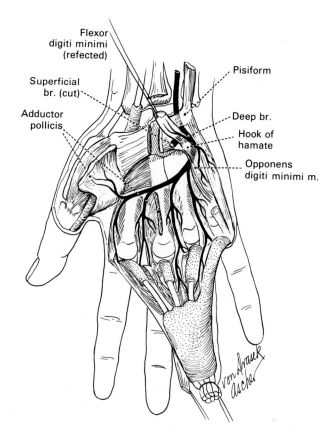

FIG. 15–20. The ulnar nerve at the wrist and its deep branch in the hand. After reflecting the palmar aponeurosis, the flexor retinaculum was divided and all flexor tendons have been pulled distally. In addition, the muscle bellies of the flexor digiti minimi and of the adductor pollicis (transverse head) have been divided and elevated to reveal the nerve deep to them.

that binds it down to the pisiform or by the other band that arches over its deep division at the hook of the hamate.

The nerve is in a vulnerable position behind the medial epicondyle. Due to deformity or previous trauma in the elbow region, or due to no known cause, the nerve may become loose and habitually dislocate from its groove. This traumatizes the nerve, leading to neuritis and sometimes paralysis. The arrangement of fasciculi within the nerve are such that those supplying the hand may be affected before the fibers that supply the flexor carpi ulnaris and the flexor digitorum profundus. When the nerve supply of the latter muscle is lost, the muscle imbalance observed in the ulnar two fingers will improve and the degree of clawing will be reduced.

Superficial and Deep Palmar Arches

The **ulnar artery** divides into a superficial and deep branch just distal to the pisiform bone. The **superficial palmar arch** is the continuation of the superficial division of the ulnar artery across the palm (Fig. 15–17). The arch is completed by the anastomosis with the superficial palmar branch of the radial artery that enters the hand through or across the thenar eminence. The arch is level with the distal border of the extended thumb and is embedded with its branches in a layer of loose connective tissue and fat between the palmar aponeurosis and the flexor tendons. Its branches are the **common digital arteries** which divide into **proper digital arteries** at the finger webs. The pulsation of the latter may be palpated along the side of the fingers against the phalanges. They are the chief source of blood to the fingers. In the palm and fingers, branches of the superficial arch run in company with the digital nerves.

The **radial artery** enters the hand between the first and second metacarpal bones through the interwall between the two heads of the first dorsal interosseous. It continues across the anterior surface of the interossei as the **deep palmar arch** and anastomoses with the deep branch of the ulnar artery (Fig. 15–17). The arch is on level with the hook of the hamate and is deep to the flexor tendons. The **palmar metacarpal arteries** arise from its convexity and anastomose in the finger webs with the common digital arteries. Digital arteries of the thumb (princeps pollicis) and to the radial side of the index finger (radialis indicis) originate separately from the deep palmar arch. All arteries are accompanied by small venae comitantes.

Smaller arterial arcades are also found on the dorsum of the hand which are fed by carpal branches of the ulnar, radial, and interosseous arteries. They are reinforced by perforating branches of the palmar metacarpal arteries. The dorsal metacarpal and dorsal digital arteries are derived from these delicate arterial arcades.

The multiple anastomoses between all vessels of the hand explain why bleeding is so profuse from lacerations in any part of the hand. Bleeding usually cannot be controlled by compression or ligation of only one major vessel. The brachial artery may have to be compressed.

ANATOMIC RELATIONSHIPS IN THE HAND

The anatomic foundation of the hand is represented by the metacarpal bones and phalanges (Fig. 15–21). Of all major structures, only the extensor tendons and the dorsal digital expansions of the fingers lie on the dorsal aspect of this foundation, everything else is contained in the palm of the hand in clearly ordered layers. Deepest are the interossei, associated with the metacarpal bones. Only a potential fascial space intervenes between this and the next layer which contains the long flexor tendons with the associated lumbrical muscles. Most superficial is the palmar aponeurosis. The vessels and nerves run in two planes. The deep branch of the ulnar nerve and the deep palmar arch lie between the interossei and the flexor tendons; branches of the median nerve and the superficial palmar arch are between the flexor tendons and the palmar aponeurosis. On each side of the palm are the muscles of the thenar and hypothenar eminences with the nerves and vessels of the thumb and little finger. The fingers contain the flexor tendons in their osseofascial tunnels and the digital nerves and vessels.

Deep and Superficial Fascia

The hand is invested by a complete layer of **deep fascia** as if it were in a glove. All cutaneous nerves, blood vessels, and lymphatics run in the **superficial fascia** which is sparse over the dorsum but in the palm and in the pulp of the fingers forms pads of fat subdivided by fibrous septa. These septa tether the skin to the deep fascia. They are particularly well developed along the skin creases and in the pulps of the fingers. The septa prevent sliding of the skin when an object is grasped. On the back of the hand, the skin slides freely over the deep fascia. It can be

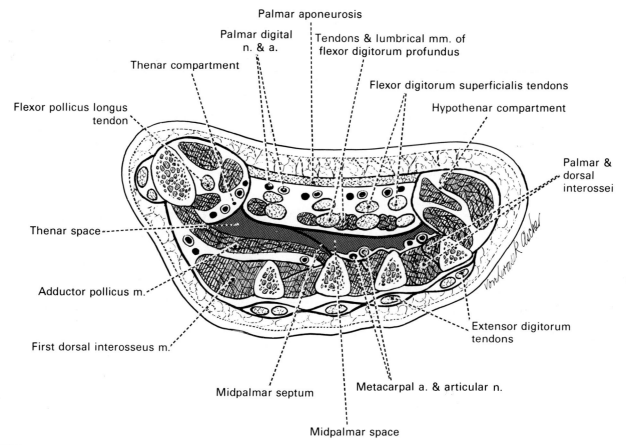

FIG. 15–21. A section of the hand across the metacarpal bones to show the anatomic relationship of various layers and the fascial spaces in the palm.

pinched up between finger and thumb and can also be lifted up by edema, hematoma or pus. In the palm and finger pulp, such effusions are well localized by the septa, and as pressure builds up in these loci considerable pain is generated. The septa have to be divided by a horizontal cut when such abscesses are drained in order to open up the discrete fascial spaces.

The Palmar Aponeurosis

In the central part of the palm, the deep fascia fuses with the palmar aponeurosis. This triangular, tendinous sheet is continuous at its apex with the palmaris longus tendon, and at its base breaks up into a pair of slips for each finger (Fig. 15–22). The slips insert into the fibrous sheaths of the flexor tendons. The aponeurosis is present, even if the palmaris longus is lacking. Most of its fibers run longitudinally but transverse fibers also exist which merge on each side with the delicate deep fascia that covers the thenar and hypothenar emi-

nences. The most distinct transverse fibers form a continuous band which becomes conspicuous across the finger webs once the skin is reflected. This structure is the **superficial transverse metacarpal ligament.** It differs from the deep ligament of the same name in that it is uninterrupted, does not attach to the palmar plates of the MCP joints, and it lies more distally and superficially, reaching almost to the free edge of the finger webs. When an MCP joint dislocates, the metacarpal head may become caught in the space between the superficial and deep transverse metacarpal ligaments. Reduction will not be possible until the metacarpal head has been eased out of the clasp of the two ligaments.

The palmar aponeurosis may undergo fibrosis and contracture, producing dense fascial bands that look like tendons. Because of the attachment of the aponeurosis to the fibrous digital sheaths, the contracture leads to flexion deformity of the fingers. This condition is called **Dupuytren's contracture** and is common in middle aged or older

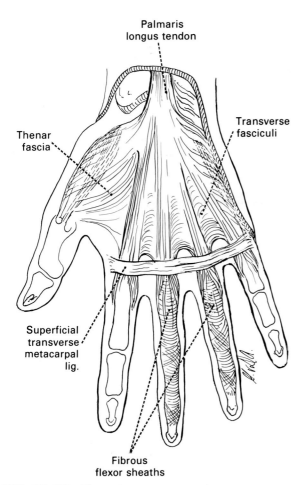

FIG. 15-22. The palmar aponeurosis.

men. It usually affects the ring and little fingers but may affect any part of the palm. The joints and tendons are normal, but the fibrous digital sheaths may be affected by the same process. The etiology of the condition is unknown.

Fascial Spaces and Septa of the Palm

Between the palmar aponeurosis and the deep fascia that covers the palmar surfaces of the interossei, the palm is filled by loose connective tissue and some fat. In this connective tissue are embedded the long flexor tendons, the lumbricals, nerves, and blood vessels. The connective tissue facilitates the sliding of these structures on one another during movements of the hand. Certain compartments are delineated in this tissue by more or less well defined septa which connect the deep surface of the palmar aponeurosis to the deep fascia of the interosseous muscles. Effusions or pus can open up

potential spaces in this loose tissue. Clinically, these spaces have become less important since antibiotics became available. Out of 1000 cases of hand injuries, in only six were the fascial palmar spaces involved (Robins).

Two such potential spaces exist in the palm of the hand: the midpalmar space and the thenar space (Figs. 15–21, 15–23). The **thenar space** is between the anterior surface of the adductor pollicis and the flexor tendons of the index finger. The long flexor of the thumb is on its lateral side. The **midpalmar space** is between the interossei and the deep surface of the tendons of the middle and ring fingers. The long tendons of the little finger run along the medial side of the space. The spaces are closed in the normal hand, are not lined by synovial membrane, and no structures run through them.

When the synovial sheaths of the digits become infected, pus may burst into the palmar spaces

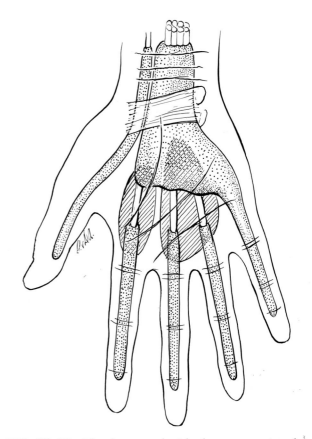

FIG. 15–23. The thenar and midpalmar spaces in relation to the synovial sheaths of the flexor tendons in the palm of the hand. The fascial spaces are shaded by lines, the synovial bursae by stippling.

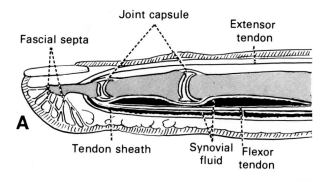

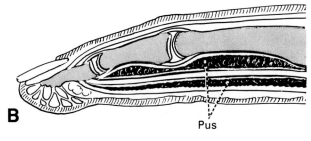

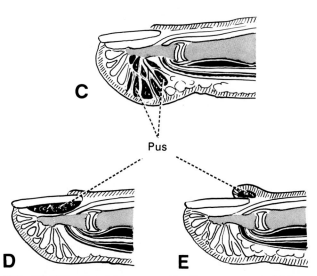

FIG. 15-24. Fascial spaces of a finger commonly involved in local infections. **(A)** Normal anatomy. **(B)** Tenosynovitis. **(C)** Felon. **(D)** Subungual abscess. **(E)** Paronychia.

from the distended sheaths. Figure 15–23 illustrates which space is likely to be involved in tenosynovitis of the various digits.

Fascial Compartments of the Fingers

Because of the susceptibility of the fingers to penetrating wounds, infection and suppuration are fre-

quently encountered in various connective tissue compartments of the fingers. Most often involved are the tissues under the nail or the nail fold, in the pulp of the finger, or the digital synovial tendon sheaths themselves. Much of the relevant anatomy has already been discussed (Figs. 15–3, 15–4, 15–10, 15–11).

The fibrous digital sheaths lined by synovial membrane extend to the base of the distal phalanx. The rest of this plahanx supports the pulp of the finger, and on its dorsal aspect the phalanx is covered by the nail (Fig. 15–24A).

When the digital synovial tendon sheaths are distended by exudate or pus (Fig. 15–14B) **(tenosynovitis)** the entire finger is swollen but tenderness is chiefly confined to the palmar aspect along the digital tendon sheaths. All joints are held in slight flexion and all movements are painful, especially extension, which stretches the inflamed synovial sheaths. To drain the sheaths the incision must avoid scarring of the fibrous sheaths on the flexor surface because that would lead to contracture. Therefore, the incision must be made on the side of the finger, dorsal to the palmar digital nerves and vessels (Fig. 15–4).

A localized **subcutaneous abscess** over the phalanges will not have such generalized signs. Its drainage must avoid infection of the synovial sheaths. An abscess in the finger pulp is known as a **felon** (Fig. 15–24C). It is drained by a transverse incision through the side of the finger which severs the fibrous septa that localized it, and avoids scar formation over the sensory surface of the finger.

Infections under the nail (Fig. 15–24D) must be opened up by incising the nail longitudinally and evulsing the smaller half of the nail. The nail will regrow as the site of nail growth is located under the nail fold. An abscess under the nail fold (Fig. 15–24E) **(paronychia)** should be treated by incising and freeing up the nail fold, and if necessary, also removing the proximal portion of the nail.

CLINICAL EVALUATION

The physician is called upon to examine the hand more frequently than any other part of the musculoskeletal system. There are several reasons for this. The physical interaction of the hand with the environment is more intimate and active than that of any other part of the body. This alacrity demands that the hand be exposed and unprotected, and as a consequence its injury rate is high. Furthermore, systemic diseases which affect joints, nerves, and arteries throughout the body often manifest their most pronounced effects in the hands because of the numerous joints and bursae, and because hand function depends on a rich innervation and blood supply. Previous chapters have emphasized that lesions located anywhere between the wrist and the cervical spinal cord are liable to produce disability which affects the hand, and in some instances, only the hand. Therefore, clinical evaluation of hand function must include assessment of the cervical vertebral column and spinal cord, the brachial plexus, and all segments of the upper limb proximal to the hand.

Symptoms

Localized pathology, as a rule, gives rise to sharply **localized pain** in the hand, the precise site and cause of which has to be determined by physical examination. **Generalized pain** in the hand is usually a sign of pathology in cervical cord segments (syringomyelia, tumor) and in the cervical spine, or it may be due to ischemia caused by peripheral vasospasm (Raynaud's disease, etc.) or compression of the arteries in the neck (p. 196) or in the arm and forearm (p. 222). In many cases, localized pain limits digital movements, but **loss of movement** can result from several painless conditions. These include ruptured or cut tendons, nerve paralysis, and contractures (Dupuytren's, collateral ligaments, interosseous muscle contracture).

Tingling or pins and needles (paresthesia) is always indicative of neuronal pathology and may be the sign of systemic disease (e.g., polyneuritis or other neuropathies). If only a single peripheral nerve is affected by compression, the symptoms are confined to its territory of distribution. However, if the cause is vascular, the paresthesia will be generalized in the hand. With bilateral symptoms, spinal cord involvement must be suspected. Likewise, complaints of **weakness, clumsiness,** or **tremor** are indications for a thorough evaluation of the central nervous system.

Physical Examination

Inspection. An injured or painful hand is supported across the chest, and the patient avoids its use during undressing.

The normal attitude of the hand is the **position of rest** in which the wrist is slightly extended, the MCP and IP joints of all fingers are partially flexed, and the thumb rests in neutral position against the index and middle fingers; the transverse metacarpal arch is quite pronounced, noticeably cupping the palm of the hand. The hand deviates from this position if some of the deep flexor tendons are cut, if the median or ulnar nerves are interrupted, (pp. 243, 244), or if the radial nerve is damaged at or above the elbow. Injury to the lower roots of the brachial plexus deprives the hand of its intrinsic muscles, leading to flattening of the metacarpal arch and to clawing, similar to that seen in ulnar nerve lesions.

Finger deformities characteristic of the more common tendon injuries have already been described (p. 238).

The hand should be inspected systematically, comparing the two sides and paying attention to the following:

On the palmar aspect:
1. Missing or supernumerary digits; excessive webbing; unusual configuration of the fingers (shortness, stubbiness, spidery slenderness, equal length, etc.). In addition to these congenital anomalies some endocrine disorders (acromegaly, myxedema, cretinism) are associated with stubby malformations of the hands.
2. Signs of atrophy in the thenar and hypothenar eminences.
3. Palmar creases, any tethering of skin in the palm or fingers.
4. Any ulcers, erythema, pallor, generalized or localized swellings. Normally, there are slight depressions over the metacarpal heads while the web spaces between them bulge gently into the palm.

On the dorsum:
1. Generalized swelling and puffiness on the dorsum of the hand suggests infection in the palm, or interference with the venous or lymphatic drainage of the limb. If present bilaterally, systemic causes of edema must be investigated.
2. Color and general appearance of the nails and the skin of the fingers. In addition to subungual and periungual inflammation and abscesses, the nails may show deformities (clubbing, spooning) associated with certain systemic diseases. Normally, there is some hair growth over the proximal phalanges. Lack of hair, cyanosis, pallor, or ulceration are suggestive signs of inadequate blood supply. The skin becomes fine and shiny in inflammatory joint disease and in atrophic conditions.
3. Swelling, deformity, and erythema of the joints. Rheumatoid arthritis produces a characteristic deformity (Chap. 22); in degenerative joint disease nodules may develop at the DIP joint (Chap. 23).

4. Exaggeration of the normal depressions between the metacarpals and extensor tendons is indicative of interosseous atrophy. The most noticeable muscle loss affects the first dorsal interosseous. Wasting of these muscles may be the result of denervation (ulnar nerve, T1 lesions) or of changes associated with rheumatoid arthritis.

Palpation. The examiner should lightly rub the back of his or her own fingers over the palmar and dorsal surface of the patient's hands. Skin temperature and moisture are best assessed and compared this way. Excessive sweating is a sign of sympathetic overactivity and so may be coldness. Dry, hot skin confirms damage to the nerve serving the cutaneous area.

All bones and joints should be palpated precisely:

1. Bones of the wrist region including the carpals.
2. All metacarpals and phalanges. Localized tenderness over any bone may be due to fracture, subperiosteal hematoma, osteomyelitis, or neoplasm. Further investigation by x-ray is indicated.
3. All MCP and IP joints should be palpated. In the flexed fingers the MCP joint line is palpable distal to the prominence of the knuckles; in the palm it is roughly level with the distal palmar skin crease.
4. The long tendons should be palpated in the relaxed palm and fingers. The physical signs of their common disorders were discussed with their anatomy.

Assessment of the Circulation. The rate at which pink color returns to the skin after a tightly clenched fist is opened is a good measure of capillary circulation. So is the rate of reversal of blanching in the nail bed after pressure is removed from the nail. Palpation of the brachial, radial, and ulnar pulses was described in Chapter 14 and so was in this chapter, the maneuver for testing the patency of the radial and ulnar arteries.

Range of Motion. Combined flexion of MCP and IP joints brings all the finger tips in contact with the distal palmar skin crease. This is the sum of approximately 90° flexion at all joints. If this amount of flexion cannot be obtained, the distance of the finger tips from the skin crease can be measured or the actual degrees of flexion can be recorded at each joint with a goniometer. Extension varies from person to person and the same applies to the flexion-extension range of the thumb. However, it should be possible to completely oppose the thumb to both the index and little fingers.

If the active range of movement is limited, the passive range must be assessed. A frequent cause of reduced MCP flexion range is contracture of the collateral ligaments. Inability to attain the neutral or an extended position at the MCP joints results from scarring and shortening of the interossei. This may be the outcome of such injuries as metacarpal fracture, burns, grease gun, and sandblast injuries of the hand. The resultant interosseous contracture produces flexion at the MCP joints and extension at the IP joints. It is not possible to extend actively or passively the MCP joints because of the shortness of the interossei. Passive flexion of the IP joints may slacken slightly the tight interosseous, and then some MCP extension may become possible.

Muscle Strength. Strength should be assessed in individual muscles and also in power grip and precision grip. In addition to testing in each finger the flexor digitorum superficialis and profundus (p. 231), the examiner should interlock his fingers with those of the patient. Normally, the fingers cannot be forced into extension. Power grip integrates other muscles with finger flexors and is best tested by the patient maximally squeezing the examiner's index and middle finger in his grip.

Opposing extension of the MCP joint by applying resistance to the proximal phalanx assesses strength of the extensor digitorum because this is the only muscle capable of extending the MCP joint.

The **strength of the interossei** is best assessed by testing abduction and adduction at the MCP joints. The patient spreads the fingers and resists the examiner's attempt to push them together. Normally, considerable resistance is encountered. Adduction power is tested by the examiner attempting to pull a card away which is firmly held between adjacent sides of the patient's two fingers.

Opposition of the thumb should be tested to the index and little fingers. For assessing the power of this movement, the patient firmly opposes the thumb against the tip of the index finger, the two digits describing a perfect circle (Fig. 15–9). The examiner interlocks his index and thumb in a similar position with those of the patient and attempts to force them through between the patient's index and thumb. This test assesses the power of precision grip, and requires the integrity of a complex set of muscles, prominent among which is the first dorsal interosseous. Furthermore, nervous pathways for proprioception and muscle coordination must also be intact.

To test the **adductor pollicis,** the patient holds a card firmly between the side of the thumb and index finger. If the adductor is intact, the thumb is stabilized with its interphalangeal joint in extension as the patient resists the examiner's attempt to pull the card away. If the muscle is weak or paralyzed, the patient will flex the interphalangeal joint and will try to retain the card by flexion power.

Tests for the abductor pollicis brevis and abductor digiti minimi have been described already (Figs. 15–6, 15–7).

Joint Stability. Collateral ligaments of the MCP and IP joints should be tested in flexion and extension. Abduction-adduction force applied to the phalanges should not elicit any movement of the IP joints in any position. Collateral ligaments of the MCP joint restrict abduction-adduction in the flexed postion (p. 229). Rupture or evulsion of the palmar plates will permit hyperextension at the affected MCP or IP joints. Tears in the extensor hood lead to instability of the IP joints which have been discussed already (p. 238).

Sensation and Integrated Functions. Cutaneous sensitivity to light touch is tested with the back of the fingers, and pin prick is used for pain perception. Two point discrimination is tested by asking the patient whether he or she feels one or two points of a bent paper clip touching the skin, as the examiner varies the distance between the points. Normally, points 2–6 mm apart can be resolved on the flexor surface, but the distance is much greater on the dorsum. It is important to remember that ischemia seriously impairs cutaneous sensitivity.

To test higher integrated sensory function, the patient should feel and identify such common objects as coins, keys and a pen, keeping the eyes closed. In case of cerebral damage, the patient may be unable to do this despite the fact that touch and pain sensation may have been unimpaired. Integrated motor and sensory function is further assessed by asking the patient to pick up a pen and sign his name.

SUGGESTED READING

Bojsen-Møller F, Schmidt, L: The palmar aponeurosis and the central spaces of the hand. J Anat *117*: 55, 1974
A scholarly reevaluation of anatomy with important contributions

Bunnell's Surgery of the Hand (Revised by J. H. Boyes), 4th ed. Philadelphia, JB Lippincott, 1964
Although this volume is intended specifically for the hand surgeon, much excellent information can be gained from it for understanding functional anatomy and for diagnosing abnormalities

Editorial: The puzzle of Dupuytren's contracture. Lancet ii: 170, 1972
Review the evidence for the etiology and pathogenesis of this common abnormality in the hand

Harris C, Rutledge GL: The functional anatomy of the extensor mechanism of the finger. J Bone Joint Surg [A] *54*: 713, 1972
The description of the dorsal digital expansion in this book is based largely on this article

Kaplan EB: Functional and Surgical Anatomy of the Hand, 2nd ed. Philadelphia, JB Lippincott, 1965
Basic anatomy is well integrated with surgical management of lesions

Kilgore ES, Graham WP, III (eds): The Hand: Surgical and Non-Surgical Management. Philadelphia, Lea & Febiger, 1977
An up-to-date volume consisting of 30 chapters contributed by several authors which encompass normal anatomy and all aspects of pathology and clinical problems commonly encountered in the hand. Chapter 2 and Chapter 3 give an interesting account of anatomy and the physical examination of the hand. Vascular, ligamentous and joint injuries, fractures, pain, etc., are treated competently in separate chapters, and all discussions take normal structure and function as a starting point

Kuczynski K: Carpometacarpal joint of the human thumb. J Anat *118*: 119, 1974
The importance of this joint was emphasized in the text. Knowledge of its precise anatomy is important in understanding hand movements and treating joint injuries

Long C: Intrinsic-extrinsic muscle control of the fingers. J Bone Joint Surg [A] *50*: 973, 1968
The paper is based on electromyographic studies and contributes much to the understanding of finger movements

Napier JR: The prehensile movements of the human hand. J Bone Joint Surg [B] *38*: 902, 1956
Descriptions of hand movement in this book are based to a considerable degree on this article

Porter J, Radivojevic M, Williams TF: Dupuytren's disease. Arch Intern Med *129*: 561, 1972

Robins HC: Infections of the hand. J Bone Joint Surg [B] *34*: 567, 1952
An extensive clinical survey of hand infections

Sunderland S: The action of the extensor digitorum communis interosseous and lumbrical muscles. Am J Anat 77: 189, 1945
Based on a series of selected cases with ulnar, median or radial nerve lesions or combinations of these lesions, the author deduces the action of various muscles responsible for finger movements. A thorough and instructive paper

16
The Hip Region and the Lumbosacral Plexus

CORNELIUS ROSSE

In contrast to the prehensile and sensory functions of the upper limb, the lower limb of man bears the entire body weight and serves the purpose of locomotion. Although the anatomy of the upper and lower limbs conforms to the same basic plan (Chap. 11), the different functional requirements of the lower limb are reflected in structural adaptations of the pelvic girdle, the hip, knee, and ankle joints, and in the architecture of the foot.

In the static, erect position, the body is usually supported on both legs but all the body weight can be transferred to one leg. During locomotion this transfer takes place from one leg to the other in the gait cycle (Chap. 19). Whether static or moving, the body must be stabilized on the supporting leg and, therefore, stability is the crucial factor at all joints of the lower limb.

The sacroiliac joints, the pubic symphysis, and some stout ligaments unite the two hip bones and the sacrum into the **bony pelvis** (see Fig. 11–2). The movements of the pelvis consist chiefly of side-to-side and anteroposterior tilts which occur at the hip joints. The pelvis transmits the body weight via the bones of the limbs to the ground. The line of gravitational force passes through a series of links made up by the hip, knee, and ankle joints and the joints of the foot (see Figs. 19–1, 19–2). The direction of pelvic tilt and the tendency of the various links to buckle will be determined by gravity's line of force in relation to the various joints. The hip is a ball-and-socket joint, and therefore the pelvis may tilt or rotate at the hip in any direction. It is important to appreciate that the function of muscle groups serving the hip is not only to initiate movement but to stabilize the hip, controlling and preventing its tilt and buckling in those positions where its ligaments alone cannot counterbalance the gravitational force.

THE PELVIC GIRDLE

At birth, the pelvic girdle consists of three bones, the ilium, ischium, and pubis. They are held together by hyaline cartilage. These three bones remain recognizable even after puberty when ossification of the cartilage converts the pelvic girdle into a single bone called the **hip bone** or **coxal bone.** Each of the bones has an acetabular portion by which it is united to the others (see Fig. 11–2) and by which it articulates with the femur. The three bones diverge from the acetabulum in different directions. Palpable parts of the ilium, ischium, pubis, and femur are of special importance because it is in reference to these bony landmarks that various degrees of pelvic tilt, deformity, and limb shortening can be determined. The proximal end of the femur, though not part of the pelvic girdle, is also conveniently considered here.

Bony Landmarks

The Ilium. Like a wing, the ilium projects upward from the acetabulum (Fig. 16–1). Its medial surface flanks the abdominal cavity and its lateral or gluteal surface gives attachment to the abductor musculature of the hip. The upper margin of the bone called the **iliac crest** is palpable all along its length. Anteriorly, it terminates in the **anterior superior iliac spine** and posteriorly in the **posterior superior iliac spine.** In most individuals, the anterior spine is visible as a prominence while the position of the posterior spine is marked by a dimple. Two smaller spines (anterior and posterior inferior iliac spines) on the anterior and posterior edges of the bone are inaccessible because of the overlying muscles.

The posterior superior iliac spines are on level

253

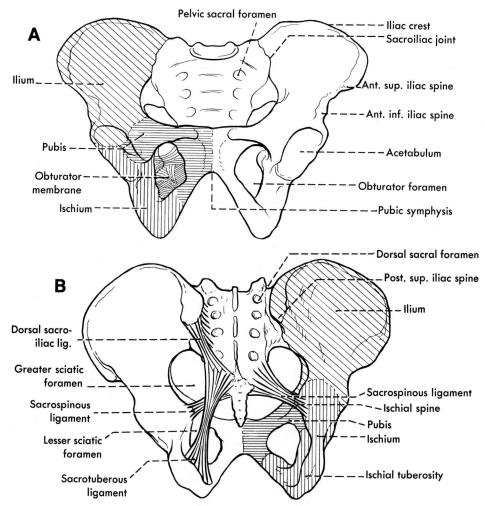

FIG. 16-1. The bony pelvis from an anterior **(A)** and a posterior **(B)** view. The three component bones of the pelvic girdle are shaded differently. (Hollinshead WH: Anatomy for Surgeons, vol 3, 2nd ed. New York, Harper & Row, 1969)

with S2 and indicate the position of the sacroiliac joints which cannot be palpated. The summit of the iliac crests is on level with the L4 spinous process. Just anterior to the summit, the **tubercle of the iliac crest** is palpable; it is on level with L5.

The Ischium. Only the most posteroinferior part of the ischium is palpable through the substance of the buttock when the hip is flexed. This is the **ischial tuberosity** (Fig. 16–1B). In the sitting position, the body is largely supported by the tuberosity. The **sacrotuberous ligament** runs from it to the sacrum, and the hamstring muscles originate from it. The **ramus** of the ischium projects forward and forms the posteroinferior boundary of the **obturator foramen**. The **ischial spine** projects back-

ward and medially from the body of the ischium. It is on level with the center of the acetabulum and can be palpated only *per rectum* or *per vaginam*. The sacrospinous ligament joins it to the sacrum (Fig. 16–1B).

The **greater sciatic notch** is formed as the posterior border of the ischium continues into the ilium. The sacrospinous ligament and sacrum convert the notch into the greater sciatic foramen (Fig. 16–1B) through which branches of the sacral plexus and internal iliac artery reach the lower limb. The **lesser sciatic notch** is inferior to the spine. The two ligaments convert it into the lesser sciatic foramen.

The Pubis. The anterior or most ventral component of the pelvic girdle is the pubis (see Fig. 16–1).

The **body** of the pubis articulates with its fellow of the opposite side across the pubic symphysis. The symphysis is in the median plane. Two rami diverge from the body; the **superior ramus** fuses with the ilium and ischium in the acetabulum while the **inferior ramus** fuses with the ramus of the ischium (conjoint ramus). The two pubic rami embrace the obturator foramen which is almost completely filled by the obturator membrane. The conjoint ramus is palpable in the perineum from the body of the pubis to the ischial tuberosity. The **pubic crest** along the superior margin of the body terminates laterally in the **pubic tubercle.** When a finger is run medially along the crease of the groin from the anterior superior iliac spine, the pubic tubercle is the first bony landmark encountered. The **inguinal ligament** connects these two bony points. It is not palpable but is important to note for future reference.

Proximal End of the Femur. The upper end of the femur consists of the head, neck, and two trochanters. Of these only the **greater trochanter** is palpable (Fig. 16–2). It is directly inferior to the tubercle of the iliac crest and is on level with the pubic tubercle. The **femoral head, neck,** and **lesser trochanter** are deeply buried in muscles, but the head may be palpated through the overlying muscles, halfway between the pubic symphysis and the anterior superior iliac spine.

Though not demonstrable by palpation, the following are important features to be noted on the proximal end of the femur: The greater trochanter projects upward from the junction of the neck and shaft, and its tip is level with the center of the femoral head. Posteromedially, the **trochanteric fossa** is between the neck and the trochanter. The lesser trochanter faces medially and backwards at the junction of the neck and the shaft. The **inter-**

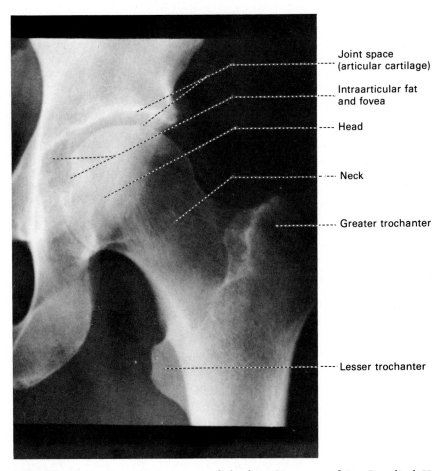

Joint space
(articular cartilage)

Intraarticular fat
and fovea

Head

Neck

Greater trochanter

Lesser trochanter

FIG. 16-2. Anteroposterior x-ray of the hip. (Courtesy of Dr. Rosalind H. Troupin)

trochanteric line runs between the two trochanters anteriorly while posteriorly the trochanters are connected by the **intertrochanteric crest.** The **quadrate tubercle** is a smooth eminence on the crest, and the rough, longitudinal **gluteal tuberosity** is inferior to the crest. The tuberosity leads into the **linea aspera** that runs down the posterior aspect of the femoral shaft. The trochanters and the other bony features mentioned designate points of muscle attachments.

The **femoral neck** is about 5 cm long and projects from the shaft medially, upward, and also forward. These angulations between the neck and shaft are important because they influence where the gravitational force line falls in relation to the hip and the knee (Ch. 19). The **angle of inclination** made by the axes of the femoral neck and shaft decreases from about 150° at birth to 126–128° in adulthood, reaching 120° in old age. A deformity due to a decrease in the angle of inclination is known as **coxa vara** (Fig. 16–8), and it essentially shortens the leg and also limits hip abduction. Because of the medial displacement of the line of force acting on the hip joint in relation to the knee, the knee will tend to be forced into valgus (bowlegs). Increase in the angle of inclination (coxa valga) lengthens the limb and mimics hip abduction contracture. Because of the relative lateral displacement of the weight bearing force line, the knee becomes predisposed to a varus deformity.

The forward projection of the femoral neck is described as the **angle of torsion.** This angle is measured between the axis of the neck and the transverse axis that passes through the femoral condyles and is normally about 12°. An increase (anteversion) or decrease (retroversion) in the angle of torsion will influence rotation of the limb at the hip and will produce a gait with "toeing in" or "toeing out," respectively. In addition, anteversion displaces the body's center of mass anteriorly in relation to the knee, predisposing to its hyperextension. Retroversion, on the other hand, will tend to produce knee flexion and will recruit the knee extensors to stabilize the joint.

Orientation of the Pelvis

Knowledge of the correct orientation of the pelvis is important not only in the physical examination but for explaining and appreciating various movements and actions of muscles. In the normal erect position the four superior iliac spines (right and left anterior and right and left posterior) lie in one and the same transverse (horizontal) plane

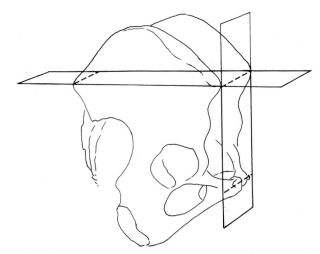

FIG. 16–3. Orientation of the pelvis: The four superior iliac spines lie in one and the same horizontal plane. The anterior superior iliac spines and the pubic tubercles are in the same vertical plane.

(Fig. 16–3). If this requirement is met, the pelvis is said to be *level* or *neutral*. In a level pelvis, furthermore, the anterior superior iliac spines and the pubic tubercles lie in the same vertical plane (Fig. 16–3).

A pelvic dip to one side is detected by inspecting the standing patient from the front and noting the deviation of the anterior superior iliac spines from their horizontal alignment. The same may be done with reference to the posterior spines. Anterior or posterior tilts are detected with reference to the alignment of the anterior and posterior superior iliac spines. Such tilts are effectively camouflaged by compensatory spinal curvatures (see Chap. 9).

Movements

Although the pelvis behaves essentially as a single bony unit, slight movements are possible between the pelvic girdle and the sacrum at the **sacroiliac joints.** The movements consist of gliding and rotational displacements, and in young people probably occur normally during locomotion. In the later months of pregnancy, the range of these movements becomes greater due to the laxity of the ligaments and of the pubic symphysis. Abnormal mobility or subluxation may be a cause of low back pain. Force may be applied to stress the joint, using the opposite femur as a lever (Fig. 16–4). If pathology in the hip joint can be excluded, pain elicited in the sacral region by the stress is indicative of disease in the sacroiliac joint.

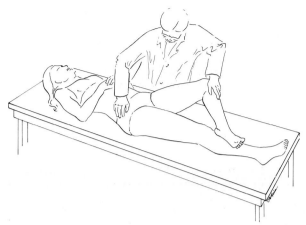

FIG. 16–4. Testing of the sacroiliac joints. The joint on the right side is stressed by pressing on the right anterior superior iliac spine and on the distal end of the left femur after the left hip has reached its limit of movement in the position shown.

As far as normal and abnormal ambulation is concerned, the important movements of the pelvis occur at the hip. The pelvis moves as a whole on the stabilized femur at the hip joint.

THE HIP JOINT

Without the stabilizing effect of surrounding muscles, the shoulder joints would dislocate if they had to sustain the weight of the body as in a handstand. The hip joint, on the other hand, is so constructed that the body weight can be supported on the femoral heads with minimal or no expenditure of muscular energy. Deeply molded articular surfaces and strong ligaments are the key factors in the stability of the hip joint.

Anatomy of the Joint

The hip is a **polyaxial synovial joint** (see Fig. 5–10) in which the closely fitting **ball-and-socket**-shaped articular facets permit movement in all directions. In comparison with the shoulder, these movements are limited by strong ligaments and interlocking articular surfaces.

Articular Surfaces. The spheroidal femoral head fits into the cup-shaped acetabulum (Fig. 16–2) and is retained in it even after the capsule and muscle attachments around the joint are severed. This is due largely to the **acetabular labrum,** the fibrocar-

tilaginous lip of the bony socket, which must be stretched or torn in order to pull the head from the acetabulum. The labrum is completed inferiorly by the **transverse ligament** of the acetabulum which bridges a notch that exists in the lower rim of the bony socket (Fig. 16–5).

With the exception of a central, small, navellike recess, the **fovea,** the femoral head is completely covered by articular cartilage. By contrast, the acetabulum is lined only by a horseshoe-shaped **lunate articular surface** which leaves a nonarticular **acetabular notch** inferiorly, and cartilage is lacking also in the center. On both bones the cartilage is thickest superiorly, where the greatest weight is borne. This may be appreciated from the depth of the joint space seen on an x-ray (Fig. 16–2). Only during squatting is the inferior aspect of the femoral head exposed to any weight bearing.

The Capsule and Ligaments. The thick, fibrous capsule encloses a voluminous joint cavity which contains the acetabular labrum, the head and neck of the femur, as well as the ligament of the head with a fat pad that surrounds it (Fig. 16–5). Th~

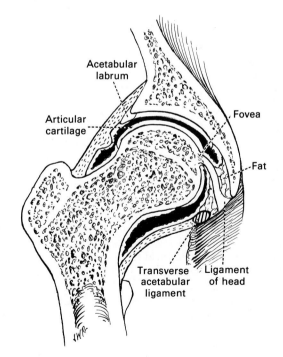

FIG. 16–5. A diagrammatic coronal section through the hip joint. Synovial membrane (not labeled) lines the capsule, covers the femoral neck, the ligament of the head, and the intraarticular fat.

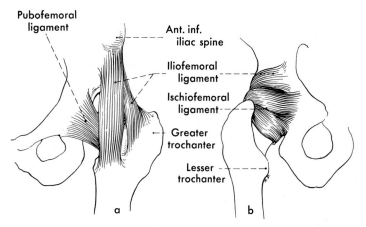

FIG. 16-6. Chief ligaments of the capsule of the hip joint from in front (**A**) and from behind (**B**). (Hollinshead WH: Anatomy for Surgeons, vol 3, 2nd ed. New York, Harper & Row, 1969)

femoral attachments are far beyond the articular margins. Anteriorly, the capsule is attached between the bases of the two trochanters along the intertrochanteric line and posteriorly to the base of the neck, excluding the trochanteric fossa from the joint cavity. It is clinically important that up to the age of 18–19 years the epiphyseal cartilage of the greater trochanter is partially, and that of the femoral head completely, intracapsular.

Although some of the circular fibers of the capsule form a thickened ring around the femoral neck *(zona orbicularis)*, the main reinforcements run longitudinally. Most important of these is the **iliofemoral ligament,** the strongest ligament in the body (Fig. 16–6). Shaped like an inverted Y, its stem attaches to the anterior inferior iliac spine, and its two arms fan out in continuity along the intertrochanteric line. This ligament is the chief factor in counterbalancing the gravitational force during relaxed standing which, since it falls behind the transverse axis of the hip joints, would tend to tilt the pelvis backwards on the femoral heads (Chap. 19). The ligament becomes maximally taut in extension and medial rotation, that is in the close-packed position of the hip. It is the chief factor which limits these ranges of movement. The **pubofemoral** and **ischiofemoral ligaments** (Fig. 16–6) limit abduction and lateral or medial rotation.

The **ligament of the head** is intracapsular (Fig. 16–5). Surrounded by a sleeve of synovial membrane, it passes from the acetabular notch and transverse ligament to the fovea. It is of doubtful importance, and it may occasionally be absent.

The Synovial Membrane. The capsule is lined by synovial membrane which reflects at the femoral capsular attachments and invests the femoral neck in a synovial sleeve (Fig. 16–5). The synovium is attached to the edges of the articular margins on both femur and acetabulum, and thus excludes the intraarticular fat, the ligament of the head, and the femoral neck from direct contact with synovial fluid. It may protrude anteriorly through a defect in the capsule between the iliofemoral and pubofemoral ligaments and may communicate with a bursa lying deep to the tendon of the iliopsoas.

Nerve and Blood Supply. Sensory (proprioception, pain) and vasomotor fibers reach the hip joint in the articular branches of the nerves that supply the prime movers of the joint. These include the **obturator** and **femoral nerves** as well as smaller branches of the sacral plexus (superior gluteal nerve, nerve to quadratus femoris). The precise distribution of these nerves has been worked out, and some have been severed in attempts to relieve hip pain.

The hip, like all other joints, receives its blood supply from a **periarticular arterial anastomosis** which is fed by the circumflex branches of the femoral artery and by the obturator and superior gluteal branches of the internal iliac artery. All intraarticular structures are dependent on this anastomosis for their blood supply, the adequacy of which is most critical for bone, and especially for the proximal femoral epiphysis during its growth.

Branches of the anastomosis pierce the capsule at its femoral attachment and surround the femoral neck as they proceed toward the head beneath the synovial membrane, supplying the underlying bone. These are the **retinacular vessels.** Before closure of the epiphyseal plate, the retinacular vessels can reach the femoral head only via the periosteum which bridges the avascular epiphyseal cartilage between the neck and the head of the femur. After closure, anastomosis is established between epiphyseal and metaphyseal vessels within the cancellous bone, but further distally there is little or no anastomosis between the nutrient artery of the shaft and the vascular bed of the neck. An inconstant small artery in the ligament of the head contributes little to the blood supply of the head and if the retinacular vessels in the periosteum are damaged, the epiphysis of the femoral head becomes predisposed to ischemic necrosis. Femoral neck fracture, dislocation of the hip, and slipping of the femoral epiphysis are all liable to injure the retinacular vessels.

The forces to which the head of the femur is subjected during weight bearing may displace the epiphysis before bony union between the head and the neck is established (Fig. 16–7). The ischemic changes result in softening and degeneration of the epiphysis, leading to abnormal growth and permanent deformity even though with time the deformed femoral head becomes revascularized (Fig. 16–8).

In many cases ischemic necrosis of the proximal femoral epiphysis occurs without any demonstrable slip of the epiphysis. This condition is known as osteochondrosis or Legg-Calvé-Perthes disease. Fracture of the femoral neck in adults may lead to bone necrosis, resulting later in collapse of the femoral head or nonunion of the fracture.

Anatomic Relations. Unlike the shoulder joint, the hip joint is not accessible to direct palpation. The capsule is surrounded on all sides by muscles. Swelling and joint distention are difficult to detect clinically.

Posterior to the joint is the gluteal region or buttock, which under cover of the massive gluteus maximus contains the abductor muscles of the hip along with a number of short muscles which surround the capsule and function as rotators (Fig. 16–14). Anteriorly, the joint is covered by the rectus femoris, iliopsoas, and pectineus (Fig. 16–13), while inferiorly the obturator externus and the adductor muscles render the joint inaccessible.

When the femur is dislocated posteriorly, it may compress or damage the sciatic nerve which lies on

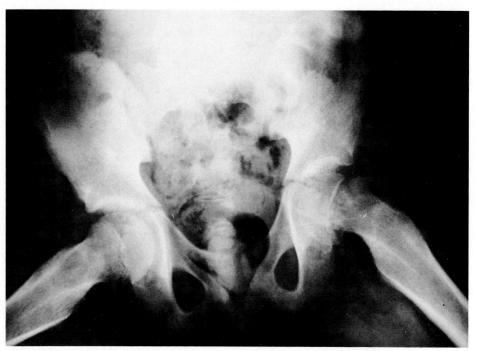

FIG. 16–7. Slipped epiphysis of the left femur. The x-ray was taken in the so-called frog-leg position with the thighs abducted and laterally rotated. Compare the normal epiphysis on the right with that on the left. Note also that union of the three components of the hip bone has not taken place in the acetabulum. (Courtesy of Dr. Rosalind H. Troupin)

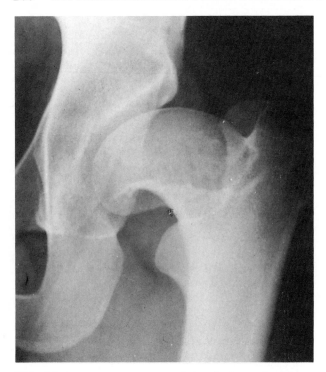

FIG. 16–8. Coxa vara in an adult which resulted from osteochondrosis of the proximal femoral epiphysis during childhood. Note the flattened, deformed femoral head, and the decreased angle between the femoral neck and shaft. (Courtesy of Dr. Rosalind H. Troupin)

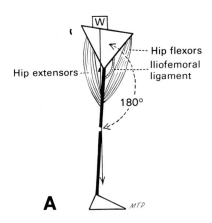

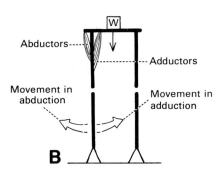

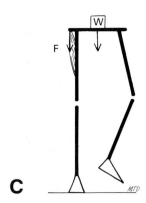

FIG. 16–9. Simplified schematic representation of the pelvis and lower limbs with the major muscle groups at the hip. **(A)** Lateral view. The pelvis is represented as a triangle. W = the body's center of mass and gravity's line of force acting from it. **(B)** Anterior view. The pelvis is represented as a bar. **(C)** Abductors of the hip on one side balance the pelvis when the opposite leg is lifted. F is the force exerted by these muscles and operates at the hip in addition to W.

the short rotator muscles underneath the gluteus maximus (Fig. 16–14). The femoral nerve and femoral artery cross the joint anteriorly lying on the iliopsoas. Because this muscle effectively guards them, they are less liable to come to harm when the femur is dislocated anteriorly.

Movements

Flexion and extension are produced by the spin of the femoral head within the acetabulum, the mechanical axis of the movements being the femoral neck. The femoral shaft serves as a lever for these movements to which the muscles attach. Abduction, adduction, medial, and lateral rotation are the result of swings and slides of the femoral head and neck. All these movements come into play during the normal gait cycle, and their limitation due to deformity, contracture, or paralysis results in abnormal gait patterns characterized by compensatory adaptations (Chap. 19). It is particularly important, therefore, to test the motion ranges at the hip. This will be dealt with before considering

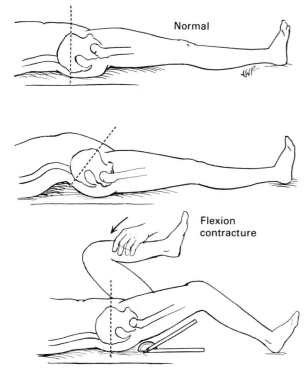

FIG. 16–10. The Thomas test for the diagnosis of hip flexion contracture. The patient is lying supine on a hard surface with hips and knees extended. If there is no contracture, the pelvis remains neutral with the anterior superior iliac spine lying vertically above the posterior superior iliac spine. If a flexion contracture is present, in order to keep the legs on the table, the patient arches his back, compensating for the forward tilt of the pelvis. To test the right hip, the left thigh is flexed passively until the anterior superior iliac spine directly overlies the posterior superior iliac spine. This places the pelvis in the neutral position and brings down the lumbar spine flat on the table. If there is a flexion contracture, the right thigh cannot remain on the table and will make an angle with it which equals the angle of the deformity.

the muscle groups responsible for these movements. The soft tissues which may limit hip movements can be appreciated with reference to the simplified schematic diagrams of Figure 16–9.

Flexion. The range of active flexion is in excess of 100° but falls short of bringing the thigh and the abdomen in contact with each other unless the lumbar spine is also flexed. The passive range of hip flexion tested in the supine patient by applying force to the flexed knee is greater. Its limitation may be due to bony deformity or to contracture of the hip extensors (Fig. 16–9A). Indeed, hip flexion is

limited when the knee is extended, which puts the hamstrings (hip extensors) under tension.

Extension. Extension is limited to about 15° but its apparent range can be increased spectacularly by extension of the lumbar spine as in an arabesque performed by a ballet dancer. The passive range of hip extension, though small, is an important requirement for normal ambulation.

The movement is limited by the length of the iliofemoral ligament and the hip flexors (Fig. 16–9A). Pathologic shortening of these muscles or of the ligament (hip flexion contracture) will reduce the range of extension, causing forward tilting of the pelvis, which displaces the gravitational force line forward. This is compensated for by an increased lumbar lordosis and produces abnormal gait. Decreased extension range (flexion contracture) is diagnosed or ruled out by the **Thomas test** (Fig. 16–10).

Abduction-Adduction. The abduction-adduction range required for normal ambulation is quite small. The femora are abducted when standing with the legs apart and are adducted when the legs are crossed over each other, a position commonly assumed during sitting.

The range of movement in abduction and adduction is limited by the ultimate length of the muscles, since ligamentous restraints of the joint in this plane are minimal. It is readily appreciated from Figure 16–9B that abduction is limited by the length of the adductors and *vice versa*. If the adductor muscle group is pathologically shortened, as in adductor contracture, not only is the range of abduction limited but a deformity also results (Fig. 16–11).

Rotation. Medial and lateral rotation of the femoral shaft result from anteroposterior swings and slides of the femoral head in the acetabulum which may occur in any position of flexion-extension. The range of rotation increases as flexion is increased due to relaxation of the ligaments. The rotation range should be tested in the flexed and extended position of the hip (Fig. 16–12).

Muscles

Functionally, the most important muscle groups around the hip are its flexors and abductors. The flexors accelerate the thigh as it is swung into motion during the gait cycle and the abductors stabilize the pelvis when the body is supported

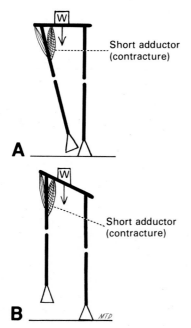

FIG. 16–11. The effect of hip adduction deformity on pelvic tilt and apparent leg length. **(A)** Contracture of hip adductors prevents the leg from achieving the neutral (vertical) position in the abduction-adduction plane. **(B)** For walking the limb must be vertical and, therefore, the pelvis must be elevated which produces a fixed tilt. An apparent shortening of the leg is the result.

only on one leg. Other prime movers include extensors, adductors, and lateral and medial rotators. More often than not a number of these muscles are called into action as antagonists to the force of gravity for controlling and preventing the movement which is the opposite to that of their own prime mover action. This may be appreciated from the simplified schematic representation of the main muscle groups around the hip (Fig. 16–9).

Flexors. A number of muscles with primary actions other than hip flexion are capable of flexing this joint because a vector component of their line of pull crosses the hip anteriorly. However, these muscles become important in hip flexion only when the chief flexors of the hip are weak or paralyzed. The chief flexors are the **iliacus** and the **psoas major** which insert on the lesser trochanter via a common tendon, having crossed the hip anteriorly (Figs. 9–21, 16–13). The iliacus originates from the pelvic surface of the ilium and can only move the hip joint. The same is true, in essence, of the psoas, despite the fact that it is attached to the last thoracic and all lumbar vertebrae. Its ineffec-

tiveness as a vertebral flexor has been considered earlier (see Chap. 9). The two muscles produce hip flexion whether the trunk or the legs are stabilized. A low level of electrical activity is present in them during relaxed standing as they assist the iliofemoral ligament in counterbalancing the force of gravity.

The **rectus femoris** (Fig. 16–13) is primarily an extensor of the knee and is the only head of the quadriceps which crosses the hip. Therefore, it is quite an effective hip flexor, especially when the knee is also flexed. The pectineus, sartorius, and all the adductors can also contribute to hip flexion.

The spinal cord segments chiefly concerned with hip flexion are L2,L3 (see Table 12–2), and they are distributed to these muscles via the lumbar plexus. Because of the developmental rotation of the limb, and because of the variety of muscles involved, the nerves to hip flexors do not conform as clearly to the basic plan of limb innervation as the nerves supplying flexors of the shoulder (see Chaps. 11 and 12). As one would expect, the psoas is innervated directly by ventral rami L1,L2,L3, but L2,L3 fibers reach the iliacus, pectineus, and sartorius via the femoral nerve which also supplies the extensors of the knee. The adductors, as expected, are innervated by the obturator nerve, formed by the anterior divisions of the lumbar plexus.

The strength of the chief hip flexors is tested by opposing the movement in a seated patient whose legs are hanging over the edge of the table or chair. The examiner should apply resistance to the distal end of the femur as the patient flexes one hip after the other, exerting maximum effort.

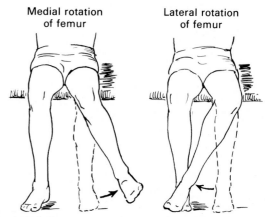

FIG. 16–12. Medial and lateral rotation of the femur with the patient sitting, that is with the hip flexed. Medial and lateral rotation should also be tested similarly with the hip extended, that is, the patient lying prone and knees flexed to 90°.

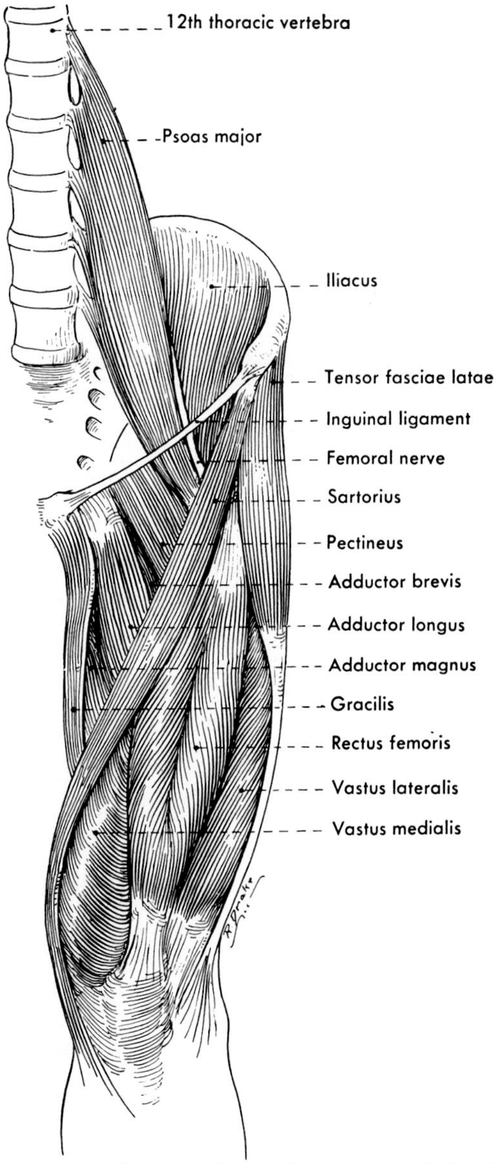
12th thoracic vertebra
Psoas major
Iliacus
Tensor fasciae latae
Inguinal ligament
Femoral nerve
Sartorius
Pectineus
Adductor brevis
Adductor longus
Adductor magnus
Gracilis
Rectus femoris
Vastus lateralis
Vastus medialis

FIG. 16-13. The muscles of the groin and thigh seen from the front. They include flexors and adductors of the hip and extensors of the knee. The femoral triangle is formed by the inguinal ligament, the sartorius, and adductor longus. (Hollinshead WH: Anatomy for Surgeons, vol 3, 2nd ed. New York, Harper & Row, 1969)

Extensors. The most powerful extensor of the hip is the **gluteus maximus** (Fig. 16–14), but it is called into action only during rapid and powerful extension or when resistance has to be overcome. In the normal gait cycle hip extension is achieved primarily by the **hamstrings** (Figs. 16–14, 17–12). Paralysis of the gluteus maximus, which is the largest muscle in the body, does not seriously compromise ambulation on level ground. The muscle is required, however, for hip extension in climbing and going upstairs and also in getting up from a squatting position. Both the hamstrings and glutei contract when the trunk is swayed forward and will continue to be active as long as the gravitational force line from the body's center of mass falls anterior to the hip. They stop contracting as soon as the trunk is restored to a vertical position above the hip.

The **gluteus maximus** originates over a wide area of the back of the bony pelvis (Fig. 16–14), including the posterior end of the iliac crest, the ilium, sacrum, coccyx, and sacrotuberous ligament. Only the deep fibers of the lower half of this thick, quadrangular muscle insert into the gluteal tuberosity of the femur; the remaining and far greater part inserts into the **iliotibial tract** which is a strong longitudinal tendonlike band in the fascia lata, the deep fascia of the thigh (see Figs. 17–1, 17–13).

The muscle extends the femur not only via its bony attachment but also through the iliotibial tract. Although the latter descends to the tibia and crosses the knee joint (p. 286), the gluteus maximus does not move the knee because the tract is fixed along its length to the femur via the lateral intermuscular septum of the thigh. Acting through the iliotibial tract, the gluteus maximus, together with the **tensor fasciae latae** controls anteroposterior tilting of the pelvis when the body weight is supported on one leg. These two muscles are recruited if the leg is slightly flexed at the hip and knee, foregoing the stabilizing effect of the ligaments at these joints. The tensor fasciae latae arises anteriorly from the lateral lip of the iliac crest and, as an anterior counterpart of the superficial portion of the gluteus maximus, inserts into the iliotibial tract. Though not mentioned earlier, the tensor fasciae latae functions as a flexor of the hip. The muscle is supplied by the superior gluteal nerve (L4,L5) and the gluteus maximus by the inferior gluteal nerve (L5,S1,S2).

The muscles attached to the ischial tuberosity are collectively known as the **hamstrings.** They make up the muscle mass of the posterior compartment of the thigh or of the ham and include the **semimenbranosus, semitendinosus, long head of the biceps femoris,** and a portion of the **adductor magnus.** With the exception of the adductor magnus, they insert below the knee and they are *flexors of the knee joint.* When their distal attachment is fixed, the hamstrings exert force on the pelvis causing *extension of the hip* because their line of pull on the ischial tuberosity is posterior to the hip joint. Which of the joints will move depends on

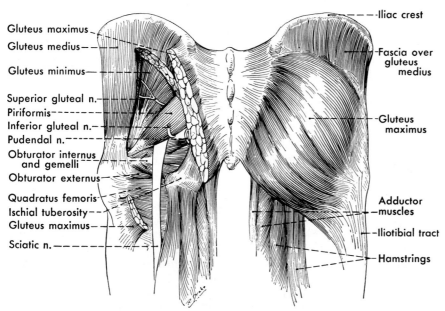

FIG. 16-14. Muscles on the posterior and lateral aspects of the hip. Most of the left gluteus maximus and part of the gluteus medius are shown removed. (Hollinshead WH: Anatomy for Surgeons, vol. 3, 2nd ed. New York, Harper & Row, 1969)

the balance of other stabilizing factors. As noted above, they are more active as hip extensors during ambulation than the gluteus maximus. They are all supplied by segments L5,S1,S2 through the tibial part of the sciatic nerve.

Abductors. The main abductors of the hip are the **gluteus medius** and **gluteus minimus** (Fig. 16–14). These two fan-shaped muscles originate on the lateral surface of the ilium (the minimus anterior and deep to the medius) and insert by separate tendons into the greater trochanter. The gluteus medius and minimus are relaxed when the body weight is supported on both legs, but otherwise they are in constant use despite the fact that abduction of the femur as such seems an unusual movement in everyday activity. During walking, the alternating contraction of the two abductors on the right and left side may be confirmed if the hands are placed over the muscles just below the iliac crests. The contraction occurs on the side of the stance leg, and its purpose is to prevent the pelvis from sagging on the opposite side. When standing on one leg, voluntary relaxation of the abductors results in tilting of the pelvis downward on the unsupported side, mimicking abductor weakness or paralysis, while voluntary increase in their contraction will tilt the pelvis upward, mimicking contracture. The importance of such pelvic tilts with respect to ambu-

lation is considered in Chapter 19. During clinical evaluation the efficiency of the abductors may be tested by observing the level of the two anterior and posterior superior iliac spines (Fig. 16–3) while the patient is standing on one leg. If the abductors are weak, the anterior or posterior superior iliac spine will sag on the opposite side (positive *Trendelenburg test*). The power of the abductors of one side may be assessed more accurately when the patient lying on the contralateral side abducts the thigh against gravity and against resistance.

Both abductors are supplied by the superior gluteal nerve (L5,S1). The tensor fasciae latae (sharing the same nerve) and the upper fibers of the gluteus maximus (supplied by the inferior gluteal nerve) can assist in abduction.

Adductors. It is not completely understood why the hip is endowed with such a large and powerful adductor musculature. The use of these muscles as prime movers is rather limited. However, the adductors seem to be activated by postural reflexes during ambulation. They stabilize the pelvis on the femora during the phase of the gait cycle when both feet are on the ground (double support); and they apparently stabilize the femur when the knee is forcefully flexed or extended. During these efforts, their contraction becomes palpable.

The group includes the **adductor longus, brevis,** and **magnus** (Fig. 16–13). These muscles arise in continuity from the body of the pubis and the conjoint ramus, the adductor part of the magnus fusing with its hamstring part attached to the ischial tuberosity. The muscles fan out laterally to insert into the linea aspera. They are all supplied by the obturator nerve (L2,L3,L4). In comparison with these large muscles, it seems hardly worth mentioning the gracilis, pectineus, and other small muscles around the hip which are also capable of producing some adduction.

The power of the adductors is assessed clinically by trying to force the extended legs apart while the patient attempts to keep the thighs together.

Rotators. Numerous muscles have a rotatory action on the femoral shaft, but only few function primarily as rotators. These are situated in the gluteal region deep to the gluteus maximus and include the **piriformis, obturator internus** with the **gemelli,** the **quadratus femoris** (Fig. 16–14), and also the **obturator externus.** All these muscles insert in or around the trochanteric fossa and rotate the femur laterally. They are strongly assisted by the gluteus maximus.

There is no corresponding group of medial rotators, and it is still disputed precisely which muscles contribute to this relatively powerful movement. The anterior fibers of the **gluteus medius** and **minimus** are undoubtedly involved and, according to electromyographic evidence, so are the adductors, despite the fact that analysis of their attachments and line of pull intuitively predicts lateral rather than medial rotation. The iliopsoas has been championed both as a medial and lateral rotator. Electromyography suggests that it does not participate significantly in rotation of the hip in either direction. However, when the femoral neck is fractured, the iliopsoas produces lateral rotation of the femoral shaft which is recognized as a sign diagnostic of the lesion.

CLINICAL EVALUATION

Throughout life, the hip is the joint most frequently affected by disease; most of its abnormalities characteristically afflict distinct age groups. Failure to establish an early diagnosis, particularly in the young, causes prolonged suffering and serious disability.

Dislocation of the hip is one of the most common congenital anomalies. Routine examination of every neonate must exclude this abnormality. In the young child, hematogenous sepsis frequently involves the hip because of its intraarticular growth plate (Chap. 23). Tuberculous arthritis is still common in children of some underdeveloped countries, though now it is rare in North America. Avascular necrosis of the femoral head (Legg-Calvé-Perthes disease) afflicts the 5 to 10-year-old age group, while a slipped femoral epiphysis characteristically is encountered between the ages of 10 and 18 years. Beyond the age of 50, the most common cause of hip pain is degenerative joint disease, which, of all joints, most frequently involves the hips. Preceding trauma or any gait abnormality will hasten the onset of this disease at an earlier age. Despite the robust construction of the hip, its dislocation and associated fractures are common in traffic accidents. Fracture of the femoral neck typically occurs in the elderly; one in every 20 women who reach the age of 65 will sustain such a fracture.

This section deals in general terms with the symptoms and physical examination of the hip region, and, of all the common types of disturbed hip function, only congenital dislocation will be considered in some detail because of its frequency and important sequelae if not diagnosed and treated at birth.

Symptoms

A painful limp is the presenting clinical picture in most acute disorders of the hip. In a child, refusal to use the limb may be the first sign noticed. Deformity unless due to acute trauma, is usually a sequela of some acute condition.

Pain caused by pathology in the hip joint is usually felt in the groin and as a rule is aggravated by weight bearing. The pain may be referred to the medial side of the thigh, or it may be felt in the knee without any complaints in the hip region. This may be explained by the overlapping innervation of the two joints (see Chap. 17) and must be borne in mind during the examination of both joints.

The patient may complain about a painful hip when there is no pathology in this joint. Groin pain may be due to femoral or inguinal hernia, to inflamed inguinal lymph nodes, or to a psoas abscess. In each case, the pain may be worse during walking. Pain may be referred to the hip region from the lumbar spine, the sacroiliac joints, or the pelvis. Such referred pain is usually felt in the gluteal region and radiates down the back of the thigh, expecially if it is of nerve root origin. Ischemia of the gluteal muscles may produce pain in the buttock during walking (intermittent claudication). This is due to blockage of the internal iliac arteries in the pelvis from which originate the superior and inferior gluteal arteries that supply the gluteal muscles.

Physical Examination

The preceding sections of this chapter dealt with palpation and testing of the various structures, as their anatomy was discussed. The purpose of this section is to describe a sequence to be followed during examination of a patient and to enlarge on some diagnostic manuevers not yet discussed.

Inspection. Examination of the hip should begin with observation of the gait. The clinical evaluation of gait is presented in Chapter 19 and will not be repeated here. For the regional examination of the hip, the patient must be disrobed save for a pelvic slip and, in women, a brassiere.

With the patient standing in the anatomic position, the following should be observed from the front, back, and side view:

1. Posture of the spine, noting especially scoliotic, lordotic, and kyphotic curves as well as deviation of the entire trunk to one or the other side. These abnormal spinal postures may be secondary to fixed pelvic deformity or to hip pain.
2. Orientation of the pelvis (Fig. 16–3), judging lateral tilt by comparing the alignment of the anterior or two posterior superior iliac spines. Anteroposterior tilt is judged by the vertical alignment of the anterior superior iliac spines and the pubic tubercles as well as by flattening or exaggeration of the normal lumbar curvature (see Fig. 9–23).
3. Posture of the legs, noting the position adopted in relaxed standing by the hip, knee, and foot. Are any of the joints flexed or hyperextended? Is the entire sole of both feet in contact with the ground? Are the legs wide apart; is there any crossover? Are both feet and both patellae facing symmetrically forward?
4. Asymmetry in the soft tissues of the thighs and buttocks. Is there any sign of atrophy? Is there symmetry in the two gluteal folds, the skin creases that delineate the buttocks from the thighs posteriorly? In infants are the skin folds of the thighs in the groin symmetrical?
5. Any swelling, redness, scars, or sinuses in the hip region.

Palpation. Palpation should proceed bilaterally, comparing the two sides and noting any swelling, tenderness, or increase in skin temperature.

1. All bony points available for palpation should be felt. These include the iliac crests with their spines, the pubic crests and tubercles, the greater trochanters, and the ischial tuberosities.
2. Muscles of the buttocks and the thighs should be compared by palpation on the two sides.
   The rest of the examination is best conducted with the patient lying on an examination table.
3. Soft tissues of the inguinal region and femoral triangle (p. 274) should be palpated, feeling for lymph nodes and for the pulsation of the femoral artery halfway between the symphysis pubis and anterior superior iliac spine. Deep to the artery is the iliopsoas and the hip joint. A swelling in this region, inferior to the inguinal ligament, is likely to be a psoas abscess rather than a distended hip joint. A psoas abscess is a sequela of tuberculous or other suppurative lesions of lumbar vertebrae, the pus from which tracks down to the thigh within the fascial covering of the psoas major. Psoas abscess is still frequently seen in those parts of the world where tuberculosis is prevalent.
4. With the hip flexed, the sciatic nerve should be palpated through the gluteus maximus. The nerve lies half way between the ischial tuberosity and the greater trochanter (Fig. 16–14). Tenderness over the trochanter may be due to inflammation of the overlying trochanteric bursa.

Ranges of Movement. The normal ranges of movement have been described earlier in the chapter. It is important to test the active and passive ranges of hip flexion, extension, abduction, adduction, and medial and lateral rotation in the flexed and extended position of the hip (Fig. 16–12). Before testing for contractures, it is best to assure that the pelvis lies square on the table permitting the legs to adopt the position dictated by any existing contracture. The Thomas test should be performed to rule out hip flexion contracture (Fig. 16–10).

Muscle Strength. The various muscle groups should be tested as described earlier in the chapter. The Trendelenburg test is an important maneuver for assessing the functional efficiency of the abductors. It should be remembered, however, that a positive Trendelenburg test may be due not only to abductor weakness but also to dislocation of the hip, coxa vara, or an ununited fracture of the femoral neck. These conditions either approximate the greater trochanter to the iliac crest or disturb the stability of the femoral head's fulcrum. All these factors, of course, result in effect in abductor inefficiency.

If weakness is present in any muscle group, the *grade* of muscle strength must be recorded (see Chap. 7) and the limb must be positioned so that the muscle works against gravity and also with the effect of gravity eliminated.

Leg Length Measurements. The supine position is the best for measuring the discrepancy between the length of the two legs. Ideally, the distance should be recorded between the head of the femur and the sole of the foot. As the head of the femur cannot be palpated, by custom the anterior superior iliac spine is used as the superior reference point, and instead of the sole of the foot the precisely identifiable medial malleolus of the

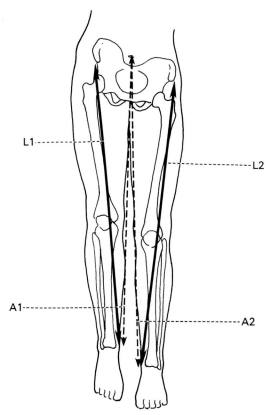

FIG. 16-15. Points of reference in measuring true and apparent leg lengths. In the case illustrated, the right leg appears shorter due to pelvic tilt, and $A_1 < A_2$, but true leg lengths are equal ($L_1 = L_2$).

tibia is chosen as the inferior reference point. This distance is known as **true leg length** (Fig. 16–15), but it is important to be aware of the fact that "true leg length" will vary for the same leg, depending on its position in the abduction-adduction plane. This is because the anterior superior iliac spine is located *lateral* to the femoral head. Adduction of the leg will increase true leg length and abduction will decrease it. Therefore, the two legs must be placed in comparable position relative to the pelvis; that is, if there is a fixed adduction deformity of the leg, the other hip must be adducted to the same angle before true leg length on the two sides can be meaningfully compared.

Shortening may be due to a short tibia or femur, to dislocation of the hip, or to coxa vara. The length of the femora may be compared by measurements between the tip of the greater trochanter and the femoral condyles, and the same can be done for the tibia using the tibial condyles and the medial malleolus as reference points. In cases of dislocation or femoral neck deformity, the relationship of the tip of the greater trochanter will be distorted relative to other bony points of the pelvis. There are several tests for detecting such deformity, although the diagnosis must be based chiefly on x-rays.

With the patient lying in the lateral position, normally the tip of the greater trochanter falls along or below the line that connects the ischial tuberosity and the anterior superior iliac spine (Nélaton's line). Dislocation and coxa vara displace the trochanter upward. Similarly, the medial extension of a line that connects the tip of the trochanter to the anterior superior iliac spine of its own side will normally intersect a similar line from the opposite side in the median plane and above the umbilicus (Schoemaker's line). A simple diagrammatic sketch can readily demonstrate that displacement of one or both trochanters in relation to the anterior superior iliac spine will distort this relationship.

If an *apparent leg length inequality* can be detected in the standing position after the true leg length of the two limbs was found to be equal by measurement, a fixed lateral pelvic tilt must exist. It is important to measure **apparent leg length** discrepancy, and for this measurement the legs of a supine patient must be placed parallel to one another and in line with the trunk. The inferior reference point remains the medial malleolus, but superiorly the measurement is taken from the umbilicus or from the xiphisternal junction (Fig. 16–15).

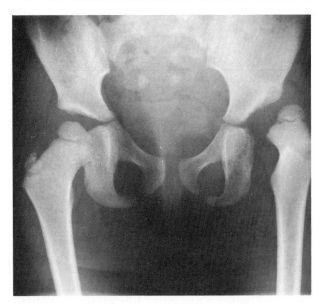

FIG. 16–16. Congenital dislocation of the hip. In the radiograph the head of the left femur is dislocated. Note the wide open acetabulum and the smaller epiphysis of the femoral head on the left compared with the right. These radiologic signs appear only some time after birth. Note also that the inferior edge of the right femoral neck forms a smooth arch together with the inferior margin of the superior ramus of the pubis. This arch is distorted on the left.

Congenital Dislocation of the Hip

The condition consists of spontaneous dislocation of the hip, occurring either before or during birth (Fig. 16–16). It is five times more common in the female than in the male. Multiple factors contribute to the etiology. Dislocation of the hip should be looked for in every newborn child. The diagnosis is established by the physical signs.

Inspection. The dislocated limb appears shortened. This may be apparent by an alteration in the number and symmetry of the skin creases in the thigh and by the difference in the level of the knees when both hips and knees are flexed with the infant supine (Fig. 16–17).

Movement. Abduction of the affected hip is limited, as the femoral head impinges on the ilium. Frequently, involuntary contraction of the adductor muscles also limits abduction. Telescoping of the femur also indicates instability and dislocation. This is elicited by grasping the knee and thigh in one hand and the pelvis in the other. If disloca-tion is present, the thigh will shorten and lengthen when the examiner pushes up and pulls down on the limb.

Ortolani's Sign. Ortolani's click sign is the most important diagnostic test for hip subluxation or dislocation in the newborn. It is usually not possi-ble to elicit the sign later than 5 days after birth; this emphasizes the importance of a careful physi-cal examination at the earliest time. The examiner grasps both thighs with the knees flexed so that his fingers follow along the femur to the greater trochanter, the thumb placed on the medial side of the thigh. The palm cradles the knee and the flexed leg. The opposite hip is fully abducted to fix the pelvis. The examiner adducts the flexed hip, pres-sing the thigh posteriorly and then abducts the hip, pulling the thigh forward. A click is palpable or audible when the head of the femur enters or leaves the acetabulum (Fig. 16–18).

THE LUMBOSACRAL PLEXUS

Like the upper limb, the lower limb is innervated through a nerve plexus derived from ventral rami of spinal nerves. This is the lumbosacral plexus, the lumbar part of which is located in the abdo-men, and the sacral part in the pelvis. The major nerves which issue from this plexus for the supply of the lower limb are derived from the **ventral rami of L2 to S3** spinal nerves (Fig. 16–19). L1 and S4,

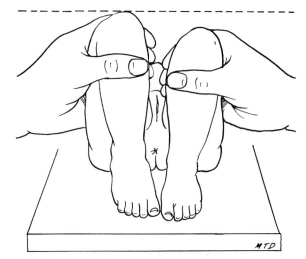

FIG. 16–17. The femur appears shorter on the side of the dislocation, because the femoral head has been dis-placed upward.

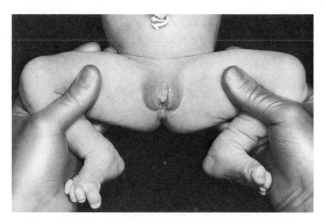

FIG. 16-18. Examination of the hips in the newborn infant for Ortolani's sign, an indication for dislocation (for description, see text). (Adams JC: Outline of Orthopedics, 6th ed. Baltimore, Williams & Wilkins, 1968)

usually included in representations of the lumbosacral plexus, supply as a rule only a limited area of skin in the inguinal and perianal regions, respectively, and have no muscular distribution in the limb. However, when the plexus is *prefixed* or *postfixed*, L1 or S4, respectively, may supply both muscle and skin in the limb.

The lumbosacral plexus, like the brachial plexus, conforms to the basic plan of a limb plexus discussed in Chapters 11 and 12. Each **root**, representing a ventral ramus, splits into an **anterior** and **posterior division** for the respective supply of the flexor or extensor compartments or their equivalents. These divisions are regrouped into the definitive, major nerves that proceed to the lower limb (see Figs. 11-7, 11-9) without the complicating interposition of trunks and cords seen in the brachial plexus (Fig. 16-19).

Types of Nerve Fibers

The lumbosacral plexus is composed predominantly of somatic nerve fibers. The **somatic efferents** are the axons of neurons in the lateral portions of the anterior horns of grey matter in spinal cord segments L2-S3. These groups of neurons are chiefly responsible for the lumbar enlargement of the cord (Chap. 10). The cell bodies of **somatic afferents** concerned with exteroceptive (pain, temperature, pressure, touch) and proprioceptive (joint position sense, muscle spindle) impulses from the lower limb are located in L2-S3 spinal ganglia. **Sympathetic efferents** control vasomotor activity and sweating in the lower limb.

They enter the plexus as postsynaptic fibers through grey rami communicantes contributed to each root of the plexus by lumbar and sacral sympathetic chain ganglia.

The presynaptic neurons for the sympathetic outflow to the lower limb are located in the lateral column of grey matter in T10-L2 segments (Chap. 10; for comparison see Fig. 13-17). All presynaptic fibers that relay to the lower limb after synapsing in lumbar and sacral sympathetic ganglia enter the sympathetic chain via white rami communicantes at or above L2 spinal nerve. Therefore, resection of the upper three lumbar sympathetic ganglia with the intervening sympathetic trunk completely deprives the lower limb of sympathetic innervation. Severe and chronic vasospasm, one of the causes of painful ischemic changes in the foot, which can lead to gangrene, (Raynaud's disease) may be eliminated by such a *lumbar sympathectomy.*

Formation

Lumbar Plexus. As soon as L2,L3,L4 roots of the lumbar plexus emerge from the intervertebral foramina, they are engulfed by the psoas major because this muscle is attached to the lateral surface of the lumbar vertebrae and also to their transverse processes. The roots split into anterior and posterior divisions within the psoas and reunite to form the branches of the plexus which emerge from the muscle along its lateral or medial border. The **femoral nerve,** formed by the posterior divisions of L2,L3,L4, descends from the plexus lateral to the muscle; the anterior divisions of the same roots unite to form the other major branch of the plexus, the **obturator nerve,** which leaves the psoas medially.

Only a portion of L4 ventral ramus contributes to the lumbar plexus; the remaining smaller part, with L5 root, forms the **lumbosacral trunk** which descends into the pelvis and feeds into the sacral plexus (Fig. 16-19). The lumbosacral trunk and the obturator nerve enter the pelvis lying on the ala of the sacrum, medial to the psoas.

Sacral Plexus. The ventral rami of S1,S2, and S3 emerge from the anterior sacral foramina and proceed laterally on the anterior surface of the piriformis. This muscle originates from the sacrum lateral to the foramina and has been seen in the gluteal region after it has left the pelvis (Fig. 16-14). The lumbosacral trunk joins the sacral roots and fuses with S1. The plexus is quite inaccessible

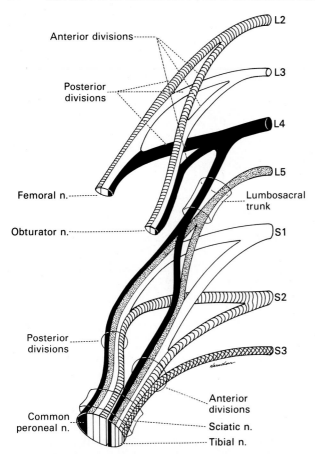

FIG. 16-19. The basic plan of the lumbosacral plexus and its major terminal branches. Each root of the plexus is designated by a different pattern of shading to illustrate the manner of its distribution.

because it lies in the posterior wall of the pelvic cavity; its anterior relations are the branches of the internal iliac artery embedded in endopelvic fat and connective tissue.

All the roots, including L4 and L5 contained in the lumbosacral trunk, split into anterior and posterior divisions (Fig. 16–19). However, the separation of these divisions is not apparent without dissection. Furthermore, anterior and posterior divisions converge laterally to form an apparently single, large nerve trunk, the **sciatic nerve,** which leaves the pelvis with the piriformis through the greater sciatic foramen. The sciatic nerve, in fact, is composed of two nerves which not infrequently issue independently from the plexus and leave the pelvis undisguised. The posterior divisions of L4,L5,S1,S2 form the **common peroneal nerve;** the corresponding anterior divisions plus the anterior

division of S3 form the **tibial nerve** (Fig. 16–19). The posterior division of S3 is represented in minor, cutaneous branches of the plexus.

Branches

In addition to the four major nerves of the lower limb mentioned so far, there are a number of small lumbar and sacral branches which supply skin and muscle in the limb. As in the brachial plexus, muscular branches innervate the girdle musculature which, in the lower limb, include the gluteal muscles together with the short rotators of the thigh.

Major Branches. The distribution of the main terminal branches of the lumbosacral plexus has been described in Chapter 11 (see Figs. 11–7, 11–9). It is useful to attach functional labels to each of these nerves when considering their anatomy.

1. The **femoral nerve** (L2,L3,L4) is the nerve of *knee extension and hip flexion* (see Fig. 17–2). It supplies a large area of skin on the anteromedial aspect of the thigh and the medial aspect of the leg and foot. Clinically, it is best evaluated by testing the power of knee extension and cutaneous sensitivity over the medial malleolus.

The femoral nerve descends from the lumbar plexus sheltered by the lateral margin of the psoas and comes to lie in the furrow between the psoas and iliacus, which it supplies. The nerve enters the thigh and it breaks up into numerous branches as soon as it passes beyond the inguinal ligament. These branches are distributed to all four heads of the quadriceps and to the pectineus and sartorius. Two to three large cutaneous branches innervate the skin anteriorly down to the knee (anterior cutaneous nerves of the thigh), and the largest branch known as the **saphenous nerve** reaches as far distally as the medial side of the metatarsophalangeal joint of the big toe. The femoral nerve supplies also both the hip and knee joints.

2. The **obturator nerve** (L2,L3,L4) is the nerve of the *adductors of the hip* and is clinically best evaluated by testing the power of adduction. Its cutaneous distribution is restricted to a small area on the medial side of the thigh above the knee.

Having descended into the pelvis along the medial side of the psoas, the nerve skirts the side wall of the pelvis and exits into the thigh through the superomedial corner of the obturator foramen. It breaks up into branches for all the adductors, the obturator externus, and the gracilis. Like the femoral nerve, it supplies the hip and knee joints.

3. The **common peroneal nerve** (L4,L5,S1,S2) is

the *chief nerve of ankle dorsiflexion* (i.e., extension) and is clinically best evaluated by testing the power of ankle dorsiflexion. Its cutaneous distribution is limited; it supplies skin on the lateral aspect of the calf and on the dorsum of the foot. The nerve separates from the tibial nerve above the popliteal fossa and its distribution in the leg much resembles that of the radial nerve and its posterior interosseous branch.

4. The **tibial nerve** (L4,L5,S1,S2,S3) is the *chief nerve of knee, ankle and toe flexion*, as well as the nerve of the intrinsic muscles of the foot. It is a complex nerve, encompassing the equivalents of both the median and ulnar nerves as well as the nerves to the hamstrings. Its clinical evaluation is complex and can be meaningful only after the regional distribution of the nerve is understood.

Its terminal branches (**medial and lateral plantar nerves**) in the sole of the foot resemble the median and ulnar nerves in the hand, both with respect to muscular and cutaneous distribution. In the calf, the tibial nerve innervates all the flexor muscles equivalent to those in the flexor compartment of the forearm. In the thigh, the nerve supplies all the hamstrings, including the hamstring part of the adductor magnus. In addition to those in the sole of the foot, its cutaneous branches supply the medial side and back of the calf as well as the lateral side of the foot.

Minor Branches. Figure 16–20 shows the minor branches of the lumbosacral plexus. The femoral branch of the **genitofemoral nerve** (L1,L2) supplies skin just distal to the inguinal ligament (the genital branch innervates the cremaster muscle, p. 175), and is the only branch of the lumbar plexus which perforates the psoas and descends to the inguinal region on the surface of the muscle. The **lateral femoral cutaneous nerve** (L2,L3) leaves the lumbar plexus laterally and enters the thigh just anterior to the anterior superior iliac spine. It supplies a large area of skin on the lateral side of the thigh as far down as the knee.

Omitted from Figure 16–20 is an occasional branch of the lumbar plexus, the **accessory obturator nerve** (which, if present, supplies the pectineus). The ilioinguinal and iliohypogastric nerves, both derived from L1, do not properly belong to the lower limb plexus, though they are customarily included among its branches.

Both anterior and posterior divisions of the sacral plexus give off muscular branches (Fig. 16–20). The **superior gluteal nerve** (L4,L5,S1) leaves the pelvis through the greater sciatic foramen, accom-

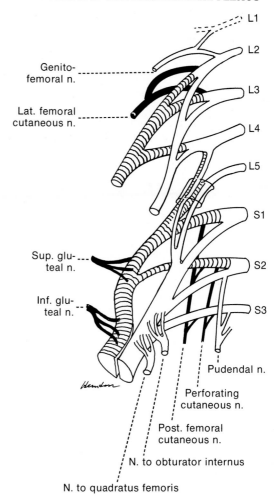

FIG. 16–20. The branches of the lumbosacral plexus. Posterior divisions are striated and minor branches derived from them are shown in black; anterior divisions and the branches derived from them are unshaded.

panied by an artery of the same name. The nerve supplies the gluteus medius, minimus, and the tensor fasciae latae. The **inferior gluteal nerve** (L5,S1,S2) follows a similar course with its artery and is spent in the gluteus maximus. The **nerve to the quadratus femoris** (L4,L5,S1) and the **nerve to the obturator internus** (L5,S1,S2,S3) supply these lateral rotators of the hip as well as two small muscles, the gemelli. The **piriformis** receives branches from the posterior divisions of S1 and S2.

Two cutaneous branches of the sacral plexus supply an extensive area of skin in the back of the thigh down to the knee. The larger is the **posterior femoral cutaneous nerve** (S1,S2,S3) and the smaller, the **perforating cutaneous nerve of the thigh** (S2,S3). The **pudendal nerve** (S2,S3,S4), included in Figure 16–20, is the *nerve of the perineum* and does not contribute to the innervation of the limb.

Clinical assessment of the minor branches of the lumbosacral plexus relies on testing the muscles and cutaneous areas supplied by them. Because of the less precise action of the muscles around the hip, this is less straightforward and clinically less critical than is the case with the minor branches of the brachial plexus.

Injuries

Gun shot wounds are the most frequent cause of discrete lesions within the lumbosacral plexus and among its branches. Dislocation of the hip, fracture of the pelvis, or pelvic neoplasms may also compromise various nerves.

SUGGESTED READING

Adams JC: Outline of Orthopedics, 6th ed. Baltimore, Williams & Wilkins, 1968
Chapter 8 describes concisely the common diseases of the hip, their diagnosis and treatment.

Haymaker W, Woodhall B: Peripheral Nerve Injuries. Philadelphia, WB Saunders, 1967
Chapters 13 and 14 present the normal anatomy of the lumbosacral plexus and illustrate the diagnosis of nerve injuries with numerous clinical cases.

Hollinshead WH: Anatomy for Surgeons, Vol 3, The Back and Limbs, 2nd ed. New York, Harper & Row, 1969
Chapter 8 deals with detailed anatomy of the hip joint and of the gluteal region. Chapter 7 discusses the formation of the lumbosacral plexus with variations and the distribution of its branches. Extensively illustrated, copious bibliography.

Hoppenfeld S: Physical Examination of the Spine and Extremities. New York, Appleton-Century-Crofts, 1976
Chapter 6 is a well-illustrated account of the physical examination of the hip region.

Joseph J: Movements at the hip. Ann R Coll Surg Engl, 56: 192, 1975
A brief and interesting treatise of some intriguing issues concerning hip function and ambulation.

Strange FS St: The Hip. Baltimore, Williams & Wilkins, 1965
This small book is mainly oriented toward the treatment of various disorders of the hip. In each instance there is a clear and pertinent consideration of structure and function as well as of diagnosis.

Trueta J: The normal vascular anatomy of the human femoral head during growth. J Bone Joint Surg [B] 39: 358, 1957
A classical paper on the subject.

17
The Thigh and the Knee

CORNELIUS ROSSE

The basic structural similarities and differences between the upper and lower limbs have been discussed in Chapter 11. The thigh of man is distinguished from the arm and from the thigh of other primates by its massive musculature, a reflection of the bipedal mode of existence. The function of this muscle mass is to extend the knees, raising the body into the upright posture, and to balance, on the tibial condyles, the femur and the pelvis which support the rest of the body. The knee is a weight-bearing joint, and, while allowing movement, it converts the lower limb into a solid pillar in the fully extended position, relying for stability only on its ligaments. In all other positions, however, muscle power is required to maintain balance at the knee during both standing and locomotion (Chap. 19). Stability is the most important consideration in the clinical assessment of the knee and this assessment is based on the sequential evaluation of the anatomic structures capable of furnishing stability.

The thigh muscles that move the knee have already been encountered in the previous chapter. The extensors are the quadriceps, consisting of the rectus femoris and the three vasti; the flexors are the hamstrings. The anatomic relation of these muscle groups to one another and to the vessels and nerves that pass through the thigh will be considered before dealing with the knee joint and with the precise actions which these muscles have on the knee.

THE THIGH

Compartments

The femur does not separate the thigh as clearly into a flexor and an extensor compartment (Fig. 17–1) as the humerus and intermuscular septa do in the arm (see Fig. 14–9). Not only is the an-teroposterior orientation of the two compartments reversed (Chap. 11) but the extensor muscles (vastus medialis, lateralis, and intermedius) almost completely surround the femur as they arise from it, leaving only the *linea aspera,* a narrow strip of bone posteriorly, for the other muscles. With the exception of the relatively small short head of the biceps femoris, the flexor muscles do not attach to the femur; they descend to the knee from the ischial tuberosity. More bulky than the knee flexors are the adductors of the hip, the homologues of which in the arm are represented only by the insignificant coracobrachialis. The adductors occupy a large medial compartment and insert into the femur (Fig. 17–1) as far distally as the adductor tubercle. A furrow running between the extensor and adductor compartments spirals down the medial side of the thigh starting at the inferior apex of the femoral triangle. The furrow is roofed over by the sartorius (Figs. 16–13, 17–1) and in this subsartorial or **adductor canal** descend the femoral vessels and the saphenous nerve. The femoral and obturator nerves are represented in the extensor and adductor compartment respectively only by their branches (Figs. 17–2, 17–3). The sciatic nerve approaches the popliteal fossa sandwiched between the hamstrings and the adductor magnus. Its tibial component distributes branches to the hamstrings including the posterior portion of the adductor magnus which originates from the ischial tuberosity (see Fig. 18–11). The other half of the sciatic, the common peroneal nerve, is destined for muscles and skin below the knee.

Fascia Lata and Intermuscular Septa. The deep fascia of the thigh, known as the fascia lata, forms a strong fibrous sheath around the thigh. It is attached superiorly along the iliac crest, the inguinal ligament, the conjoint ramus, ischial tuberosity, sacrotuberous ligament, and the sacrum, and inferiorly to the bony points around the knee. Just below the inguinal ligament the fascia lata roofs over the femoral triangle. Here, branches of the femoral artery, tributaries of the femoral vein, and lymph vessels pass through the **saphenous opening** which is an aperture in the fascia lata. At the back of the knee, the fascia lata roofs over the popliteal fascia and changes its name to popliteal fossa.

A lateral and a medial intermuscular septum extend from the fascia to the linea aspera, separating the extensor compartment from the hamstrings laterally and from the adductors medially. No definite septum exists between the hamstrings and adductors (Fig. 17–1).

The **iliotibial tract** which receives the insertions of the gluteus maximus and the tensor fasciae latae is a strong tendinous reinforcement in the fascia, and spans the length of the thigh from the iliac crest to the lateral condyle of the tibia.

The Femoral Vessels

The femoral artery and vein are the continuation of the external iliac vessels, and behind the knee they become the popliteal artery and vein. The femoral artery enters the **femoral triangle** midway between the symphysis pubis and the anterior superior iliac spine as it emerges from underneath the inguinal ligament, which forms the base of the triangle (Fig. 16–13). The artery leaves the triangle at its apex, which is formed at the meeting point of the sartorius and adductor longus. The changing relationship of the femoral artery to the femoral vein as they descend through the triangle is a reflection of the developmental rotation of the limb. Starting out in a medial position at the triangle's base, the vein winds behind the artery as the two vessels approach the apex. This relationship is retained throughout the **adductor canal** in which the artery and vein run toward the medial condyle of the femur. In this subsartorial canal the vessels lie between the vastus medialis and the adductor muscles (Fig. 17–1). About a hand's breadth above the knee joint the artery and vein incline posteriorly and enter the popliteal fossa passing through a hiatus in the tendinous fibers of the adductor magnus.

In the femoral triangle the femoral nerve is lateral to the artery before it breaks up into its branches. Two of these, the saphenous nerve and the branch to the vastus medialis, accompany the femoral vessels in the adductor canal.

A number of small branches are given off by the artery in the femoral triangle for the supply of the groin and the external genitalia. Other small branches supply the neighboring muscles in the adductor canal. The femoral artery gives off its largest and most important branch, the **profunda femoris artery**, in the femoral triangle. This artery,

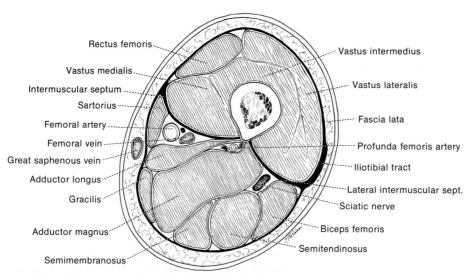

FIG. 17-1. A transverse section through the middle third of the thigh drawn to show schematically the division of the musculature into compartments and to illustrate the position of the femoral and profunda femoris vessels. The thickness of the fascia lata, intermuscular septa, and iliotibial tract are exaggerated.

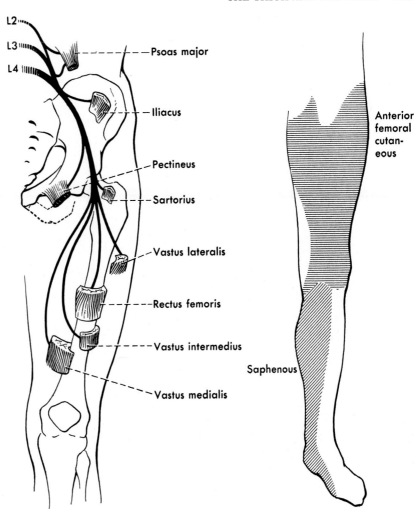

L2
L3
L4

Psoas major

Iliacus

Pectineus

Sartorius

Vastus lateralis

Rectus femoris

Vastus intermedius

Vastus medialis

Anterior femoral cutaneous

Saphenous

FIG. 17-2. Muscular and cutaneous distribution of the femoral nerve. (Hollinshead WH: Anatomy for Surgeons, vol. 3, 2nd ed. New York, Harper & Row, 1969)

and not the femoral, is the chief source of blood for the thigh musculature. The **lateral** and **medial circumflex arteries** branch off the profunda and encircle the proximal end of the femur. They participate in the circumtrochanteric anastomosis and through the thigh musculature send branches as far down as the knee (descending branch of the lateral circumflex). The profunda femoris itself descends posterior to the floor of the adductor canal (Fig. 17-1) and is separated from the femoral artery by the adductor longus. In addition to other muscular branches, so-called **perforating arteries** arise from the profunda throughout its course which perforate the adductor magnus passing through small tendinous foramina in its attachment to the linea aspera. The perforating arteries

distribute blood to muscles in the posterior compartment.

The femoral vein receives numerous muscular tributaries, and in the femoral triangle the **profunda femoris vein** and the **great saphenous vein** empty into it.

Intermittent Claudication. The femoral artery and its branches are frequently affected by atherosclerosis. Atheroma may seriously limit or completely block blood flow, producing ischemia in the muscles, especially during exercise, which manifests itself by pain. The pain develops during walking and is rapidly relieved by rest. The condition is known as intermittent claudication.

If the profunda femoris artery is blocked, pain

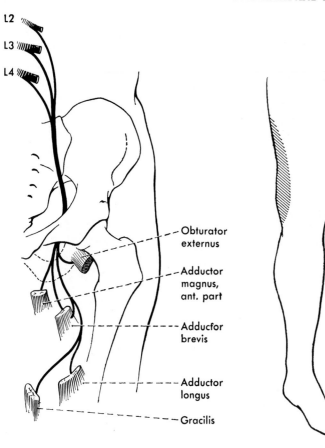

Obturator externus

Adductor magnus, ant. part

Adducfor brevis

Adductor longus

Gracilis

FIG. 17-3. Muscular and cutaneous distribution of the obturator nerve. (Hollinshead WH: Anatomy for Surgeons, vol. 3, 2nd ed. New York, Harper & Row, 1969)

develops during walking in the thigh muscles. Blockage of the femoral artery distal to the origin of the profunda leads to intermittent claudication in the calf. If the artery is blocked more proximally, symptoms develop in the calf sooner than in the thigh.

THE KNEE

The knee is the largest joint in the body. Its anatomy and mechanics are quite complex. Normal function and its derangement can only be appreciated by knowing the anatomy of all constituent structures. Most knee disorders encountered in clinical practice result from injury. The mechanism of injury gives the clue to the structures most likely involved. Most of the structures are accessible by palpation or can be tested clinically. It should, therefore, be possible to make an anatomic diagnosis in practically all knee injuries.

The knee joint consists of two articulations which are closely integrated. The distal end of the femur articulates with the tibia at the **tibiofemoral joint** and with the patella at the **patellofemoral joint.** The fibula is excluded from the knee joint (see Fig. 11–4A) and articulates independently with the lateral condyle of the tibia at the **superior tibiofibular joint.**

Anatomic Landmarks

The **patella** is prominent in the extended knee. Reference to x-rays of the knee (see Fig. 8–8) will emphasize that the patella rides higher than generally appreciated, and its inferior tip is at least 1 cm proximal to the tibiofemoral joint line. With the quadriceps relaxed, the relatively flat patellofemoral articular surfaces (see Fig. 8–8F) permit manual, side-to-side displacement of the patella. However, because the patella is essentially a sesamoid bone in the tendon of the quadriceps, it becomes fixed when the muscle contracts or when the knee is flexed. Isometric contraction of the quadriceps in an extended knee throws into prominence the stout tendon of the muscle. The segment of this tendon proximal to the patella is known as the **quadriceps tendon,** while its distal segment between the patella and the **tuberosity of the tibia** is designated as the **ligamentum patellae** (or patellar ligament).

The expanded ends of the distal femoral and proximal tibial epiphyses, known as the **medial** and **lateral condyles** of each bone, are best examined with the knee flexed. Running the hand down the medial side of the thigh, the first bony point reached is the **adductor tubercle** on the femoral condyle. Proceeding further distally, first the **medial epicondyle** and then the articular margin of the femoral condyle are reached. The latter is separated by a narrow gap from the articular margin of the medial condyle of the tibia. The articular margins on both bones may be traced with precision anteriorly and posteriorly. The femoral articular margin leads anteriorly to the patella, that of the tibia to the ligamentum patellae. The space between the diverging anterior margins of the medial condyles is occupied by an intraarticular fat pad, which is also palpable on the lateral side of the ligamentum patellae between the diverging margins of the two lateral condyles. In the depth of these spaces the **menisci** may be identified by firm, deep palpation. The edge of these semilunar cartilages may be felt slipping in and out between the tibial and femoral articular margins as the tibia is rotated medially and laterally. The menisci are palpable along each side of the joint, though they cannot be discerned as distinct structures along the joint line.

The **head of the fibula** is visible and palpable posterolaterally on the lateral condyle of the tibia. Just above it, across the joint line, the **lateral epicondyle** is palpable as a tubercle on the femoral condyle. Posteriorly, the contents of the popliteal fossa preclude precise bony palpation. The tendons of the hamstrings are useful landmarks on either side of this space, especially if the muscles are isometrically contracted or if knee flexion is opposed. The tendon of the biceps attaches to the head of the fibula, and on the medial side the overlapping tendons of the semitendinosus and semimembranosus can be distinguished.

Anatomy of the Joint

The knee is a compound synovial joint which functions as a hinge. However, in addition to the prevailing flexion-extension produced by the rolling of the tibiofemoral articular surfaces on one another,

tibiofemoral gliding or translation also take place. The latter movements are more pronounced in the knee and contribute more to the flexion-extension range than in any other hinge joint. This gliding is responsible for the constantly changing position of the hinge axis and also for a significant degree of tibiofemoral rotation. The up-and-down gliding of the patella on its sellar femoral articular surface (see Fig. 8–8F) is integrated with tibiofemoral flexion and extension and needs no further discussion. The tibiofemoral articulation, on the other hand, has to be understood in some detail.

Articular Surfaces. Interposed between the medial and lateral condyles is a pair of semilunar cartilages or menisci which prevent direct contact between much of the tibial and femoral articular facets. Nevertheless, the configuration of these surfaces is a determining factor as far as the movements are concerned.

The **intercondylar notch** separates the two femoral condyles posteriorly like two limbs of an inverted U (Fig. 17–4). The anterior conjoined portion of the articular surfaces accommodates the patella, while the limbs of the U, including their rounded, posterior ends, articulate with the menisci and the tibia. On both condyles, the tibial and patellar surfaces are separated by shallow but distinct grooves, better marked on the cartilage then on the bones (Fig. 17–5). The patellar surface is larger on the lateral condyle and includes the prominent **trochlea.** The tibial surface is greater, however, on the medial condyle, the importance of which will become clear in the discussion of the close-packed position of the knee.

The **intercondylar eminence** is interposed between the two condylar articular facets of the tibia (Figs. 17–4, 17–5). The two facets upon which the menisci rest are entirely separate. Posteriorly, articular cartilage extends over the smooth lip of the lateral condyle but otherwise the articular surfaces are confined to the tibial plateau.

Capsule and Its Ligaments. Unlike most synovial joints, the capsule of the knee does not form a closed fibrous sleeve around the joint. The typical arrangement is present only medially and laterally where the thin fibrous capsule bridges the joint space between femoral and tibial articular margins. Even here, this simple arrangement is complicated by the capsule's attachment to the circumference of the menisci. Portions of the capsule above and below their meniscal attachment are known as the **coronary ligaments.** These "liga-

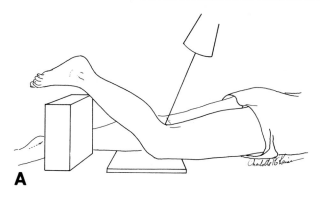

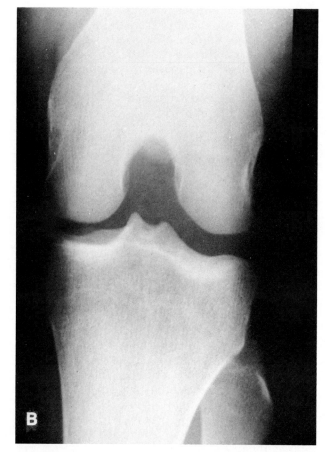

FIG. 17-4. X-ray of the knee taken in a slightly flexed position (**A**) to optimally reveal the condylar articular surfaces, the nonarticular femoral intercondylar notch, and tibial intercondylar eminence (**B**). Note that the femoral articular surfaces are convex from side to side while the tibial surfaces are slightly concave; the menisci are invisible; the apex of the patella can just be seen in the intercondylar notch; the fibula is some distance below the tibiofemoral joint line. (Courtesy of Dr. Rosalind H. Troupin)

ments'' are thin and loose and permit the necessary sliding and twisting of the menisci during joint movement. On the lateral femoral condyle the fossa in which the tendon of the popliteus is attached (Fig. 17–7D) is enclosed within the capsule and so is part of the muscle.

Posteriorly, the capsular attachment does not follow the articular margins. On the femur it continues from one condyle to the other enclosing the intercondylar notch within the capsule (Fig. 17–6C). There is a gap in its tibial attachment which provides a hiatus for the exit of the popliteus muscle from the joint (Fig. 17–6C). The edge of the capsule which arches over the muscle is known as the **arcuate ligament.**

Anteriorly the capsule is deficient (Fig. 17–6A). The deficiency is closed by the quadriceps tendon, the patella, and ligamentum patellae. The fibrous capsule fuses on each side with these structures, enclosing a large, irregular space within the joint. This space is filled largely with intraarticular fat. The capsule is substantially reinforced on each

side of the patella and ligamentum patellae by tendinous fibers derived from the quadriceps, which, instead of inserting into the patella, join the ligamentum patellae directly. These aponeurotic expansions fuse with the capsule and are known as the medial and lateral **patellar retinacula.**

The capsule is reinforced also posteriorly as well as on each side. The posterior reinforcement is derived largely from a tendinous expansion of the semimembranosus and is known as the **oblique ligament.** The lateral and medial reinforcements are intrinsic to the capsule and represent the **deep** or **capsular component of the tibial and fibular collateral ligaments.**

Accessory Ligaments. The major ligaments of the knee are independent of its capsule. One pair, the proper tibial and fibular collateral ligaments, are outside and the other pair, the cruciate ligaments, are inside the joint.

The **medial** or **tibial collateral ligament** is a broad, flat band extending from the medial

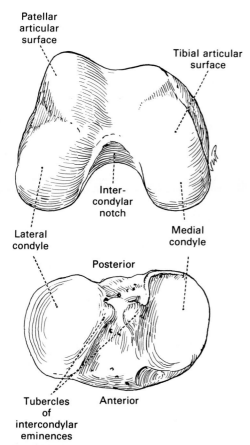

Patellar articular surface

Tibial articular surface

Inter-condylar notch

Lateral condyle

Medial condyle

Posterior

Tubercles of intercondylar eminences

Anterior

FIG. 17–5. Articular surfaces of the femur and tibia. Note the grooves on the lateral and medial condyles of the femur which separate the tibial and patellar articular surfaces. The anterior prominence of the lateral condyle is the trochlea.

epicondyle of the femur to the tibia 4 in. below the joint line. The ligament is believed to be the vestige of the tendon of the ischial or hamstring part of the adductor magnus, which inserted into the tibia before that tendon became anchored to the adductor tubercle. Along its posterior edge the ligament fuses with the deep or capsular component of the collateral ligament which has already been described with the capsule (Fig. 17–7D). Via this fusion the medial meniscus is tethered to the tibial collateral ligament. The **lateral** or **fibular collateral ligament** is cordlike and runs between the lateral femoral epicondyle and the tip of the fibula. It probably represents the vestige of the attachment of the peroneus longus to the femur. It has no connection with either the deep, capsular portion of the collateral ligament or with the lateral meniscus. Both tibial and fibular collateral liga-

ments become taut in full extension but their chief function is to provide side-to-side stability to the knee joint.

The **cruciate ligaments** inside the joint run in a criss-cross fashion between the tibia and the femur. Their main function is to prevent anteroposterior displacement of the two bones upon one another. In full extension both cruciate ligaments are tight, and they also impart side-to-side stability to the knee. The ligaments are named in accord with their tibial attachments. The **anterior cruciate ligament** is attached to the *anterior* part of the intercondylar eminence (Fig. 17–6) and passes backward into the intercondylar notch to attach far posteriorly to the lateral condyle of the femur. The **posterior cruciate ligament** is attached to the *posterior* part of the intercondylar eminence (Fig. 17–6) and passes forward in the intercondylar notch to attach to the medial condyle of the femur.

The Menisci. These are two fibrocartilaginous, semilunar-shaped wedges which partially divide the joint cavity and deepen the shallow articular facets of the tibia (Fig. 17–7). Their concave inner margin is very much thinner than their convex peripheral rim which fuses with the capsule (see Fig. 8–11A). The upper and lower surfaces of the menisci are in contact with the articular cartilage of the femoral and tibial condyles respectively, and both surfaces are moistened by synovial fluid. Both menisci are anchored via their anterior and posterior horns to the intercondylar eminence. The lateral meniscus also gains attachment posteriorly to the medial condyle of the femur via the **meniscofemoral ligaments,** and therefore its movements are guided by the movements of the femur. Its mobility is enhanced by the **popliteus muscle** which gives a muscle slip to the cartilage as it passes out of the joint (Fig. 17–7). The muscle can pull the mensicus backward over the smooth edge of the lateral tibial condyle, which is covered with articular cartilage. The medial meniscus is more fixed and is more widely open than the lateral meniscus. The tibial collateral ligament attached to it at the joint line is partly responsible for its restricted mobility (Fig. 17–7).

The menisci are penetrated by nerves derived from the capsular plexus but they are avascular except for their most peripheral zone which is fused with the capsule. When the menisci are torn there is pain but no intraarticular hemorrhage, and because of the avascularity, they do not heal. A torn meniscus has to be resected and as a rule it regenerates as an ingrowth from the capsular connective tissue.

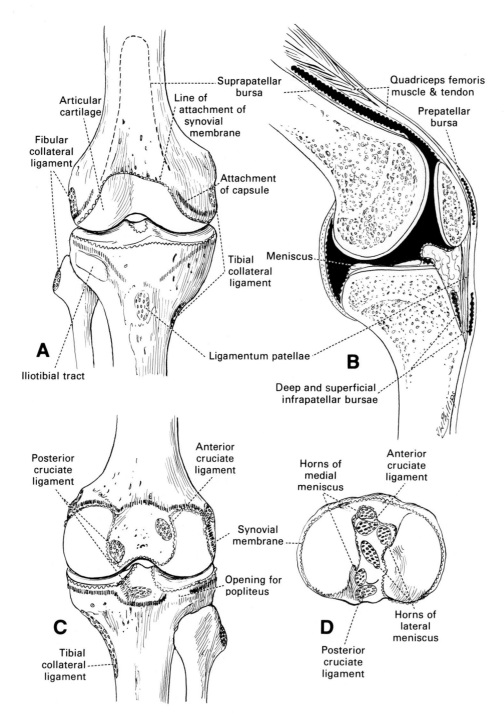

FIG. 17–6. Attachments of the synovial membrane, capsule, and ligaments to the femur and tibia seen anteriorly **(A)**, posteriorly **(C)**, and superiorly **(D)**. In **B**, a sagittal section slightly to one side of the joint midline shows the extent of the synovial cavity and some of the bursae around the knee.

Synovial Membrane and Bursae. The attachment of the synovial membrane follows closely the articular margins (Fig. 17-6). Synovium lines the capsule and covers all intraarticular structures except the mensici. The cruciate ligaments, the popliteus muscle, and a large fat pad behind the ligamentum patellae are therefore intracapsular but extrasynovial. As the membrane is draped over the fat it is raised up into an **infrapatellar fold** presenting a ridge over which the two limbs of the U-shaped synovial cavity communicate with each other. The extrasynovial space between the limbs of the U is occupied by the cruciate ligaments in the intercondylar notch. At the anterior conjoined portion of the cavity the synovial membrane sweeps upward from its femoral attachment to cover the anterior surface of the femur, then a hand's breadth above the patella it reflects forward onto the quadriceps tendon and attaches to the superior margin of the patella (Fig. 17-6). The large cul-de-sac created in this fashion is the **suprapatellar bursa** or **pouch** (Fig. 17-8). Posteriorly, a much smaller extension of the synovial cavity is interposed in the form of a bursa between the popliteus muscle and the tibia as that muscle exits from the joint.

There are numerous other bursae around the knee which normally do not communicate with the joint, although quite often some of them may do so. The bursae are clinically important in the differential diagnosis of swellings around the knee. The most important of these bursae are associated with the patella and the patellar ligament. The **prepatellar bursa** lies between the skin and the patella. The **superficial** and **deep infrapatellar bursae** lie superficial and deep to the ligamentum patellae, respectively. Posteriorly there are bursae associated with muscle attachments around the knee (semimembranous, medial, and lateral heads of the gastrocnemius). There is a bursa around the fibular collateral ligament separating it from the biceps tendon and the joint capsule. A bursa lines also the pocket between the free anterior part of the tibial collateral ligament and the capsule. Lower

FIG. 17-7. Dissections to show the interior of the knee (From the Hunterian Museum, Royal College of Surgeons, London) (**A**) Anterior view. (**C**) Superior aspect of the tibia. (**B** and **D**) Posterior views. Note the relative positions of all ligaments and the popliteus muscle with its attachment to the lateral meniscus. The arcuate ligament marks the limit of the joint capsule over the muscle. (Last RJ: Anatomy, 5th ed. London, Churchhill, 1976)

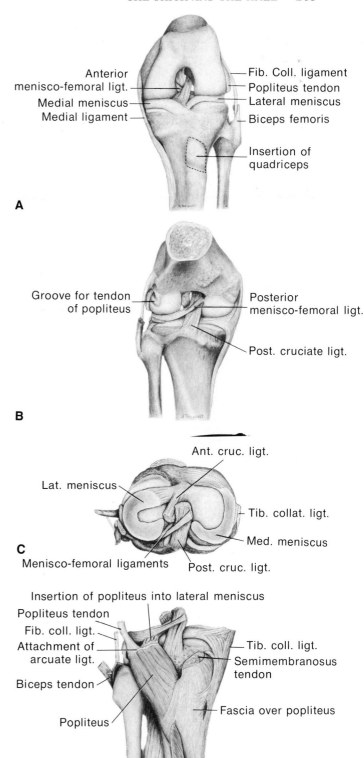

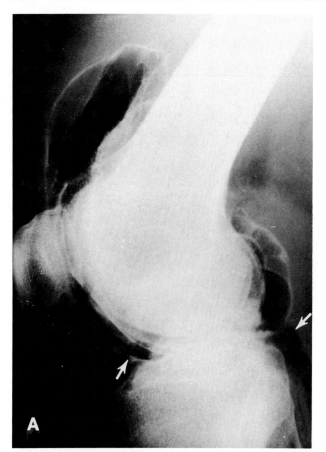
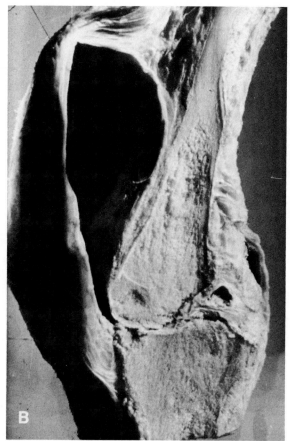

FIG. 17–8. (A) Pneumoarthrogram of the normal knee. Introduction of a small amount of contrast medium which sticks to the surface of the synovium was followed by injection of about 25 cc of air. In this lateral x-ray the extent of the synovial cavity is revealed. Note the spacious suprapatellar bursa and the posterior extent of the two limbs of the U-shaped cavity, the profiles of which overlap in this projection. Part of the infrapatellar fold is visible **(anterior arrow).** The popliteus bursa is filled with air and is revealed as a radiolucency **(posterior arrow). (B)** A specimen from the Hunterian Museum (Royal College of Surgeons, London) showing in a sagittal section (cut to one side of the patella) a distended suprapatellar bursa. The knee shows degenerative changes with some degree of ankylosis.

down a complicated bursa intervenes between the tendons of insertion of the semitendinosus, sartorius, and gracilis (bursa anserina).

Effusions into the Knee

In the normal extended knee, the patella is in contact with the femur and depressions are visible on either side of the patella. A large effusion in the joint obliterates these depressions and elevates the patella. This elevation can be confirmed by ballottement of the patella against the femoral condyles (Fig. 17–9). In moderate effusions the patella may not be elevated. To elevate the patella, fluid has to

be displaced from the suprapatellar pouch and the side of the joint cavity by compression before ballottement (Fig. 17–10). This maneuver will not elevate the patella in small effusions. To demonstrate a small effusion, the fluid must be milked into the depression on one side of the patella. Then such an effusion may be demonstrated by transmission of the fluid or a fluid impulse by percussion from one side of the patella to the other.

Blood and Nerve Supply

An arterial anastomosis is formed around the knee which is fed chiefly by genicular branches of the

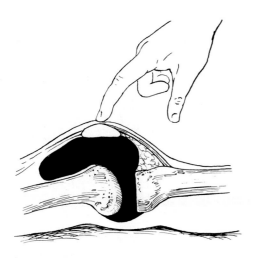

FIG. 17–9. Ballottement of the patella in testing for the presence of a large effusion into the joint.

popliteal artery. The paired superior and inferior **genicular arteries** skirt the femoral and tibial condyles and supply the bone as well as the joint. Their anastomosis is reinforced by descending and ascending genicular branches derived from the femoral and tibial arteries, respectively. An unpaired middle genicular branch of the popliteal artery supplies mainly the contents of the intercondylar notch.

The knee joint is supplied by several nerves and some of these also innervate the hip joint. This explains why pain is so readily referred from a diseased hip to the knee. The general rule is that the nerves that supply the prime movers also innervate the joint. Accordingly, the femoral nerve supplies the knee via its branches to the vasti and via the saphenous nerve; one or more large branches are contributed to the knee by the tibial nerve, the chief nerve of the flexors. In addition, both the obturator and peroneal nerves send branches to the knee joint.

Movements

In full flexion the rounded articular surface on the posterior aspect of the femoral condyles is in contact with the tibial plateau and the menisci. In this position the articular surfaces are maximally incongruent and permit a wide range of accessory movements as well as active rotation of the tibia. As the tibia is extended more and more anterior parts of the femoral articular surfaces come in contact with the tibia and the menisci. Because the curvature of the two femoral condyles is neither equal nor circular, the resultant movement is a composite of the tibia's sliding and rolling (see Fig. 5–11) on the femoral condyles in a forward direction. This takes place when the knee is extended with the foot off the ground. During weight bearing the tibia is stabilized and the femur rolls on it in a forward direction. Concomitant with the forward roll, the femur has to slide backward on the tibia in order to maintain contact and achieve increasing congruence between the articular surfaces.

Maximum stability of the knee is attained in full extension because close packing of the joint is obtained in this position (p. 86). The chief requirement of close pack is maximal congruence of the articular surfaces. Because the tibial articular facet does not extend as far forward on the lateral as on the medial femoral condyle (Fig. 17–5), congruence is attained sooner between the lateral condyles than between the medial condyles. When the lateral condyles are close-packed, the tibia and femur are in a straight line and the anterior edge of the lateral meniscus has reached the groove on the femoral condyle which separates its tibial and

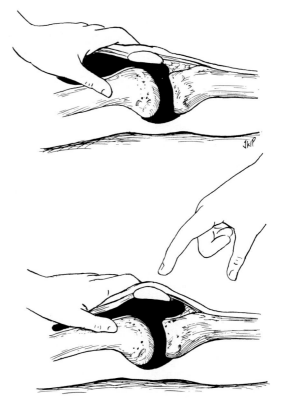

FIG. 17-10. When there is a moderate effusion, fluid from the suprapatellar bursa has to be displaced before ballottement of the patella can be performed.

patellar facets. This is not the case on the medial side. In order to bring the edge of the medial meniscus to the anterior limit of the tibial articular surface of the femoral condyle, either the tibia or the femur has to *rotate*. If the femur is stabilized the tibia will spin and slide in a lateral direction, or if the tibia is stabilized, the femur will spin and slide medially. This element of rotation during the final phase of knee extension is essential for close-packing or *locking* the knee. In this position no accessory movements are permitted nor is there any possibility for active rotation of the tibia. The capsule and all ligaments of the joint are maximally taut and the knee is converted into a solid pillar.

The rotation associated with extension is *conjunct rotation*, the inevitable outcome of extension determined by the shape of the articular surfaces. No rotator muscles are called into action to effect the required tibial or femoral spin. The conjunct rotation is produced by the knee extensors which are incapable of rotating the femur or the tibia actively and independent of extension.

Before flexion can begin the knee has to be *unlocked* by reversing the conjunct rotation of extension. For this, a specific force is required which is furnished by the popliteus muscle. The popliteus can medially rotate the tibia or laterally rotate the femur, depending on which bone is stabilized. This rotation restores the joint into loose pack, and flexion or active rotation may proceed.

The menisci play a passive but important role in movements of the knee. The flexion-extension component of movement takes place mainly between the femoral condyles and the menisci; the latter adapting their shape to the curvature of the advancing femoral condyles. The rotation component of the movement occurs chiefly between the menisci and the tibia, the menisci moving with the femur.

Muscles

The bulk of the thigh muscles consists of the prime movers of the knee (Fig. 17–1) which in addition to producing knee flexion and extension are important in stabilizing the joint when it is in loose pack. A number of thigh muscles capable of exerting force across the knee can also move the hip (rectus femoris, hamstrings, sartorius, gracilis, gluteus maximus, and tensor fasciae latae via the iliotibial tract). These muscles evidently play a role in coordinating movement between the two joints and via

postural reflexes recruit appropriate muscles for stabilizing the joints and balancing the trunk at the hip and knee.

Extensors. The **quadriceps** is the extensor of the knee. Three of its four heads, the **lateral, medial,** and **intermediate** vasti (Figs. 17–1, 17–11) originate from the anterior aspect of much of the shaft of the femur. The **rectus femoris,** the fourth head, arises from the iliac bone and consequently also flexes the hip. Acting in unison via the quadriceps tendon, the patella, and ligamentum patellae, the four heads extend and stabilize the knee. The muscle is tonically contracted when full extension of the knee is maintained with the foot off the ground. But if the fully extended knee supports the body weight, the quadriceps is completely relaxed. However, flexion of the weight bearing knee reflexly recruits the quadriceps for stabilizing the joint. Quadriceps contraction is readily palpable not only during rising from a seated position (knee extension) but also during the reverse act which is accompanied by progressive knee flexion.

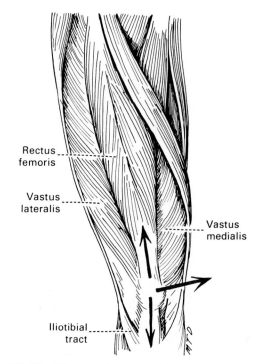

FIG. 17–11. The quadriceps. The rectus femoris conceals the vastus intermedius. The patella is stabilized by muscle balance. Note the insertion of some fleshy fibers of the vastus medialis into the medial side of the patella.

The quadriceps is best demonstrated by opposing knee extension with the patient supine or seated on the edge of the examination table. The strength of the muscle can be built up by lifting weights with the foot. An athlete can lift one third of his body weight through 90°.

The extensor muscle mass is innervated by branches of the femoral nerve (Fig. 17–2). The segments involved are L2, L3, and L4 with predominance of L4. The knee jerk (see Chap. 12) tests the integrity of these segments; chiefly that of L4.

Flexors. The chief flexors of the knee are the semimembranosus, semitendinosus, and biceps femoris, collectively known as the hamstrings. All these muscles arise from the ischial tuberosity (Fig. 17–12). Their extensor action on the hip has already been considered (see Chap. 16). It depends on other muscles whether the hip or the knee or both joints will be moved by hamstring contraction. The **semimembranosus** inserts posteromedially into the condyle of the tibia and into the knee joint capsule; the **semitendinosus** passes beyond the medial condyle and attaches a hand's breadth below the joint line together with the gracilis and sartorius. The latter two muscles are not counted among the hamstrings, but can assist in knee flexion. The ischial portion of the **biceps femoris** is known as its *long head*, and it is joined by the *short head* which originates from the linea aspera. The biceps inserts into the head of the fibula, its tendon splitting around the fibular collateral ligament.

The tendons of the hamstrings were identified among the anatomic landmarks around the knee. Their strength can be tested by opposing knee flexion, best performed with the patient lying prone. The hamstrings are supplied by the tibial component of the sciatic nerve (Fig. 18–11), but the short head of the biceps is innervated by the common peroneal nerve. The chief segmental supply of the knee flexors is from L5 and S1.

Muscles of the leg which attach to the femoral condyles assist in knee flexion. These include the gastrocnemius, popliteus, and plantaris. They also are innervated by the tibial nerve.

Rotators. In the loose-packed position of the knee the tibia can be rotated medially and laterally. With the knee locked, the rotation occurs at the hip. Medial rotation of the tibia or the femur is produced by the semimembranosus, semitendinosus, sartorius, and gracilis, while the biceps femoris and popliteus are lateral rotators.

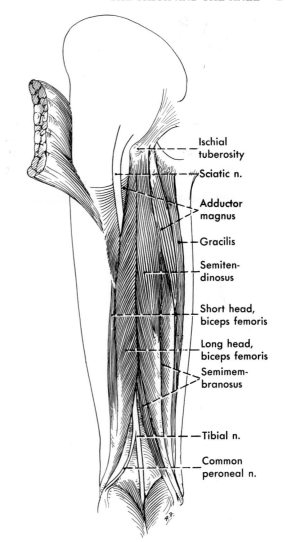

FIG. 17–12. Muscles of the posterior compartment of the thigh. The hamstrings flex the knee and extend the hip. (Hollinshead WH: Anatomy for Surgeons, vol. 3, 2nd ed. New York, Harper & Row 1969)

Stability of the Knee Joint

Joint stability is crucial for the function of the knee. Bony factors of stability in this joint are negligible. Consequently, the integrity of ligaments and muscles is indispensable.

In relaxed standing the force of gravity maintains the knee in extension (see Fig. 19–2). In this position the joint is dependent on its ligaments for stability. The reinforced posterior part of the capsule and the anterior cruciate ligament are the chief factors in checking hyperextension, but the tension in all ligaments is increased in this extended position. The clinical evaluation of ligamentous integrity is described later in this chapter.

As soon as the weight-bearing knee is flexed, muscle is called into action to stabilize the joint. Even a few degrees of flexion are accompanied by contraction of the quadriceps. A powerful quadriceps can maintain stability in the knee despite considerable laxity of ligaments. Wasting or weakness of this muscle results in instability of the knee, described by the patient as a feeling of insecurity or the knee giving way.

Stabilization of the patella is a crucial factor in the quadriceps mechanism. Since the femoral shaft articulates with the tibia at an angle, the pull of the quadriceps tends to displace the patella laterally. Lateral displacement of the patella is prevented by 1) the prominent trochlea of the lateral femoral condyle (Fig. 17–5) and 2) the attachment of the vastus medialis into the medial border of the patella (Fig. 17–11).

In the flexed position of the weight bearing knee the femoral condyles have a tendency to slip forward on the tibial plateau (Fig. 8–8D). The popliteus together with the anterior cruciate ligament oppose this tendency. Especially important is the **iliotibial tract** which is attached to the anterior surface of the lateral tibial condyle (Fig. 17–6) and transmits force to the knee from the gluteus maximus and tensor fasciae latae. This stout tendonlike band becomes prominent when weight is borne on the flexed knee (Fig. 17–13). The pelvis with the femur is balanced on the sloping tibial plateau by the gluteus maximus and tensor fasciae latae via the iliotibial tract.

Injuries to the Knee

Injuries of the knee are common. The most frequently damaged structures are ligaments and menisci. The ligaments are torn when force from an external source is applied to the knee, while injury of the menisci usually results from forces generated within the individual.

Major violence is needed to completely rupture a ligament, and most often only partial tearing of the fibers occurs. The direction of the force applied to the knee determines which ligament bears the brunt of the impact.

The **tibial collateral ligament** is most frequently injured by a force applied to the outer side of the joint while the foot is weight bearing. If the knee is

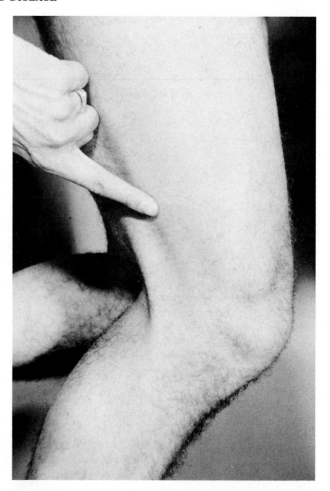

FIG. 17-13. The iliotibial tract, seen anterior to the biceps tendon, is an important structure in stabilizing the flexed knee when it is supporting the body weight.

extended in such an injury, the anterior cruciate ligament is also tightened, and if sufficient force is imparted it may also rupture. In a tibial ligament rupture, the medial meniscus may lose its ligamentous attachment and become displaced into the joint cavity. The rupture of tibial collateral and anterior cruciate ligaments with detachment of the medial meniscus is not uncommon. Isolated injury may also occur in the **anterior** or the **posterior cruciate ligament** from hyperextension force when the foot is fixed to the ground. In these injuries the posterior capsule is also torn. In children and adolescents, avulsion of a piece of bone on the anterior part of the intercondylar eminence to which the cruciate ligament is attached may occur rather than the ligament rupture. In the case of a complete rupture, surgical repair of the torn ligament is indicated because the knee relies on its ligaments for stability. Partial tears should be treated by immobilization in a plaster cast for 4 to 8 weeks.

Meniscus injuries can be diagnosed in the majority of cases by the history alone, provided an accurate account of the mechanism of the injury can be given by the patient.

During extension, tension is first built up in the anterior cruciate ligament, which then guides the rotation of the femur. When movement occurs suddenly while the limb is weight bearing, the menisci may get caught between the femoral and tibial condyles, and a meniscal tear results. The lateral meniscus, due to its controlled mobility, enjoys a much greater degree of protection then the medial meniscus, and it is seldom damaged. The medial meniscus is most commonly torn when it is caught between the condyles of the femur and tibia. This usually occurs when the weight bearing limb is flexed at the knee with the tibia fixed in lateral rotation.

At the time of injury the subject may be aware of something tearing or giving in the joint, but pain, frequently accompanied by a nauseous sensation, is the prominent clinical feature. Swelling due to an effusion, often blood-tinged, follows rapidly. Full extension of the knee may be prevented by displacement of the torn meniscus between the articular surfaces. The joint is then said to be locked, a term not to be confused with that applied to describe the close-packed position of the normal knee.

Although there are a number of physical signs produced by different types of tears, the most useful physical sign of a torn meniscus in the acute state is accurately localized joint line tenderness. The meniscus is palpable over most of its margin. Once the firm diagnosis of a torn meniscus is made, the meniscus should be removed. The presence of a torn meniscus will eventually lead to degenerative joint disease because of the incongruity it produces.

CLINICAL EVALUATION

In addition to the high rate of mechanical injury, the knee is prone to almost every type of inflammatory as well as degenerative joint disease. Furthermore, the metaphyseal regions of the femur and tibia at the knee are common sites of osteomyelitis and neoplasia. The clinical features of these diseases are discussed with their pathology in the appropriate chapters. This section deals with the regional symptoms and signs of disease and mechanical injury in the knee, and its aim is to present a systematic approach to evaluating all anatomic structures in the knee region. In clinical practice the selection and sequence of diagnostic maneuvers must be guided, of course, by the history. For example, testing of the cruciate and collateral ligaments in an acutely inflamed, painful knee would not only be uninformative, but is emphatically contraindicated. The history of the complaints is important in the diagnosis of all types of disease in the knee, but is of particular significance in cases of injury. The mechanism of injury gives the most important clue to the structures damaged.

Symptoms

Complaints about the knee include pain, instability (giving way), clicking, restricted movement or locking of the joint, swelling, deformity, and stiffness.

In nontraumatic cases the onset and character of the **pain** must be pursued as outlined in Chapter 7. The history may suggest the diagnosis and will indicate whether the cause is likely to be in bone or in the joint tissues. Local causes of knee pain can almost always be diagnosed by physical examination. Pain may be referred to the normal knee from compressed lumbar spinal nerves or, more commonly, from a diseased hip. It is well to remember that knee movement may exaggerate the pain in both instances because it may stretch the compressed nerve roots or because of the hip movement associated with most habitual movements of the knee.

In adolescence and young adulthood local causes of joint pain peculiar to the knee are *osteochondritis dissecans* and *chondromalacia of the patella*, both of unknown etiology. In the former, necrosis of a patch of articular cartilage and subchondral bone on the femoral condyle give rise to pain and discomfort felt usually after exercise. The necrotic segment eventually separates, becoming a loose body in the joint. In chondromalacia, a deep seated pain in the knee (often worse during long periods of sitting with knees bent) is caused by roughening, fibrillation, and degeneration on the patello-femoral cartilage surfaces.

Weakness and wasting of the quadriceps predisposes to a feeling of insecurity or to an actual **giving way** of the knee. This complaint is usually a sequela of a knee injury treated with prolonged immobilization. With a weak quadriceps the knee will feel insecure even if all the ligaments have healed adequately. There may be a congenital or acquired posttraumatic tendency for the patella to subluxate or dislocate. Many patients are only aware of an insecurity in the knee and are vague about the actual cause. When weight bearing on the flexed knee, the patient may be caught off guard, and the patella dislocates laterally, requiring manual replacement. Pain and joint effusion are associated with these incidents.

Lax ligaments and a weak quadriceps predispose to **clicking** of the knee but clicks occur commonly in many normal joints and there is no pain associated with them. The sounds are generated in the patellofemoral joint or by the movement of the menisci. Painful grating or clicking sounds indicate degenerative joint disease or a damaged meniscus.

All painful inflammatory joint lesions and tense effusions restrict movement, but **locking** of the joint in some degree of flexion occurs with meniscal tears and loose bodies. In meniscal tears extension is restricted and the knee can usually be flexed from the locked position. Movement is restricted in all directions when a loose body is caught between the condyles. Pain and effusion due to synovial irritation are usually present in both instances.

The complaint of **stiffness** must be defined in association with pain in various types of arthritis. Stiffness will also develop after periods of immobilization following an injury. With programmed exercise such stiffness will wear off unless there is excessive scarring of the tissues in and around the knee.

Physical Examination

For proper evaluation, both thighs, knees, and legs must be bare; the patient should be wearing shorts or a pelvic slip.

Inspection. In cases of trauma gross deformity around the knee will suggest major ligamentous or bony injury. In routine physical examination the patient should be inspected standing in the anatomic position and the following should be noted:

1. Alignment of the femur, tibia, and patella. Mild degrees of knock-knee (genu valgum) and bowlegs (genu varum) are common in children and normal growth usually corrects the deformities unless they are excessive. In such cases congenital causes or rarefying diseases of bone (e.g., rickets) must be evaluated. These deformities may be the outcome of epiphyseal plate injuries, malunion of fractures around the knee, and abnormal posture in the feet and at the hips. Hyperextension deformity (genu recurvatum) results from muscle imbalance, growth abnormalities, or unhealed ligamentous injuries. All these deformities distort the mechanics of the joint, displace the normal relation of the line of gravitational force in relation to the knee, and predispose to degenerative joint disease. The alignment of the patella with the foot should be noted and for all deformities the two sides should be compared.

2. The level of the two patellae and of the popliteal skin creases should be compared in relaxed standing. It should be noted whether or not both knees are straight when the soles of the feet contact the ground.

3. Contour of the soft tissues in the thigh and around the knee. Attention should be paid to symmetry in the bulk of the quadriceps, especially the patellar fibers of the vastus medialis. The muscle should be compared relaxed and in isometric contraction, keeping the knees extended. Quadriceps atrophy is a cardinal sign of a diseased knee. The normal hollows at the sides of the patella and ligamentum patellae should be noted, as should abnormal swellings. The latter are better scrutinized with the patient seated or lying on the examination table.

4. Redness, discoloration, sinuses, and scars.

5. The knees should be inspected with the patient walking, paying attention to the phases of the gait cycle as described in Chapter 19.

Palpation. 1. Skin temperature and texture should be felt gently over a painful and swollen joint.

2. Unless there are contraindications, all accessible anatomic structures should be palpated, noting tenderness, swelling, or breach in continuity. The section on Anatomic Landmarks has described a sequence for palpation and this should be followed in a physical examination. The following are additional useful points in diagnosing the cause of pain.

a. Both patellar and femoral surfaces of the patellofemoral joint may be examined if the patella is manually displaced laterally or medially, while the quadriceps is kept relaxed. In chondromalacia of the patella and in osteochondritis dissecans the diseased surfaces may be demonstrated.

b. The tibial tuberosity may be tender, swollen, and hypertrophied in children due to trauma and inflammation of its epiphyseal cartilage. This

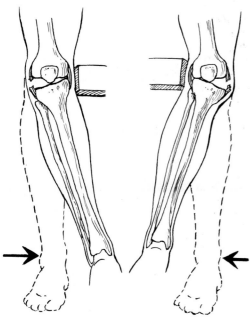

FIG. 17-14. Method of testing the collateral ligaments of the knee.

must be distinguished from a tender metaphysis, which is suggestive of osteomyelitis.

c. The edges of the menisci should be palpated along the joint line starting anteriorly on either side of the patellar ligament. Tenderness is suggestive of meniscal tear.

d. Such tenderness must be distinguished from that due to partial tear in the collateral ligaments. The anterior edge of the tibial collateral ligament is not discernible but it does not extend further forward than the vertical line drawn from the adductor tubercle. The fibular collateral ligament is lax in the flexed knee but adduction of the tibia in this position will tighten it. Sufficient adduction (varus) force will be applied to the knee by resting the flexed leg on the opposite knee. The ligament can then be felt as a tense cord above the head of the fibula.

3. Roughness of the articular surfaces should be tested by eliciting crepitus. This may be done by passively moving the patella on the femur or the tibia on the femur, in the latter instance keeping one hand cupped over the patella. A grating sensation, often audible, may be due to degenerative joint disease, chondromalacia, or osteochondritis dissecans. Loose bodies may also produce crepitus.

4. The tissues responsible for diffuse swelling should be determined by palpation. Malignant primary bone tumors around the knee may present as a hot, diffuse tender swelling, as may osteomyelitis of the tibia and femur when inflammation has spread to the superficial tissues. The diagnosis of joint effusions has already been discussed. The thickness of the synovial membrane should be assessed by feeling the tissues over the relaxed knee above and below the patella. Hypertrophied synovium in a rheumatoid joint has a characteristic, thickened doughy texture.

5. The identity of localized swellings may be determined by palpation. Exostoses are common around the knee (see Chap. 29). They are hard and continuous with bone. Distended bursae are cystic and fluctuation is demonstrable in them. They may communicate with the joint synovial cavity. Their anatomic location is important in differential diagnosis of swellings around the knee (p. 282).

6. The contents of the popliteal fossa should be palpated.

Range of Movements and Muscle Strength. Flexion of the knee is normally limited by contact between the calf and the thigh. In full extension, the angle between the tibia and femur is slightly greater than 180° in women, and slightly less than 180° in men. Both active and passive ranges must be tested and the presence of contractures must be evaluated. Testing the strength of the prime movers was described earlier in the chapter.

Joint Stability. Both collateral and both cruciate ligaments must be tested. In assessing ligamentous integrity, the muscles must be relaxed. To test the collateral ligaments the knee must be slightly flexed. This eliminates the stabilizing effect of the cruciate ligaments on the extended knee. The tibial collateral ligament is tested by grasping the patient's ankle with one hand and using the other

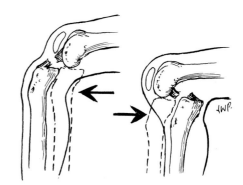

FIG. 17-15. Method of testing the cruciate ligaments of the knee (anterior and posterior drawer sign).

hand as a fulcrum at the knee. Abduction force is applied at the ankle, attempting to produce a valgus deformity of the knee. The lateral collateral ligament is tested by attempting to produce a varus deformity (Fig. 17–14). Complete tear of the ligaments results in separation of the femoral and tibial articular margins. Incomplete tear produces pain confirmed by tenderness over the ligament.

The anterior cruciate ligament is tested by attempting to displace the tibia anteriorly on the femur with the knee flexed to about 90° and the foot stabilized. The proximal end of the tibia is grasped and pulled forward. If the anterior cruciate ligament is torn, a forward displacement of the tibia will occur (drawer sign). Integrity of the posterior cruciate ligament is tested in an identical manner by posterior displacement of the tibia (Fig. 17–15).

SUGGESTED READING

Adams JC: Outline of Orthopedics, 6th ed. Baltimore, Williams & Wilkins, 1968
Chapter 9 deals concisely with the more common diseases and injuries of the knee

Brantigan OC, Voshell AF: The mechanics of the ligaments and menisci of the knee joint. J Bone Joint Surg [B] *23*: 44, 1941
This and the following reference are papers with excellent functional considerations of ligaments of the knee joint.

Brantigan OC, Voshell AF: The tibial collateral ligament: its function, its bursae and its relation to the medial meniscus. J Bone Joint Surg [B] *25*: 121, 1943

Cailliet R: Knee Pain and Disability. Philadelphia, FA Davis 1973
A well-organized, clearly written, handy book which, after dealing with the functional anatomy of the knee, discusses the diagnosis and treatment of painful and disabling conditions that affect the knee.

DePalma AI: Diseases of the Knee. Philadelphia, JB Lippincott, 1954
A well-written, comprehensive book on the knee. The main emphasis is on diagnosis and surgical management of diseases and injuries of the knee but excellent description of functional anatomy is also included.

Hollinshead HW: Anatomy for Surgeons, Vol 3, The Back and Limbs, 2nd ed. New York, Harper & Row, 1969
Chapters 8 and 9 give a well-referenced, complete description of the anatomy described in the present chapter.

Hoppenfeld S: Physical Examination of the Spine and Extremities. New York, Appleton-Century-Crofts, 1976
Chapter 7 presents a well-illustrated, clearly written, step-by-step account of the physical examination of the knee. Identification of all anatomical structures is well presented.

Morrison JB: The mechanics of the knee joint in relation to normal walking. J Biomechanics *3*: 51, 1970
A concise discussion of knee mechanisms.

18
The Leg, Ankle, and Foot

CORNELIUS ROSSE

The leg and foot are built on the same basic plan as the forearm and hand. Although morphologically equivalent structures are readily recognized in the upper and lower limbs, there are important differences in the organization of these structures which reflect the different functional needs in the hand and the foot. The emphasis is on freedom and versatility of movement in the upper limb, whereas in the lower limb it is on weight bearing and propulsion for locomotion. Accordingly, the aim in the treatment of disability affecting the hand and the foot is to preserve and restore the anatomy necessary to meet these different functional needs.

The anatomic description of the leg and foot in this chapter relies extensively on comparisons with the forearm and hand. As explained in Chapter 11, rotation and extension during development position the lower limbs for weight bearing in the erect stance. In contrast to the forearm, the flexor aspect of the leg faces posteriorly and its extensor aspect anteriorly. Likewise, the sole of the foot looks backward, whereas the palm of the hand looks forward. Furthermore, the foot assumes a position at right angles to the leg. Therefore, *flexion of the foot is qualified as plantar flexion and extension is often referred to as dorsiflexion.* In the anatomic position the first or preaxial digit of the hand (thumb) is on the lateral margin, while the preaxial digit of the foot (hallux or big toe) is on the medial margin of the limb.

SKELETON AND BONY LANDMARKS

The skeleton of the leg consists of two parallel bones, the tibia and fibula, which correspond to the radius and ulna, respectively. Unlike the arrangement at the elbow and wrist, the fibula is excluded from the knee joint but forms an integral part of the mortiselike, concave articular surface at the ankle (Fig. 18–1).

The **tibia** is subcutaneous anteriorly. Its two condyles have been described and examined in Chapter 17. The anteromedial surface is palpable under the skin (Fig. 18–9) from the tibial tuberosity to the **medial malleolus.** Of the **fibula,** only its upper and lower thirds are directly palpable. The latter terminates as the **lateral malleolus.** The tip of the lateral malleolus is at a lower level than the medial malleolus (Fig. 18–1).

The seven bones of the **tarsus** are not arranged as clearly into proximal and distal rows as the carpal bones. Only one of them, the **talus,** articulates with the tibia and fibula (Figs. 18–1, 18–5). Because of the malleoli, the talus is hardly accessible to palpation. Its large trochlear surface is accommodated in the tibiofibular mortise; its anterior round head fits into the concavity of the navicular; and its inferior surface rests on the calcaneus (Fig. 18–2). The talar neck is situated between the head and the trochlea and can be palpated just anterior to the fibular malleolus, especially when the foot is plantar flexed and inverted. It does not yield to pressure, demonstrating a close fit between the malleoli.

The bulk of the **calcaneus** represents the backward projecting heel, the surfaces of which can be explored by palpation. Two other points are useful landmarks on the calcaneus: 1) Just inferior to the talar neck the upper surface of the calcaneus is palpable through the soft tissues of the dorsum of the foot. The bony depression filled by the soft tissues is the **sinus tarsi** which is the lateral aperture of a bony tunnel, known as the **tarsal canal.** The tarsal canal separates the nonarticular portions of the talus and calcaneus. Just in front of

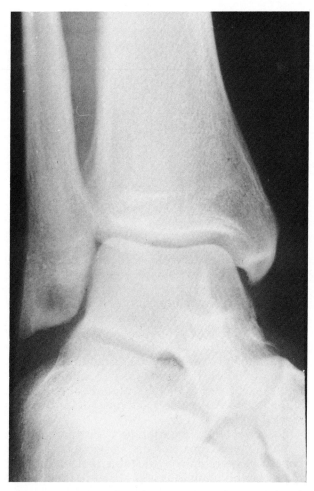

FIG. 18-1. The ankle joint. The x-ray was taken with the axis of the ankle joint parallel to the film to show the configuration of the articular surfaces. (Courtesy of Dr. Rosalind H. Troupin)

the sinus tarsi, the calcaneus articulates with the cuboid. 2) A finger breadth below the tip of the medial malleolus, the **sustentaculum tali** can be identified as a buttress projecting medially from the calcaneus. As its name implies, it supports the talus.

The **navicular** is identifiable by its tubercle, which is 3.5 cm. anterior to the medial malleolus, on level with the sustentaculum. In the interval between the sustentaculum tali and the navicular is the **spring ligament** and the talus is in contact with all these structures.

The position of the talus is noteworthy. It is surrounded by the joints which are the chief determinants of foot movements. In addition to the ankle or talocrural joint, these are the subtalar joint directly below and the talocalcaneonavicular joint in front and anteroinferiorly.

The distal row of tarsal bones consists of three cuneiforms and the cuboid. The **cuneiforms** are in line with the three medial rays of the foot and articulate with the corresponding metatarsals as well as with the navicular. In the living foot they cannot be discerned separately. The **cuboid** is in line with the lateral two metatarsals. Its relationship to the calcaneus has been noted. The cuboid is palpable immediately proximal to the prominent tuberosity of the fifth metatarsal which overlaps the cuboid as it projects backward from its base (Fig. 18–2B).

The arrangement of the metatarsals and phalanges is similar to that of the corresponding segments of the hand skeleton. The chief difference is that the metatarsal bone of the big toe is not independent of its fellows and enjoys no special privilege for independent movement. Through the thickness of the foot, all metatarsals and phalanges can be grasped between finger and thumb. In the sole of the foot the head of the first metatarsal rests on and articulates with two sesamoid bones.

Segments of the Foot Skeleton

It is customary and expedient to refer to segments of the foot rather than individual bones when describing movements and deformities. The segments are the forefoot, midfoot, and hindfoot. These terms, omitted from the anatomic nomenclature, are largely self-explanatory and are used rather loosely. The **hindfoot** consists of the talus and calcaneus, while the **forefoot** is made up of the metatarsals and phalanges. The navicular, cuboid, and cuneiforms comprise the **midfoot**. During the stance phase of ambulation (see Chap. 19), body weight is transferred from the hindfoot to the forefoot. In this process the midfoot and the forefoot become converted into a rigid lever as the propulsive force is imparted to the ground at push-off. The greatest amount of intrinsic foot movement takes place between the hindfoot and midfoot. The joints involved are the talonavicular and calcaneocuboid joints, which together are spoken of as the **transverse tarsal** or **midtarsal joint.**

JOINTS

Before describing individual joints, it is helpful to clarify the various movements possible in the foot. For understanding the dynamic mechanisms of the

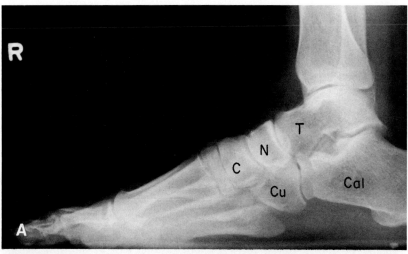

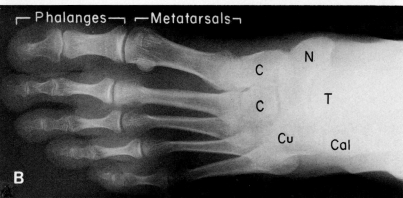

FIG. 18-2. X-rays of the foot. **(A)** Lateral view, weight bearing. **(B)** Superior view, weight bearing. T = talus; Cal = calcaneus; N = navicular; Cu = cuboid; C = cuneiform. Because of overlapping contours only two of the three cuneiforms are labeled. Note the two sesamoid bones at the head of the first metatarsal. (Courtesy of Dr. Rosalind H. Troupin)

foot, not only the joints but the ligaments and intrinsic and extrinsic muscles have to be taken into consideration. The behavior of the foot during ambulation will therefore be discussed later in the chapter.

Movements of the Foot

In the neutral or anatomic position the foot makes a 90° angle with the tibia. **Plantar flexion** increases and **dorsiflexion** decreases this angle. The motions occur principally at the ankle joint, and the axis passes through the tips of the two malleoli. Due to the different level of these bony points, the axis slopes backward, downward, and laterally. Because of this deviation from the horizontal, the foot will deviate from the sagittal plane during plantar flexion and dorsiflexion. Plantar flexion is associated with some **toeing in** and dorsiflexion with **toeing out.** Toeing in and out may be produced also by tibial rotation or fixed tibial tor-

sion, but not by abduction-adduction at the ankle. The talocrural joint permits only flexion and extension.

Inversion and **eversion** are movements which turn the sole of the foot inward and outward, respectively. This side-to-side rotation of the foot takes place at the subtalar and transverse tarsal joints around a roughly anteroposterior axis which deviates somewhat from the sagittal plane. Both the heel and the forefoot partake in these movements. During inversion and eversion the heel deviates medially and laterally from its neutral position in which the calcaneus is vertically aligned with the midline of the tibia (Fig. 18–3). The deviation of the forefoot is gauged by the line of the second metatarsal in relation to the tibia (Fig. 18–4).

Since the axis of inversion and eversion is not strictly in the sagittal plane, in addition to the rotation movement, the forefoot is **adducted** during inversion and **abducted** during eversion (Fig.

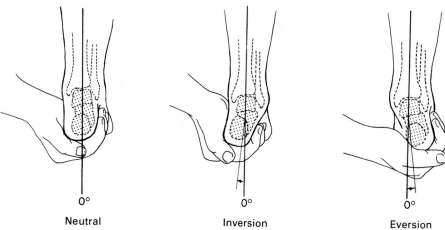

FIG. 18–3. Inversion and eversion of the heel. In the neutral position the vertical axis of the heel is aligned with the longitudinal axis of the tibia. (Joint Motion, Method of Measuring and Recording. Chicago, American Academy of Orthopedic Surgeons, 1965)

18–4). These movements occur chiefly at the transverse tarsal joint. Active abduction or adduction of the forefoot is not possible independent of inversion and eversion. What appear to be abduction and adduction of the whole foot, especially when the heel is used as a fulcrum, are due to tibial or femoral rotation.

Yet another pair of movements is associated in the foot with inversion and eversion. These movements are **supination** and **pronation.** In contrast to the radioulnar movements designated by the same terms in the forearm, supination and pronation of the foot are the result of displacement of the metatarsals in relation to one another. The movements involve the transverse tarsal joint and joints distal to it. The foot cannot be actively pronated and supinated independent of inversion and eversion. In the neutral position, the heads of the metatarsals are in the same horizontal plane (in contact with the ground). Supination (associated with inversion) elevates the head of the first metatarsal and depresses the head of the fifth. Pronation (associated with eversion) has the opposite effect.

Although the first time round it is simplest to consider these movements with the foot off the ground, it is more important to understand them in the planted, weight-bearing foot and in the gait cycle. Instead of producing toeing in and toeing out, the obliquity of the ankle axis will impose rotation on the tibia as it travels over the talus in plantar and dorsiflexion with the foot fixed. Standing on a sloping surface with parallel feet, one foot

higher than the other, requires inversion of the lower and eversion of the upper foot. Standing on a wedge placed under the metatarsal heads from the medial side puts the forefoot into supination. Putting the wedge under the metatarsals from the lateral side pronates the foot.

Tibiofibular Joints

The tibiofibular joints differ radically from the radioulnar joints which permit pronation and supination of the head. Movement of any significant degree is prevented between the tibia and the fibula by the **inferior tibiofibular joint.** This is the only syndesmosis in the entire appendicular skeleton. Its function is to fix the distal end of the fibula in a groove on the lateral aspect of the tibia. This fibrous joint is essential for the integrity of the ankle joint. The fibrous tissue which bridges the narrow gap between the two bones for a distance of 3.5 cm is the **crural tibiofibular interosseous ligament.** Its short, strong fibers run from the tibia to the fibula and stop short of the ankle joint, a small distance proximal to its articular margins. The interosseous ligament, distinct from the interosseous membrane and much stronger, is the key structure in preventing separation of the two bones by forces applied to the lateral malleolus via the talus and the calcaneus. The ligament is so strong, that when these forces are excessive (e.g., in an eversion injury) the fibula will break proximal to the ligament rather than the ligament rupture. The tibiofibular syndesmosis is reinforced by thinner and weaker ligaments placed superficially on the front and back of the joint. These are the **anterior** and **posterior tibiofibular ligaments,** which tear more easily.

The interosseous ligament acts as a fulcrum between two lever arms. Minor rotational displacements of the malleolus, the short arm of the lever, are magnified at the proximal end of the fibula. The **superior tibiofibular joint** is a synovial joint, the flat surfaces and thin capsule of which allow for a greater amplitude of movement.

Ankle Joint

Articular Surfaces. The ankle or **talocrural joint** is a hinge joint. The talar articular facet is the **trochlea** which is convex superiorly in an anteroposterior direction (Fig. 18–2A) and becomes relatively flat where it extends down on each side of the talus to articulate with the malleoli (Figs. 18–1, 18–5). The trochlea resembles more closely a tangential slice of a truncated cone than a slice of a cylinder (Fig. 18–6). The apex of the imaginary cone points medially and therefore the tibial malleolar facet of the trochlea is smaller than the fibular facet (Fig. 18–1). Correspondingly, the medial curvature of the trochlea has a smaller radius than its lateral curvature.

The tibiofibular or crural socket into which the trochlea is received is customarily described as a mortise. A cast of this mortise would duplicate all contours of the trochlea. There is better congru-ence between the articular surfaces than in any other joint. A good fit is maintained through the whole range of plantar flexion and dorsiflexion, and in no position is there any lateral play or accessory movement permitted in the mortise. This has been proven to be so, contradicting the widely held opinion that the talus is loose in plantar flexion and tight in dorsiflexion. The distance between the malleoli does not increase when the ankle is dorsiflexed, although a small amount of lateral rotation of the fibular malleolus may be permitted by the obliquity of the tibiofibular interosseous ligament. Rigid surgical fixation of the tibiofibular syndesmosis by screws or other means does not limit the range of dorsiflexion.

The obliquity of the joint axis discussed in the preceding section and the conical shape of the talocrural articular surfaces fully explain the mechanisms of ankle flexion and extension and account also for most of the toeing in and toeing out associated with these movements.

Ligaments. The thin fibrous capsule which surrounds the joint is reinforced on each side by collateral ligaments. The ligaments are attached to the tip of each malleolus, and each has components which span not only the ankle joint but the talocalcaneal joints as well (Fig. 18–5). By virtue of their calcaneal attachments, these bands stabilize both the ankle and talocalcaneal joints and play a role in integrating motion between them.

The medial collateral ligament is known as the

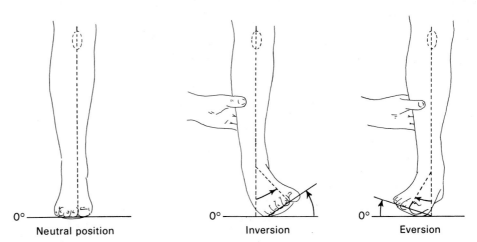

| 0° | 0° | 0° |
| Neutral position | Inversion | Eversion |

FIG. 18–4. Inversion and eversion of the forefoot. In the neutral position the line of the second metatarsal is aligned with the midline of the tibia. Inversion is associated with adduction and eversion with abduction of the forefoot. (Joint Motion, Method of Measuring and Recording. Chicago, American Academy of Orthopedic Surgeons, 1965)

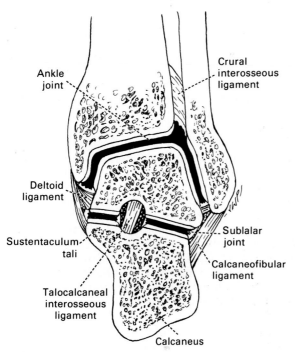

FIG. 18–5. Coronal section through the ankle joint showing the tibiofibular syndesmosis, the ankle joint with its collateral ligaments, and the subtalar joint with the talocalcaneal interosseous ligament.

deltoid ligament because it fans out in delta shape from the margins of the tibial malleolus to attach in continuity from the navicular in front to the calcaneus and talus behind. The ligament is robust and consists of deep and superficial portions (Fig. 18–5). The deep fibers (anterior tibiotalar ligament) attach to the nonarticular medial surface of the talus overhung by the malleolus. The superficial portion is made up of tibionavicular, tibiocalcaneal, and posterior tibiotalar fibers which merge with one another. Some fibers also attach to the spring ligament, filling in the gap between the navicular and the sustentaculum tali.

The **lateral collateral ligament** consists of three discrete bands: the anterior and posterior talofibular ligaments, counterparts of similar fibers on the medial side, and the much longer, cordlike **calcaneofibular ligament** which passes from the tip of the malleolus downward and backward.

The collateral ligaments give side-to-side stability to the ankle. Plantar flexion is limited by the anterior talofibular and tibiotalar ligaments and dorsiflexion by the posterior counterparts. Tibiocalcaneal and calcaneofibular ligaments also

stabilize the talocalcaneal joints. These are the ligaments of the ankle which are prone to rupture in inversion and eversion injuries. In such injuries the malleoli may also fracture. This is particularly true of the medial malleolus which may be evulsed rather than the deltoid ligament rupture. Ligaments of the tibiofibular syndesmosis discussed already, are, of course, crucial for the integrity of the crural socket.

The Subtalar and Transverse Tarsal Joints

Articular Surfaces and Movements. Inversion and eversion movements take place around the talus and involve synchronously the subtalar and transverse tarsal joints. The subtalar joint func-

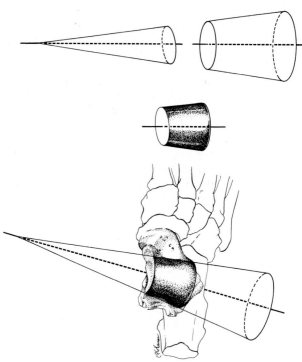

FIG. 18–6. Schematic representation of the trochlea of the talus. The trochlear articular surface resembles a segment of a truncated cone, the apex of which points medially and forward. For this reason the articular surface for the medial malleolus is smaller than that for the lateral malleolus and, for the same reason, medial and lateral curvatures of the trochlea have different radii. Note also that medial and lateral facets of the truncated cone are cut at different angles. The axis of the cone coincides with the axis of the talocrural joint. (Adapted from Inman VT: The Joints of the Ankle. Baltimore, Williams & Wilkins, 1976)

tioning as a link between the talus and the calcaneus permits inversion and eversion of the heel. The transverse tarsal joint functions as a link between the hindfoot and the midfoot and extends the inversion-eversion movement range produced by the subtalar joint. The transverse tarsal joint itself consists of two anatomically separate articulations, the talocalcaneonavicular and the calcaneocuboid joints. Independent movements are not possible in any of these three joints.

The **subtalar joint** is directly below the talocrural joint. The concave talar and convex calcaneal articular facets are reciprocally shaped. Talus and calcaneus move in relation to one another like two members around a mitered hinge (Fig. 18–7), the axis of which inclines backward, downward, and laterally. Rotation of the horizontal member is evident as inversion-eversion, while rotation of the vertical member is evident as tibial rotation. The latter is an important component of movement at the ankle, the mechanisms of which are beyond the scope of the present discussion.

The subtalar joint is a determinative joint of the foot and influences movement at the transverse tarsal joint. The **talocalcaneonavicular** portion of the transverse tarsal joint has ball and socket-shaped surfaces and rotation of the midfoot

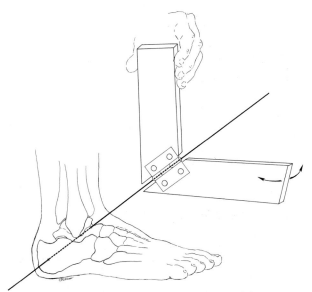

FIG. 18–7. The subtalar joint compared to a mitered hinge. The axis of the joint and the hinge are indicated. Swinging of the horizontal member of the hinge in a medial and lateral direction mimics inversion and eversion of the calcaneus respectively. (Adapted from Inman VT: The Joints of the Ankle. Baltimore, Williams & Wilkins, 1976)

primarily takes place here. The talar head and the inferior surface of its neck represent the ball, while the composite socket is made up of the navicular, the superior surfaces of the spring ligament, and the sustentaculum tali. The functional integration of calcanean movements at the subtalar joint with movements of the midfoot becomes self-evident as soon as it is appreciated that the spring ligament unites the calcaneus (hindfoot) and the navicular (midfoot) into this socket. Movements at the **calcaneocuboid joint,** the lateral half of the transverse tarsal articulation, are an inevitable outcome of calcaneal movements and of the lack of appreciable independent movement within the midfoot. Figure 18–8 explains how the transverse tarsal joint adds a pivotal element to midfoot movements in inversion and eversion.

Eversion of the heel and the associated pronation of the foot render the transverse tarsal joint particularly mobile, permitting passive flexion, extension, abduction, adduction, and rotation between the hindfoot and forefoot. However, inversion of the heel and the associated supination of the forefoot apparently lock the transverse tarsal joint, because all movements between the hindfoot and forefoot now become restricted. In the gait cycle, elevation of the heel off the ground (heel-off) is associated with heel inversion, and the transverse tarsal joint becomes close packed in a like manner, converting a pliable foot into a rigid lever.

Ligaments. The subtalar joint and lateral and medial components of the transverse tarsal joint are enclosed by independent fibrous capsules lined by synovial membrane. In addition to the spring ligament and the tibiocalcaneal and calcaneofibular portions of the collateral ligaments of the ankle, there are a number of other important ligaments associated with these joints. The **talocalcaneal interosseous ligament** occupies the tarsal canal and separates the subtalar from the talocalcaneonavicular joints, reinforcing both. The **cervical ligament** in the sinus tarsi is attached to the neck of the talus and the upper surface of the calcaneus. More anteriorly in the sinus, one limb of the **bifurcate ligament** runs between the calcaneus and the navicular (dorsal calcaneonavicular ligament, of much less consequence than its plantar counterpart, the spring ligament) and the other limb between the calcaneus and cuboid (dorsal calcaneocuboid ligament). The plantar counterpart of the latter (plantar calcaneocuboid ligament) is more important and is known as the **short plantar ligament.**

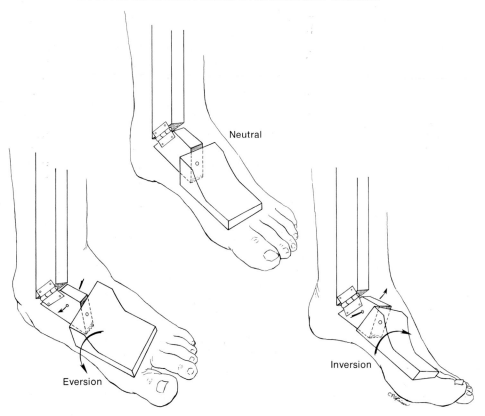

FIG. 18–8. Schematic representation of the movements of the calcaneus and forefoot in inversion and eversion. The horizontal member of the mitered hinge represents the calcaneus which moves as explained in Figure 18–7. The midfoot and forefoot skeleton is represented by a stylized block which is linked to the hindfoot via the transverse tarsal joint. Pivoting of the block on the hindfoot in a medial and lateral direction increases the range of eversion and inversion. In this model associated movements of adduction and abduction are disregarded. (Adapted from Inman VT, Mann RA, in Inman VT (ed): DuVries' Surgery of the Foot, 3rd ed., St. Louis, Mosby, 1973)

Joints of the Midfoot and Forefoot

Intertarsal joints distal to the transverse tarsal articulation possess more or less plane surfaces and so do the tarsometatarsal joints. Numerous plantar and dorsal interosseous ligaments secure the bones to one another and reinforce the capsules of these synovial joints. The anatomy of the metatarsophalangeal joints resembles that of the metacarpophalangeal joints in the hand. Between the metatarsal heads the **deep transverse metatarsal ligament** connects the thick plantar ligaments or plates of these joints (the arrangement is similar to that shown in Figs. 15–2, 15–3), and some fibers of the ligaments attach also to the base of the proximal phalanx and the metatarsal head. The range of extension is greater at these joints than the range of flexion. The anatomy of interphalangeal joints corresponds to that in the hand.

MUSCULAR COMPARTMENTS OF THE LEG

The muscles which provide movement at the ankle and tarsus are arranged in compartments in a similar manner to the prime movers of the wrist and carpus. As in the forearm, these compartments house also the long flexors and extensors of the toes, but the orientation of the compartments is reversed. The flexors occupy the posterior compartment or the calf, and the extensors are located anteriorly (Fig. 18–9). Laterally, a third compart-

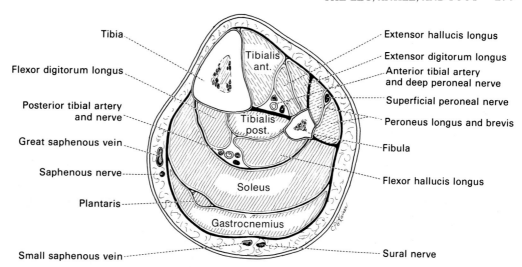

FIG. 18-9. Transverse section of the leg.

ment is present for which there is no counterpart in the forearm, and it contains the peroneal muscles. Each of these compartments is supplied by its own nerve; the tibial nerve serves the flexor compartment, the deep peroneal nerve the extensors, and the superficial peroneal nerve supplies the long and short peroneal muscles. The muscular and cutaneous distribution of these nerves is illustrated in Figures 18–11 and 18–13, and reference should be made to them as each functional group of muscles is discussed.

Prime Movers of the Ankle

Corresponding to the radial and ulnar flexors and extensors of the wrist, there is in the appropriate compartments a pair of primary plantar flexors and a pair of dorsiflexors for the ankle.

Plantar Flexors. The two heads of the **gastrocnemius** originate from the two femoral condyles and are functional analogues of the two wrist flexors. Their muscle bellies fuse into a common tendon, which lower down is joined by the soleus (Figs. 18–10 and 18–12). The **soleus** lying deep to the gastrocnemius corresponds morphologically to the flexor digitorum superficialis in the forearm and, like that muscle, originates from both bones of the leg. However, the destination of the soleus for the sole of the foot is interrupted by the backward projecting heel, and, therefore, via the massive **calcanean** or **Achilles tendon,** it inserts together with the gastrocnemius into the posterior surface of the

calcaneus. Acting together as the **triceps surae,** the three muscle bellies represent the most important motor unit which provides the impetus for propulsion. The segmental innervation of these plantar flexors is by S1 and S2 (see Table 12–2) via branches of the tibial nerve (Fig. 18–11). Their power can be tested by opposing plantar flexion, or better, by observing elevation of the heel during the attempt of standing on the toes. If a patient instructed to hop up and down on his toes with one foot, lands flatfooted, weakness of the triceps surae must be suspected. The ankle jerk objectively tests the integrity of the muscle and the nervous pathways.

The **plantaris** resembles the palmaris longus, but its tendon is not continuous with the plantar aponeurosis, because the muscle, like the soleus, is captured by the heel.

Other muscles which pass behind the axis of the ankle joint can plantar flex the foot, however, since they do not make use of the heel as a lever arm, they are less powerful and less effective. These muscles include the tibialis posterior, the peroneus longus and brevis, as well as the long digital flexors.

Dorsiflexors. The tibialis anterior and the peroneus tertius represent the primary dorsiflexors of the ankle, but the joint can, of course, be dorsiflexed also by the digital extensors which cross it (Fig. 18–12). The **tibialis anterior** is the most bulky muscle in the anterior compartment. It originates from the tibia and interosseous membrane and inserts into the medial cuneiform and the base of the first metatarsal. The **peroneus ter-**

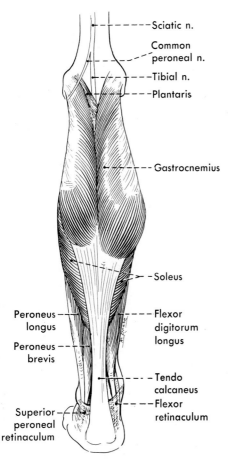

FIG. 18–10. Some of the muscles of the calf seen from the back. (Hollinshead WH: Anatomy for Surgeons, vol. 3, 2nd ed. New York, Harper & Row, 1969)

tius (misnamed because it is not in the peroneal compartment) is actually part of the muscle belly of the digital extensor. However, its tendon inserts into the base of the fifth metatarsal, restricting the muscle's action to ankle dorsiflexion. The segmental supply of both dorsiflexors is chiefly from L4 and L5 (see Table 12–2) via branches of the deep peroneal nerve (Fig. 18–13). The muscles can be tested by opposing dorsiflexion. The tendon of the tibialis anterior is the first prominent tendon anterior to the medial malleolus.

Extrinsic Flexors and Extensors of the Toes

Flexors. Since the superficial digital flexor represented by the soleus does not reach the digits there is only one common extrinsic digital flexor in the calf, the **flexor digitorum longus** (Figs. 18–9, 18–10). The muscle corresponds to the flexor digitorum profundus in the forearm. As in the forearm, the **flexor hallucis longus** is a separate muscle. The flexor digitorum arises from the tibia and the flexor hallucis from the fibula. The tendons of both muscles negotiate the heel on the medial side and enter the sole of the foot behind the medial malleolus. The tendons are invested in synovial sheaths and are retained in place by the flexor retinaculum (Fig. 18–10) which is much thinner than the corresponding structure at the wrist. The tendons insert into the distal phalanges and the anatomic arrangement of synovial and fibrous flexor sheaths in the toes through which the tendons pass is similar to that of the fingers. Both muscles are served by the tibial nerve (Fig. 18–11); the segments are S1 and S2 (see Table 12–2).

Extensors. The **extensor digitorum longus** and **extensor hallucis longus** in the anterior compartment are supplied by the deep peroneal nerve (Fig. 18–13), chiefly by segments L5 and S1. Both originate from the fibula (Fig. 18–9) and insert into the toes via the dorsal digital expansions analogous to those in the fingers. In front of the ankle the tendons are retained in place by the extensor retinacula (Fig. 18–12) and are enclosed in synovial membrane.

Inverters and Everters

In the leg there are no muscles which correspond to supinators and pronators of the forearm since such movements do not exist in the lower limbs. Eversion is a movement peculiar to the foot and it is produced by the **peroneal muscles.** The peroneus longus and brevis arise from the fibula, pass behind the lateral malleolus, lateral to the axis of the subtalar joint (Figs. 18–7 and 18–12). The brevis inserts into the base of the fifth metatarsal, but the longus enters the sole of the foot in a groove of the cuboid and crosses the sole before it inserts into the base of the first metatarsal and the bones around it. The peroneus tertius can assist in eversion because its line of pull is also lateral to the subtalar axis. The longus and brevis are supplied by the superficial peroneal nerve (L5,S1).

The principal inverter of the foot is the **tibialis posterior** and it is substantially assisted by the **tibialis anterior.** The tibialis posterior is the deepest muscle in the flexor compartment (Fig.

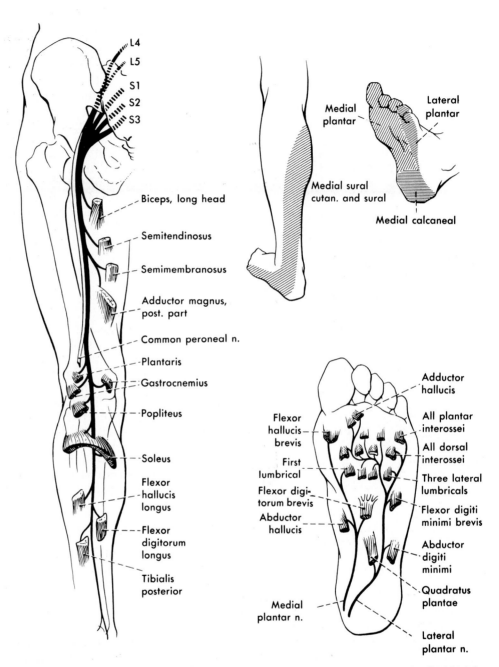

L4
L5
S1
S2
S3

Biceps, long head

Semitendinosus

Semimembranosus

Adductor magnus,
post. part

Common peroneal n.

Plantaris

Gastrocnemius

Popliteus

Soleus

Flexor
hallucis
longus

Flexor
digitorum
longus

Tibialis
posterior

Medial
plantar

Lateral
plantar

Medial sural
cutan. and sural

Medial calcaneal

Adductor
hallucis

All plantar
interossei

All dorsal
interossei

Three lateral
lumbricals

Flexor digiti
minimi brevis

Abductor
digiti
minimi

Quadratus
plantae

Lateral
plantar n.

Flexor
hallucis
brevis

First
lumbrical

Flexor digi-
torum brevis

Abductor
hallucis

Medial
plantar n.

FIG. 18-11. Muscular and cutaneous distribution of the tibial nerve. (Hollinshead WH: Anatomy for Surgeons, vol. 3, 2nd ed. New York, Harper & Row, 1969)

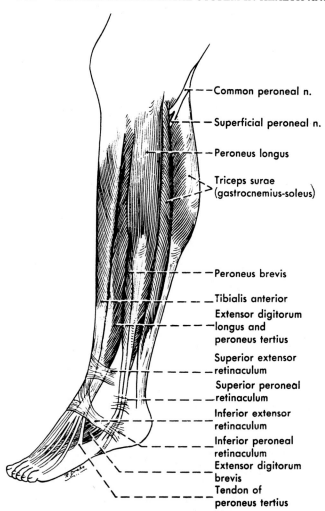

Common peroneal n.

Superficial peroneal n.

Peroneus longus

Triceps surae
(gastrocnemius-soleus)

Peroneus brevis

Tibialis anterior

Extensor digitorum
longus and
peroneus tertius

Superior extensor
retinaculum

Superior peroneal
retinaculum

Inferior extensor
retinaculum

Inferior peroneal
retinaculum

Extensor digitorum
brevis

Tendon of
peroneus tertius

FIG. 18-12. Lateral view of the muscles of the leg.
(Hollinshead WH: Anatomy for Surgeons, vol. 3, 2nd ed.
New York, Harper & Row, 1969)

18-9). It arises from the tibia, fibula, and the interosseous membrane. Its tendon enters the foot
behind the medial malleolus, passing on the medial side of the subtalar axis before it inserts into
the tuberosity of the navicular and other bones
around it. The tibialis posterior is supplied by the
tibial nerve, the most important segments in inversion are L4 and L5 (see Table 12-2).

It can be readily deduced from the attachments
of the muscles that the tibialis anterior and posterior will supinate the foot at the transverse tarsal
joint, whereas the peroneus longus, brevis, and
tertius will pronate it.

Deep Fascia and Intermuscular Septa

Intermuscular septa delineate the compartments
which contain the functional muscle groups discussed in the preceding section (Fig. 18-9). These
septa extend from the fibula to the deep fascia
which forms a rather firm investment of the leg.
Muscle contraction and relaxation generate a
pumplike effect within the compartments which
forces venous blood upward in the venae comitantes of the anterior tibial, posterior tibial, and
peroneal arteries. Valves prevent backflow in these
deep veins which receive blood also from the superficial veins connected to them by communicating veins. The muscular pump generates flow from
superficial to deep veins as long as the valves in the
communicating veins remain competent. Should
the valves in the communicating veins become in-
competent, blood will be forced by the pump from
deep to superficial veins, predisposing to
varicosities and to varicose ulcers due to increased
venous and capillary pressure.

The fascial confines are responsible for increasing intracompartmental pressure when there is
any swelling of tissue deep to the leg's investing
fascia. Swelling is a frequent complication of fractures and the anterior compartment is most often
endangered (anterior compartment syndrome). Ischemic necrosis of the muscles similar to that seen
in the forearm soon results unless the deep fascia is
incised to relieve pressure. Signs of increasing intracompartmental pressure include pain and loss
of sensation in the distribution of the nerve which
is compressed in the compartment.

Nerves and Vessels of the Compartments

The **tibial nerve** is deep in the posterior compartment and descends with the **posterior tibial
artery** between the flexor digitorum longus and
flexor hallucis longus (Figs. 18-9, 18-11). Nerve
and artery terminate by dividing into medial and
lateral plantar branches behind the medial malleolus. The **common peroneal nerve** winds around
the neck of the fibula, and in the peroneal compartment it divides into superficial and deep
peroneal nerves (Fig. 18-13). The **superficial
peroneal nerve** descends in that compartment un-
accompanied by an artery and terminates by supplying the skin on the dorsum of the foot. The **deep
peroneal nerve** pierces the intermuscular septum
and descends through the anterior compartment
among its muscles. It is joined by the **anterior tib-**

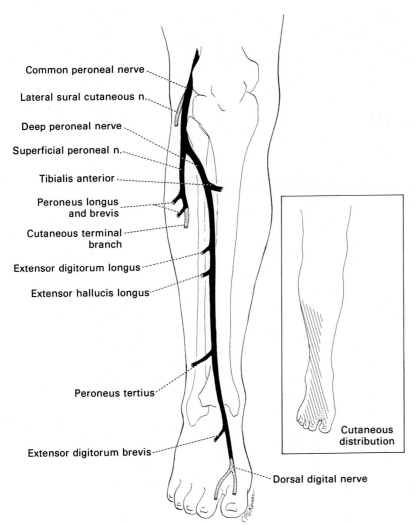

Common peroneal nerve

Lateral sural cutaneous n.

Deep peroneal nerve

Superficial peroneal n.

Tibialis anterior

Peroneus longus
and brevis

Cutaneous terminal
branch

Extensor digitorum longus

Extensor hallucis longus

Peroneus tertius

Extensor digitorum brevis

Dorsal digital nerve

Cutaneous
distribution

FIG. 18–13. Muscular and cutaneous distribution of the deep and superficial peroneal nerves.

ial artery which enters this compartment from the popliteal fossa through a hiatus at the superior edge of the interosseous membrane.

THE FOOT

Plantar Aponeurosis and Plantar Fascia

The superficial fascia forms a tough and thick padding over the sole of the foot whereas it is sparse on the dorsum. The plantar aponeurosis springs from the calcaneus and as it fans out toward the toes, it sends fiber bundles to the dermis and septa into the depth of the sole. As in the hand, an intermuscular or marginal septum springs from each side of the aponeurosis and demarcates the intrinsic muscles of the first and fifth digits from a central compartment which is occupied by the flexor tendons and lumbricals. Over the ball of the foot additional sagittal septa connect the plantar aponeurosis to the fascia that covers the interosseous muscles and to the deep transverse metatarsal ligament. In this manner, tunnels are created which transmit the flexor tendons, lumbricals and some of the digital nerves. Cushions of connective tissue sprouting from these septa and fat pads protect these structures from compression (Fig. 18–14) which the ball of the foot sustains during the heel-off to toe-off phases of the gait cycle (see Chap. 19). Superficial fibers which proceed from the aponeurosis into the

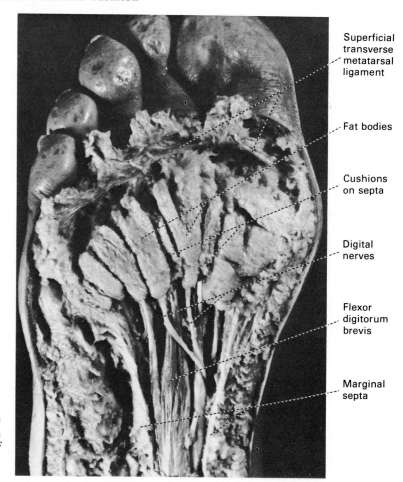

Superficial transverse metatarsal ligament

Fat bodies

Cushions on septa

Digital nerves

Flexor digitorum brevis

Marginal septa

FIG. 18-14. Dissection of the sole of the right foot. The plantar aponeurosis has been removed. (By kind permission of F Bojsen-Møller, KE Flagstad, and The Journal of Anatomy, London)

interdigital spaces and span between fibrous flexor sheaths of adjacent toes become taut when the toes are extended, as happens at push-off. In this manner the aponeurosis and skin becomes fixed over the ball of the foot. But when the metatarsal heads first contact the ground just before weight transfer to the forefoot, the toes are in the neutral position and this permits the skin to slide freely over the metatarsal heads.

Intrinsic Muscles

The topography and nomenclature of the intrinsic muscles correspond to that in the hand even though many of the muscles are ineffective in performing the movements proclaimed by their names. Their chief function is maintenance of the architecture in the *dynamic foot*.

As in the hand, there is a superficially placed **abductor** for the big toe and the little toe, and deep

to them there is, for each, a **short flexor.** Opponens muscles are lacking in the foot and have probably merged with the short flexors. The **flexor hallucis brevis** consists of two heads and so does the **adductor hallucis** which resembles the adductor of the thumb. The fused tendons of the short muscles of the hallux contain a sesamoid bone on each side before they insert into the proximal phalanx (Fig. 18–2B). The metatarsal head actually rests on the two sesamoid bones when the ball of the big toe contacts the ground.

In the central compartment of the sole the deepest muscle layer consists of the **dorsal and plantar interossei.** They are positioned to abduct and adduct the toes respectively in reference to the second digit, the line of which represents the axis of the foot. Their origins, insertions, and actions are similar to their counterparts in the hand. By simultaneously flexing the metatarsophalangeal joints and extending the interphalangeal joints, they transfer some of the weight from the metatarsal heads to the toes. Their strength can be gauged by observing a slight elevation of the metatarsal heads when the patient is asked to press on the ground firmly with all his toes, keeping the heel also in contact with the ground.

Unlike in the hand, there is an intrinsic digital extensor in the foot. The **extensor digitorum brevis** arises from the area of the sinus tarsi, its fleshy belly gives rise to five tendons which join the dorsal digital expansion of each toe.

The flexor digitorum brevis, flexor accessorius, and lumbricals are also intrinsic to the foot; however, they are better considered together with the long flexor tendons.

Long Flexor Tendons and Associated Muscles

The counterpart of the flexor digitorum superficialis in the leg was identified as the soleus. In the foot the **flexor digitorum brevis** represents the muscle. It originates from the inferior surface of the heel and is the most superficial muscle underneath the plantar aponeurosis. The tendons of the **flexor digitorum longus** and **flexor hallucis longus** pass deep to it as they enter the sole just below the medial malleolus. The insertion and the arrangement of tendons within the digital fibrous flexor sheaths corresponds to that seen in the fingers.

Entering from the medial side, the line of pull of the long digital flexor is oblique across the foot, tending to abduct the toes as well as to flex them. A small muscle, the **flexor accessorius** (also known as the quadratus plantae) corrects this obliquity. This muscle arises from the calcaneus deep to the flexor digitorum brevis and inserts into the posterior margin of the yet undivided flexor digitorum longus tendon. Deep to this tendon passes the long flexor tendon of the hallux, and as the two tendons cross, they become anchored to one another by a substantial tendinous slip. Deep to both tendons passes the tendon of the **peroneus longus,** crossing the cuneiform bones on its way toward the base of the first metatarsal.

The **lumbrical muscles** arise from the tendons of the flexor digitorum longus as they do from the profundus tendons in the palm.

Nerve and Blood Supply of the Foot

The sole of the foot is supplied by the medial and lateral plantar nerves, terminal branches of the tibial nerve (Fig. 18–11). Motor innervation to the intrinsic muscles is derived mainly from S2 segment. The **medial plantar nerve** corresponds closely to the median nerve in the hand and it serves all the intrinsic muscles of the big toe, except its adductor, and supplies the flexor digitorum brevis (as the median nerve supplies the flexor digitorum superficialis). It terminates in plantar digital nerves, the cutaneous distribution of which corresponds to that of the median nerve. The **lateral plantar nerve** corresponds to the ulnar nerve in the hand and it serves all intrinsic muscles except those supplied by the medial plantar nerve and the extensor digitorum brevis. (The latter is innervated on the dorsum of the foot by the deep peroneal nerve.) The nerve crosses to the lateral side of the sole between the flexor digitorum brevis and flexor accessorius, and in addition to the muscles it supplies skin on the lateral one and one-half toes.

The cutaneous innervation of the dorsum of the foot is chiefly from the superficial peroneal nerve (Fig. 18–13). The deep peroneal nerve supplies only adjacent sides of the first cleft. The saphenous nerve supplies skin along the medial edge and the sural nerve along the lateral edge of the foot. The precise cutaneous distribution of nerves to the foot is of less importance than in the hand, but familiarity with the dermatomes is essential in the diagnosis of lesions of the spinal cord and nerve roots (Chap. 12).

Arterial blood reaches the foot via the terminal branches of the anterior and posterior tibial arteries, and these two systems anastomose with one another freely through the first intermetatarsal space. The anterior tibial artery continues past the ankle joint as the **dorsalis pedis artery** whose pulsation is palpable over the cuneiforms. It has several branches on the dorsum of the foot but most of its blood is fed into the sole. The artery resembles the radial artery on the back of the wrist.

The pulsation of the posterior tibial artery is visible and palpable behind the medial malleolus just before it divides into the **medial** and **lateral plantar arteries.** These vessels accompany the nerves similarly named, and after supplying the muscles feed into plantar metatarsal and digital arteries. The lateral plantar artery, having crossed to the lateral side of the foot, forms the **plantar arch** which terminates by anastomosing with the dorsalis pedis artery in the first interosseous space.

Assessment of the circulation of the foot is important clinically. This should be based not only on the palpable pulses but on the rapidity of capillary filling after the skin or nail bed of the toes has been temporarily blanched by pressure.

Architecture of the Foot

The skeletal pieces of the foot are so shaped that when they are held together they form a twisted plate (Fig. 18–15). The anterior edge of the plate represented by the metatarsal heads is horizontal and is in contact with the ground. Posteriorly the edge of the plate is vertical and coincides with the vertical axis of the heel. The edges of such a twisted plate, of necessity, describe arcs, one more pronounced than the other. In the foot, the lower arc is lateral and the higher arc is medial. In a long foot these arcs are less pronounced than in a short foot.

Intrinsic movements between the bones of the foot tend to increase or decrease the degree of the twist in the osteoligamentous plate. Standing with the feet wide apart untwists the foot and this is the result of inversion and supination. Standing with the feet together increases the twist, and standing with crossed legs maximally exaggerates it. In the latter position, the feet are everted and pronated. The medial and lateral arcs in the twisted foot are clearly recognizable as arches. By comparison, an untwisted foot appears flat. Inspection of the footprint with the feet wide apart, together, or crossed over will confirm this.

Traditionally, the foot has been described as an arched structure, the two feet placed side by side resembling a dome. In such a description, a **transverse arch** of the largest span is said to be present across the bases of the metatarsals. In each foot, a **medial** and a **lateral longitudinal arch** are also recognized. The anterior pillar of the medial arch is taken to be the medial three metatarsals, the cuneiforms, and the navicular, and the posterior pillar is represented by the calcaneus. The lateral arch consists anteriorly of the lateral two metatarsals and the cuboid, and posteriorly, of the calcaneus. The medial arch is surmounted by the talus, which transmits to the two pillars most of the body weight via the subtalar and talocalcaneonavicular joints. A part of this force is transmitted to the lateral arch via the subtalar joint. These terms retain their uesfulness but the dynamic concept of a twisted plate is closer to reality than the architectural units of a rigid edifice.

Maintenance of Foot Architecture. The shape of the bones themselves is responsible for the existence of the twisted plate and consequently also for the arches. The maintenance of foot architecture, however, depends on the structures which hold the bones together and provide joint stability in the resting, weight bearing, and striding foot. Ligaments play the chief role. They are so positioned that they not only retain the bones in alignment but permit changes in the degree of the twist. Ligaments alone are responsible for maintaining the arcs in the twisted plate of the relaxed foot and also in the weight-bearing static foot. The medial and lateral arches of the foot will be maintained without recruiting any muscles, intrinsic or extrinsic, when up to 400 pounds of weight are applied to the knees of seated subjects. The more important ligaments are shown in Figure 18–16. The plantar calcaneonavicular or **spring ligament** ties together the anterior and posterior pillars of the medial arch. The **long plantar ligament** spans from the calcaneus to the cuboid and to the bases of the lateral metatarsals, reinforcing the lateral arch. The **short plantar ligament,** deep to it, plays a similar role, but other ligaments are also important. The **plantar aponeurosis** spans the distance between the anterior edge of the twisted plate and the lower end of its vertical posterior edge (Figs. 18–15, 18–16).

As soon as the weight distribution is shifted within the foot skeleton by movement, muscles are recruited. These include both extrinsic and intrinsic muscles. Of the extrinsic muscles the **tibialis posterior** and **peroneus longus** are the most important. In the gait cycle after heel strike, the lateral part of the forefoot makes first contact with the ground (the foot is inverted and supinated). Then, as the weight is transferred to the ball of the big toe, the foot increasingly pronates and everts. The tibialis posterior and peroneus longus work in concert during the stance phase when weight is being transferred to the forefoot and control the shift of the forefoot from supination into pronation. Both muscles also help to stabilize the leg on the

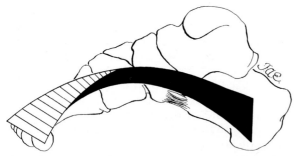

FIG. 18–15. The osteoligamentous framework of the foot represented as a twisted plate. (Adapted from Mac-Connaill MA, Basmajian JV: Muscles and Movements, Baltimore, Williams & Wilkins, 1969)

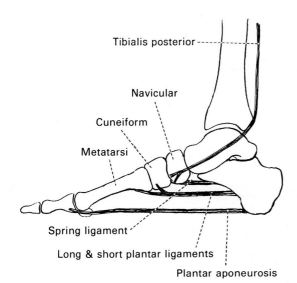

Tibialis posterior

Navicular

Cuneiform

Metatarsi

Spring ligament

Long & short plantar ligaments

Plantar aponeurosis

FIG. 18-16. Schematic representation of the most important structures responsible for the maintenance of the longitudinal arches of the foot. For simplicity's sake, all ligaments are shown in the same sagittal plane and are seen from the same medial side.

dynamic foot. Contraction of the long digital flexors stabilizes the toes when the body weight is borne only on one foot. The intrinsic flexors contribute to this function. The abductors and short flexors are in an ideal location for stabilizing and supporting the medial and lateral arches. They relieve the ligaments of undue strain in the loaded, moving foot. The plantar aponeurosis becomes tensed by dorsiflexion of the toes and this also supports and increases the arches, especially after the heel has been lifted off the ground.

Foot Deformities

In those societies where shoes are worn, nearly 50 percent of mankind suffers from some structural abnormality of the feet. A minor proportion of deformities is due to congenital causes, the early diagnosis of which is important for preventing permanent disability. Of these, only the most common type of clubfoot will be discussed. Flatfoot (pes planus), pes cavus, and hallux valgus with the associated bunion are selected for discussion from the deformities acquired after birth.

The precise etiology of many deformities remains unknown. Skeletal defects are less common than muscular imbalance. Although the architecture of the foot is primarily maintained by its ligaments, muscle imbalance due to spasticity or paralysis resulting from upper or lower motor neuron disease or from myopathies invariably leads to foot deformity, because the ligaments eventually yield to the unbalanced deforming forces. The initially supple deformities eventually become fixed due to contracture of the muscles or abnormal bony development during growth. Congenital and acquired deformities may be altered during the growth period. However, treatment of foot deformities must not be neglected after the growth period, even if the cause of the deformity is incurable, because the tendency remains for the bones and the soft tissues to adapt to the deforming forces. Without treatment the deformity may become worse.

Types of Deformity. The more common foot deformities are:

Equinus, in which the foot points downward and is fixed in the position of plantar flexion.

Calcaneus, in which the heel points downward and the foot is fixed in dorsiflexion.

Varus, in which the entire foot deviates toward the midline of the body at a number of joints distal to the ankle joint (inversion, adduction, supination).

Valgus, in which the foot deviates in a direction opposite to the varus (eversion, abduction, pronation).

Pes planus (flatfoot), in which the arches are flattened.

Pes cavus, in which the arches are exaggerated.

The various deformities often occur in combination. An example of a complex deformity is clubfoot.

Clubfoot. Although in general usage the term means a deformed foot, in medical practice clubfoot has come to be restricted to designate the most common type of congenital foot deformity, **talipes equinovarus.** The foot is in equinus (plantar flexed), often due to underdevelopment or contracture of the calf muscles. The forefoot is inverted, adducted, and supinated, due in many cases to underdevelopment of the peroneal muscles. The heel is also inverted.

With such a deformity, the child will bear his body weight on the base and shaft of the fifth metatarsal. The condition should be diagnosed at birth. The foot may appear to be in equinovarus even in a normal infant, but this posture readily yields to passive manipulation, and before the age of one year the foot can be passively dorsiflexed to

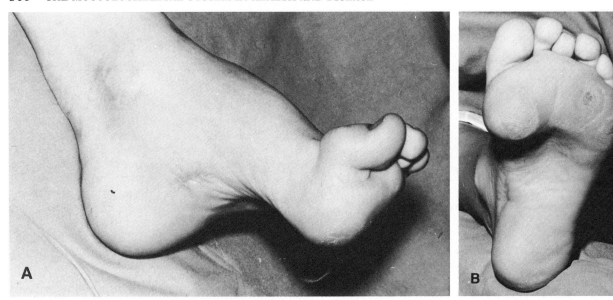

FIG. 18–17. Pes cavus showing the exaggerated arch and clawed toes **(A)** and the callosities over the metatarsal heads **(B).**

the extent that its dorsum and the little toe nearly touch the anterior surface of the tibia. In a talipes equinovarus deformity this cannot be attained. In cases of bilateral deformity, spina bifida with associated spinal cord anomalies should be looked for. The deformity will become permanent due to misshapen tarsal bones unless treatment is instituted. Treatment consists of putting the foot into appropriate splints and casts. If these fail, or in neglected cases, surgical correction is the method of choice.

Flatfoot. As explained earlier, untwisting of the osteoligamentous foot plate reduces or eliminates the arches. There are no defined criteria for distinguishing a pathologic from a normal flatfoot. Only one out of a thousand people with flat feet develop symptoms.

In a flatfooted subject there is increased mobility of the bones. The head of the talus may rest on the ground. The forefoot is pronated and generally abducted. There is more toeing-out. During walking there is greater muscular activity in an attempt to maintain or restore the arches. The interplay of the tibialis posterior and peroneus longus in stabilizing the foot is particularly important. Rupture of the tibialis posterior tendon promptly results in flattening of the arches, and this should be suspected when unilateral flatfoot develops suddenly.

A flexible flat foot need not be regarded as abnormal and should not be treated unless symptoms

develop. When such a patient stands on the toes, the medial longitudinal arch is restored in the foot through the windlass action of the aponeurosis and the contraction of the long and short toe flexors. In a rigid flat foot this is not the case. Rigid flatfoot may result from congenital fusion of the tarsal bones or from spasticity or contracture in the peroneal muscles. If eversion of the heel is associated with the flat foot, the calcaneus tendon will be thrown out of alignment with the vertical axis of the heel. This will slacken the tendon. For this reason the tendon will shorten with time, eventually preventing in the weight-bearing foot inversion of the heel and the restoration of the arches.

Pes Cavus. In a short foot the longitudinal arches are more exaggerated than in a long foot. Abnormally high arches are due either to congenital causes or to muscle imbalance, usually resulting from neurologic disorders. Exaggeration of the arches compromises the foot more than flattening of its arches. Pes cavus is usually associated with clawing of the toes (Fig. 18–17). This deformity excludes them from taking their normal share of weight off the metatarsal heads.

The exaggerated arch is usually produced by lowering the metatarsal heads in relation to the hindfoot. This displaces the toes dorsally, particularly if the deformity is associated with paralysis of the interosseous muscles. The metatar-

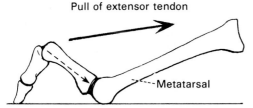

FIG. 18–18. Mechanism of metatarsalgia due to displaced tendons of the toes. The **solid arrow** indicates the direction of pull not only of the extensor digitorum but also of the displaced intrinsic muscles and of the flexor digitorum.

sophalangeal joints will be hyperextended and the unopposed pull, or later the contracture, of the digital extensors depresses the metatarsal heads further via the force vector transmitted along the hyperextended proximal phalanx (Fig. 18–18). If the interossei are intact, their displaced tendons in relation to the metatarsophalangeal joint axis will have a similar effect. In addition to the body weight, these excessive forces provide the explanation for the metatarsalgia and the hard, extensive callosities over the ball of the foot which are usually associated with pes cavus (Fig. 18–17B). The clawed toes also suffer from pressure sores and corns because of abnormal friction from the shoe. Degenerative joint disease in the tarsus is a common sequela of pes cavus.

Hallux Valgus. A study in the 1950s revealed that as much as one-third of the shoe-wearing population exhibits some lateral deviation of the big toe at the metatarsophalangeal joint. Hallux valgus is more common in women, and wearing of shoes with high heels and pointed toes is undoubtedly the most important cause in the majority of cases. The deformity does occur, however, where the etiology is clearly different.

Valgus deviation of the toe is almost always associated with varus deviation of the first metatarsal which renders its head medially prominent (Fig. 18–19). Friction and trauma lead to hypertrophy, distension, and inflammation of a subcutaneous bursa overlying the medial side of the metatarsal head. This soft tissue swelling is the **bunion,** but sometimes the complex of bony deformities is also included under this name. The angulation at the metatarsophalangeal joint produced by the hallux valgus and metatarsus varus changes the line of pull of the short muscles attached to the proximal phalanx, and this is revealed on x-rays by the displacement of the sesamoid bones which move to the lateral side of

the metatarsal. It is evident that these muscles, as well as the extrinsic flexor and extensor which bowstring in the angle between the two bones, will tend to increase the deformity. The deformity requires surgical correction for which there are numerous procedures.

CLINICAL EVALUATION

A large section of the population seeks medical advice because of complaints in the foot. Many of

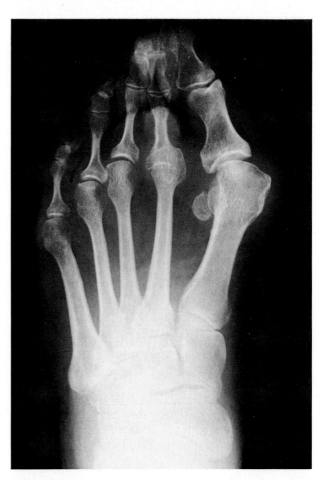

FIG. 18–19. Hallux valgus deformity. Note that in addition to the valgus deformity at the first metatarsophalangeal joint, there is pronounced metatarsus varus, the metatarsal head is hypertrophied and rotated medially, the sesamoid bones are displaced laterally into the first intermetatarsal space. The latter is due partly to the rotation of the metatarsal along its long axis and partly to the displaced line of force exerted by the intrinsic muscles of the hallux. (Courtesy of Dr. Rosalind H. Troupin)

these foot problems can be related to interference with the unique function and architecture of the foot, but the foot and ankle are also subject to diseases which affect the musculoskeletal system elsewhere. Inflammatory joint diseases involve the ankle and tarsal joints as well as the joints of the toes. Degenerative joint disease is less common in the ankle but does occur in the subtalar and transverse tarsal joints and in the metatarsophalangeal joint of the big toe. Osteomyelitis and benign and malignant neoplasms may all involve the bones of the leg and foot. Many neurologic and muscle disorders present with symptoms and signs in the feet or with abnormalities of the gait, and such systemic diseases as diabetes mellitus and arteriosclerosis generate serious problems in the feet. Acute and chronic trauma is responsible for disability in a high proportion of cases.

Because the anatomy of the leg and foot is so accessible to examination, it should be possible to make a diagnosis in practically all cases, based on the history and physical examination. The evaluation of a patient with foot problems should, however, consider the whole patient and include a general examination when so indicated. The following account concentrates on the chief symptoms confined to the leg and foot and presents a routine for the evaluation of the functional anatomy of the region. The leg and foot must also be examined as a dynamic unit because they are important constituents of the locomotor system. Some of their abnormalities are revealed only in the gait cycle.

Symptoms

Complaints about the leg, ankle, and foot include swelling, deformity, instability, paresthesias, cramps, and ulcers, but the most important symptom is pain. If the **pain** is due to localized pathology, the patient can usually indicate the site precisely, and the structure involved is identifiable by examination. In most instances of localized as well as generalized pain, the history of onset and character of the pain suggest the nature of the pathologic process (see Chap. 7). In each case it must be ascertained what the relationship of the pain is to standing and walking. Generalized pain in the calf or anterior part of the leg may develop after unusual or sustained exercise. The pain may be due to tender, swollen muscles (muscle strain) and may progress to a genuine anterior compartment syndrome (p. 302), or microscopic cortical

fractures in the tibia (shin splints) may be responsible for it. Unaccustomed, prolonged standing or walking can generate foot strain involving ligaments, muscles, and bones of the foot. A metatarsal bone, usually the second, may fracture (march fracture) under these circumstances. A painful calf may be the first symptom of phlebitis or myositis. Inadequate blood supply to the muscles gives rise to the characteristic pain of intermittent claudication (p. 275). Severe ischemia generates burning pain in the foot during rest, particularly at night. Such pain may be generalized, or if due to ischemia of a peripheral nerve rather than the tissues of the foot, it may conform to the distribution of the nerve. The pain may be relieved by cooling and dependency of the foot.

Pain in the leg and foot may also be due to nerve root compression or nerve entrapment in the region of the knee, under the retinacula around the ankle, or between the metatarsal heads. The causes of localized foot pain are best dealt with in relation to the regional examination of the foot. Arthritis in the ankle and subtalar joints generates diffuse pain in the heel region which may sometimes be referred to the calf.

Localized **swellings** in the foot usually present with pain. The pain is caused either by the lesion itself or by pressure on it. Patients with heart failure complain of bilateral swelling of the ankles. Venous or lymphatic obstruction produces similar, sometimes unilateral, swelling. The swelling is painless and pits under firm pressure.

Painful, paroxysmal tetanic contractions or **cramps** of the plantar and calf muscles have no identifiable cause in the majority of cases. The cramps may be related to overuse or fatigue, but they usually seize the muscle at rest or during the night. Carpopedal spasms are a feature of hypocalcemic tetany (see Chap. 3), but in this condition the cramps are not confined to the foot and there are other signs of neuromuscular hyperexcitability present.

Some congenital **deformities** may not reveal themselves until the child begins to walk, when they present as gait abnormalities. Adult patients often only complain of deformity in the feet and toes when abnormal pressures produce pain.

Ulcerations of the leg, foot, and toes have multiple local and systemic causes. The lesions are, as a rule, associated with pain unless the underlying cause includes neuritis or peripheral neuropathy. Painless ulcers of the foot are characteristic of diabetic neuropathy and tabes dorsalis.

Physical Examination

Inspection. Socks and stockings should be removed from both feet, and if the history suggests more than a minor lesion localized to the foot, the spine, pelvis, hips, thighs, and knees should also be examined with the patient standing and walking.

First, the patient sits on the edge of the examination table, legs and feet hanging free. The following observations should be made:

1. Vertical alignment of patella with the first interosseous or interdigital space. Significant deviation of the foot axis from the sagittal plane suggests tibial torsion or valgus or varus deformity of the forefoot.
2. The relaxed foot should hang in slight plantar flexion unless there is bony deformity, contracture, or spasm in the leg muscle.
3. The medial longitudinal arch should be recognizable except in children of less than 2–3 years of age, in whom the arch is padded by fat.
4. All five toes should be straight or only slightly bent and there should be no overriding, clawing, valgus, or varus deviation.
5. The sole of the foot should be inspected, and generalized and localized swellings and erythema should be noted on the sole and dorsum. Callosities, warts, ulcers, and varicosities should be looked for.
6. Lack of hair, cyanosis, or pallor are suggestive of inadequate blood supply.

The patient should stand, preferably on a platform, and the medial arches of the two weight-bearing feet should be inspected and the alignment of the vertical axis of the heel with the calcaneus tendon should be noted. Should the foot be flat, it is important to observe whether or not the heel is everted. In a flat-footed subject the examiner or the patient should passively extend the big toe to observe whether or not the medial longitudinal arch becomes restored through the windlass action of the plantar aponeurosis. Then the patient should be required to rise on tiptoes which should produce inversion of the heel and an increase in the longitudinal arch.

Next, one weight-bearing foot should be observed while the opposite leg is lifted. In the normal foot this results in pronation. The patient should be requested to rotate his body from one side to the other while standing on one leg. Medial and lateral rotation of the tibia will produce alternating pronation and supination of the normal foot.

Palpation. All bony points of the leg and foot, described under landmarks, should be systematically palpated, looking for tenderness and bony abnormalities. These landmarks should aid in the location of lesions in bones, joints, and soft tissues. The following regions should be carefully palpated:

1. **The heel region.** Above the heel, the calcaneus tendon may be tender because of minor tears due to overuse, or the connective tissue around it may be inflamed. The tendon may be completely ruptured and a gap may be palpable. Tendon rupture should be confirmed by suddenly squeezing the calf muscles with the patient in the kneeling position. Normally this produces slight plantar flexion, but no movement will occur if the tendon is torn.

   A deep and a superficial bursa is associated with the insertion of the calcaneus tendon on the back of the heel, and the bursae may become inflamed. Tenderness on the plantar surface of the calcaneus may be caused by bony spurs which are palpable or by strain and inflammation in the plantar aponeurosis and its calcaneal attachment.
2. **The hollow of the sole of the foot.** Strain of the plantar aponeurosis and of the intrinsic muscles of the foot results in tenderness along the medial arch. This is particularly pronounced when pressure is applied to the hollow of the foot while the toes are passively extended. Tenderness immediately proximal to the tuberosity of the navicular is suggestive of a strained spring ligament.
3. **The ball of the foot.** Pressure on the metatarsal heads, neuroma of digital nerves, and calluses are responsible for tenderness in this area. In metatarsalgia, usually the head of the second metatarsal is most painful.

   The circulation should be assessed by feeling skin temperature and texture, by verifying pulses, and by determining the rate of capillary filling.

Range of Motion. In eliciting active and passive ranges of movement, note must be taken of whether or not the limiting factor is pain. Movement should be separately tested at the ankles, subtalar, transverse tarsal, and metatarsophalangeal joints.

The obliquity of the ankle axis should be determined by locating the tips of the malleoli. The axis runs through these two points and the more oblique it is the more toeing in will occur after heel strike.

To test the range of plantar flexion and dorsiflexion, one hand grasps the heel and the other stabilizes the foot. Ankle movement is elicited by moving the heel. The two sides should be compared. There is considerable variation in range from individual to individual but there should be at least 15° dorsiflexion and 20° plantar flexion.

Inversion and eversion is tested by stabilizing the leg above the ankle with one hand and moving the heel with the other. It is useful to test active movement at the ankle and subtalar joints while the foot is held by the examiner without trying to restrict the motion.

The transverse tarsal joint is tested by applying a varus or valgus force to the forefoot with one hand while the other hand stabilizes the heel. A few degrees of abduction and adduction should be obtained. The toes should be flexed, actively and passively. Normally, 70 to 90° of extension is present at the metatarsophalangeal joint of the big toe.

A quick test of active ranges of motion can be done by asking the patient to take a few steps walking on his toes, on his heels, and with the foot inverted and everted. These tests also give an impression of muscle power in the various functional groups.

Joint Stability. The collateral ligaments of the ankles should be palpated for tenderness and so should the anterior tibiofibular ligament. To test the stability of the ankle, the leg should be grasped with one hand and the heel with the other. If the foot can be pushed forward in the ankle mortise, the anterior talofibular and/or tibionavicular ligaments are probably torn. Excessive inversion and eversion indicate tears in the deltoid or calcaneofibular ligaments.

Grasping the foot in one hand and supinating it permits a free range of movement in the foot skeleton, if the heel is everted at the same time with the other hand. Pronation of the forefoot and inversion of the heel locks the joints and reduces motion between the tarsal and metatarsal bones.

Muscle Strength and Neurologic Examination. Walking on the toes, heels, and lateral and medial edge of the foot gives a rough and ready test of muscle strength. The strength of each muscle group should also be tested by resisting the movement they produce. These maneuvers were described earlier in the chapter. It is important to test the strength of the tibialis anterior, the toe extensors, the triceps surae, the tibialis posterior, and the intrinsic muscles of the foot.

In the neurologic examination the nerves and segmental values should be kept in mind when the various muscle groups are tested. The ankle jerk should be elicited by tapping the calcaneus tendon while the foot is relaxed. Slight, passive dorsiflexion of the foot is advantageous because it stretches the tendon. Skin sensation over the dermatomal areas should be tested (see Chap. 12).

Observation of the Foot During Walking. The patient should walk barefoot and also wearing his shoes. His shoes should be inspected separately. Familiarity with phases of the gait cycle is a requirement for a meaningful examination (see Chap. 19).

Observation should begin with noting the heel of one foot striking the ground. As the rest of the sole contacts the ground, the forefoot gradually pronates, transferring weight to the first metatarsal head. When the heel is raised, it promptly inverts and the metacarpophalangeal joints more and more extend. The weight is now supported on the pronated forefoot. It should be recalled that the osteoligamentous footplate is most rigid when the heel is inverted and the foot is pronated. Just before push-off the foot supinates and inverts, causing the head of the first metatarsal to be lifted off the ground slightly in advance of all the others. During these movements there should not be any slipping or rotation of the ball of the foot.

The shoes provide information about the behavior of the foot in ambulation. There should be noticeable wear posterolaterally on the heel and under the ball of the foot medially. The creases in the upper part of the shoe across the metatarsal heads should be straight. Note should be taken of supports, pads, inlays, or metal tabs over areas of abnormal wear.

SUGGESTED READING

Adams CJ: Outline of Orthopedics. Baltimore, Williams & Wilkins, 1968
Chapter 10 briefly and clearly discusses the common abnormalities and diseases of the leg, ankle and foot.
Cailliet R: Foot and Ankle Pain. Philadelphia, FA Davis 1968
A readable, well-illustrated, concise text dealing with functional anatomy, diagnosis and treatment of many disorders in the ankle and foot.
Hicks JH: The three weight bearing mechanisms of the foot. In Evans FG (ed): Biomechanical Studies of the Musculoskeletal System. Springfield, IL, Charles C Thomas, 1961

An interesting account of the biomechanics of the foot. Introduces the significance of the plantar aponeurosis in maintenance of the arches.

Hollinshead WH: Anatomy for Surgeons, Vol 3, The Back and Limbs, 2nd ed. New York, Harper & Row, 1969
Chapter 9 presents the detailed anatomy of all structures of the leg, ankle and foot with extensive bibliography.

Hoppenfeld S: Physical Examination of the Spine and Extremities. New York, Appleton-Century-Crofts, 1976
Chapter 8 gives a detailed, step-wise, well-illustrated account of the physical examination of ankle and foot.

Inman VT (ed): DuVries' Surgery of the Foot, 3rd ed. St. Louis, CV Mosby, 1973
Chapter 1 presents a clear description of the biomechanics of the ankle and foot closely tied to anatomical and physiological principles. Chapter 2 describes the physical examination of the foot and ankle based on the biomechanics of the joints.

The book contains well-illustrated chapters on congenital and acquired deformities and other abnormalities of the foot.

Inman VT: The Joints of the Ankle. Baltimore, Williams & Wilkins, 1976
An interesting and analytical reevaluation of the anatomy and biomechanics of the ankle and subtalar joints. A thorough and scientific analysis based on measurements and model building.

Jones, WF: Structure and Function as Seen in the Foot. London, Bailliere, Tindall and Cox, 1944
A classical treatise on the foot.

MacConnaill MA, Basmajian JV: Muscles and Movements. Baltimore, Williams & Wilkins, 1969
Chapters 5 and 13 introduce the concept of the twisted osteoligamentous lamina of the foot and explain much of the functional anatomy of the foot using this concept.

19
Normal and Pathologic Ambulation

WALTER C. STOLOV

Ambulation can be defined in a broad sense as the type of locomotion by which the body is translated on a surface from one point to another. Ambulation is essential for the maintenance of life in all species of animals except those which rely exclusively on swimming or flight. In the human, a bipedal pattern of ambulation is acquired during infancy, and the actual or impending loss of this skill generates great stress at all subsequent periods of life. Therefore, patients who perceive any abnormality in their pattern of ambulation, be it acute or gradual in onset, invariably seek medical attention.

When injury or pathologic changes compromise upright posture or interfere with normal ambulation, a variety of compensatory mechanisms is called into action in the musculoskeletal system, which strives for maintaining function. These adaptations manifest themselves as abnormal gait patterns, and are invariably less efficient and more costly in terms of energy than the normal mechanisms. When abnormal gait is observed, the most striking feature is the manner in which these compensatory adaptations are being used, while the underlying pathology may be completely concealed. It is necessary, therefore, to analyze and understand the compensatory mechanisms which are called into operation by specific abnormalities in order to establish a diagnosis. This will be possible only if the physician is familiar with the normal mechanisms of posture and with the dynamics of normal gait. The understanding of energy requirements for these functions is germane to the analysis of gait abnormalities, and therefore this chapter deals first with energy factors of relaxed standing and ambulation.

ENERGY REQUIREMENTS

Relaxed Standing

The relaxed standing posture in humans is a relatively low energy activity. The energy requirement for relaxed standing in a 70 kg adult is 1.8 Kcal/min compared to 1.0 Kcal/min for the supine position. Walking at a rate of 3 mph requires 4.3 Kcal/min. The achievement of near effortless equilibrium in relaxed standing in normal subjects results from an effective counterbalancing of the forces of gravity by the restraining action of ligaments, especially at the hip and knee.

Figure 19–1 indicates the gravitational force line during relaxed standing as it acts through the center of mass. The line lies in the median plane and runs anterior to the thoracic vertebrae, through the body of S2 vertebra, behind the hip joint, and in front of the knee and ankle joints. Figure 19–2 shows schematically the relationships of the body's center of mass at S2 and the gravitational force line from the center of mass. Ligaments play a major role, but the maintenance of equilibrium in relaxed standing requires continuous contraction of the extensors of the neck and the triceps surae, as well as intermittent low level activity in the lumbar part of the erector spinae. The abdominal muscles, quadriceps, gluteus maximus, hamstrings, and hip abductors are, however, essentially relaxed.

Figure 19–3 illustrates how balance is achieved at the hip and knee by the restraining force of the ligaments without invoking muscle contraction, and how at the ankle joint active participation of the soleus and gastrocnemius is required to

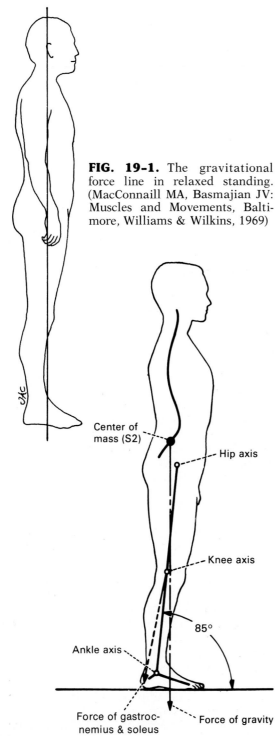

FIG. 19-1. The gravitational force line in relaxed standing. (MacConnaill MA, Basmajian JV: Muscles and Movements, Baltimore, Williams & Wilkins, 1969)

Center of mass (S2)

Hip axis

Knee axis

85°

Ankle axis

Force of gastrocnemius & soleus

Force of gravity

FIG. 19-2. In the relaxed, standing posture the gravitational force line through the center of mass falls behind the hip joint, in front of the knee joint, and in front of the ankle joint. In the lower limbs active muscle contraction for balance is required, but only in the gastrocnemius-soleus muscles.

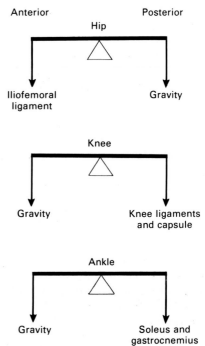

Anterior   Posterior
Hip

Iliofemoral   Gravity
ligament

Knee

Gravity   Knee ligaments
and capsule

Ankle

Gravity   Soleus and
gastrocnemius

FIG. 19-3. Schematic representation of forces acting to maintain balance in relaxed standing. Hip: iliofemoral ligament anteriorly balances the force of gravity posteriorly. No active muscle contraction is required. Knee: ligaments and capsule provide the restraining force posteriorly which balances the gravitational force anteriorly. No active muscle contraction is required. Ankle: gravitational force anteriorly is balanced by the contraction of the gastrocnemius and soleus posteriorly.

achieve balance. It is easy to see that if the passive range of hip or knee extension and of dorsiflexion of the ankle become restricted, additional muscular activity will be required to maintain the upright posture. Further, alteration of the normal thoracic and lumbar curvatures of the spine will also add to energy consumption required to maintain balance. This is readily illustrated by considering a patient with hip and knee flexion deformity who also has a kyphotic vertebral column (Fig. 19–4). The force of gravity through the center of mass in such a patient falls anterior to the hip joint and posterior to the knee joint. In such a situation, the extensor musculature of the hip and knee must also contract to prevent the hip and knee from collapsing (Fig. 19–5, compare with Fig. 19–3). Consequently, standing would require an increased expenditure of energy and could no longer be considered a low energy activity.

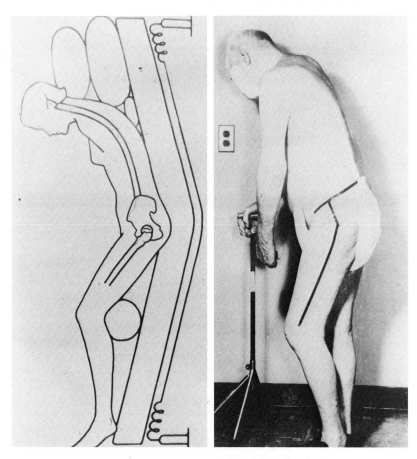

FIG. 19-4. A patient with kyphosis and hip and knee flexion deformity due to prolonged confinement to bed in the posture indicated by the drawing. The patient's hip and knee are in maximum possible extension. To prevent the hip and knee from collapsing, the extensors of both joints must contract. (Kottke FJ, in Krusen, FH (ed): Handbook of Physical Medicine and Rehabilitation, 2nd ed. Philadelphia, WB Saunders, 1971)

Ambulation

Ambulation on level ground may be viewed as a forward translation of the center of mass. For movement to occur, an external force must be applied. The external force is in essence the friction generated between the foot and the ground as the leg "pushes off." This force is generated by the hip extensors and plantar flexors of the ankle. When there is no frictional resistance between the foot or shoe and the ground (e.g., when attempting to walk on a greased floor or on slick ice), no forward movement will take place.

One might expect that the most efficient way to move would be one in which the center of mass is translated along a line parallel to the ground, mimicking the progress of a wheel (Fig. 19–6). By so doing, vertical displacements of the center of mass would be avoided and no added energy would be required to elevate the body mass against gravity. In normal ambulation, however, the center of mass does oscillate up and down (Fig. 19–6). Walking with the center of mass parallel to the ground would require the hip and knee to be in flexion, and

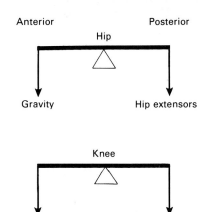

FIG. 19-5. Schematic representation of forces acting to maintain balance in relaxed standing by a patient with hip and knee flexion deformity as illustrated in Figure 19–4. Compare with the forces in Figure 19–3. **(A)** Hip: the force of gravity is now anterior and is balanced by the contraction of the hip extensors posteriorly. The iliofemoral ligament is no longer in action. **(B)** Knee: the force of gravity is now posterior and is balanced by contraction of the knee extensors anteriorly. The ligaments of the knee are no longer in action.

consequently the gravity force line through the center of mass would lie anterior to the hip and posterior to the knee. Considerable added energy would be needed because hip and knee extensors would now have to contract to prevent the hip and knee from collapsing.

Normal, relaxed ambulation on level ground for minimum energy expenditure is a compromise between the extra energy required for elevating the center of mass and the energy needed to maintain the hips and knees flexed. The sinusoidal curve which the center of mass in effect traces has a total vertical amplitude of about 5 cm.

A normal subject engaged in comfortable unhurried but directed ambulation automatically assumes a speed where the overall energy expenditure expressed in calories/min is a certain minimum (Fig. 19–7). Energy consumption increases when speed increases beyond this rate, and actually it also increases when speed is consciously reduced. The latter requires the use of muscles to retard and reduce leg swing below its natural pendulum rate.

The energy cost of ambulation can be expressed as calories/meter/kg, which gives a measure of the efficiency of ambulation. Figure 19–8 compares such measurements for normal subjects and several pathologic states, and reveals the following energy effects of pathologic ambulation when compared with the normal:

1. A pathologic pattern results in a lower speed for comfortable, minimum energy ambulation.

2. For a given speed, pathology results in a greater expenditure of energy.

3. The most efficient energy expenditure for a pathologic ambulator occurs at a lower speed than that for a normal person.

THE GAIT CYCLE

During forward progression, specific movements at the hip, knee, and ankle joints bring about vertical oscillations in the body's center of mass during locomotion. The movements require specific contraction of various muscle groups of the lower limb during the different phases of the gait.

Phases of the Gait Cycle

At any time a limb is either in contact with the ground (stance phase), or it is in the air (swing phase). The duration of the gait cycle for any one limb extends from the time the heel contacts the ground (heel strike, HS) until the same heel contacts the ground again. **Stance phase** begins with HS and ends with the toe leaving the ground (toe-off, TO). **Swing phase** begins with TO and ends with HS. Stance phase occupies 60 percent and swing phase 40 percent of a single gait cycle. Figure 19–9 depicts a full gait cycle for the left and right leg along the same time axis. The figure shows that a period of **double support** (DS) exists when both limbs are in stance phase. This period accounts for about 15 percent of the cycle in normal, comfortable walking, and extends from the onset of HS of

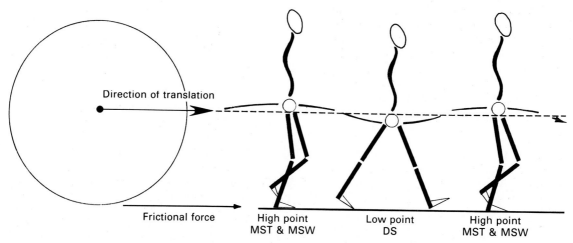

Direction of translation

Frictional force

High point
MST & MSW

Low point
DS

High point
MST & MSW

FIG. 19–6. Schematic comparison of the progression of a wheel and normal bipedal ambulation. In the latter, the center of mass describes a sinusoidal curve while the wheel's center of mass is translated parallel to the ground.

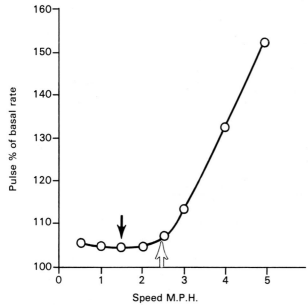

FIG. 19-7. Energy consumption as a factor of the speed in straight line walking. Energy consumption is expressed as percent increase in pulse rate over the basal rate. The white arrow indicates the comfortable speed assumed spontaneously. The black arrow represents walking rates if the leg swings as a free pendulum and corresponds to true minimum energy costs. The energy cost of comfortable speed is slightly greater than the minimum in order to give the limbs straight line direction (mean values obtained from 14 normal subjects).

one limb to TO of the other. As the speed of walking increases, the duration of the DS period shortens. Running is defined as a pace at which DS is no longer present.

The first portion of stance phase extends from HS to foot-flat (FF). **Mid-stance** (MST) lasts from FF to heel-off (HO), all of the foot being in contact with the ground. The last period of stance is from HO to TO. Swing phase consists of an initial period of *acceleration* beginning with TO, while the second half of swing is a period of *deceleration* which ends with HS. **Mid-swing** (MSW) is the transition period between acceleration and deceleration.

Center of Mass Oscillation

The high point of the center of mass is reached during MST and its low point occurs during DS (Fig. 19-6). Any pathology that increases the vertical distance between high and low points increases

the energy cost of ambulation, and at the same time decreases the speed of comfortable walking. The high point is controlled by two specific movements: one takes place at the hip and the other at the knee, while the low point is influenced by one at the hip alone. The two determinants of the high point are pelvic tilt and knee flexion in MST, while the low point is determined by pelvic rotation. In addition, the center of mass oscillates also horizontally as the body is supported alternately by each stance leg.

Pelvic Tilt in MST. When one leg is in stance phase, the pelvis sags on the side of the swinging leg. The result of this pelvic tilt is that the center of mass rises less than if the tilt had not taken place (Fig. 19-10). The pelvic movement can be viewed in effect as adduction of the stance leg at the hip, which occurs despite the fact that hip abductors are contracting. The hip abductors control the degree of the tilt, the extent of which is 4–5°.

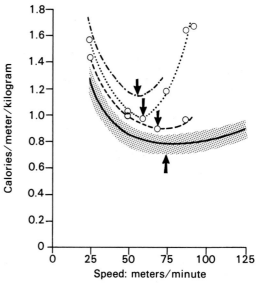

FIG. 19-8. Energy expenditure in normal and pathologic ambulation. **Heavy curve:** average energy expenditure in cal/m/kg of normal subjects walking at various speeds. **Stippled area:** approximately one standard deviation. The other lines show the energy expenditure by patients with gait abnormalities. The arrows represent the natural walking speeds. With increasing pathology, the most comfortable speed shifts toward lower values and the energy costs increase. (Bard G, Ralston HJ: Arch Phys Med Rehab 40:415, 1959)

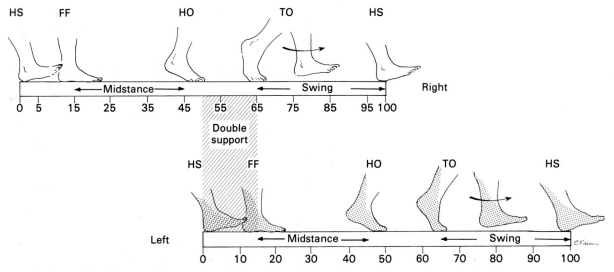

FIG. 19-9. The phases of the gait cycle shown on the same time axis for left and right legs.

Knee Flexion in MST. The high point of the center of mass is further reduced by flexion of the knee in MST. The knee is in 15° flexion at this point. The hip is also flexed (Fig. 19–11). Contraction of the hip and knee extensor muscles is therefore required because the gravitational line now falls anterior to the hip and posterior to the knee axis.

Pelvic Rotation. As the advancing leg reaches HS it places its own anterior superior iliac spine ahead

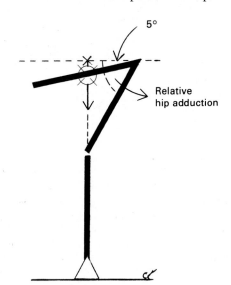

FIG. 19-10. Pelvic tilt during MST reduces the high point of the center of mass from X to ⊗. In the schematic diagram the tibia, femur and pelvis are represented by solid bars.

of that on the contralateral side, where the leg is coming into HO. The vertical projection of the limb length is higher with pelvic rotation than if pelvic rotation did not occur (Fig. 19–12). The result of the rotation is that the center of mass falls less during DS than if the rotation had not taken place. Pelvic rotation has the added effect of producing a longer stride length for the same amount of hip flexion of the advancing leg and hip extension of the retreating leg (Fig. 19–13). About 5° of pelvic rotation occurs.

Lateral Sway and Arm Swing. In addition to vertical oscillation of the center mass, *lateral sway* or side-to-side oscillations also occur with each step. This motion is necessary to bring the gravitational force line over the stance limb (Fig. 19–14). Lateral sway to each side is maximal at MST. The total amplitude of side-to-side movement of the center of mass is about 5 cm. Like the pelvic tilt, it also produces relative adduction of the stance hip. Lateral sway will increase if the base of support increases. The **base of support** is the distance between the two heels as they cross each other, and may vary from 10–20 cm. The degree of normal adduction of the femoral shaft and the angle between the femoral shaft and the tibia determine the size of the base (Fig. 19–14).

While **arm swing** does not influence center of mass oscillations, it does coordinate with pelvic rotation and leg advance and occurs in specific relation to them. Both pelvic rotation and leg advance impart an angular momentum to the lower

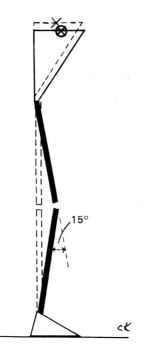

FIG. 19–11. Knee flexion in MST further reduces the high point of the center of mass from X to ⊗.

half of the body. The conservation of angular momentum principle requires that the total body angular momentum must be zero, since it is zero prior to the initiation of ambulation. Arm swing imparts angular momentum in a direction reverse to that of the lower half of the body. This should be clear from Figure 19–15 which illustrates arm swing in relation to leg advance. The vertebral column undergoes rotatory stresses as a result of these reverse rotations. The lumbar spine is stressed in a direction opposite to that of the thoracic spine.

Joint Movements and Muscle Action

Muscle activity and joint movements concerned with ambulation are best understood by analyzing the substages of the stance and swing phase in the gait cycle. The periods to be considered in the **stance phase** are: 1) HS to FF; 2) FF to MST, 3) MST to HO, 4) HO to TO (the push-off period); and in **swing phase**: 1) TO to MSW (acceleration) and 2) MSW to HS (deceleration). During these periods muscle groups contract either to give or reduce momentum to the advancing limb or they counterbalance gravitational forces and the forces imparted by the ground to the limb.

Heel Strike to Foot Flat. At the time of HS the hip is flexed about 25°, the knee is fully extended and the ankle is in neutral position midway between plantar and dorsiflexion. Heel strike generates a reactive force from the ground. This reactive force creates a moment to drive the hip into greater flexion and it also tends to flex the knee. The same force drives the foot into plantar flexion, bringing the sole in contact with the ground (FF). To check and control this tendency for flexion, extensor muscles of all three joints have to contract. At the hip this includes the gluteus maximus and the

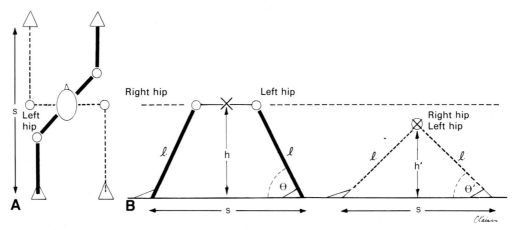

FIG. 19–12. Effect of pelvic rotation in reducing the fall in the center of mass at DS. **(A)** Top view showing stride length, S, with **(straight line)** and without **(dotted line)** pelvic rotation. **(B)** Side view showing height of center of mass (h) with pelvic rotation and without rotation (h'). h = $\ell\sin\theta$ and h' = $\ell\sin\theta$.

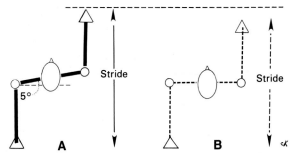

FIG. 19-13. Stride length with (**A**) and without (**B**) pelvic rotation with the same amount of hip flexion and extension.

hamstrings; at the knee the quadriceps which contracts as it is lengthening (eccentric contraction), allowing the knee to flex 20°, at the ankle the contracting dorsiflexors (extensor digitorum longus, extensor hallucis longus and tibialis anterior) allow 15° of plantar flexion. Quadriceps contraction is largely responsible for absorbing the jarring "shock" of heel strike, while the ankle dorsiflexors prevent slapping of the foot on the ground as they contract while they elongate. **Contraction of the extensor musculature in effect prevents continued flexion under the body weight and guards against collapse of the limb.**

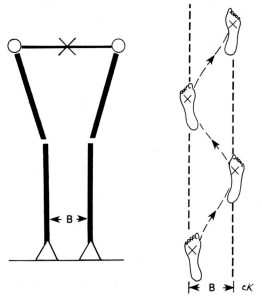

FIG. 19-14. Horizontal oscillations of the body's center of mass (lateral trunk sway) as the body is alternately supported on each stance leg. The extent of the sway is determined by the base of support.

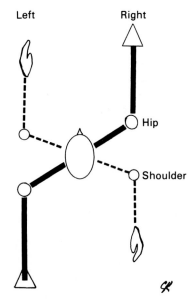

FIG. 19-15. Arm swing coordinates with leg advance. Forward arm swing matches contralateral leg advance.

Foot Flat to Mid-Stance. After attaining FF, the body moves forward over the planted foot, reaching the position of MST where weight is supported by the stance leg. This forward movement eliminates flexion at the hip and plantar flexion at the ankle, dispensing with the contraction of their extensors, but 15° flexion is retained at the knee. Therefore, the weight bearing knee has to be supported by the quadriceps which now shortens as it contracts.

Two additional groups of muscles are called into action at MST as a consequence of the body weight being supported by the stance leg. These are the abductors of the hip and plantar flexors of the foot. By the time of MST, the opposite leg has been lifted off the ground and the force of gravity tilts the pelvis down on the side of the swing leg. The hip abductors of the stance leg (gluteus medius and minimus, tensor fasciae latae) are called into action to control and counterbalance hip adduction which results from the pelvic tilt (Fig. 19–16). Plantar flexors (gastrocnemius, soleus, tibialis posterior, flexor digitorum longus, peroneus longus) are recruited in MST to counterbalance the reactive force from the ground which, following attainment of FF, forces the foot into dorsiflexion as the body moves forward over the ankle. Dorsiflexion of up to 15° is achieved at the end of MST.

With attainment of FF, all segments of the limb begin a relative lateral rotation. The tibia laterally rotates on the femur, the femur on the pelvis and the pelvis rotates with respect to the vertical axis. This lateral rotation continues until TO.

Mid-Stance to Heel-Off. As the body continues its forward momentum while the foot is still flat on the ground, gravity's line of force, acting from the center of mass, falls increasingly forward, generating a reactive force from the ground which further extends the hip, knee, and the ankle. By the time HO is reached, the hip is extended 10–15° without any active participation of its own extensors. In fact, the iliopsoas is called into action to counterbalance the extension force. As gravity's line of force is now anterior to the knee, quadriceps contraction is eliminated. In the foot, the ground reaction forces shift forward toward the metatarsal heads, increasing the dorsiflexion moment. As a consequence, the contraction of plantar flexors gathers strength and peaks as the heel is lifted (HO), providing the foward propulsive force needed for push-off. The gastrocnemius, being a flexor of the knee as well as of the ankle, prevents

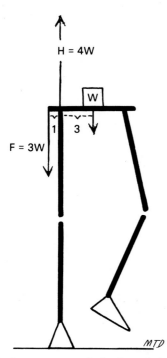

FIG. 19–16. Contraction of the hip abductors of the stance leg minimizes downward tilt of the pelvis on the side of the swing leg. Hip compression force on the side of the stance leg is nearly four times body weight. For instance, in a patient weighing 165 pounds, 660 pounds compression force would be acting at the hip when he stands on one leg as during stance phase. F = hip abduction force; H = hip compression force; W = body weight.

attainment of complete extension at the knee. Since the pelvis is still supported on one leg, hip abductors remain active during this phase.

Heel-Off to Toe-Off. This is the push-off phase and the last period of stance. The main thrust for forward propulsion occurs during this period. It also is the phase of double support, for the contralateral limb is commencing its own HS to FF period (Fig. 19–9).

The hip begins to move in the direction of flexion, the adductor muscles assisting the iliopsoas as they anticipate the first phase of swing. The most striking changes occur at the knee and ankle. During this phase the almost completely extended knee flexes to 40°, and in response to the reacting force (transmitted from the metatarsal heads) which flexes the knee, the quadriceps again begins its contraction. The ankle moves from 15° dorsiflexion at the commencement of HO to 35° plantar flexion at TO. As the toe is lifted, the calf muscles relax and activity in the hip abductors also ceases.

Toe-Off to Mid-Swing. This is the first stage in swing phase, the period of acceleration of the advancing leg. The required forces are generated by flexors of the hip. The iliopsoas is active throughout, until MSW is reached, at which point it relaxes. After TO, the knee continues its flexion passively as the thigh is accelerated by the hip flexors. The ankle is actively dorsiflexed. The continuation of hip and knee flexion, and dorsiflexion of the ankle at MSW "shorten" the leg to allow clearance of the ground.

With TO all segments of the limb commence the reversal of the lateral rotation attained after FF in the stance phase. This medial rotation continues from TO until the same leg reaches FF again. The pelvis rotates 5°, the femur 9° with respect to the pelvis, and the tibia another 9° with respect to the femur. The total medial rotation is 23°, but with fast walking it may increase to 35°.

Mid-Swing to Heel-Strike. The hip joint gains only a few additional degrees of flexion before HS. Its flexion is slowed by contraction of the hamstrings. The knee joint ceases to flex and it rapidly moves from 65° flexion to full extension at HS. The rapid knee extension results mostly from pendulum action and is slowed by eccentric contraction of the hamstrings. Full knee extension is achieved as HS commences. This is the only point in the gait cycle where the knee is fully extended. The ankle joint is held in the neutral position by the dorsi-

TABLE 19–1. Range of Motion Requirements For Normal Ambulation

Hip flexion–extension	45°
Total lateral–medial rotation of all segments	23°–35°
Hip Adduction	4°–8°
Knee flexion–extension	65°
Ankle dorsiflexion	15°
Ankle plantar flexion	20°

flexors until HS. The force requirement of the dorsiflexor group is less during swing than during the HS–FF phase of stance.

SUMMARY. Table 19–1 gives the ranges of motion at different joints required for normal, comfortable ambulation on level ground. An abnormal gait pattern will result if structural abnormalities of joint surfaces, capsules, ligaments, or muscles that cross the joints are sufficient to reduce motion below the ranges indicated.

Table 19–2 summarizes the main muscle actions and their timing in the gait cycle. Knowledge of these factors permits interpretation of abnormalities secondary to muscle weakness and range of motion losses common to many musculoskeletal disorders.

NEURAL CONTROL OF LOCOMOTION

The gait cycle as described above implies the existence of a nervous system capable of smoothly turning on and off various flexor and extensor muscle groups at the right time, coordinating the upper and lower limbs for reciprocal action, modifying the speed of ambulation, and adjusting to the demands of various terrains. A master program somewhere in the CNS might be postulated as a controlling single computer, or given the various inhibitory and excitatory spinal reflexes operative on contralateral and ipsilateral muscles (see Chap. 4), it might be suggested that all ambulation is simply an activity triggered and sustained by various spinal reflexes.

Ablation and stimulation experiments in animals, and more recently functional human studies employing reversible "lesions," have demonstrated that neither of the above two hypotheses accounts sufficiently for the neural control of ambulation, and a more complex series of influences is necessary to explain the observed phenomena. At the heart of the current theoretical construction is the existence of **pattern generators** in the spinal cord (Fig. 19–17) that are genetically determined. A pair of these exists for the legs in the lumbosacral cord and a pair for the arms in the cervical cord. These pattern generators are conceived of as having subunits for flexors and extensors, or possibly subunits for each joint of the limb. The generators are programmed for turning on the appropriate alpha and gamma motor neurons in their proper sequence. For setting the pattern of reciprocal limb movements, interneuronal connections are required which feed inhibitory and excitatory signals from one limb generator system to all the others based on what phase any one limb may be in at the time.

The activity of the limb pattern generators is believed to be determined by a central command system located in the midbrain which most likely operates via the reticulospinal tract. The command system sets each of the four limb generators to the same level of activity, and via their interneuronal connections, the generators coordinate changes in their own activity to produce the phasic pattern required for ambulation. In addition, the four pattern generators receive nonspecific input from the periphery which may independently trigger a level of activity. In the decorticate cat sustained noxious stimulation of its tail induces or speeds up walking movements. Likewise in the human, similar nonspecific noxious or threatening stimuli may be capable of directly setting the generators without first requiring cerebral interpretation and secondary resetting of the command system.

Additional postulated influences in setting the level of generator activity are so-called specific peripheral inputs from specific receptors. The hip joint capsule has been suggested as a location for specific receptors capable of setting the level of generator activity. Consider the situation of a person walking down a hill stumbling over something and about to fall foward. In such a situation, rapid

TABLE 19–2. The Main Muscle Functions Necessary for Normal Ambulation

Muscles	Gait Cycle Action
Quadriceps	HS to MST
	TO to MSW
Gluteus maximus	HS to MST
Gluteus medius and minimus	HS to TO
Tibialis anterior and peroneals	HS to FF
	TO to HS
Gastrocnemius and soleus	MST to TO
Iliopsoas and adductors	TO to MSW
Hamstrings	MSW to HS

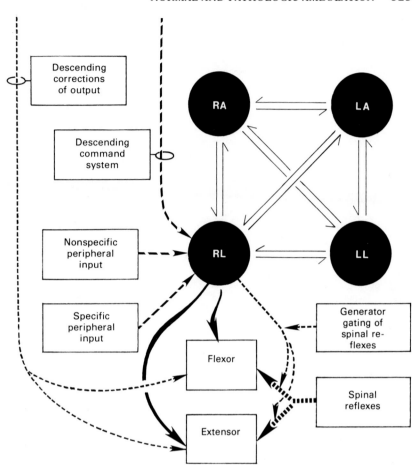

FIG. 19-17. Neural control of locomotion. The four pattern generators for each limb have interneuronal connections. The various inputs and outputs are illustrated only for the pattern generator of the right leg (RL). The right arm (RA), left arm (LA) and left leg (LL) generators would receive similar inputs. For explanation see text.

stepping occurs to abort the fall by bringing the base of support back under the center of mass. The specific input in this example is believed to be derived largely from receptors in the hip triggered by the hip movement at the impending fall. Impulses from the receptors then set the pattern generators to a higher level of activity, resulting in accelerated phasic movements of fast stepping.

This theory of the neural control of locomotion requires that the limb pattern generators directly stimulate the alpha and gamma motor neurons of the extensors and flexors of their respective limbs in the proper sequence to achieve the muscle contractions required for the gait cycle. The theory allows for two additional influences on the output of the generator systems capable of varying the amount or amplitude of alpha and gamma discharge that is triggered by the pattern generators. These are the descending pathways and the spinal reflexes. The rubrospinal tracts facilitate flexion and inhibit extension, while the vestibulospinal

tracts exert a reciprocal effect. The spinal reflexes in this scheme allow for load compensations. Changes in loads that alter spindle afferent and tendon organ discharge stimulate their respective reflex responses and modify the appropriate alpha and gamma discharge. Spinal reflexes, like some of the descending pathways, modify the output of the pattern generators and are not involved in setting the level of their activity. It is possible that the generators themselves have the ability of opening and closing different spinal reflex pathways.

Figure 19–17 summarizes the current status of the theory of neural control of locomotion. Modifications and corrections are certain to occur in this relatively new area of investigation.

GAIT DESCRIPTION

When a physician observes an abnormal gait, the sorting of simultaneously occurring events can pre-

A. CADENCE
    1. Symmetrical?
    2. Rhythmic?

B. TRUNK
    1. Fixed deviation   Lt   Rt?
    2. Lurch   Lt Rt?
       during stance of Rt or Lt leg?

C. PELVIS
    1. Fixed tilt? Lt?
              Rt?

    2. Drop? Lt?
           Rt?

D. BASE
    1. Stable?   Normal?
       Broad?   Narrow?
    2. Variable?
       Consistent?
       Inconsistent?

E. PAIN
    1. Where?
    2. When?

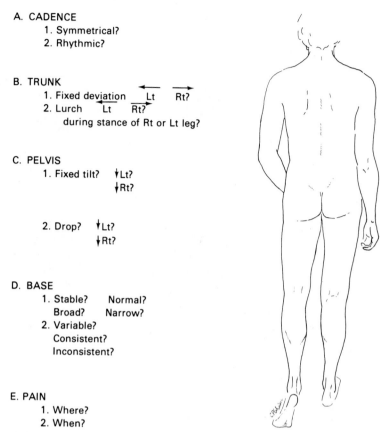

FIG. 19–18. Gait description. Major points of observation in front and back view.

sent a problem, unless the patient is observed in a systematic and disciplined manner. The description of the normal gait cycle and the classes of gait abnormalities which will be described below suggest a logical system of observation and recording which is also the most useful for analysis.

A patient is best observed with a minimum of clothing. Observations should be conducted where the space available is sufficiently long so that the patient can walk at his usual, most comfortable rate. Enough privacy should be assured so that self-consciousness should not interfere with the usual pattern. The patient should be observed walking in his usual shoes as well as barefoot. Both these activities occur in most people in the course of their daily life. Inspection of old shoes for the wear pattern is helpful. Ambulation should be observed from the side as well as from the front and back. All abnormalities should be recorded with reference to specific phases of the gait cycle separately for the right and left leg.

If **pain** is experienced during walking, the patient should signal its onset or indicate when it is more severe, so that its position in the gait cycle can be identified. The anatomic location of the pain is also important, but it should not be assumed that the seat of pathology is necessarily at the same site.

The **speed** should be noted as well as the **cadence,** paying particular attention to whether or not the time spent in the stance phase is equal on the two sides. The **symmetry** with regard to the left and right sides determines the unilaterality or bilaterality of the problem. **Reproducibility** of any abnormality with each gait cycle adds further to understanding.

In addition to the above general observations for pain, cadence, symmetry, and reproducibility, the following specific observations should be made 1) trunk lurches, 2) abnormal pelvic tilts, 3) stride lengths, 4) the base, and 5) the character of the heel strike, mid-stance, push-off, and mid-swing. Arm swing is also observed, although it is less informative. Some of these observations are best made while viewing the patient from the side and the others from a front or back view.

Front and Back View

Figure 19–18 summarizes the observations to be made in this view.

1. Front or back views give information about **trunk lurches** to either side during stance phase. Fixed scoliotic deformities are seen from the back and they are present both during stance and swing.
2. Exaggerated **pelvic tilts** must be watched for and can be highlighted by markers placed over both anterior and both posterior superior iliac spines. A belt snugly tightened below the iliac crests in the supine position will help to appreciate pelvic movement during locomotion.

The pelvis may dip on the contralateral side at each stance phase, or it may become elevated on the side of the swing leg. If a pelvic tilt or elevation is fixed, the deformity will not change whether the leg is in stance or in swing.

3. **Widening of the base** is readily detected by observing the distance between the feet at mid-stance-mid-swing. Sufficient *decrease in the base* can occur to produce foot or leg contact during swing with the leg crossing over or scissoring after mid-swing. The degree of **foot clearance** during mid-swing may be viewed from the front as well as from the side.
4. Phasic pain, cadence, symmetry, and reproducibility of any abnormality is observed and recorded.

Side View

Figure 19–19 summarizes the observations to be made from this view.

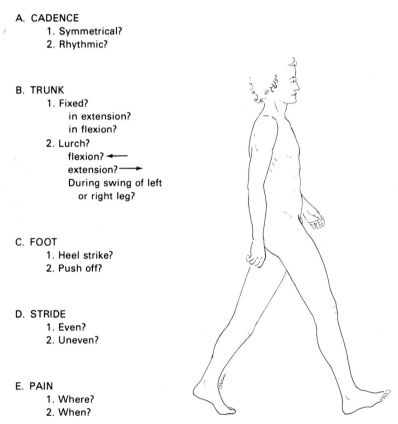

A. CADENCE
    1. Symmetrical?
    2. Rhythmic?

B. TRUNK
    1. Fixed?
        in extension?
        in flexion?
    2. Lurch?
        flexion? ←
        extension? →
        During swing of left
        or right leg?

C. FOOT
    1. Heel strike?
    2. Push off?

D. STRIDE
    1. Even?
    2. Uneven?

E. PAIN
    1. Where?
    2. When?

FIG. 19-19. Gait description. Major points of observation in side view.

1. Forward and backward **trunk lurches** are revealed in this view. Fixed kyphotic or lordotic curvatures of the spine are evident both during stance and swing, but lordosis may be phasic, visible only during stance. Trunk lurches may be secondary to foward or backward rotations of the pelvis about a transverse axis. Backward pelvic tilt is more difficult to detect.
2. Asymmetries in **stride length** are easy to observe. It is difficult to judge whether or not stride length is symmetrically short for both legs.
3. The nature of **heel strike** and the subsequent flexion of the knee are best observed in the side view.
4. The loudness of the sounds made at FF are also easy to relate visually to the gait cycle. Full contact of the sole of the foot at MST coupled with relative ankle dorsiflexion is also perceivable. It is more difficult to resolve a separate HO occurring just before TO, but viewing from the back may be helpful.
5. The degree of knee flexion and ankle dorsiflexion during mid-swing generally pose no observation problems.
6. The presence of phasic pain, cadence, symmetry, and reproducibility of abnormalities have to be confirmed in the side view as well.

GAIT ABNORMALITIES

It was noted at the beginning of this chapter that the most striking feature of abnormal gait is the compensation mechanism used for maintaining the most efficient method of locomotion while the underlying pathology more often than not is concealed. A **limp** is a deviation from the normal pattern of the gait cycle required to maintain ambulation in the face of the deficit. Analysis of this deviation leads to the diagnosis of the causal factor.

Gait abnormalities are causally derived from five classes of problems: 1) pain, 2) muscle weakness, 3) reduced range of passive joint movement, 4) CNS disturbances (which may also include weakness), and 5) functional inhibition.

In gait abnormalities caused by **pain,** the compensatory pattern adopted is the one which removes or diminishes the discomfort. The resultant pattern is known as an **antalgic gait.** In gaits secondary to **muscle weakness,** the compensatory pattern is largely but not exclusively the one which alters the location of the center of mass of the body with respect to the base of support **(paralytic gait).**

In situations where the **passive range of motion** is limited by structural factors in articular surfaces, ligaments, the capsule, or in the muscles that cross the joints, the compensatory mechanism usually exaggerates the motion ranges required by unaffected joints **(structural gait).** Compensations for **CNS problems** are more complex and are not as effective. They may involve attempts at adjusting the center of mass as well as increases in motion range. However, because a well functioning CNS is required for such adjustments, these adaptations are not effective. The resultant gait pattern is described as **neurologic gait. Functional inhibition** of the CNS may be conscious or subconscious. The term **hysterical gait** is usually applied to the subconscious variant, and **malingering** to conscious inhibition. Compensation mechanisms may be nonexistent, bizarre, or obvious (e.g., canes, crutches, wheelchair). The basic urge for maintaining normal ambulation may be superceded by psychological and emotional stress. The patient may withdraw from the stressful situation by exhibiting total inability or severe derangement of locomotion. This, in effect, relieves him or her from having to deal with the stressful circumstances. Furthermore, the patient may derive an important "secondary" gain when nonambulatory. The decision whether functional inhibition is conscious or subconscious is often difficult to make. Moreover, functional inhibition may be superimposed on organic pathology.

The following sections deal with some of the most common classes of abnormal gaits. The gait abnormalities associated with these are expressed and explained in terms of the principles of gait description presented in the previous section. Only the more important abnormalities are dealt with, however.

Antalgic Gaits

All antalgic gaits have several characteristics in common. Jarring is avoided, hence heel strike is usually absent. Stance phase on the affected side is reduced, hence contralateral swing phase is also shortened, which explains the reduced stride length on the contralateral side. The duration of swing phase, of course, determines stride length.

Midline Vertebral Pain. The gait pattern is symmetrical. Cadence is slow and the patient walks in a guarded manner. Trunk rotation is inhibited, resulting in reduced or absent pelvic tilt in midstance and pelvic rotation about a vertical axis, as well as arm swing. These inhibitions impart a guarded character to the gait. The stride lengths are short and heel strike is absent. If the pathology is associated with the vertebral bodies, the trunk leans backward throughout stance and swing, to minimize paraspinal muscle contraction. The latter would increase vertebral compression forces. If the pathology is posterior to the vertebral bodies, the trunk leans forward throughout the gait cycle.

Unilateral Back Pain. All the above features are the same as for midline pain except trunk posture. In soft tissue lesions, the trunk leans toward the affected side during stance and swing to reduce tension. In intervertebral disk disease with nerve root irritation, the trunk may lean toward the unaffected side during stance and swing to reduce intradiskal pressure, or it may lean toward the involved side to relax the tense nerve roots.

Hip Pain. The gait is asymmetrical, stance phase on the affected side is reduced, HS is absent, and toe walking prevails during stance. The hip is kept in flexion, abduction, and lateral rotation. This posture relaxes the ligaments of the hip and reduces joint tension. Flexion of the hip leads to knee flexion, and ankle plantar flexion. Flexion of all three joints characterizes all portions of the stance phase. Inhibition of hip medial rotation results in pivoting on the metatarsal heads of the affected side just before TO, and the base is widened during swing phase. For clearance of the limb during swing, pelvic elevation rather than downward tilt prevails. A trunk lurch toward the affected leg during stance completes the picture. The trunk lurch shifts the center of mass toward the affected side. This turns off hip abductor contraction in the stance leg and reduces the compression forces at the hip (Figs. 19–16, 19–20).

Knee Pain. A knee joint flexed at 25° provides the largest capsular volume and the least tension, if effusion is present. The ankle is plantar flexed in order to equalize "leg length" and hence only the toe contacts the ground throughout stance. Even without effusion, a painful knee will be kept flexed. An absent HS requires plantar flexion for metatarsophalangeal contact to occur with the ground. This shifts the gravitational force line anterior to the knee axis and creates an extension moment, therefore, minimizing the need for quadriceps contraction. Consequently, compression of the knee will be reduced by the same principle as the one which decreases hip compression forces by a lateral trunk lurch.

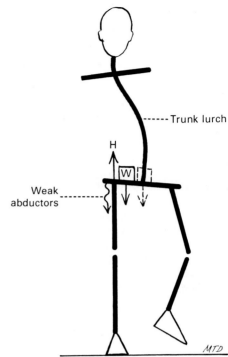

FIG. 19-20. Trunk lurch toward the painful hip of the stance leg shifts the center of mass (W) nearer to the hip and thus the force required of the abductors for balancing the pelvis becomes reduced (compare with Fig. 19–16). Therefore, the hip compression force becomes reduced proportionately. In hip abductor muscle weakness a similar trunk lurch compensates for the absence of hip abductor forces to maintain the pelvis level.

Ankle Pain. The usual range of ankle motion is reduced. The most comfortable angle is assumed throughout stance and swing. HS to FF phase may occur without plantar flexion. Instead, knee flexion after heel strike will be exaggerated and will compensate. HO may occur early after mid-stance to reduce relative dorsiflexion, and the heel may not rise as high before TO as normally, in order to reduce plantar flexion. There is asymmetry, and the stance phase is reduced as in all other unilateral lesions.

Foot Pain. Patterns depend on the location of discomfort. Lesions in the heel will eliminate heel strike and promote toe contact during stance. Metatarsal or phalangeal pain will eliminate HO, inhibit push-off, reduce forward thrust, and exaggerate hip and knee flexion during the first half of swing. Discomfort in the medial longitudinal arch also affects push-off. Contact with the ground may be restricted to the lateral border of the foot which is most convincingly revealed by the wear pattern of the shoes.

Neurologic Gait

Spasticity. The pathologic gait of spastic patients is due to exaggerated stretch reflexes coupled with reflex inhibition of antagonists. There may also be an element of disturbance in extensor-flexor coordination. However, reciprocal leg movement is established by spinal pattern generators. Adductor tonicity is usually present whether the basic spasticity is extensor or flexor.

Unilateral extensor spasticity is usually associated with upper motor neuron weakness of the hip abductors and therefore the trunk lurches toward the affected side during stance phase as in the paralytic gait with hip abductor weakness (p. 331). Pelvic elevation during swing of the affected leg is usually necessary for the swing leg to clear the floor. Heel strike is absent due to spasticity of plantar flexors which is coupled with upper motor neuron weakness of the ankle dorsiflexors. Midstance may be characterized by hyperextension of the knee secondary to spastic plantar flexors. Swing phase is characterized by absent or greatly reduced knee flexion due to quadriceps spasticity. Absent knee flexion coupled with a plantar flexion posture during swing contributes to circumduction which is associated with pelvic elevation. The affected leg advances with a short stride length and the base will be narrow. The leg may cross over due to adductor muscle spasticity.

In **unilateral flexor spasticity** ambulation may not be possible if the strength of the quadriceps is also reduced, because this results in an unstable knee during stance. If ambulation is possible, forward trunk lurch may be present. Both the affected and unaffected limb may show decreased stride length; the latter because leg advance requires hip extension range of motion on the contralateral side, which is restricted by the flexor spasticity. Heel strike may be absent and the base may be narrow with cross over.

Spastic gaits generally show slow cadence, asymmetry, particularly if the spasticity is unilateral, and abnormal patterns reproduce with each cycle.

Cerebellar Dysfunction. While reciprocal leg movements may be present due to the intact pattern generators, interference with cerebellar function abrogates precision and coordination in the gait. Leg placement will be variable and reproducibility will be lost. Each step, therefore, may be different as far as base and stride length are concerned. Deviation may also appear from the straight line of progression, reminiscent of acute alcoholic intoxication. The base will be wide to compensate for the balance disturbance but the compensation is often not effective. Stance phase may show a fully extended knee throughout, because a fully extended knee does not require quadriceps contraction. The cadence may not be slowed because a deliberate slow down exaggerates the problems of coordination.

Position Sense Impairment. Loss of position sense is usually symmetrical and so is the abnormal pattern. As long as vision remains good, the abnormal pattern will reproduce itself from cycle to cycle. The main compensation is a broadening of the base to increase the area of support. Foot contact may be accentuated for added sensory feedback. Heel strike may be absent to maintain a larger area of contact throughout stance.

Dysfunction of Basal Ganglia. Parkinson's disease is the most common pathology. It affects the basal ganglia bilaterally and the gait abnormality is also bilateral. Reproducibility is present and the cadence is faster rather than slower. The basic posture is one of trunk flexion, hip flexion, knee flexion, and ankle plantar flexion. Available joint motion is reduced throughout due to rigidity. Therefore, arm swing, pelvic tilt, pelvic rotation, and knee flexion are all greatly reduced. Load compensation is often nonexistent. The gait pattern is almost the same regardless of the terrain. Rapid compensatory adjustments do not occur in response to changes in the position of the center of mass. Therefore, falls are frequent. Adjustments are difficult for preventing a backward fall. Heel strike is usually absent, stance phase may be restricted to toe contact, and strides are short. The toe may be dragged during swing phase. The gravitational force line through the center of mass falls anterior to the base of support. This produces *festination*, an increase in speed, as the patient "chases after his center of mass" until he runs into an obstacle or is stopped by an attendant.

Paralytic Gait

Isolated paralytic gait patterns were more common prior to the control of poliomyelitis. They are still seen, of course, in the middle aged and elderly patients who contracted the disease in the 1950s or earlier. Isolated paralytic gait disturbances still occur due to acute trauma, nerve compression syndromes, spinal nerve root lesions, and peripheral mononeuritis. Quite often, however, paralytic disorders of various types coexist with gait patterns provoked by pain, limited range of motion, or even neurologic disturbances. This section discusses the patterns seen in seven of the more important paralytic conditions; and for the purpose of clarity, it is assumed that each condition is occurring unilaterally and in isolation. With these provisos, all the conditions produce asymmetrical, reproducible, and slower than normal locomotion.

Hip Flexor Weakness. Hip flexors are the accelerators in swing, and therefore only swing phase of the affected limb will be disturbed. Stance phase is unaffected. The trunk lurches backwards and toward the sound side. This accelerates the thigh on the affected side and promotes leg clearance during swing. Pelvic elevation may occur. Reduced hip acceleration at the beginning of swing and at midswing results in reduced knee flexion and the stride will be short on the affected side.

Hip Extensor Weakness. Hip extensors contract after heel strike, therefore, if paralyzed, abnormality appears during stance of the affected limb and begins with heel strike. A backward trunk lurch occurs and persists throughout stance to maintain the gravitational force line behind the hip axis, locking the hip in extension (Fig. 19–3). The knee usually remains in full extension during stance.

Hip Abductor Weakness. During stance phase of the affected side, the pelvis will dip to the side of the swing leg by more than the usual 5°. Lateral trunk lurch toward the affected side (stance leg) compensates for the weakness, because with the lurch a reduced hip abductor force is required to maintain a level pelvis (Fig. 19–20). Minimal abductor weakness is usually uncompensated because the trunk does not lurch, rather an excessive pelvic tilt is tolerated. A compensated gait includes trunk lurch and occurs with severe weakness. A contralateral cane eliminates trunk lurch (Fig. 19–21). In both compensated and uncompensated gait there will be exaggerated hip and knee flexion on the side of the sound limb at midswing, if the pelvic tilt is greater than the normal 5°.

Knee Extensor Weakness. The pattern in knee

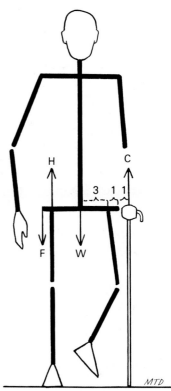

FIG. 19–21. Effect of a cane on the compression forces at the hip contralateral to the side of the cane. If a patient weighing 165 lb leans on the cane with a force of 60 lb, the force operating at the contralateral hip may be calculated as follows (W = body weight; F = abduction force; H = hip compression force; C = force acting on the cane):
Clockwise moment = Counterclockwise moment
$$W \times 3 = F \times 1 + C \times 8$$
$$165 \times 3 = F + 60 \times 8$$
$$F = 15 \text{ lb}$$
Vertical forces up = Vertical forces down
$$H + C = W + F$$
$$H + 60 = 165 + 15$$
$$H = 120 \text{ lb}$$
Comparison with Figure 19–16 shows that a force of 60 lb applied to the cane reduces the hip compression force from 660 to 120 lb.

extensor weakness may be hardly noticeable in level ground ambulation. The patient is at risk mainly after heel strike when the knee normally flexes while the quadriceps contracts. Action of hip extensor and plantar flexor muscles at heel strike can hold the knee in extension and sustain it in extension throughout stance. The gluteus maximus executes this function nicely via the iliotibial tract. A forward trunk lurch at heel strike also compensates adequately because it moves the center of mass force line anterior to the knee axis. Some patients place their hand on their thigh at heel strike and stance to assist the knee in the extended position. The absent quadriceps action will produce excess knee flexion during swing phase and the heel may rise quite high, particularly with fast walking.

Knee Flexor Weakness. Weakness of the hamstrings causes a loss of deceleration at the end of swing phase, and full knee extension remains unchecked just before heel strike. The unchecked leg produces an "overshoot" and a hard heel strike. During late stance, the knee remains in full extension until toe off because the reactive knee extension force from the floor is unopposed. These two abnormalities of gait contribute to progressive *genu recurvatum* ("back knee").

Ankle Dorsiflexor Weakness. If strength is still sufficient to lift the weight of the foot during swing only stance phase is disturbed. The HS to FF phase occurs rapidly and with an audible slap. If dorsiflexor paralysis is complete, there will be no heel strike and the first contact is made with the toes or with the entire foot. Furthermore, swing phase is associated with increased hip or knee flexion to clear the foot ("steppage gait").

Ankle Plantar Flexor Weakness. At the end of the stance, heel-off does not occur and the forward propulsive force is greatly diminished. The foot leaves the ground as a unit. The absence of heel-off promotes full knee extension in late stance. Hip flexion may be increased to lift off the leg as swing begins.

Structural Gait; Reduced Range of Passive Joint Movement

The terms *deformity* and *contracture* are frequently applied with an appropriate adjective to designate limitation of motion. **Contracture** usually refers to limitation caused by soft tissues, while **deformity** means limitation due either to soft tissue or bone. **Ankylosis** means the joint is consolidated due to fusion of the bones (bony ankylosis) or to excessive fibrosis (fibrous ankylosis).

An adjective pertaining to movement usually precedes these terms and designates the motion or position favored. It is the *opposite* motion which is restricted. Thus, **flexion deformity means a limitation of extension.** Quite incorrectly, the term contracture is sometimes used when the limitation is due to bony deformity. This use should be avoided.

This section discusses gait abnormalities in which deformity limits movement at hip, knee, and ankle. The term deformity rather than contracture will be used because it includes limitation of motion due to bony or soft tissue factors or to both. The problems of unequal leg length are also discussed since this abnormality also falls in the structural group. All the examples are unilateral deficits and, hence, are asymmetrical. Reproducibility and a reduced cadence characterize all these gaits.

Hip Flexion Deformity. Reduced hip extension results in a reduced stride length of the *unaffected* limb. MST of the affected limb may show increased knee flexion. Toe walking or early HO during stance occurs with large flexion deformities. Reduced hip extension is compensated for by lumbar lordosis after midstance. If the back is not supple, a foward trunk lurch may appear instead.

Hip Extension Deformity. Stride length is reduced on the *affected* side. Lumbar flexion occurs at heel strike if the back is supple because of the upward pelvic rotation. If the back is not supple, the trunk lurches backward at heel strike. In order to clear the foot during swing of the affected leg, knee flexion or pelvic elevation may be exaggerated.

Hip Adduction Deformity. Figure 16–11 shows the pelvic elevation of the affected side that must occur during stance and swing of the affected leg. An associated functional scoliosis convex to the opposite side is compensatory to keep the center of mass over the limb, particularly in stance. A trunk lurch toward the affected leg in stance may also occur. A narrow base with a tendency to scissor as the affected limb swings through may be observed intermittently. The apparent leg length will be shorter as a consequence of the contracture. This is alleviated by toe walking throughout stance, coupled with exaggerated hip and knee flexion on the sound side.

Hip Abduction Deformity. With loss of hip adduction the pattern is almost identical to that seen in hip adduction contracture except that the opposite limb is affected. Thus, the pelvis is elevated on the sound side during stance and swing, toe walking is seen on the sound side during stance, and the functional scoliosis is convex toward the affected side. The difference is in the base. In hip abduction deformity the base tends to be broad rather than narrow.

Hip Rotation Deformity. Loss of both medial and lateral rotation results in decreased stride lengths on both sides. During the stance phase the foot pivots in a lateral direction on the affected side. This rotation takes place during the FF to TO period.

Knee Flexion Deformity. Lack of full knee extension reduces the stride length of the affected leg. Heel strike may not occur and the heel may remain off the ground during stance as if the leg were short. The forward propulsive thrust is weakened because of the inability to achieve the degree of knee extension required at push-off. If the short leg effect is severe (e.g., 30° of flexion deformity) the sound limb may show increased hip and knee flexion during swing.

Knee Extension Deformity. Limitation of knee flexion is most apparent during swing phase. Pelvic elevation and limb circumduction clear the foot off the ground. The sound leg maintains only toe contact during stance, assisting clearance of the affected leg.

Ankle Plantar Flexion Deformity. Absence of dorsiflexion results in an absent heel strike. Toe contact persists throughout stance, which forces knee extension and may lead to genu recurvatum. The force of forward thrust at toe-off is diminished. Hip and knee flexion is exaggerated during swing (steppage gait) to clear the plantar flexed foot.

Leg Length Inequality. If the legs are of unequal length, the vertical amplitude for the oscillation of the center of mass becomes greater. Compensations adopted are those that attempt to achieve an equal effective leg length in order to reduce this vertical oscillation. If the shortening is 3–4 cm. or more, heel strike on the affected leg is absent and toe walking prevails throughout stance with full knee extension. Stride length of the shorter leg is reduced, and during stance the longer limb swings through with increased hip and knee flexion to clear the foot. Stance phase of the longer leg also shows increased hip and knee flexion. For shorter inequalities, heel strike may occur as stance begins but heel-off appears early after mid-stance. The pelvis drops on the short side when heel strike occurs and remains tilted throughout stance. The trunk shifts to the affected side.

Functional Inhibition Gait

"Hysterical" gaits can take many forms. The patterns that vary widely with each gait cycle are usually easy to detect. The patient may reel, move bizarrely from side to side, stop in stance phase balancing on one leg with shaking limbs and flailing arms. The patient may lunge toward walls, tables, or other people to hold on to tightly. Rarely does an injurious fall occur.

Those patterns that reproduce with each gait cycle are more difficult to detect, particularly if they begin "legitimately" with an injury or disease. If the pattern persists for a sufficient length of time, secondary changes confuse the analysis. Atrophy, vasomotor instability, and edema may be seen, all secondary to disuse. A high index of suspicion should prevail when neurologic and musculoskeletal examination does not seem to match the observed gait abnormality, and when the source for associated pain cannot be defined. Electrical stimulation of nerves and needle electromyographic examination of muscle can help immeasurably in clarifying apparent weakness. Strength testing usually shows quick or rachety release when resistance is applied, and twitchlike voluntary efforts when the patient is asked to contract involved muscles.

Some of the more common reproducible patterns include:

1. Full knee extension through stance
2. Knee buckling just before heel strike of the opposite limb
3. A dropped foot during swing
4. Absent heel strike and absent heel-off
5. Toe walking during stance
6. Foot inversion during stance
7. Use of hands on the anterior aspect of the thigh during stance
8. Use of hands to help the leg through during swing
9. Full contact of the foot on the floor during swing associated with markedly reduced stride length and rotation of the foot and hip
10. Reduced duration of stance phase of the involved leg
11. Use of cane or crutch on the side of the affected leg

SUGGESTED READING

Bard G, Ralston HJ: Measurement of energy expenditure during ambulation with special reference to evaluation of assistive devices. Arch Phys Med Rehabil 40: 415, 1959
An experimental analysis of the energy expenditure during ambulation at various velocities. Normal subjects, amputees, and crutch walkers are included.

Grillner S: Locomotion in vertebrates: central mechanisms and reflex interaction. Physiol Rev 55: 247, 1975
Review of the animal studies which led to the theory for pattern generators.

Herman RM, Grillner S, Stein PS, Stuart DG (eds): Proceedings of International Conference on Neural Control of Locomotion. In Advances in Behavioral Biology, Vol 18. New York, Plenum, 1976
A compendium of studies and discussions on neural control of ambulation in the human.

Klopsteg PE, Wilson, PD: Human Limbs and Their Substitutes. New York, McGraw-Hill, 1954, p. 437
One of the better discussions of angular motions and muscle activity at the various joints during ambulation.

Saunders JB DeC M, Inman VT, Eberhart HD: The major determinants in normal and pathological gait. J Bone Joint Surg [A] 35: 543, 1953
The basic initial analysis of the center of mass oscillation during ambulation as determined by point motions

Steindler A: Kinesiology. Springfield, IL, Charles C Thomas, 1955
Pages 655–691 give a good basic description of pathologic gaits.

20
Congenital Defects of the Musculoskeletal System

STERLING K. CLARREN, JANE G. SCHALLER

Congenital defects (birth defects) of the musculo-skeletal system include those bony and muscular abnormalities that are determined during intrauterine life as well as those that develop after birth and are secondary to other congenitally determined causes. Congenital defects of the musculoskeletal system represent a large and heterogenous group of anomalies that result from multiple biochemical and biomechanical disorders. These may be found in isolation or associated with other musculoskeletal diseases. They may also coexist with congenital anomalies of other organ systems.

Musculoskeletal defects are an important cause of morbidity and mortality in both children and adults. Accurate understanding of these abnormalities is important in determining the full scope of a patient's problems, appropriately treating the disorder, and in counseling the family.

ETIOLOGY AND PATHOGENESIS

Congenital defects of the musculoskeletal system, like other anomalies, can be etiologically classified as primary or secondary malformations, disruptions, or deformations. Such a classification is useful in anticipating possible associated anomalies as well as for predicting the long-term outcome, which is discussed later in this chapter. Most defects can now be classified through this system, although the genetic and environmental causes of many of these defects remain unknown.

Primary Malformations

Defects that occur early in gestation, when the skeleton and the limbs are forming, are clas-sified as primary malformations. The critical period spans embryonic stages XII to XXII, approximately between day 26 and 51 of gestation. In many primary limb malformations, both bone and muscle primordia are affected and there may be partial or complete failure of limb formation (amelia, aplasia, hypoplasia) or the limb may be abnormally formed (dysplasia). Such defects are usually obvious at birth. The tissues that remain may be quite normal histologically and biochemically, yet they may be assembled to produce a grossly abnormal limb. Such is the case in radial ray agenesis, where skeletal and soft-tissue elements of one or more rays of the hand or foot are completely missing (see Fig. 8–4A). On the other hand, the abnormality may be in the structure of the tissues as in achondroplasia, where all gross anatomical units of the limbs are present. Other primary limb anomalies permit relatively normal initial limb formation. Defects in bone, such as osteogenesis imperfecta, or in muscle, such as the muscular dystrophies, may be entirely concealed during the newborn period and only become manifest much later in life.

Limb malformations have been associated with all types of genetic inheritance patterns. Autosomal dominant, recessive, sex-linked, and polygenic modes have all been linked to specific isolated types of limb malformations and to generalized syndromes that involve the limbs. Extragenetic material, such as found in trisomy 18 or trisomy 21 syndromes, have characteristic malformations of the hands and feet that are often useful clues in making the correct overall diagnosis.

Environmental agents are also known to cause primary limb malformations. This was tragically exemplified by the drug thalidomide. Ingestion of

335

this drug by a pregnant woman from day 38 to 42 of gestation resulted in partial or complete failure of limb development (phocomelia). No other environmental agents are known to produce similar devastating limb anomalies, but ethanol, antiepilepsy drugs, and some other agents produce mild limb anomalies as part of more general malformation syndromes.

Secondary Malformations

Anomalies of the bones, joints, or muscles that result from intrinsic malformations in other embryonic tissues or systems are classified as secondary congenital malformations. Most secondary musculoskeletal malformations are attributable to primary malformations in the nervous system or to intrinsic metabolic disturbances. Secondary malformations may be apparent at birth or they may be recognized some time later.

Lower motor neuron lesions within the fetal spinal cord can lead to neurogenic muscle atrophy. The resulting muscular imbalance within and around a fetal joint may then lead to diminished joint movement. Resultant joint damage and stiffness is called arthrogryposis. Such abnormalities are most commonly encountered in infants with meningomyelocele (Chap. 9).

Upper motor neuron lesions are attributable to primary malformations of the brain or to destructive brain lesions caused by anoxia, vascular accident, metabolic processes, or infection and may lead to postnatal limb spasticity that results in eventual joint fixations or dislocations.

Congenital hypothyroidism, vitamin D deficiency, and other metabolic processes may lead to secondary bony dysplasia. Early diagnosis in these circumstances is imperative, because early intervention can often restore full function.

Disruptions

Intrauterine events that partially or completely destroy the limb after it has completed its normal embryogenesis are called disruptions. A common disruption is caused by a band constriction. There is still some debate over the origin of these bands. Most observers presently believe they develop from amniotic strands that become detached from the amniotic wall and wrap around the fetal limb. As the limb grows in circumference the amniotic strands become increasingly constricting and the structures distal to the band may become hypoplastic, dysplastic or completely amputated.

A different kind of disruption may be caused by infections. Rubella, syphilis, toxoplasma, and other organisms are known to produce bony changes in the fetal skeleton which are apparent radiologically. *In utero* vascular accidents caused by embolic phenomena have recently been proposed as another cause for disruption in fetal limb morphogenesis.

Deformations

Abnormalities that occur late in gestation, after week 30, and are produced by extrinsic compressive forces are classified as deformations. They are manifest as aberrant molding of otherwise normal fetal tissues.

The usual accommodation of the fetal head in the pelvic cavity of the mother (vertex presentation) during late gestation maximizes the uterine space and permits the fetus to stretch and maintain reasonably functional limbs. Increased compressive forces may lead to deformities in the cephalic position but other positions are more likely to give rise to deformities. Uterine constraint is more likely in first born infants when the uterine muscle tone is greatest; or in any pregnancy if the fetus is unusually large or if there is diminished amniotic fluid. Additional structures occupying intrauterine space may also restrict fetal movement. Examples are multiple fetuses and uterine fibroids. A bicornuate uterus may have similar restricting effects. Compression may also be generated outside the uterus from strong abdominal muscles, a prominent lumbar spine, or a small, bony pelvis.

The most common congenital deformities are the various types of clubfoot, namely talipes, metatarsus adductus, and calcaneovalgus (see Chap. 18). Many cases of muscular torticollis and dislocated hip are also from constraint. Occasionally, congenital scoliosis and genu recurvation may also be considered deformations.

INCIDENCE

One in almost every 10 live-born humans has some congenital defect warranting concern. About half of these abnormalities can be detected in the newborn period; the rest declare themselves at variable times, though generally during childhood. The overall incidence of congenital defects of the musculoskeletal system is not known, and only estimates can be made. Significant malformations and disruptions of the limbs occur in about 1 in 250 live births and account for about 4 percent of total birth defects. Deformities of the limbs occur in perhaps 1 in 50 infants and account for at least 20 percent of all congenital anomalies.

Malformations from genetic causes may have a predilection for certain racial groups. Many malformations affect one sex more than the other. Unfortunately, a comprehensive discussion of these specific high-risk groups for limb malformations goes beyond the scope of this chapter.

Deformations may also occasionally have a sexual or racial predilection, although they are not directly caused by genetic factors. Congenital dislocated hip, for example, occurs at least four times more frequently in females than males (see Chap. 16). It is more common in whites than blacks. It more often involves the left side, if unilateral. There are physiologic differences that account for these variations.

1. The female fetus seems to have more ligamentous laxity than the male, making deformity more likely.

2. The fetus has been shown to typically lie with its left side towards the mother's back, regardless of cephalic or breech presentation. In this posture, the left upper leg is constrained by the maternal lumbar spine and is more likely to remain adducted, predisposing to its dislocation.

3. The Negroid pelvis is generally more spacious than its Caucasian counterpart and hence is less constraining.

DIAGNOSIS AND MANAGEMENT

For the first few days after birth, a baby can usually be folded into the uterine position. Infants with deformities can usually be folded into an atypical bundle, which reconstitutes their abnormal fetal posture. While a normal newborn would usually object to such unusual positioning, the deformed baby will prefer this posture and will often cry in protest when stretched into a more usual newborn position. By placing the baby in his preferred uterine position, the deformities in question can be understood, and associated deformities may be anticipated. For example, a baby with metatarsus adductus has a higher than average chance of having dislocated hips.

In general, deformed babies have no increased risk of having malformations. The only notable exception to this is Potter's syndrome, where extensive renal anomalies lead to oligohydramnios, which produces uterine constraint.

Disruptions can often be distinguished from malformations by the nonembryonic pattern of the anomaly. Sometimes, however, it is difficult to distinguish these types of abnormalities. Disruptions from amniotic bands generally occur in isolation, while disruptions from infection or infarction may be associated with other problems.

Finding any malformation should stimulate the examiner to carefully search for other malformations. The bibliography at the end of this chapter refers to texts that present known patterns of malformations.

Initial classification of anomalies along these lines is important not only in directing the rest of the physical examination, but in successfully managing the patient and counseling the family as well.

Early Correction

Deformations usually resolve spontaneously or can be corrected with *early* bracing, which molds via mild pressure towards the more desired form. If, for example, constraint has led to dislocated hip, and this is recognized at birth, prompt treatment with an abductor splint can result in total resolution. If the abnormality goes untreated until later in childhood, a return to a completely normal hip may never be possible, even with surgery.

Malformations and disruptions are often more difficult to treat than deformations both from the functional and cosmetic point of view. Long-term medical and surgical treatment is often required. A dislocated hip secondary to meningomyelocele, for example, may look clinically and radiographically similar to a hip dislocated by constraint. In this case, however, the hip is dislocated because of intrinsic muscle imbalance rather than extrinsic constraining. Generally splinting alone will not restore function; surgery is often needed and a perfect result is difficult to achieve.

Prevention of Secondary Deformities

Deformities not present at birth are likely to occur in persons with abnormal bones, for example, osteogenesis imperfecta and vitamin–D–resistant rickets, or in those with muscle imbalance, as in meningomyelocele, muscular dystrophy, and cerebral palsy. External support (bracing), exercise to develop the weak muscles, and the transfer of muscles to provide better balance frequently prevents serious bone deformities, joint subluxations, or dislocations. In such instances, the patient must be carefully followed throughout his growth phase.

Family Counseling

Early family counseling is important to help the family adjust to the problems of the patient and to guide in the planning of future children. Parents of infants with deformities can generally be assured that their child will improve through simple, conservative forms of therapy and will be fully functional in time. Parents of infants with major malformations or disruptions need to be told of the long-term, generally chronic, nature of the child's problem. Medical and social counseling for such parents is an ongoing task as the parents slowly come to understand the full nature of their child's problems.

Usually families also want to know if the abnormalities found in the youngster could recur. In general, deformations do not recur unless the mother has an anatomic abnormality (i.e., fibroids, bicornuate uterus, prominent lumbar spine). Similarly, disruptions usually do not recur. Malformations of either genetic or teratogenic origin may recur. In cases of malformations, accurate syndrome diagnosis and careful family histories are necessary to accurately predict the risk of recurrence.

Treatment Directed Toward the Whole Patient

In treating a patient with a congenital malformation, it is important to consider other associated anomalies as well as the patient's psychologic and social adjustment to his condition. An appropriate course of management can only be determined after a comprehensive understanding of the patient's medical problems and his adjustments to them. For example, major surgical corrections are not warranted in infants with lethal congenital malformations. Treatment so extensive that it would totally interfere with the normal

social development of the child may also be contraindicated.

Treatment Directed to Adaptations for Living

In many instances deformities are not correctable. Counseling and support to the child and family thus become vital aspects of management. The family must learn to accept the child and develop his strengths while minimizing his disabilities. The child should be encouraged to develop as normally as possible with the maximum amount of self sufficiency.

SUGGESTED READING

Bergsma D, Leuz W (eds): Morphogenesis and Malformations of the Limb. National Foundation–March of Dimes, Birth Defects: Original Article Series, Vol. 13, No. 1. New York, Alan R Liss, Inc, 1977
Nineteen articles by experts in the field consider such aspects of congenital limb anomalies as chemical and genetic factors, chromosomal aberrations, critical period of limb development, pathogenic mechanisms of skeletal dysplasias and classification of limb malformations.

Rubin P: Dynamic Classification of Bone Dysplasias. Chicago, Year Book Publishers, 1964
This work details the embryology and development of bone and malformations that may occur during the process of bone modeling.

Smith DW: Recognizable Patterns of Human Malformation. 2nd ed Philadelphia, W. B. Saunders, 1976
This work details over 200 malformation syndromes and is invaluable as an aid to the identification of syndromes and associated anomalies.

Smith DW: Compendium on shortness of stature. J. Pediatr 7: 463, 1967
Short stature is a skeletal abnormality of overall size, often occurring in conjunction with other specific musculoskeletal malformations. This work presents an extensive collection and description of known syndromes associated with congenital short stature in humans.

Swinyard CA (ed): Limb Development and Deformity: Problems in Evaluation and Rehabilitation. Springfield, Charles C Thomas, 1969
This collection of articles deals with normal and anomalous limb development, known causes of limb abnormalities in humans, and the management of such conditions.

Warkany J, Kalter H: Congenital malformations. New Engl J Med 265: 993–1001 and 1046–1052, 1961
This excellent, general work defines and discusses what is meant by "congenital malformations," presents speculation about factors which may cause them, and summarizes such etiologic factors as genetic abnormalities, chromosomal abnormalities, and environmental factors.

21
Metabolic Bone Disease

ABNER GOLDEN

Bone is a living, actively metabolizing tissue. Throughout life, it is constantly being remodeled by the resorption of existing calcified bone and concurrent new bone formation. These two processes are normally in close balance. Metabolic bone disease represents a significant departure from this balance, resulting in a decrease in skeletal mass (osteopenia), or an increase in total mineralized bone (osteosclerosis). With few exceptions, metabolic bone diseases affect the entire skeleton, albeit not equally in all parts of the body.

This chapter reviews the dynamics of bone formation and bone resorption, deriving a classification of metabolic bone disease based on disturbances of each of these phases. Detailed consideration will then be given to the two most important metabolic bone diseases observed in this country—renal osteodystrophy and osteoporosis. The chapter closes with a brief discussion of Paget's disease of bone. Although not usually considered a metabolic bone disease, its clinical manifestations and morphologic findings reflect a markedly altered rate of bone turnover and remodeling.

THE REMODELING OF BONE

Three distinct phases in the remodeling of bone are recognizable; the secretion of bone matrix (osteoid), the accretion of bone salt, and the resorption of mineralized bone. The younger the bone, the more rapid the rate of turnover. In general, there is a net increase in skeletal mass till the age of about 50 years, then a steady decline.

Matrix Secretion

The constant remodeling of bone is in response to the stresses placed on the skeleton. It is also the basis for the development of the haversian system of secondary osteons that characterize mature compact bone (see Chap. 2). The significance of stress as the most important, and perhaps the only, direct stimulus to new bone matrix formation is illustrated by the rapidity of loss of skeletal mass observed in astronauts during periods of living in a weightless environment. Impairment of osteoblastic collagen secretion (or its maturation) in response to stress is observed in generalized malnutrition, in severe vitamin C deficiency, and in patients with Cushing's syndrome or those receiving prolonged corticosteroid therapy. Each of these conditions is associated with deficient protein synthesis. Other factors affect bone remodeling, either directly or indirectly. Growth hormone is essential to normal skeletal development, particularly to epiphyseal growth, and excessive secretion of this hormone leads to gigantism or acromegaly. Gonadal hormones, particularly testosterone, generally stimulate new bone formation, although they also hasten the closure of epiphyses, thus limiting longitudinal growth. Thyroid hormone increases the turnover rate of bone and favors resorption. Corticosteroids, in addition to altering collagen synthesis, interfere with mineral absorption from the intestinal tract.

Bone Mineralization

Mineralization of newly formed bone matrix requires certain minimal concentrations of calcium and phosphorus in the extracellular fluid, but it occurs over a rather broad range of values. Although it has proven empirically useful to speak of a Ca × P product, it has no biologic or biochemical significance. The mechanism of mineralization of bone is poorly understood. It is not clear why the collagen of bone is normally mineralized, whereas that of other body tissues is not. While characteristics of the ground substance may be critical to this process, it is likely that the physical properties of the collagen fibrils themselves, particularly their banding, favor the nucleation of hydroxyapatite. In any event, the pattern of mineralization closely follows the organization of collagen fibrils, a prerequisite to the strength of mature bone.

Bone Resorption

The resorption of bone is intimately related to and dependent upon calcium homeostasis. Since 99 percent of body calcium is in the skeleton, bone is the only readily available source of mineral to maintain normal levels in the blood and extracellular fluid. Exchanges of mineral between bone and extracellular fluid occur continuously at the interface between bone surfaces and their surrounding hydration shells. This is a simple and rapid physicochemical mechanism. Cellular mechanisms of maintaining calcium homeostasis involve resorption of mineralized bone by osteoclasts, and to a lesser degree, by osteocytes.

Parathyroid Hormone, Calcitonin, and Vitamin D

The several hormones involved in calcium homeostasis invariably affect the structure of bone. **Parathyroid hormone** is rapidly synthesized and secreted in response to a fall in the level of ionized calcium in the circulation. This hormone, which has a half-life of but a few minutes, stimulates osteoclastic and osteocytic resorption of bone, and increases renal phosphate excretion. Since both bone matrix and minerals are resorbed, there is elevation of serum calcium and hydroxyproline, and both may appear in the urine. As soon as the serum ionized calcium level returns to normal, the synthesis and secretion of parathyroid hormone return to baseline levels.

Calcitonin is secreted by the parafollicular cells of the thyroid gland. Although not directly antagonistic to parathyroid hormone, calcitonin acts on bone so as to inhibit bone resorption. It is secreted in response to an elevation of serum ionized calcium. Parathyroid hormone and calcitonin thus constitute a relatively simple control mechanism, responding directly and rapidly to altered serum calcium levels. The serum level of inorganic phosphorus has no direct bearing on the secretion of parathyroid hormone and calcitonin, although it can affect calcium balance by its relationship to vitamin D metabolism.

Vitamin D is responsible for calcium (and phosphorus) transport from the intestinal tract. It also plays a permissive role in the calcium mobilizing action of parathyroid hormone on bone, and indeed, itself directly stimulates resorption. Before it is biologically effective, however, it must be acted upon by the liver to form 25-hydroxycholecalciferol, and then converted to the hormone $1,25(OH)_2$-cholecalciferol in the kidney. The rate of secretion of this hormone is regulated by the blood levels of ionized calcium and inorganic phosphorus. Decreased calcium levels lead to an increased synthesis of $1,25(OH)_2$-cholecalciferol by stimulating secretion of parathyroid hormone. Decreased circulating phosphorus levels also stimulate $1,25(OH)_2$-cholecalciferol synthesis, but this action is unrelated to and independent of the parathyroid glands.

CLASSIFICATION OF METABOLIC BONE DISEASE

Most metabolic bone diseases can be regarded as quantitative alterations of one or more of the three component phases of normal bone turnover; osteoid secretion, mineralization of bone matrix, and cellular resorption of mineralized bone. The term **osteopenia** denotes an overall loss of mineralized bone mass; **osteosclerosis,** an increase. The former can result from impaired osteoid synthesis, failure to mineralize normal osteoid, or from accelerated resorption. Osteosclerosis can be the product of excessive matrix formation, or failure of normal bone resorption.

Osteoporosis designates a group of conditions characterized by atrophy of bone. In many, there is a disorder of connective tissue or protein metabolism reflected in a failure to produce normal bone matrix. That matrix which is formed is normally calcified, and resorption of bone continues at a normal or reduced rate. In others, osteoporosis appears to be the result of a low grade but persistent increase in bone resorption. The serum calcium and inorganic phosphorus values are normal. Serum alkaline phosphatase and urinary hydroxyproline excretion are generally normal or slightly reduced, reflecting a low turnover rate of bone.

Osteomalacia results from disordered mineral metabolism such that there is failure of crystallization of bone salt in osteoid. When this occurs prior to the closure of epiphyses, the term **rickets** is applied. The resulting weakness of the adult or growing skeleton makes it highly susceptible to stress, and excessive amounts of osteoid are produced. Serum values are low for calcium, inorganic phosphorus, or both, but alkaline phosphatase is elevated.

Osteitis fibrosa is the bone disease resulting from a greatly accelerated rate of osteoclastic (and probably osteocytic) resorption of bone. It is almost always related to increased secretion of parathyroid hormone. When osteitis fibrosa results from primary hyperparathyroidism (e.g., parathyroid adenoma), the serum calcium is high, the inorganic phosphorus low. The alkaline phosphatase is markedly elevated, reflecting acceleration of both new bone formation and resorption. When the bone changes are due to renal failure and secondary hyperparathyroidism, elevation of serum phosphorus and depression of serum calcium are the rule.

Increased matrix formation is the mechanism leading to osteosclerosis in disorders of growth hormone secretion and in the healing of osteomalacia. Decreased bone resorption is the mechanism in hypoparathyroidism.

Table 21–1 presents a classification of metabolic bone disease. It is not meant to be complete,

TABLE 21–1. Classification of Metabolic Bone Disease

I. OSTEOPENIA

A. Osteoporosis
Senile osteoporosis
Immobilization
Shoulder–hand syndrome
Osteogenesis imperfecta
Malnutrition
  Scurvy
  Protein deficiency
Endocrine disorders
  Cushing's syndrome
  Corticosteroid therapy
  Hyperthyroidism
  Ovarian dysgenesis

B. Osteomalacia
Renal failure
Malabsorption syndromes
  Gluten enteropathy
  Nontropical sprue
  Chronic pancreatitis
  Cystic fibrosis
Vitamin D deficiency
Renal tubular acidosis
Anticonvulsant therapy
  (phenytoin)

C. Osteitis fibrosa
Renal failure
Primary hyperparathyroidism
Vitamin D intoxication
? Bone resorbing substances secreted by some neoplasms

II. OSTEOSCLEROSIS

A. Increased matrix production
Acromegaly
Renal failure
Osteofluorosis

B. Reduced resorption
Hypoparathyroidism
Osteopetrosis

rather it illustrates the points made in this chapter. Note that renal failure is listed in three locations. The reason for this will become clear in the discussion of renal osteodystrophy.

RENAL OSTEODYSTROPHY

Renal osteodystrophy is a complex metabolic bone disturbance observed in association with chronic renal failure. Now that many patients with end-stage kidney disease are kept alive for years on dialysis, this bone disorder has become commonplace and constitutes one of the most difficult and frustrating aspects of renal failure to manage. It causes severe bone pain, frequently aggravated rather than alleviated by hemodialysis. The findings in bone consist of a variable mixture of osteomalacia, osteitis fibrosa, and osteosclerosis.

Pathogenesis

At least two mechanisms may be involved in the pathogenesis of the bone changes. As nephrons are lost in progressive renal disease, there is retention of inorganic phosphorus which leads indirectly to a decrease in blood calcium. The parathyroid glands secrete increased amounts of parathyroid hormone which returns the blood calcium to normal through resorption of bone, and lowers the blood phosphorus by inhibiting its resorption in the proximal renal tubules. A new equilibrium is reached, with essentially normal calcium and phosphorus levels, but at the expense of continuously increased parathyroid function and the development of osteitis fibrosa.

Although the above mechanism may play a significant role, particularly in early renal failure, a far more important explanation is based on the failure of the chronically diseased kidney to complete the hydroxylation of cholecalciferol. Loss of this function may be the result of elevated tissue levels of phosphorus in the renal cortex. The result is markedly decreased intestinal transport of calcium, and impairment, at least at first, of the calcium mobilizing effect of parathyroid hormone. New osteoid is not mineralized. The bones become more subject to stress, and increasing amounts of osteoid are deposited, appearing as thick seams on the surface of older mineralized lamellae. The bones tend to become bowed and deformed, particularly the long bones of the limbs. When the disorder occurs in children, there is marked disturbance of endochondral bone formation at the epiphyseal plate, with massive accumulation of

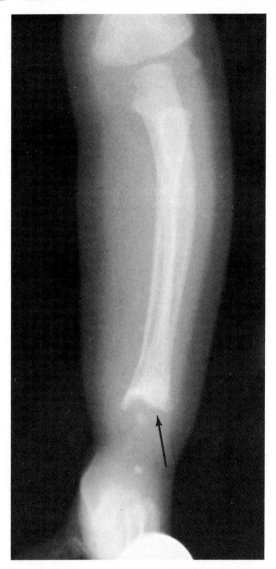

FIG. 21-1. Rickets in a four-month-old infant. There is striking cupping and fraying of the metaphysis and widening of the epiphyseal plate by the accumulation of uncalcified osteoid (arrow). The long bones show mild bowing and are poorly mineralized. These changes are frequently prominent in infants and children with renal failure and osteodystrophy. (Courtesy of Dr. Arthur Lieber)

unmineralized osteoid together with many chondrocytes (Fig. 21–1). Prolonged hypocalcemia leads to secondary hyperplasia of the parathyroid glands, and the bones begin to respond to massive secretion of parathyroid hormone. There is then superimposition of the changes of osteitis fibrosa on those of osteomalacia. Osteoclasts are numerous and actively resorb bone trabeculae, and there is progressive fibrosis of the marrow spaces in areas of resorption. Osteoid remains, however, since osteoclasts cannot resorb the unmineralized matrix.

The reason for the development of osteosclerosis in renal osteodystrophy is not clear. It has been related to qualitative changes in bone formation that yield predominantly woven rather than lamellar bone. Another possible explanation is intermittent improvement in intestinal calcium transport, permitting mineralization of many areas of osteoid accumulation.

Problems in Management

Patients with renal osteodystrophy on hemodialysis are very difficult to control. Withdrawal of any calcium from the blood aggravates the bone disease, whereas adding to the calcium level often results in extraskeletal soft tissue calcification. Renal osteodystrophy may remain a serious problem after homotransplantation. The parathyroid glands in renal failure secrete many, many times the normal amount of parathyroid hormone, and in time lose their responsiveness to changes in the blood calcium. Following transplantation, the parathyroid glands may continue to secrete excessive amounts of parathyroid hormone for months or years before resuming normal physiologic function. This worsens the osteitis fibrosa, and exposes the transplanted kidney to serious injury from excessive calcium excretion, effects that frequently necessitate subtotal parathyroidectomy.

Considerable success has attended the administration of $1,25(OH)_2$-cholecalciferol to patients with renal osteodystrophy. There is increased intestinal calcium transport, suppression of parathyroid hormone secretion, and improvement in the morphology of bone. Large doses may be required, however, and have at times induced severe hypercalcemia.

OSTEOPOROSIS

Osteoporosis is atrophy of bone. Cancellous bone becomes porous and consists of markedly thinned bony trabeculae. Cortical bone is also much thinner than normal, the loss taking place from the endosteal surface (Fig. 21–2).

Osteoporosis is undoubtedly the most widespread metabolic bone disease. It has many causes,

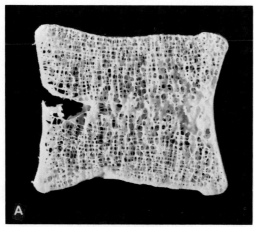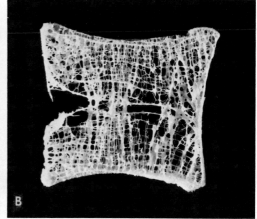

FIG. 21-2. Sections of vertebral bodies from a normal woman aged 25 **(A)** and from an 82-year-old woman with osteoporosis **(B).** There is marked thinning and a decrease in number of bone trabeculae. (Courtesy of Dr. D. P. Jenkins)

some of which are included in Table 21–1. Several mechanisms may be responsible for the bone changes. In senile osteoporosis and in scurvy, there is a defect in osteoid secretion or maturation that results in little new bone formation, while resorption continues at a normal or reduced rate. Loss of the major stimulus to bone formation, i.e., stress, accounts for the osteoporosis of immobilization. In Cushing's syndrome and in patients receiving corticosteroids, there may also be deficient osteoid production, but an increased rate of resorption appears more critical. Increased resorption is also the mechanism of osteoporosis in hyperthyroidism. In these circumstances, the rate of resorption is only slightly increased over normal, and accumulation of osteoclasts is not seen on histologic examination.

Senile Osteoporosis

Senile osteoporosis is the most common form of this disorder. It affects women predominantly, becoming manifest about 10 years after the menopause, but it is also recognizable in some 20 percent of men over 65 years of age. The lower vertebral bodies are usually most involved, and back pain is a predominent symptom. Changes in long bones, ribs, and pelvis occur later, usually in patients with more severe involvement. Shortening and compression fractures of the spine are frequent, and most fractures of the femoral neck in the aged are attributable to osteoporotic changes.

Roentgenographic studies show demineraliza-tion and kyphotic deformity of the spine, and the vertebrae assume a "cod fish" appearance due to expansion of the intervertebral disks (Fig. 21–3).

Senile osteoporosis is resistant to therapy. Although a deficiency of estrogen is commonly accepted as causative in postmenopausal women, the administration of anabolic hormones has little beneficial effect. Increasing dietary mineral intake has not proven worthwhile, not surprisingly since no disturbance of mineral metabolism is demonstrable in these patients. Attempts to decrease bone resorption by the therapeutic use of calcitonin are currently under investigation. Placing normal stress on the skeleton through exercise may prove important, at least in preventing severe disease.

PAGET'S DISEASE OF BONE

The etiology of Paget's disease of bone (osteitis deformans) is unknown, but it is probably not a metabolic bone disease. No disturbances of mineral or protein metabolism have been demonstrated. The disease may involve one or many bones, but rarely involves the entire skeleton.

The morphologic findings reflect a greatly accelerated remodeling process. The disorder appears to start as a focal area of osteoclastic resorption, and then spreads to involve most or all of the affected bone. Osteoclastic resorption is massive and associated with fibrosis of the marrow space. There is also extensive new bone formation, but

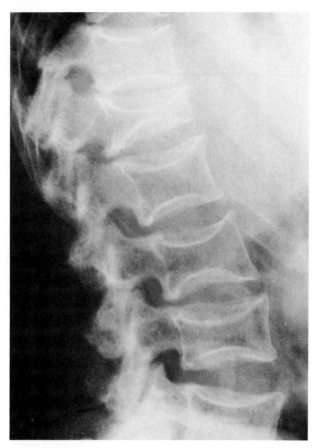

FIG. 21–3. Lower thoracic and lumbar vertebrae of a 67-year-old woman with osteoporosis. Bone density is greatly reduced and the vertebral bodies show the characteristic cod fish appearance. (Courtesy of Dr. Rosalind H. Troupin)

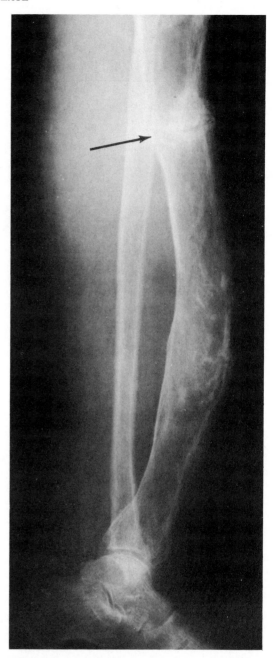

FIG. 21–4. Paget's disease. There is marked widening and bowing of the tibia, and a pattern of mixed osteoblastic and osteolytic changes. A transverse fracture (arrow) shows some healing. (Courtesy of Dr. Olcay S. Cigtay)

the very rapid turnover results in abnormal structure (Fig. 21–4). The trabeculae and cortical bone are thickened and irregular in conformation, and present a mosaic appearance on histologic examination due to prominent cement lines. Although quantitatively increased, bone is physically weak, readily fractured, and deformed by stress placed on the skeleton. A prominent finding is greatly increased vascularity, so that an involved bone will be warm to palpation, and with polyostotic involvement high output congestive heart failure may occur. It is tempting to interpret Paget's disease as due to increased vascularity of bone, but conclusive evidence is wanting.

Paget's disease is a disorder of middle and advanced age. Some 3 percent of individuals over 40 years of age have significant disease demonstrable by roentgenographic examination. The bones most frequently involved are those most subject to stress; vertebrae, pelvic bones, long bones of the limbs, and the skull. Although deformity is usually the principal manifestation, bone pain may be severe. Deafness can result from involvement of the temporal bones and the auditory canals. Patients with Paget's disease usually have normal serum levels of calcium and phosphorus, but the often extreme elevation of serum alkaline phosphatase attests to the rapid turnover of bone.

One must be alert to two important complications of Paget's disease. Some 2 percent of individuals develop malignant bone tumors, most often osteogenic sarcoma. The latter is a disease of the young. Its occurrence in older individuals is almost entirely restricted to those with Paget's disease. The second complication is related to placing patients with this disorder on bed rest. The reduced stress on the skeleton greatly diminishes new bone formation, but osteoclastic resorption continues apace, and severe, at times fatal hypercalcemia may result.

Therapy of Paget's disease has been disappointing. Recent studies have employed the antibiotic mithramycin, which inhibits bone resorption, or synthetic calcitonin.

SUGGESTED READING

Bartter FC: Bone as a target organ: toward a better definition of osteoporosis. Perspect Biol Med *16*: 215, 1973
A concise consideration of factors of importance in the pathogenesis of osteoporosis.
DeLuca HF: Vitamin D endocrinology. Ann Intern Med *85*: 367, 1976
A review of the metabolism of vitamin D, its role in calcium and phosphorus homeostasis, and in the pathogenesis of renal osteodystrophy.
Harris ED Jr, Krane SM: Paget's disease of bone. Bull Rheum Dis *18*: 506, 1968
A brief summary of the incidence, pathology, clinical manifestations and complications.
Haussler MR, McCain TA: Basic and clinical conccepts related to vitamin D metabolism and action. N Engl J Med *297*: 974, 1041, 1977
A review of the implications of recently acquired understanding and vitamin D metabolism on the pathogenesis of many disorders of mineral metabolism and renal function.

22
Inflammatory Joint Disease

JANE G. SCHALLER,   PETER A. SIMKIN

Arthritis, derived from the Greek *arthron* (joint) and *itis* (inflammation), is the term which appropriately describes inflammatory joint disease. The **primary site of inflammation in arthritis is the synovial membrane.** This chapter first discusses inflammatory diseases of joints in general terms before considering rheumatoid arthritis, ankylosing spondylitis, and gout in some detail as examples of arthritis. Septic arthritis, also a type of inflammatory joint disease, is dealt with separately in the next chapter.

Etiology

Inflammation of the synovial membrane occurs in response to various types of noxious stimuli in the synovial tissue or joint cavity, including infectious agents or foreign substances. Degenerative joint disease, although frequently called osteoarthritis, is not primarily a disease of synovial inflammation (Chap. 24). Rheumatoid arthritis is the most common type of inflammatory joint disease. In this, as well as in other inflammatory connective tissue diseases associated with arthritis (such as acute rheumatic fever, systemic lupus erythematosus, ankylosing spondylitis), the stimulus or stimuli which cause and perpetuate synovial inflammation have yet to be identified. In gout and pseudogout, crystals of uric acid and calcium pyrophosphate, respectively, are the agents which incite synovial inflammation; however, full explanations for their presence in the synovial cavity remain to be found. The etiologic agents are unknown in ankylosing spondylitis as well as in the additional related types of spinal arthritis (spondyloarthropathies). Some examples of arthritis with their stimuli for inflammation are listed in Table 22–1.

Pathogenesis

Synovium. In the synovium, as in other tissues, inflammation is characterized by increased permeability of blood vessels, increased vascularity, and accumulation of inflammatory cells. The mediators of such inflammatory responses vary and have not been fully delineated in any form of arthritis; however, lysosomal enzymes, consumption of complement, activation of kinins, and many other factors have been implicated. In some types of arthritis, products of the inflammatory response or of the basic disease may perpetuate synovitis, as may be the case with certain rheumatoid factors in some cases of rheumatoid arthritis. Some of these factors have already been mentioned in the general discussion of inflammation (Chap. 6).

Inflamed synovial tissue becomes edematous and hyperplastic with the formation of excess amounts of synovial fluid or synovial effusions. Numerous synovial villous projections become conspicuous and can nearly fill the joint cavity. If synovial inflammation continues unchecked, invasion of articular cartilage and bone may destroy the affected joint.

Synovial Fluid. Synovial effusions are a characteristic feature of inflammatory joint disease. The inflammatory joint fluid differs from normal synovial fluid in its larger volume, its increased content of serum proteins, its increased number of cells, and usually, in its decreased viscosity. The change in viscosity may be appreciated by simply dripping the fluid from a syringe. Normal fluid will string out for two or more inches while the less viscous inflammatory fluid will not. The clarity of synovial fluid depends primarily on its content of

347

white blood cells, and it ranges from the crystal clear normal fluid to gross purulence in severe septic arthritis. Fluid aspirated from normal joints does not clot spontaneously, but fluid obtained from inflamed joints does. Clotting may occur because the microvascular changes of inflammation permit fibrinogen, not normally present in synovial fluid, to enter the joint cavity. The precipitate formed by adding normal synovial fluid to dilute acetic acid is characteristically discrete and firm in appearance (mucin clot test). In most types of inflammatory joint disease this precipitate or clot is friable. The glucose level of joint fluid is normally close to that of plasma but may be significantly lower in various disease states. Examination of the joint fluid is often helpful in diagnosing various forms of arthritis (Table 22–2). In particular, fluid evaluation is essential to the diagnosis of septic arthritis and is of great importance in gout.

Cartilage. The critical period for cartilage destruction varies with different kinds of arthritis. In septic arthritis, cartilage destruction is a relatively early event occurring after a few days of unchecked joint inflammation; in rheumatoid arthritis it is usually late, occurring only after months or even years of unchecked joint inflammation. In systemic lupus erythematosus, cartilage destruction rarely occurs at all, even though arthritis may continue for years. Explanations for these different patterns of cartilage destruction in the different types of arthritis are not known. In joints severely affected by arthritis, sufficient destruction of cartilage may occur to cause total obliteration of the joint, resulting in fusion of the adjacent bony surfaces (ankylosis) (Fig. 22–1).

Clinical Manifestions

Joint inflammation is characterized by one or more of the cardinal signs of inflammation: calor (warmth), rubor (redness), dolor (pain), and tumor (swelling). Symptoms and physical findings in arthritis are directly related to the inflammation in the joint. Affected joints may be swollen, warm, erythematous, tender, and painful with consequent loss of motion. Deformity, dislocation, severe loss of motion, or complete fusion may be found in advanced disease. Wasting of muscles adjacent to affected joints is common in both early and advanced disease. When inflamed joints are

TABLE 22–1. Inflammatory Stimuli in Various Inflammatory Joint Diseases

Disease	Inflammatory Stimulus
Septic arthritis	Bacteria (e.g., pyogenic, tuberculosis)
Viral arthritis	Viruses (e.g., rubella, mumps) Immune complexes of viral antigens with specific antibodies
Gout	Sodium urate crystals
Pseudogout	Calcium pyrophosphate crystals
Trauma, hemophilia	Tissue injury and blood
Rheumatoid arthritis	Unknown
Other inflammatory connective tissue diseases	Unknown

TABLE 22–2. Characteristics of Joint Fluid in Some Types of Arthritis*

Condition	Appearance	Representative Cell Count/mm³	% Neutrophils	Fluid/Serum Glucose Ratio	Microscopic Characteristics
Normal	Serous	0–200	< 25	1	None
Inflammatory disease					
Bacterial infection	Cloudy	> 100,000	> 75	< 1	Bacteria
Tuberculosis	Cloudy	25,000	50	1 or <,1	Bacteria
Gout	Variable	10,000	60–70	1	Urate crystals
Rheumatoid arthritis	Variable	20,000	75	1 or < 1	None
Degenerative joint disease	Clear	< 2,000	< 25	1	Cartilage debris

*Although these findings may be helpful in establishing a diagnosis, they are only representative and vary from patient to patient.

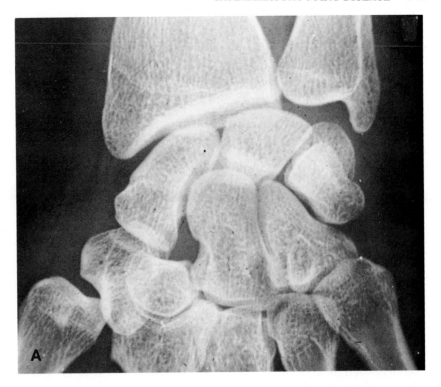

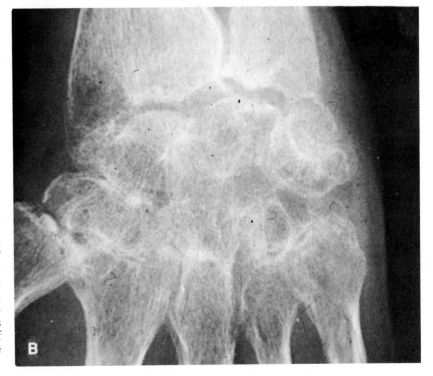

FIG. 22-1. Radiographs of a normal wrist **(A)** and of a wrist severely affected by rheumatoid arthritis **(B)**. **(A)** shows clear cortical margins of all bones, normal bone density and architecture, and normal "joint space" in all joints. In **(B)** there is a generalized demineralization and almost complete loss of bone architecture. The "joint space" is reduced or completely lost, and fusion of small bones has occurred (ankylosis). Erosion of bone is seen as interruptions in the cortical margin.

not used throughout their normal range, joint capsule and even skin about inflamed joints may shorten and tighten, leading to fixed loss of joint motion or joint contracture.

In identifying the disease state causing arthritis in the individual patient, the history and physical findings of the patient must be carefully evaluated. The duration of arthritis, the number and distribution of affected joints, and associated symptoms and signs are all important. For example, the patient with septic arthritis usually has fever and acute arthritis in one joint; the patient with rheumatoid arthritis most often has chronic arthritis of multiple peripheral joints; and the patient with ankylosing spondylitis generally has chronic arthritis that affects the spine.

Laboratory Tests

There are very few laboratory tests diagnostic of arthritis. Pathognomonic findings include organisms in the joint fluid or synovium in septic arthritis, urate crystals in the synovial fluid in gout, and calcium pyrophosphate crystals in the synovial fluid in pseudogout. Radiographs of affected joints may be useful in diagnosis and classification of types of arthritis and in providing useful information about the extent of joint damage. Various blood tests may also provide useful information, but none are diagnostic. Diseases causing arthritis often affect other organ systems as well, and recognition of such extraarticular manifestations is important in diagnosis. For example, acute rheumatic fever may be associated with carditis, characteristic skin rash, or subcutaneous nodules as well as with arthritis.

Management

In the treatment of arthritis, the first crucial objective is to determine the basic disease process. To prevent permanent joint damage, the cycle of inflammation must be interrupted before destruction of articular cartilage occurs, since this is essentially an irreversible event. Many kinds of arthritis fortunately are mild and regress spontaneously before the occurrence of permanent joint damage. This is true, for example, in acute rheumatic fever and the viral arthritides. If known, the inflammatory stimulus causing the arthritis can be removed with specific treatment (for example, appropriate antibiotic therapy in septic arthritis or therapy to lower the serum urate level in gout). In rheumatoid arthritis and other inflammatory connective tissue diseases, the primary stimulus of inflammation is not known and therefore no specific therapy is possible. In such diseases, drugs with antiinflammatory properties (such as salicylates) are the mainstay of medical therapy. Other measures, including physical therapy, attention to socioeconomic considerations, and sometimes surgery, are also important in the treatment of arthritis.

RHEUMATOID ARTHRITIS

Definition

Rheumatoid arthritis is a systemic inflammatory disease with primary manifestations in the joints. There is no recognized etiologic agent, and therefore no specific diagnostic test or therapy is currently available. The diagnosis is made on clinical grounds. All patients share the common property of chronic arthritis; however, a wide spectrum of nonarticular manifestations may also occur. The disease in children differs in many respects from that in adults. Indeed, it is probable that more than one disease is included in what we now call rheumatoid arthritis.

Incidence

Rheumatoid arthritis is a common disease, affecting an estimated 3–5 million Americans. Various population studies have reported a prevalence rate of about 3 percent in women and 1 percent in men. The disease affects people of all ages. The peak age at onset is between 30 and 40 years of age. Rheumatoid arthritis is usually not a familial disease, although predisposing genetic factors have been recognized.

Etiology

A number of contributing factors have been implicated in the pathogenesis, but the cause or causes of rheumatoid arthrits remain unknown. Many investigators have attempted to isolate and identify infectious agents, but thus far no causal organism has been found. Much research has concentrated on immunologic phenomena with emphasis on the occurrence of rheumatoid factors. These serum proteins, usually macroglobulins, are found in 80 percent of adults with rheumatoid arthritis. They have been shown to be antibodies against a specific portion of the patient's own immunoglobulin. They may be produced locally in rheumatoid synovium as well as in lymphoid tissues, and it is probable that rheumatoid factor contributes to the synovitis of some patients by

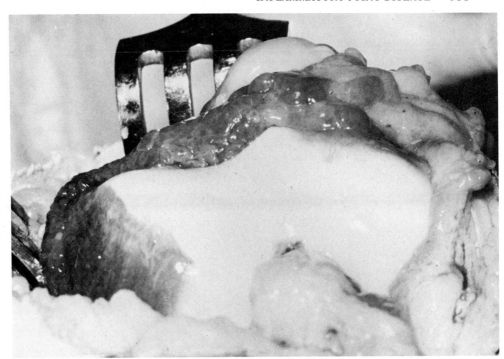

FIG. 22-2. Photograph of a knee joint attacked by rheumatoid arthritis. The joint has been opened surgically. The articular cartilage on the femoral condyle is exposed and is seen to be surrounded by hypertrophic, hypervascular synovium. The rheumatoid pannus is invading the articular cartilage from the medial and lateral sides.

the mechanism of immune complex formation. Unfortunately, rheumatoid factors are also found in other disease states and they are not diagnostic of the disease. Nor can they be considered an etiologic factor in rheumatoid arthritis.

Pathogenesis

The major target organ for rheumatoid involvement is the synovial tissue. Inflammatory disease may be present wherever synovium is found. The disease is thus not limited to synovial joints, but may also occur in tendon sheaths and bursae. Affected synovium shows marked inflammatory changes, including increased vascularity, edema, and infiltration by chronic inflammatory cells with collections of lymphocytes and plasma cells. This proliferative synovium is characterized macroscopically by enlarged projections of synovial tissue. When it becomes invasive and spreads over the cartilage of the joint, it is known as **rheumatoid pannus** (Fig. 22-2). As the disease advances, the inflamed synovial tissue may cause destruction of cartilage, bone, ligaments, and tendons. The histopathology is illustrated in Figure 22-3.

Subcutaneous rheumatoid nodules have a fibrinoid center surrounded by chronic inflammatory cells arranged radially or in a palisade. These subcutaneous nodules occur over pressure points, particularly about the elbows, the metacarpophalangeal joints, and the toes (Fig. 22-4).

Clinical Manifestations

Rheumatoid arthritis varies from a relatively short-lived inconvenience to a severe, progressive, incapacitating disease which may shorten life expectancy. Its course may be one of unpredictable remissions and exacerbations. Permanent remission occurs in a substantial number of patients. A few patients have inexorable, unremitting disease.

Although rheumatoid arthritis is primarily a disease of joints, its extraarticular manifestations include fever, weight loss, malaise, muscle wasting, lymphadenopathy, hepatosplenomegaly, as well as cardiopulmonary and ocular inflammation. A particularly serious complication is rheumatoid vasculitis, with resultant cutaneous ulcers, peripheral neuropathy, and necrosis of digits. Extraarticular manifestations in children may be particularly distinctive, and include high fever and severe systemic disease or chronic ocular inflammation (iridocyclitis).

The clinical findings in rheumatoid arthritis vary greatly. Any synovial joint may be involved although those of the thoracic and lumbar spine are generally spared. The disease often affects multiple joints in a symmetrical fashion, but some patients have asymmetrical disease in only a few

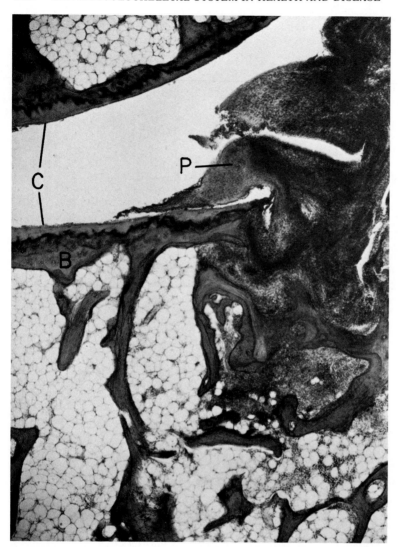

FIG. 22-3. Photomicrograph of a histologic section of an interphalangeal joint attacked by rheumatoid arthritis. The articular cartilage (C) of the two articular surfaces is separated by the joint cavity. The cartilage is somewhat thinned and its surface is roughened. The rheumatoid pannus (P) is seen on the right. It is in the process of invading and destroying cartilage and bone (B). (Hematoxylin and eosin × 20) (Courtesy of M. Mannik, M.D.)

joints. Bilateral involvement of small joints of the hands is characteristic (Fig. 22-5).

Rheumatoid arthritis is characterized by its chronicity. Once established in a given joint, inflammation usually lasts for at least several months and sometimes for many years. Affected joints may be swollen, tender, stiff, and painful. Wasting of muscles adjacent to such joints is common. Joint and muscle stiffness after inactivity is characteristic of rheumatoid arthritis and is most notable when the patient arises in the morning (morning stiffness). Such stiffness characteristically requires at least 30 minutes to work out and often lasts for several hours. In many patients rheumatoid arthritis is relatively mild and remission occurs before extensive joint dam-

age has taken place. In advanced rheumatoid arthritis, chronic deformities, including contractures, subluxation, ankylosis (Fig. 22-1), and gross local distortion of joints may be found (Fig. 22-5B). Different individuals show somewhat different reactions to the disease, with varying tendencies for development of joint instability, joint contracture, or progressive resorption of bone (Fig. 8-5A, 22-1B).

Laboratory Tests

Although there are no specific diagnostic tests, several studies may be useful in establishing the diagnosis. Rheumatoid factor is demonstrated by agglutination of gamma-globulin-coated particles (for example, latex, bentonite, sheep red cells) by the patient's serum containing rheumatoid factor. Eighty percent of adults with rheumatoid arthritis have positive serum tests for rheumatoid factor, whereas only about 10 percent of children with what is called rheumatoid arthritis have such positive tests. The erythrocyte sedimentation rate is usually elevated during periods of active disease, but this test only reflects the presence of active inflammation and has no diagnostic usefulness. Mild anemia is common during active disease. About 25 percent of patients with rheumatoid arthritis also have positive tests for antinuclear antibodies.

Synovial fluid findings may be helpful in the diagnosis (Table 22–2). The fluid is usually somewhat turbid, and yellow to greenish in color. The viscosity is poor and the white cell count is elevated, due predominantly to neutrophils. The synovial fluid sugar levels may be undetectably low, a characteristic shared only with septic arthritis. Synovial fluid levels of complement may be lowered, and rheumatoid factor tests may be positive.

X-ray changes may be helpful in the diagnosis. The earliest change is that of soft tissue swelling about affected joints. Localized periarticular demineralization of bone (osteoporosis) is another early finding (Fig. 8–5A). Periostitis may be found adjacent to affected joints. Destruction of cartilage, as in other forms of arthritis, is reflected by a narrowing of the "joint space." Localized bony erosions may be appreciated as early losses of the cortical margin of the bone. In advanced cases, extensive joint destruction occurs (Fig. 22–1) and characteristic deformities of rheumatoid arthritis are easily appreciated.

Management

The principal therapeutic objectives in rheumatoid arthritis are control of the inflammatory process and preservation of musculoskeletal function. A number of antiinflammatory agents may be helpful in the control of inflammation. The mainstay of medical treatment of rheumatoid arthritis is salicylate therapy. Other drugs sometimes used to control rheumatoid inflammation include various antiinflammatory agents (e.g., indomethacin, phenylbutazone, ibuprofen, tolmetin, naproxen, fenoprofen), injectable gold salts, the antimalarial agents (chloroquine and hydroxychloroquine),

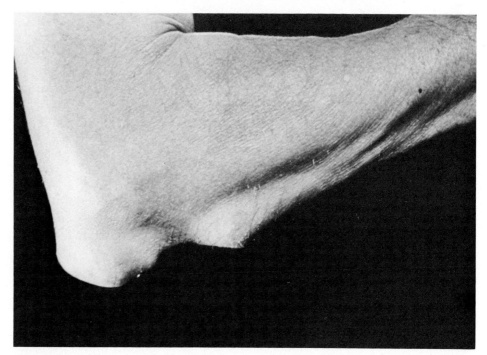

FIG. 22–4. Rheumatoid nodules. The olecranon process and the extensor surface of the forearm are the most characteristic sites for these lesions. (Courtesy of The Arthritis Foundation)

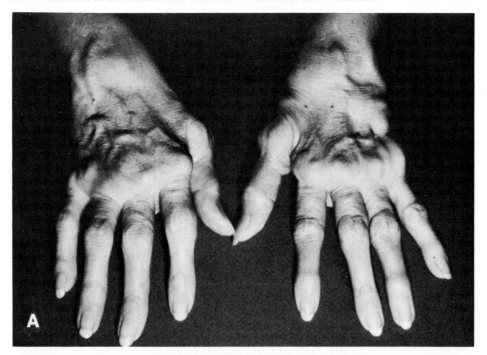

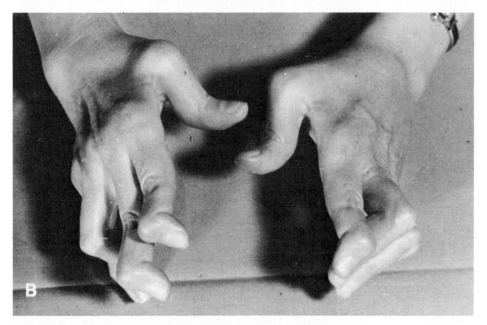

FIG. 22-5. Rheumatoid arthritis involving the hands. **(A)** Active phase of the disease. There is synovitis in the wrist, metacarpophalangeal, and proximal interphalangeal joints producing symmetrical swelling in the two hands. **(B)** Typical deformities in the hands resulting from severe rheumatoid arthritis. Note the atrophy of the interossei, boutonnière and swan-neck deformities in the fingers due to disruption of the dorsal digital expansion and the palmar plates, as well as flexion contractures of the distal interphalangeal joints.

corticosteroids, and penicillamine. Each of these drugs has serious potential toxicity and must be given only with close medical supervision, bearing in mind that the therapy should never be worse than the basic disease.

Maintenance of joint function is important in rheumatoid arthritis, as in other articular disorders. Preservation of range of motion of the joints must be emphasized. Regular range of motion exercises will usually preserve mobility if instituted early in the disease, and may restore mobility in the presence of established contractures. Strengthening exercises may prevent disuse atrophy and restore wasted muscles. Heat in the form of a hot bath is often effective in alleviating joint and muscle stiffness.

Surgery may play an important role in treatment and rehabilitation of the rheumatoid patient. Surgical procedures in certain joints may reduce pain or deformity and thus lessen disability. Surgical removal of inflamed synovium (synovectomy) is sometimes used to retard joint damage in selected joints. Severely damaged joints, particularly hips and knees, can now be replaced with total joint prostheses.

Chronic diseases such as rheumatoid arthritis have an important impact on the psychologic, social, and economic aspects of the patient's life and that of his or her entire family. Consideration of the whole patient is of paramount importance in therapy. Understanding, continuing support, and encouragement contribute greatly to therapy.

ANKLYOSING SPONDYLITIS

Definition

The term *spondylitis* denotes inflammation of the spine. Ankylosing spondylitis is a type of arthritis which characteristically affects joints of the lumbar, thoracic, and cervical vertebrae and also the sacroiliac joints. In the spine, both synovial and nonsynovial joints are involved in the inflammatory process which extends also into the associated ligaments. Peripheral joints are also affected in many patients. The diagnosis is made on clinical grounds and can only be regarded as definite if radiographic changes can be shown in the sacroiliac joints as well as in the spine, the latter associated with loss of motion. A number of other arthritis syndromes associated with spinal arthritis resemble ankylosing spondylitis and this group of syndromes is designated by the term **spondyloarthropathies.** These arthritides include Reiter's syndrome, psoriatic spondylitis, and the spondylitis of inflammatory bowel disease.

Incidence

Ankylosing spondylitis is a relatively common type of arthritis and may exist in mild forms in a significant proportion of the population. In its full blown form it is a disease of young men with peak incidence of onset between the second and fourth decades. Clinically recognized disease is much more prevalent in males than females, with six or eight males for every female. Ankylosing spondylitis frequently affects several members of the same family. Recent evidence suggests that significant genetic factors are operative in ankylosing spondylitis and the other spondyloarthropathies. Ninety-five percent of patients with clinical ankylosing spondylitis possess the histocompatibility antigen HLA B27, one of the many cell surface antigens which determine the tissue types of humans. This antigen is present in only about 6 percent of the general North American population. A similar but somewhat less striking association with HLA B27 exists for the other spondyloarthropathies. These fascinating observations suggest that in some way there is a genetic predisposition for ankylosing spondylitis; this predisposition may be related to immune response genes which exist in close proximity to the histocompatibility genes on the sixth chromosome.

Etiology

The basic causes of ankylosing spondylitis and the other spondyloarthropathies remain largely unknown. However, some clues are available. These include the documented occurrence of the spondylitis of Reiter's disease following gastrointestinal or venereal infections. Such observations suggest that in some way a particular infection has caused a chronic rheumatic syndrome in a susceptible patient. Identification of the genetic predisposition of some individuals for spondylitis has permitted further observations. It has been shown that those individuals who contract gastrointestinal infections with *Yersinia enterocolitica*, a bacterium of the plague family, and also carry HLA B27 are at high risk to incur postinfectious arthritis when compared to similarly infected individuals without B27. This again suggests that genetically predisposed hosts may be at risk for developing arthritis after certain environmental insults.

Pathogenesis

The major target organs for inflammation in ankylosing spondylitis are the synovium, the joint capsule and associated ligaments. Inflammation affects the synovial joints of the spine and also leads to calcification of interspinous and capsular ligaments with the formation of bony bridges (syndesmophytes) between adjacent vertebrae. The intervertebral disks and associated ligaments also become inflamed and later may calcify. The sacroiliac joints are characteristically affected and so is the symphysis pubis and the sterno-manubrial joint in many patients. Histology of sacroiliac joints reveals chronic inflammation. There is a marked tendency for fibrosis and anky-losis in ankylosing spondylitis, particularly in the sacroiliac and spinal joints and also in the hips. The histology of synovium in affected peripheral joints is similar to that in rheumatoid arthritis. How-ever, the synovitis of peripheral joints other than the hips is often less destructive than that of classic adult rheumatoid arthritis. Subcutaneous rheu-matoid nodules are not associated with ankylosing spondylitis. A peculiar type of aortitis resembling syphilitic aortitis occurs in some patients late in the disease. The heart conduction system may also be affected by this inflammation. Many patients also suffer from ocular inflammation at varying times during the course of the disease. This takes the form of acute, but self-limited iridocyclitis.

Clinical Manifestations

The hallmark of ankylosing spondylitis is spinal arthritis. This usually begins in the low back with symptoms of pelvic girdle stiffness and pain which is often severe at night and is relieved by moving about. Such episodes of pain and stiffness may be intermittent and recurrent over a period of years or may become persistent and chronic. Pain and stiffness generally affect the spine in an ascending fashion. Pain is sometimes severe and incapacitat-ing. On the other hand, some patients lose signifi-cant amounts of spinal mobility while suffering little discomfort. Pain may also be felt in distribu-tion areas of the sciatic nerve. Ten to twenty-five percent of spondylitis patients present first with arthritis in one or a few peripheral joints, especial-ly in the lower limb. The spinal involvement of ankylosing spondylitis may progress relentlessly

to cause a stiff spine which lacks mobility in all directions or may arrest with varying degrees of loss of back mobility. Early physical findings sug-gestive of ankylosing spondylitis include tender-ness over the sacroiliac joints, pain on stressing of the sacroiliac joints (Fig. 16–4), pain on motion of the lumbar spine, paravertebral muscle spasm, and limitation or loss of lumbar flexion (Fig. 22–6). Rotation and lateral flexion of the spine may also be lost. Permanent spinal deformity results if good posture is not maintained.

Chest expansion may be reduced secondary to involvement of the costovertebral articulations. This should be documented by measuring the chest expansion during full inspiration and expira-

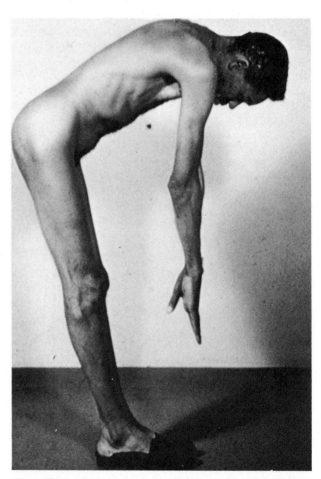

FIG. 22-6. Ankylosing spondylitis. When the patient attempts to flex the spine the lumbar region instead of assuming a smooth kyphotic curvature remains straight and rigid due to ankylosis of the lumbar intervertebral joints. (Courtesy of the Arthritis Foundation)

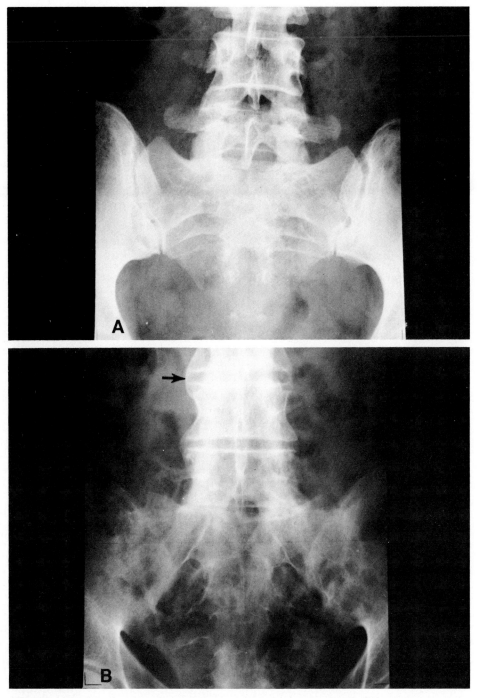

FIG. 22-7. Comparison of the radiologic appearance of the sacroiliac joints and the lower lumbar spine in a normal individual **(A)** and in a patient suffering from anky-losing spondylitis **(B).** Note the obliteration of the sacroiliac joints due to inflammation and fusion, as well as the bamboo appearance of the lumbar spine with ossification of the superficial laminae of the annulus fibrosus **(arrow).** Note also that vertebral arch joints can be readily defined in **A** while this is not possible in **B.** Vertebral arch joints are characteristically involved in ankylosing spondylitis. (Courtesy of Dr. Rosalind H. Troupin)

tion. There may be pain and tenderness about joints of the sternum or the costal cartilages. The neck may become involved, generally after the lumbar and thoracic spine. Symptoms and signs of hip, shoulder, and other peripheral joint disease may be present when these joints are involved and the Achilles tendon may become inflamed, causing heel pain. Temporomandibular joint arthritis is also associated with ankylosing spondylitis. Peripheral arthritis may be transient, but it may persist and progress, especially in the hip.

Acute iridocyclitis occurs in about 25 percent of patients some time during the disease, and heart block or aortic insufficiency due to aortitis develops in about 5–10 percent of patients late in disease.

Laboratory Tests

There are no diagnostic laboratory tests. As in rheumatoid arthritis, erythrocyte sedimentation rates may be elevated and mild anemia may be present during periods of active disease. Tests for rheumatoid factors and antinuclear antibodies are almost always negative. Synovial fluid findings from peripheral joints are not diagnostic, simply showing sterile inflammation.

Radiographs are of great help in the diagnosis. Radiographic sacroiliitis must be documented before the diagnosis can be made; such radiographic changes generally occur within the first several years of disease (Fig. 22–7). Radiographic sacroiliac changes include loss of clear distinction of sacroiliac joint margins, erosions, and sclerosis. At first the joint space may appear widened, but later the joint space narrows and may become obliterated. Radiographic changes in the thoracolumbar spine occur relatively late and consist of calcification of paraspinal ligaments leading ultimately to the typical *bamboo spine*. Radiographs may also show damage to other joints, particularly the hips.

GOUT

Definition

Gout is a form of arthritis initiated by the presence of sodium urate crystals within the joint. Although it usually begins as a single, acute, self-limited attack, gout may become chronic and be complicated by deposition of urate crystals in the subcutaneous tissue, cartilage, bone, and kidney. Uric acid precipitation within the renal collecting system leads to stones in many gouty patients.

Incidence

Gout is a rather common joint disease, and its prevalence in adult men may exceed 2 percent of the population. The normal serum uric acid level in men (5.4 mg/100 ml) is considerably higher than that found in women and is close to the theoretic saturation point of serum (7 mg/100 ml). It is presumably because of this difference that the prevalence of gout in men is some nine times higher than in women.

Etiology and Pathogenesis

Injection of monosodium urate crystals into knees of normal or gouty individuals produces typical episodes of gout. Injections of similar crystals such as calcium pyrophosphate induce identical attacks. In spontaneous disease the few initial crystals formed may serve to seed the synovial fluid, thus leading to formation of many more crystals and amplifying the inflammatory process. The majority of patients with elevated serum urate level (hyperuricemia) do not have gout and are unlikely to develop gout. The poor correlation between hyperuricemia and gouty arthritis, however, suggests that there are other important factors which act either as systemic *solubility factors* or as local *precipitating factors*, and thus contribute to the pathophysiology of gout in affected individuals.

Hyperuricemia results from overproduction and/or defective excretion of urate.

Rare but well characterized enzyme defects lead to the overproduction of urate in some individuals. In addition, proliferative diseases such as polycythemia vera, psoriasis, and myelogenous leukemia cause an overproduction of urate, presumably as a byproduct of the increased synthesis of nucleic acids. However, enzyme defects have not been identified in the majority of individuals who overproduce urate and do not suffer from proliferative diseases.

The renal handling of serum urate is strangely complex for a metabolic waste product. Serum urate is freely filtered at the glomerulus and then is almost entirely reabsorbed in the proximal tubule. The same tubule, however, resecretes urate into the collecting system and the majority of uric acid which appears in the urine consists of this secreted fraction. In renal retention of urate, the most common explanation is a defective secretory system. Secretion of urate is impaired by a number of drugs, including all effective diuretics, low doses of aspirin, and the antituberculous agent pyrazinamide. In addition, high concentrations of the normal metabolites lactate and β-hydroxybutyrate also are associated with impaired secretion of urate. As in the problem of overproduction, however, the majority of individuals with impaired elimination of urate have no recognizable reason for this defect.

Regardless of whether hyperuricemia results from overproduction of urate, from renal retention, or from a combination of the two, when the saturation point of the body fluids is exceeded, crystallization may occur with ensuing gouty arthritis.

Clinical Manifestations

Classically, gout presents with acute arthritis of the metatarsophalangeal joint of the great toe (podagra). In western populations, at least 75 percent of gouty individuals will have acute gout in this joint at one time or another. The usual victim is a middle-aged man, and his attack may often be precipitated by physical or emotional stress. Some patients experience a transient prodrome, which enables them to anticipate the attack. Once an attack has started, the pain builds rapidly, culminating within 24 hours in a pain "so exquisite and lively . . . that it cannot bear the weight of the bed clothes nor the jar of a person walking in the room." This timeless description was left to us by the 17th century physician Thomas Sydenham, who himself suffered from gout.

There may be substantial associated systemic findings including fever, anorexia, malaise, and peripheral leukocytosis. It is not surprising that these findings together with a red, hot, severely inflamed joint often lead to an erroneous diagnosis of infection.

Untreated episodes gradually resolve over a week or more and leave the joint entirely asymptomatic until the next attack. After the first episode, the patient may go for years before experiencing a second attack. Attacks tend to occur, however, with increasing frequency and may involve more than one joint at a time. Without effective treatment, the disease often leads to chronic symptoms. Chronic patients often have nodular lesions which are known as **tophi.** These lesions are often subcutaneous with the most common sites being within the cartilage of the ear and over bony prom-

inences, such as the olecranon process and the knuckles. Similar lesions may be found within articular cartilage, bone, tendons, and the kidney. Histologically, tophi are composed of conglomerates of long urate crystals which may be surrounded by an inflammatory reaction including foreign body giant cells.

Laboratory Tests

The most important single laboratory study in the diagnosis of gouty arthritis is the evaluation of synovial fluid (Table 22-2). Demonstration of sodium urate crystals in the fluid is diagnostic of gout. Although the crystals may occasionally be seen on ordinary microscopy, adequate examination demands polarizing microscopy. This simple procedure may readily be performed with any laboratory microscope. When the polarizers are positioned at right angles to each other so that all directly transmitted light is excluded, urate crystals may be seen as bright, narrow rods, frequently occurring within cells. The crystals measure up to 10μ in length (Fig. 22-8). An elevated serum urate concentration is of limited diagnostic value because of the high prevalence of asymptomatic hyperuricemia. A low value, however, may be use-

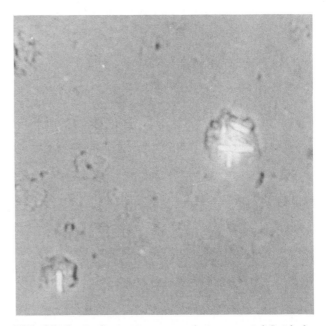

FIG. 22-8. Sodium urate crystals in synovial fluid obtained from a joint affected by acute gout. Crystals occur primarily within white cells and are best seen (as in this photograph) under polarized light.

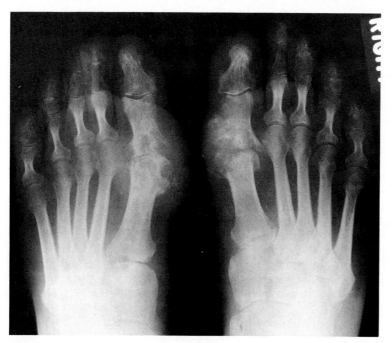

FIG. 22-9. Radiograph of the feet of a patient with tophaceous gout. The peculiar tropism of gout for the first metatarsophalangeal joint is well demonstrated. Increased soft tissue density and bony destruction at these joints are secondary to deposits of sodium urate crystals.

ful in excluding the diagnosis of gout. Assessment of urinary uric acid excretion is of value in identifying the rare gouty individual (approximately 5 percent of patients) who is a marked overexcreter of uric acid. All such individuals are overproducers of uric acid, and they are a subset of patients who are particularly susceptible to uric acid stones and other renal complications. Other laboratory studies are of little help. The radiograph of gouty joints is characteristic in advanced cases (Fig. 22–9) but is of little value in early diagnosis.

Management

Acute attacks of gout can usually be aborted with any one of a number of antiinflammatory agents, including colchicine, indomethacin, phenylbutazone, or occasionally corticosteroids. The classic agent, colchicine, appears to be effective because it interferes with the ingress of neutrophils into the joint. The cycle of inflammation is thereby interrupted and the arthritis subsides. Between attacks the prophylactic use of colchicine or other agents is of value in diminishing the frequency of episodes. When these measures do not control gout or when complications such as tophi or renal stones are present, then the serum urate level should be lowered. This may be accomplished by the use of uricosuric agents, which interfere with tubular reabsorption of filtered urate in the kidney and thereby increase the renal excretion of urate. An effective alternative is allopurinol, an agent which interferes with the production of urate and thereby lowers the levels both of serum and of urine uric acid. With these measures, satisfactory clinical results can be achieved in almost all patients.

SUGGESTED READING

Cruickshank B: Pathology of ankylosing spondylitis. Clin Orthop 74: 43, 1971
The commencement of the disease with changes in the sarco-iliac joints is described and these changes are followed in spinal joints. Comparison is made with the pathology of rheumatoid arthritis.

Harris ED Jr, DiBona DR, Krane SM: Collagenases in human synovial fluid. J Clin Invest 48: 2104, 1969
A careful investigation of one of the enzymes which may play a role in the onset and progression of rheumatoid lesions.

Hollander JL (ed): Arthritis and Allied Conditions, 7th ed. Philadelphia, Lea & Febiger, 1966
The most thorough and extensive reference work in the field of arthritis and rheumatic disease.

Hollander JL, Rawson AJ: Gamma globulin, rheumatoid factors and rheumatoid arthritis. Bull Rheum Dis *18*: 502, 1968
A persuasive summary of experiments implicating immunologic mechanisms in the pathogenesis of rheumatoid arthritis. The Bulletin on Rheumatic Diseases is available free through the Arthritis Foundation.

Kellermeyer RW: Inflammatory process in acute gouty arthritis. III. Vascular permeability-enhancing activity in normal human synovial fluid; induction by Hageman factor activators; and inhibition by Hageman factor anti-serum. J Lab Clin Med *70*: 372, 1967
An interesting presentation of evidence implicating Hageman factor activation as the initiator of the inflammatory process in gout.

Kelly WN, Greene ML, Rosenbloom FM, Henderson JF, Seegmiller JE: Hypoxanthine-guanine phosphoribosyl-transferase deficiency in gout. Ann Intern Med *70*: 155, 1969
A comprehensive review of the best characterized biochemical lesion leading to hyperuricemia and gout.

Primer on the Rheumatic Diseases. New York, Arthritis Foundation, 1973
A concise review of diseases presenting with arthritis.

Available free through the Arthritis Foundation, 1212 Avenue of the Americas, New York, NY 10036.

Schaller JG, Hanson V Conference Chairmen: Proceedings of the First American Rheumatism Association Conference of the Rheumatic Diseases of Childhood. Arthritis Rheum [Suppl] *20*(2): 145, 1977
A comprehensive collection of recent papers discussing all aspects of childhood arthritis, both practical and theoretical. Several papers deal with juvenile rheumatoid arthritis.

Schaller J, Wedgwood RJ: Is juvenile rheumatoid arthritis a single disease? A review. Pediatrics *50*: 940, 1972
The review considers the disease taking into account pathogenesis and clinical manifestations.

Sigler JW, Blum GB, Duncan H, Ensign DC: Clinical features of ankylosing spondylitis. Clin Orthop *74*: 14, 1971
A concise presentation of the characteristic clinical features of the disease.

Simkin P: The pathogenesis of podagra. Ann Intern Med *86*: 230, 1977
This short paper postulates a relationship between joint trauma, degenerative changes and gout. An anatomical explanation is proposed for the frequent involvement of the metatarsophalangeal joint of the great toe.

Stanbury JB, Wyngaarden JB, Fredrickson DS: The Metabolic Basis of Inherited Disease. New York, McGraw-Hill, 1966
Includes reviews of several genetic connective tissue diseases and an especially thorough discussion of gout.

23
Bacterial Infections of Bones and Joints

D. KAY CLAWSON

Osteomyelitis is the infection of bone, and septic arthritis is the infection of joints. These are essentially the same pathologic processes as infection of other tissues. Significant differences arise, however, as a result of the unique architecture of these tissues. An understanding of osteomyelitis requires an appreciation of the blood supply to bone and of the role played by dead bone in perpetuating the infectious process. In the case of septic arthritis the capacity to resolve the inflammatory process is limited by the presence of a closed joint cavity and a lack of blood supply to intraarticular tissues. Both osteomyelitis and septic arthritis may be divided into acute and chronic forms.

ACUTE OSTEOMYELITIS

Definition

Acute osteomyelitis represents the stage of seeding the bone with bacteria and the establishment of an area of inflammation. Without early treatment or an effective defense response, the acute phase of inflammation in bone leads to the formation of pus. The accumulation of pus may produce pressures sufficient to impair the local blood supply rapidly, leading to bone death. This sets the stage for chronic osteomyelitis which may last a lifetime.

Incidence

The incidence of this disease is decreasing annually in western civilization due to early treatment with antibiotics. The chronic forms occurring because of late diagnosis and inadequate early treatment are still a major national health problem.

The disease affects all age groups, but the classic acute form is found in children. Males are affected slightly more frequently than females and morbidity is greater in the lower socioeconomic groups. The prognosis is excellent if early and adequate treatment is instituted. If treatment is delayed, the chronic form with its persistent infection and drainage may produce serious growth disturbances or profound functional loss of the joint or of the whole limb.

Etiology

Bacterial infection of bone may be 1) hematogenous in origin as the result of a bacterial septicemia, 2) the complication of an open fracture by direct contamination from the outside, 3) the complication of a surgical operation on bone, or 4) the result of direct extension from soft tissue infection such as an ulcer. Irrespective of the route of infection, the most common offending organism in all age groups is *Staphylococcus aureus*. **Acute osteomyelitis classically occurs in the metaphysis of the long bones of children and is hematogenous in origin.** In the adult, osteomyelitis more commonly results from other routes of infection.

Pathogenesis

Approximately 25 percent of the patients with osteomyelitis give a history of a recent infectious process (respiratory, ear, or cutaneous). A history of preceding minor injury is common, but its role in the pathogenesis has not been substantiated.

The bacteria reach the metaphyseal bone and settle in the sinusoids of the bone marrow. An inflammatory process follows, with hyperemia,

363

edema, and the accumulation of neutrophils. Thrombosis of small blood vessels may result from the inflammatory process. The blood supply to the affected bone is further compromised by increasing local pressure because the process is taking place within rigid-walled cancellous spaces (Fig. 23–1). *In the absence of treatment, bone death occurs in about 72 hours.* Dead bone is recognized by the absence of cells in the lacunar spaces and is known as **sequestrum** (Fig. 23–2). The pressure within the bone may be raised to the extent that edema fluid and pus are forced through the haversian and Volkmann's canals to elevate the periosteum. Once the periosteum is elevated, cortical bone is isolated from its blood supply. As the inflammatory exudate egresses, the bacteria are forced into the minute vascular channels of the bony cortex. *This dead bone, seeded with bacteria, then acts as a permanent reservoir for bacterial growth and invasion. No antibiotic is able to penetrate the depth of the sequestrum;* hence antibiotics cannot eradicate the infection once this stage has been reached.

In certain joints the growth plate cartilage is partly or completely intraarticular (shoulder and hip joints). In such joints, osteomyelitis can extend from the metaphysis into the joint producing an associated septic arthritis. In most instances involvement of the adjacent joint is unusual because the joint capsule and the epiphyseal plate serve as a barrier to the extension of infection (Fig. 23–1). The presence of an effusion in the joint adjacent to the affected metaphysis is not unusual in osteomyelitis, but this joint fluid is sterile *(sympathetic effusion)*. It is important to realize that the epiphysis itself is not a primary focus of osteomyelitis and that most epiphyses have a vascular supply separate from that of the adjoining metaphysis (Fig. 7–5).

The age of the patient suffering from hematogenous osteomyelitis conditions the behavior of the infectious process. In infants, especially the newborn, the disease process tends to be rampant, with extensive destruction of the entire shaft of a bone. Secondary joint invasion is common. In the child from 1 to 16 years of age, in whom the majority of growth plates in long bones are active, the metaphyses are the sites of predilection, and direct joint involvement is rare. In adults, there is no epiphyseal growth plate and extensive spread from the metaphysis to the shaft, as well as into the joint through the epiphysis, may occur.

Clinical Manifestation

Symptoms. The patient with acute osteomyelitis is usually extremely ill, with high fever, malaise, lethargy, and often vomiting. This disease must always be suspected in an ill, irritable child with a fever of unknown origin. Systemic symptoms are particularly prominent during bacteremia at the time of bone seeding. If the child complains of pain over a bone, the diagnosis is readily suspected, however, pain will often be diffuse and the child will merely refuse to walk or to use the limb. The physical examination of all ill children with fever of unknown origin should include careful evaluation of the limbs and *point tenderness over the metaphyses of long bones* must be specifically looked for. Early in the course of the disease such tenderness may be only mild, but it later becomes exquisite.

Signs. In the early phase of the disease, the crucial physical sign is **point tenderness over the metaphysis** of a long bone. Examination of the metaphysis must be meticulous. The presence of erythema and swelling is a late physical sign appearing only after extraosseous expansion of the disease. The affected area will usually be splinted by reflex spasm of the surrounding musculature. Point tenderness over the metaphysis in an ill, febrile child is sufficient to make the diagnosis even before positive bacteriologic evidence or radiographic findings are available. All too often, the severely ill child with septicemia and toxemia may show no local signs suggestive of a focus of bone infection.

Laboratory Tests

During the phase of septicemia, bacteria may be cultured from the blood. Unfortunately, positive cultures are found in only 50 percent of cases. Blood cultures should be repeated on several occasions with each spiking temperature. If point tenderness is identifiable over a metaphysis, aspiration or biopsy of this area will usually allow for isolation of the offending organism. Laboratory findings which suggest bacterial infection include a moderate to high erythrocyte sedimentation rate and moderate leukocytosis with a predominance of neutrophils. However, if the acute septicemia has been partially treated with antibiotics and the condition is moving towards a more chronic form, the white blood count may be within normal limits.

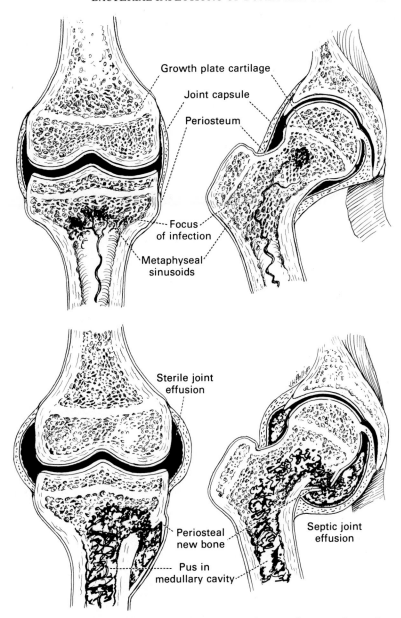

FIG. 23-1. Two stages of acute osteomyelitis in bones where the metaphysis is extracapsular (at the knee shown on the left) and where it is intracapsular (at the hip shown on the right). The two upper figures illustrate the establishment of the focus of infection in the metaphyseal sinusoids with accompanying thrombosis of small blood vessels. The lower figures illustrate the stage reached 2 to 3 weeks later. Note the elevated periosteum, the subperiosteal new bone formation, and the joint effusion. Where the metaphysis is extracapsular, the effusion remains sterile, but where it is intracapsular, the effusion as a rule is infected.

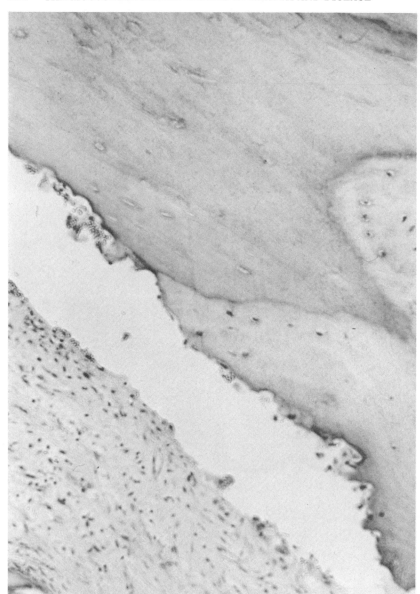

FIG. 23–2. Photomicrograph of dead and living bone from an area of chronic osteomyelitis. The sequestrum occupies the upper portion of the section: osteocytes are absent from the dead bone and are missing also from the few lacunae at the lower edge of the sequestrum where it abuts against newly formed bone. The dense fibrous tissue seen in the lower left of the field is infiltrated by chronic inflammatory cells and is typically present in association with chronic inflammatory lesions.

During the first 10–14 days of the illness, there are no radiographic changes. The earliest definite radiographic sign is periosteal new bone formation that occurs after the periosteum has been lifted by the escaping pus from the medullary cavity. This is usually not demonstrable until the 10th to the 14th day (Fig. 23–3).

A radionuclide **bone scan** (see Chap. 8) is sensitive to early metabolic and vascular changes of bone and may be useful in identifying areas of osteomyelitis within the first day or so after the onset of the symptoms (Fig. 23–4). Bone scan is of great value in confirming the early diagnosis of osteomyelitis long before routine radiographs reveal any changes. Nevertheless, it should be abundantly clear that in the *crucial first days of hematogenous osteomyelitis the diagnosis depends on the clinical features.* Bone scanning and appropriate bacterial cultures may support the diagnosis. Failure to recognize osteomyelitis early can result in extreme morbidity and occasionally mortality. As few as three days of unrecognized or untreated disease can set the stage for chronic osteomyelitis.

Management

Optimal treatment is based on *early diagnosis* when appropriate antibiotics will *cure* the disease. Appropriate antibiotic treatment should ideally be initiated within 72 hours of the onset of symptoms. The disease can usually be cured at this stage with no sequela. Management of the acutely ill child should, therefore, include two or three blood cultures, an aspiration or needle biopsy of an area of point tenderness in the metaphysis, and the immediate institution of antibiotics. It is important not to delay antibiotic therapy by waiting for a bacterial diagnosis. It is beyond the scope of this chapter to discuss the choice of antibiotic therapy when the causative organisms cannot be immediately identified. One of the references listed at the end of the chapter is devoted to this problem. Adequate dosage of the antibiotic should be administered parenterally. Treatment should be continued until there is no evidence of systemic disease, point tenderness disappears, and the sedimentation rate returns towards normal. This usually requires at least three weeks of antibiotic therapy.

Significant pus formation must be removed sur-

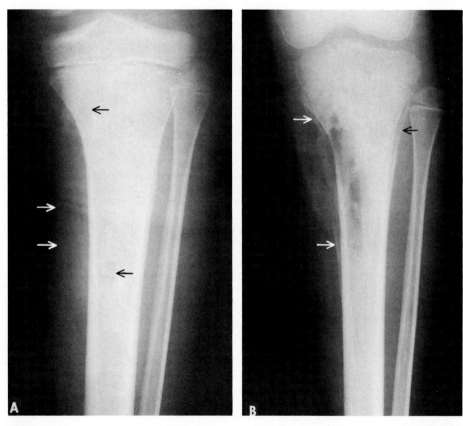

FIG. 23-3. Radiographs of the knee region in a 12-year-old boy with acute osteomyelitis of the proximal end of the tibia. In **A,** taken approximately 8 days after the establishment of the septic focus in the metaphysis, **black arrows** point to two areas of bone with decreased radiodensity, which probably represent the initial site of infection in bone. The structure of bone is not crisp, the fuzziness being due most probably to inflammatory exudate in the bone. **White arrows** point to the outline of a soft tissue swelling around the metaphysis. **B,** taken 2 weeks later, shows extensive irregular areas of radiolucency in the metaphysis and upper part of the diaphysis. The periosteum has been elevated by pus extensively around the circumference of the metaphysis (indicated by **arrows**) and subperiosteal new bone formation is taking place.

gically. If pus is sufficient to elevate the perio-steum, surgical decompression will hasten the resolution of the disease process and frequently prevent further destruction of bone and its blood supply. In addition to the direct treatment of the infectious processes, the associated dehydration, electrolyte disturbances, and nutritional altera-tions must be also corrected.

CHRONIC OSTEOMYELITIS

Definition

Chronic osteomyelitis represents the stage of bone infection where the infected dead bone has become surrounded by dense, relatively avascular fibrous tissue (Fig. 23–2).

Incidence and Etiology

In the United States chronic osteomyelitis is most commonly seen as a sequela of open fracture or operative treatment on the spine or the long bones. Unfortunately, it is still seen also as sequela of inadequately treated, acute, hematogenous osteomyelitis. Once established, chronic bone infection is very difficult to eradicate, regardless of treatment. *Staphylococcus aureus* is still the most common pathogenic organism, but virtually every type of bacterium and fungus has been im-plicated as a cause of chronic osteomyelitis, and mixed infection is not infrequent. The usual his-tory is one of recurrent flares of activity with ab-scess formation and drainage through sinus tracts, followed by periods of quiescence which may last for many years. The disability associated with the disorder depends on the extent and location of involvement.

FIG. 23–4. **(A)** X-ray of the right shoulder of a 9-year-old child 5 days after onset of illness and fever of unknown cause. It is difficult to discern any abnormality. **(B)** Following intravenous administration of technetium-99, a bone scan reveals that, in addition to sites of hemopoietic red bone marrow, there is a hot spot in the proximal diaphysis of the right humerus (**arrow,** the patient is viewed from the back) revealing an asymmetric, abnormal focus of increased metabolic and vascular activity. **(C)** X-ray of the same patient two weeks later shows that despite the fact that treatment was instituted on day 5, a substantial amount of bone death has occurred. There is gross distortion of the normal bony architecture associated with pus formation, periosteal elevation, and new bone formation paralleling the cortex **(arrows).** (Courtesy of Dr. Rosalind H. Troupin)

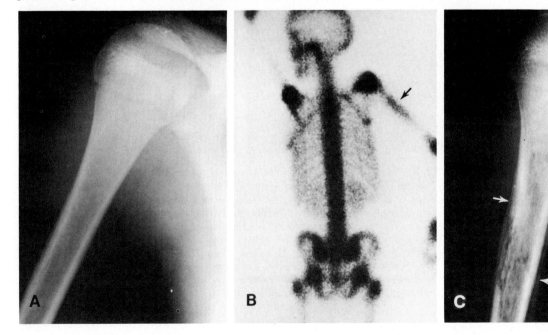

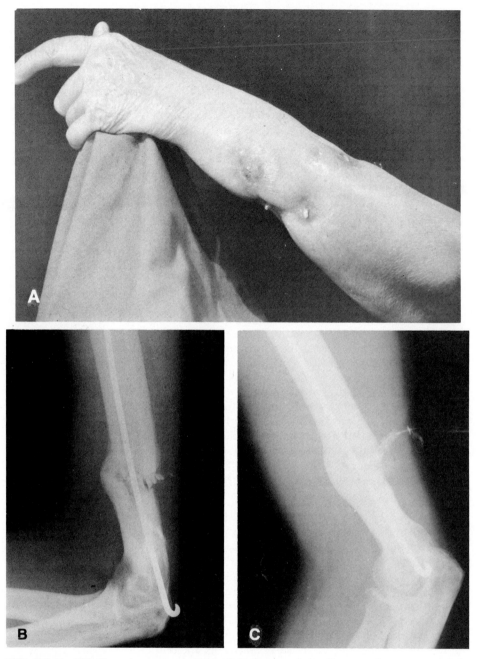

FIG. 23-5. (A) Chronic osteomyelitis of the bones of the forearm showing multiple sinus tracts with chronic pus drainage. (B) Chronic osteomyelitis of the distal humerus in a different patient following fracture and internal fixation. Small pieces of sequestrum are seen to lie within the sinus tract, demonstrated by a sinogram in **C.**

Pathogenesis and Pathology

As the pus from the acute infection forms and increased pressure develops, the haversian system and Volkmann's canals become invaded by bacteria, and the bone loses its blood supply. Once this stage is reached, bacterial activity may continue indefinitely. It has been shown experimentally that even extremely high doses of antibiotics are unable to penetrate more than a millimeter or two into dead bone, hence, it is almost impossible to eliminate the nidus of chronic infection without radical surgery. As the body's defenses mount, a wall of granulation tissue develops around the focus of infection. This tissue later becomes a dense, relatively avascular scar, forming an almost impenetrable shell around the sequestrum. With time, sinuses develop, through which pus drains from the infected tissue to the surface of the skin (Fig. 23–5).

If the disease is well walled off there may be no systemic signs of infection for many years. Following operative procedures or trauma to the area, the infection may, however, flare once again to an acute form. Occasionally a flare-up of a chronic osteomyelitis with systemic symptoms, abscess formation, and eventual drainage will occur without a known inciting cause. Chronic osteomyelitis can only be cured permanently through eradication of the reservoirs of infection in dead bone, tissue space, or infected avascular scar tissue.

Clinical Manifestations and Laboratory Findings

The diagnosis of chronic osteomyelitis is usually evident from the history of intermittent attacks of cellulitis (inflammation of the soft tissues), abscess formation, drainage, and the existence of sinus tracts. Laboratory studies frequently show a persistently elevated erythrocyte sedimentation rate, although this may return to normal when the process is well walled off. The white blood cell count remains normal except during periods of bacteremia associated with fever. The clinical findings are variable. At times, patients may have full function with no bone tenderness. Frequently, a deep ache is present, and occasionally there is severe pain associated with muscle spasm and splinting. Radiographic evaluation shows areas of bone loss and new bone proliferation (Fig. 23–6).

Management

Cure of chronic osteomyelitis requires surgical eradication of all infected, dead bone and its associated scar tissue. This must be accomplished under antibiotic treatment using large doses of the appropriate bactericidal antibiotic. The management of a patient must weigh the difficulty which obtaining a cure presents against the consequences of allowing the disease to run a chronic course. If the disease is in a site that can be surgically approached for removal of all the dead bone and associated scar tissue, it is worth attempting this treatment. The procedure is usually carried out with preoperative, intraoperative, and postoperative antibiotics. Continuous irrigation and suction drainage are sometimes necessary to eliminate the dead space after surgical removal of the diseased tissue and to provide egress for any dead tissue or bacteria that can not be removed at the time of surgery. Antibiotics must be administered

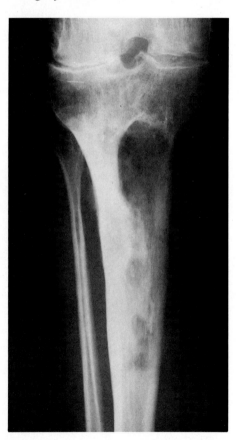

FIG. 23-6. Chronic osteomyelitis of the tibia. The extensive sclerosis and the presence of abscess cavities in the metaphysis and diaphysis are pathognomonic of the disease. The knee joint shows changes of degenerative joint disease most likely secondary to disease resulting from the long standing osteomyelitis.

for 3–6 weeks until the sedimentation rate has returned to normal. If it appears impossible to eradicate the infection surgically, the patient is treated symptomatically while maintaining drainage of the sinuses. Intermittent courses of antibiotics have to be reinstated from time to time when systemic symptoms reappear.

The complications of chronic osteomyelitis left untreated include secondary seeding of the infection, amyloidosis, pathologic fracture, and malignant transformation (squamous cell carcinoma) in the sinus tract (Fig. 23–7).

ACUTE SEPTIC ARTHRITIS

Etiology

Septic arthritis may affect any age group, but is more frequently seen in infants and young children and in patients suffering from diabetes mellitus or rheumatoid arthritis. The bacteria may enter the joint from 1) hematogenous spread, in which case several joints may be involved, 2) direct extension from adjacent osteomyelitis, or 3) penetrating injury by foreign body or from diagnostic or therapeutic joint puncture. As in osteomyelitis, *Staphylococcus aureus* is the most common offending organism except in infants from 1 month to 4 years of age where *Hemophilus influenzae* is found most frequently. Tuberculous arthritis, still common in many parts of the world, is now relatively rare in North America. Almost any organism, however is capable of producing septic arthritis. In more recent years, gonococcal infection has become a frequent pathogen in septic arthritis.

Pathogenesis

The bacteria in hematogenous septic arthritis lodge in the synovial membrane. Even when there is direct bacterial inoculation into the joint cavity, within 72 hours most of the bacteria will be found in this membrane.

The inflammatory response is seen primarily in the synovial membrane, which becomes thicker as it is infiltrated with inflammatory cells. This hyperplastic synovial membrane invades the articular cartilage starting at the joint margins. As in rheumatoid arthritis, such changes are soon followed by cartilage destruction. The mechanism of cartilage destruction is not known. Proteoglycans are lost first, thus exposing collagen fibrils. These exposed collagen fibrils are further eroded by wear and by enzymatic activity of various collagenases.

The inflammatory process in the synovial membrane results in a joint effusion which may vary from a slightly turbid fluid to frank pus. Loculation of pus may occur in synovial recesses and seriously interfere with the effectiveness of treatment.

If septic arthritis is untreated for several days, joint destruction usually occurs and pathologic dislocation or subluxation may take place. These complications are most often seen in the septic hip joint, where early diagnosis and adequate treatment are particularly difficult. If the body defenses and the response to treatment are inadequate, spontaneous fusion or fibrous ankylosis may occur between the articulating bones. Septic arthritis, particularly of the tuberculous type, has a distinct tendency to go on to smoldering chronic infection with recurrent flares of activity. Even when adequately treated, a septic joint may become normal by all accepted clinical and radiographic criteria only to undergo eventual degenerative joint disease. This is an expression of the cartilage damage incurred during the acute stage.

Clinical Manifestations and Laboratory Findings

In evaluating all forms of acute arthritis, it is essential to exclude septic arthritis. The diagnosis is established by aspiration of the joint effusion (see Table 22–2). Organisms should be identified by smear and culture of the synovial fluid. Inasmuch as the bacteria may become intracellular or found within the synovial membrane, it is often useful to obtain a synovial biopsy for bacterial culture and histology if the diagnosis is uncertain. This is particularly true in tuberculous arthritis. In carrying out joint aspiration, the needle must not transgress a surrounding area of cellulitis or osteomyelitis. This would introduce sepsis into an otherwise sterile effusion. Other laboratory findings are similar to those of acute osteomyelitis. Radiographs may show only a joint effusion with capsular distention and displacement of adjacent fat shadows. Only late in the course of the disease, with destruction of the articular cartilage, do the radiographs show "joint space" narrowing or erosion of the subchondral bone and joint subluxation (Fig. 23–8).

Differential Diagnosis of Acute Osteomyelitis and Septic Arthritis

The differential diagnosis between septic arthritis and osteomyelitis is frequently difficult. In septic

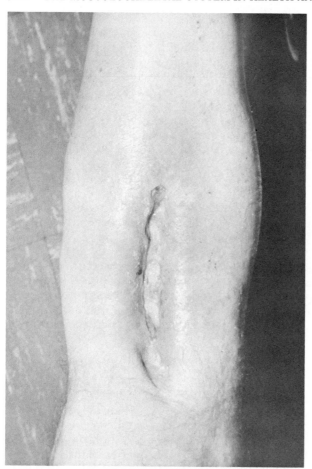

FIG. 23–7. Chronic drainage of tibial osteomyelitis to the back of the knee and calf. Dead bone is visible in the depth of the ulcer. The induration and the appearance of the edge of the ulcer are indicative of malignant transformation.

arthritis, however, it is unusual for the patient to submit to passive joint movement, whereas the child with osteomyelitis often allows joint movement provided it is performed gently. Furthermore, in osteomyelitis there is point tenderness over the metaphysis rather than over the joint itself. Other causes of acute arthritis such as gout, rheumatic fever or rheumatoid arthritis must be differentiated. Cellulitis, especially over the proximal end of the long bone, may be difficult to distinguish from osteomyelitis. When cellulitis is secondary to osteomyelitis, the disease is well advanced and other diagnostic criteria should be evident.

Management

Treatment is based on early diagnosis, identification of the offending organism, and institution of appropriate, systemic antibiotic therapy. Local treatment to the joint should consist only of aspiration of pus. Aspirations must be repeated as often as necessary to ensure proper decompression of the joint. If the aspirate is thick pus, it is helpful to irrigate the joint with sterile saline. This should be done with a large needle and only under operating room sterile conditions. Open drainage of the joint is indicated only where the reaccumulation of fluid cannot be closely followed (as in the hip joint) or where it is impossible to evacuate the pus fully due to recesses or loculation. Instillation of antibiotics directly into the joint is inappropriate since all known antibiotics cross the synovial membrane. Moreover, the antibiotic injected into a joint can act as a foreign substance, thus increasing the inflammatory process. It must be remembered that the articular cartilage has been damaged and is more pliable. The joint should, therefore, be protected and motion should begin in traction, without bearing weight until the joint has fully recovered and the individual has a normal range of motion and good muscle power.

CHRONIC SEPTIC ARTHRITIS

The classic form of chronic septic arthritis is **tuberculous arthritis,** but any inadequately treated, acute, septic arthritis may become chronic. Tuberculosis may affect a joint by extension from an adjoining bone or by primary synovial involvement. Its onset is insidious and creeps up on the patient like "a thief in the night." The outstanding physical finding is the striking atrophy in the surrounding musculature, which appears out of proportion to the severity of the disease. Management of chronic septic arthritis is based on the use of appropriate antibiotics plus surgical removal of the hyperplastic tissue and joint pus. The prognosis for joint function is poor.

Special Considerations

1. Patients with **hematologic disorders,** and particularly those with sickle cell disease, are prone to develop bone infection. *Salmonella* was once considered to be the usual offending organism but it has now been shown that while this organism is

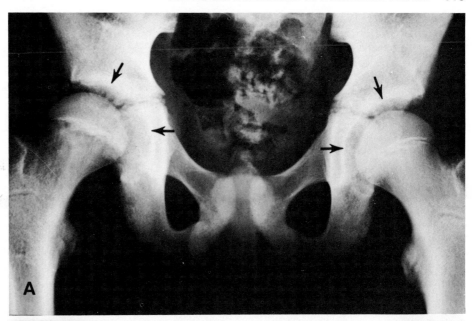

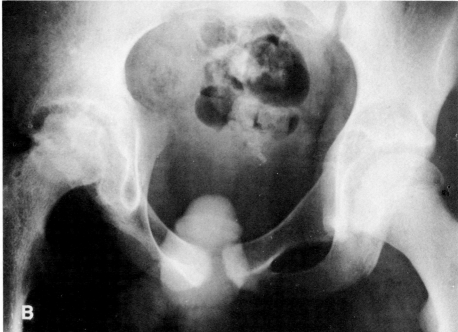

FIG. 23–8. Septic arthritis of the right hip in a 12-year-old boy. **(A)** At the early stage separation of the articular surfaces is due to joint effusion under tension. The depth of the "joint space" can be compared on the two sides with the aid of the arrows which point to the profile of the bony acetabular articular surface. **(B)** Late stage of the disease shows striking destruction of joint tissues, including the acetabular cortex, the femoral head and neck, and even osteolysis of the lesser trochanter due to extraarticular extension of the inflammatory process. Ankylosis is inevitable in this joint. (Courtesy of Dr. Rosalind H. Troupin)

still common, all types of bacterial osteomyelitis may be seen in patients with blood dyscrasias.

2. Intervertebral disks of the spine are a frequent site of a low grade inflammatory process often described as **diskitis.** While not all diskitis has been shown to be infectious in nature, it probably represents a low grade infection. The onset of diskitis is usually insidious. Small children may just refuse to walk, whereas older children and adults will complain of increasing low back or leg pain. In the adult, genitourinary infection or operative manipulation may be antecedent events, as may intravenous administration of drugs. *E. coli* and a variety of other organisms have been implicated. Physical findings include back splinting, pain on back motion, and paravertebral muscle spasm. Over the ensuing two or three weeks, the disk space as seen on x-rays will be noticeably narrowed, confirming the diagnosis. The erythrocyte sedimentation rate is often elevated; the white blood cell count is usually within normal limits. If the individual is not acutely ill, treatment can consist of plaster or brace immobilization. If fever is present, an attempt to establish a bacterial diagnosis by needle biopsy of the invertebral disk may be indicated, especially in older children and adults. In infants and children, the prognosis is excellent with resolution of the symptoms and eventual restoration of disk height, often without antibiotic therapy. In adolescents and adults, a bacterial etiology is more common and the prognosis must remain more guarded. The disk will usually not reform. If an abscess is suspected, it should be surgically drained and all necrotic disk material or dead bone removed. In such instances, spinal fusion may be necessary.

SUGGESTED READING

Clawson DK, Dunn AW: Management of common bacterial infections of bones and joints. J Bone Joint Surg [A] 49: 164, 1967
A concise account of the salient pathologic, radiographic and clinical features of osteomyelitis and pyogenic arthritis, including their treatment.

Goldenberg DL, Brandt KD, Cohen AS, Cathcart ES: Treatment of septic arthritis. Arthritis Rheum 18: 83, 1975
A good evaluation of various types of treatments.

Hansen ST, George RC, Clawson DK: Orthopedic infections. In Kagan BM (ed): Antimicrobial Therapy. Philadelphia, WB Saunders, 1974, p 321
This brief paper is concerned with the treatment of septic arthritis and osteomyelitis and discusses the antibiotic therapy of choice when the causative organisms have not been immediately identified.

Treves S, Khettry J, Broker FH, Wilkinson RH, Watts H: Osteomyelitis: early scintigraphic detection in children. Pediatrics 57: 173, 1976
This article describes the value of bone scan.

Trueta J: Osteomyelitis. In Trueta J: Studies of the Development and Decay of the Human Frame. Philadelphia, WB Saunders, 1968, p 255
A brief but interesting description of osteomyelitis covering pathogenesis, clinical course, and sequelae.

Wadvogel FA, Medoff G, Schwartz MN: Osteomyelitis: a review of clinical features, therapeutic considerations and unusual aspects. N Engl J Med 282: 198, 260 and 360, 1970
This series of articles presents an excellent account of the disease.

24
Degenerative Joint Disease

PETER A. SIMKIN

Degenerative joint disease is characterized by a localized noninflammatory deterioration of articular cartilage. The deterioration is associated with intrinsic changes in cartilage structure and metabolism influenced by aging, heredity, erosion, endocrine factors, deposition of abnormal materials, and other poorly understood factors. Acute or repetitive trauma is a well recognized contributing factor in the pathogenesis. Although changes in cartilage are in all cases primary, clinical and radiographic features are largely determined by secondary alterations in bone. This condition, often referred to as **osteoarthritis**, is not a true arthritis, since inflammation is not the primary event in this disease.

Incidence

Degenerative joint disease is by far the most common of all musculoskeletal disorders, occurring in more than 40 million Americans. There is no racial or sexual predilection for the disease. The highest correlation is with advancing age. Although the disease is progressive, changes occur slowly and symptoms may be few. Most patients tolerate degenerative joint disease surprisingly well, and the patient with early disease can be reassured that he is unlikely to become incapacitated. A significant number of patients, however, eventually become disabled.

All joints may be involved by this process, with most morbidity resulting from involvement of the spine, hips, and knees. Though exposed to similar weight-bearing stress, the ankle is rarely affected.

Etiology

The etiology of degenerative joint disease is not known. A number of factors, however, clearly play a part in the pathogenesis.

Trauma. Trauma is the most significant identifiable cause of degenerative joint disease. Chronic repetitive trauma to the articular cartilage may result from instability or incongruity of a joint; for example, an unstable knee or a subluxed hip. Normal joints subject to unusual repetitive trauma show an increased tendency to degenerate; for example, the elbow of a baseball pitcher. Acute injuries, especially to the knee, may also lead to degenerative joint disease which may not become manifest until years after the injury.

A causative role for repetitive impulse loading has been suggested by recent experimental studies. Sudden impacts across joints are normally transmitted directly into the subchondral trabecular bone (see Fig. 5–4). When such forces are excessive or are unduly repetitive, there will be trabecular fractures which on healing will lead to thickening of the trabeculae. This process must then result in stiffening of the subchondral bone with an impaired ability to absorb the forces applied across the joint. This loss of subchondral spring will necessarily increase the stress on the articular cartilage with ensuing acceleration of surface wear and tear. A considerable body of experimental evidence supports this hypothesis although the extent of its contribution to the overall picture of degenerative joint disease remains uncertain.

One of the most severe forms of traumatic degenerative joint disease occurs in joints deprived of sensory innervation. Degenerative changes occur early and progress rapidly in these joints, presumably because of faulty alignment permitted by the absence of pain. The classic example of this is the Charcot joint of tertiary syphilis.

Heredity. Genetic factors are clearly significant in inbred strains of mice which suffer from degenerative joint disease. In man the best example is that of **erosive osteoarthritis**. In this condition, de-

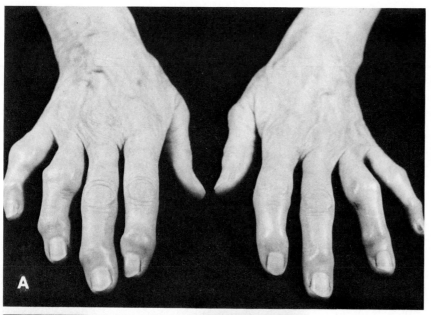

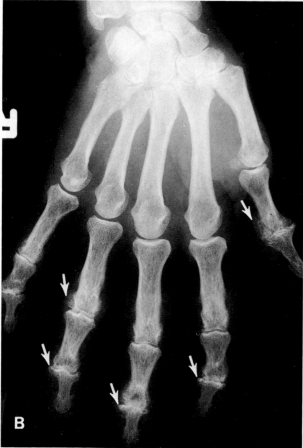

FIG. 24-1. Erosive osteoarthritis of the hands. **(A)** The distal interphalangeal joints are deformed by Heberden's nodes and there is bilateral involvement of the fourth and fifth proximal interphalangeal joints. Note, however, that in contrast to the rheumatoid hands in Figure 22–5A, the wrists and metacarpophalangeal joints are spared. (Courtesy of The Arthritis Foundation) **(B)** X-ray of the hand of a different patient suffering from erosive osteoarthritis. Note the osteophytes underlying Heberden's nodes at the distal interphalangeal joints, and other bony spurs that occur independent of nodes in the thumb and the proximal interphalangeal joint of the ring finger. The wrist, intercarpal, and carpometacarpal joints are normal. (Courtesy of Dr. Rosalind H. Troupin)

generative disease characteristically involves the proximal and distal interphalangeal joints, as well as the carpometacarpal joints of the thumb. There is a very high familial incidence and the process usually involves women at the time of menopause. It is in this condition that small, paired nodules occur over the dorsum of the distal interphalangeal joints. These lesions are known as Heberden's nodes (Fig. 24–1).

Age. The role of aging in degenerative joint disease is clearly present but poorly understood. Radiographic and histologic evidence of degenerative joint disease is almost universal by the eighth decade. Whether these lesions arise from primary biochemical changes in cartilage or are the legacy of years of accumulated trauma is not known.

Past History of Arthritis. In many instances degenerative changes represent the legacy of past inflammatory episodes. This occurs after healed infection of joints and is often seen in inactive rheumatoid arthritis. The damaged cartilage is then subjected to accelerated wear. Whether enzymes play a similar role in the initiation of erosion and continuation of idiopathic degenerative joint disease is not clear.

Miscellaneous. A number of metabolic diseases lead to deposition of foreign materials within the cartilage which then appear to accelerate its degeneration. Among these are hemosiderin in **hemochromatosis,** homogentisic acid in **alkaptonuria,** and calcium pyrophosphate in **chondrocalcinosis.** Cartilage is also subject to endocrine influences, and degenerative changes may result from endocrine imbalance. The most notable example of this is **acromegaly.** Nutritional deficiencies may represent another major factor in degenerative joint disease. In Chapter 5 the role of synovial fluid in the nutrition of articular cartilage was discussed. Diffusion of nutrients is greatly enhanced by compression and decompression of the cartilage. Any local factor interfering with the diffusion or supply of nutrients may contribute to degenerative joint disease. Degenerative joint disease may be induced experimentally by a period of prolonged compression followed by usage. Cartilage will degenerate if it is isolated from the articular surface with which it is usually in contact. This is observed clinically in the hip joint, where the earliest changes occur on non-weight-bearing areas of the articular surface of the femoral head.

Pathogenesis

The structure and function of articular cartilage were discussed in Chapter 5. Cartilage must remain resilient in order to absorb and distribute the forces which are applied across joints. To retain its minimal friction articular cartilage must maintain a smooth and unbroken surface. Once surface changes have occurred, friction is increased and a vicious cycle of accelerated wear and cartilage destruction is underway. In early degenerative joint disease there is roughening of the cartilaginous surface, with flaking parallel to the superficial layer of collagen fibers. Further fibrillation of the surface area then occurs, and clefts may penetrate the depth of the cartilage. Despite localized proliferation and increased metabolic activity of chondrocytes, there is loss of water and proteoglycans reflected by loss of metachromasia in histologic sections. The early and late changes of cartilage in degenerative joint disease are compared with normal cartilage in Figure 24–2. These microscopic changes are accompanied by **gross thinning of the cartilage,** which becomes roughened, dull, and opaque. As the cartilage is worn away, there is **proliferation of the underlying bone,** which may ultimately develop a smooth, marbled appearance after its exposure. This bony proliferation also extends laterally beyond the joint margins, presenting as spurs or **osteophytes. Cystic areas** also commonly form in the subchondral bone for reasons which remain uncertain. One theory is that these lesions result from the very high pressures which develop in synovial effusions during vigorous use of diseased joints. According to this concept, cysts develop where pressure and synovial fluid are transmitted through cartilaginous fissures into the underlying cancellous bone.

Clinical Manifestations

The most common symptom of degenerative joint disease is an aching pain in the region of the joint. The pain is exacerbated by activity and largely relieved by rest. The pain, however, characteristically recurs after prolonged rest and may be especially severe at night. On physical examination there is little or no evidence of inflammation, but a

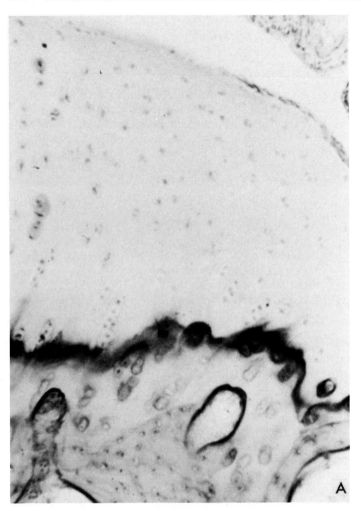

FIG. 24–2. Photomicrographs of histologic sections of articular cartilage in the normal and in degenerative joint disease. **(A)** Normal articular cartilage. **(B)** Early degenerative changes in cartilage. **(C)** Marked degenerative changes in cartilage. The surface is smooth in **A,** with normal distribution of chondrocytes. In **B,** there is flaking of the cartilage parallel to the surface with areas of softening in the matrix. Deep fissures are seen in **C,** with focal proliferation of chondrocytes. (× 200) (Courtesy of The Arthritis Foundation)

moderate effusion may be present. A localized grating feeling of the joint on motion (crepitus) is characteristic. There may be spasm of muscles around involved joints. Significant limitation of motion is often present and may not be recognized by the patient. Symptoms are usually insidious in onset and progress gradually. Acute symptoms also occur and may be associated with well-localized pain and tenderness. Such episodes are frequently caused by local trauma impinging on osteophytic processes.

Laboratory Tests

The synovial fluid, reflecting the lack of inflammation, has a low white blood cell count and those cells present are predominantly mononuclear (Table 22–2). The viscosity is normal, the protein content is low, and the fluid does not clot. The synovial fluid may contain significant amounts of particulate debris which is presumably derived from the cartilage.

Radiographic changes include characteristic narrowing of the "joint space" and an underlying bony reaction (Fig. 24–3). This is reflected as sclerosis of the bone with formation of osteophytes. Bone cysts may be quite large. There is a poor correlation between radiographic findings and symptoms.

As would be expected from the localized nature of this disease, there are no significant changes in other laboratory tests such as blood chemistries or hematologic studies.

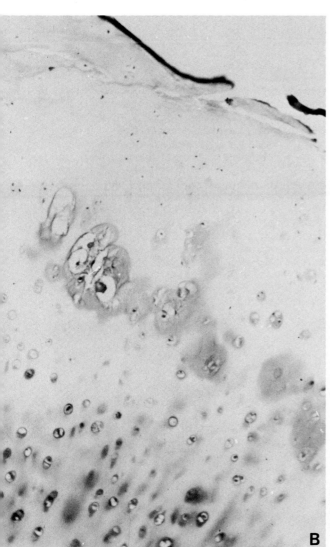

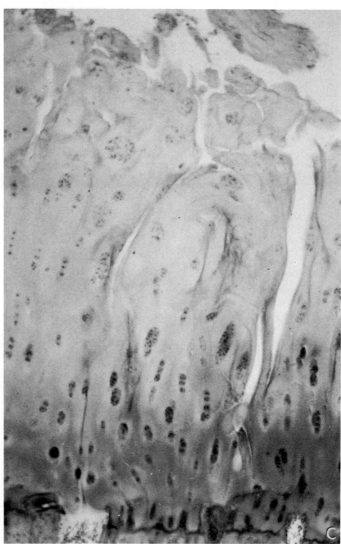

(continued)

Management

Articular cartilage possesses very limited capacity for repair and there are no known methods to effectively renew damaged cartilage by medical means. Therapeutic goals in degenerative joint disease are therefore primarily limited to relief of pain and retarding progression of the degenerative process.

Relief may be achieved with aspirin and other analgesics and rest of the joint. The use of heat relaxes associated muscle spasm. Abnormal joint wear may be substantially alleviated by attention to proper posture and the use of exercises to improve joint stability. In selected cases surgery may be indicated to improve the distribution of weight within a joint (osteotomy) or to create an artificial joint (arthroplasty or prosthetic replacement).

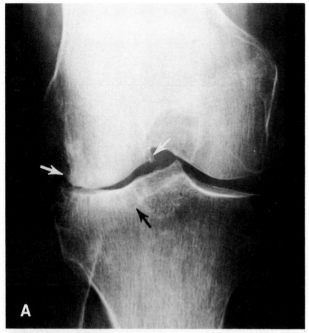

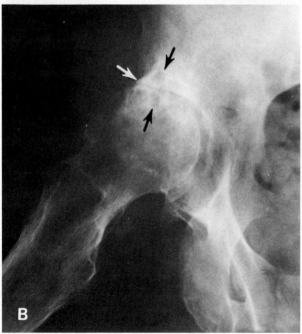

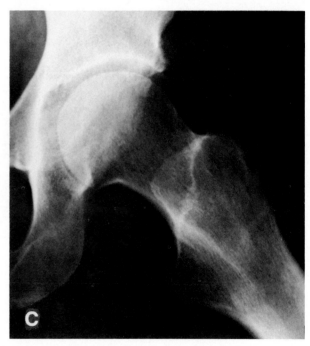

FIG. 24-3. X-rays of a knee (**A**) and a hip (**B**) showing different degrees of degenerative joint disease. In **A** the joint between the medial condyles shows no abnormality. However, there is narrowing of the "joint space" between the lateral condyles. There is sclerosis adjacent to both tibial and femoral articular surfaces; radiolucency in the tibia suggests cysts (**black arrow**), and osteophytes project like spurs from the edges of the femoral condyle (**white arrows**). Comparison of the hip in **B** with a normal hip shown in **C** illustrates the cardinal radiologic features of advanced degeneration. Both hips are in the frog-leg position with the thigh abducted and laterally rotated. Compare the depth of the joint space, especially superiorly, the sclerosis, and the mottled appearance of the bone in **B** due to cysts (**black arrows**). An osteophyte projects from the sclerosed lip of the acetabulum (**white arrow**). (Courtesy of Dr. Rosalind H. Troupin)

SUGGESTED READING

Mankin JH: The reaction of articular cartilage to injury and osteoarthritis. N Engl J Med *291*: 1285 and 1335, 1974
A thorough review emphasizing metabolic and biochemical changes in damaged cartilage.
Pathogenesis of osteoarthrosis. Lancet ii: 1131, 1973
A concise, well-referenced review of proposed mechanisms for degenerative joint disease as "joint failure" which may occur either by overloading normal cartilage or through intrinsic defects in the cartilage itself.
Radin EL: Mechanical aspects of osteoarthritis. Bull Rheum Dis *26*: 862, 1976
A clear exposition of the concept that repetitive impulse loading of joints leads to increased stiffness of subchondral bone with a secondary increase in the mechanical stress to articular cartilage.

25
Disorders of Tendons and Bursae

D. KAY CLAWSON

Inflammation and degeneration in tendons and dense connective tissue are responsible for a significant amount of morbidity in the musculoskeletal system. Extraarticular synovial membrane in bursae and tendon sheaths is subject to all the inflammatory diseases of synovial joints (Chap. 22) but in addition, bursae, tendons and their synovial sheaths are affected by a number of pathologic processes which do not involve joints. Inflammation of the synovial membrane of bursae and tendon sheaths is called **bursitis** and **tenosynovitis.** Inflammation of tendons is called **tendinitis.** These terms are often incorrectly interchanged. Inflammation in these structures may occur secondary to specific diseases (for example, infections and rheumatoid arthritis) or may result from chronic trauma or idiopathic degeneration. These conditions are sometimes associated with complete or incomplete tendon rupture.

The true incidence is unknown, since *bursitis* is a household word used for a variety of common, painful afflictions about joints. Bursitis and tendinitis are seen in adults of all ages; however, the conditions are more prevalent in the 35 to 55 age group. Women are affected more often than men. The prognosis is excellent if the condition is accurately diagnosed and appropriate treatment is instituted.

TENDINITIS AND TENOSYNOVITIS

Etiology and Pathogenesis

Tendons undergo disuse atrophy and degeneration with aging similar to other tissues. Since they are relatively avascular, they have a lower metabolic turnover and are less capable of repair than the more vascular structures. Any tendon can develop tendinitis or tenosynovitis. However, the condition is seen most commonly in three sites:

1. Where a tendon crosses a joint at an angle (for example, long head of the biceps at the shoulder; abductor pollicis longus and extensor pollicis brevis at the wrist)

2. Where the tendon is subjected to unusual forces (for example, common origin of the forearm flexors and extensors on the humeral epicondyles)

3. Where sharp angulation of the tendon fibers occurs at the site of insertion (for example, supraspinatus tendon at the shoulder)

At these sites degeneration is accelerated and rupture is not uncommon. Tendons subject to chronic trauma sustain microscopic and macroscopic tears. The reparative process is associated with the presence of inflammatory and multinucleated giant cells, and often leads to the deposition of calcium salts at the reparative sites. The condition is then called **calcific tendinitis.** The calcium salts may accumulate in considerable quantities and may burst into an overlying tendon sheath or bursa, producing **calcific tenosynovitis** or **bursitis** (Fig. 25–1). Bursae and tendon sheaths may also be affected by rheumatoid arthritis and infection. The histopathology then resembles the intraarticular synovial lesions in each of these conditions. Degenerative or inflammatory changes may result in a compromise between the size of the tendons and the fibrous sheath through which they pass. This condition is called **stenosing tenosynovitis.**

Clinical Manifestations

Owing to a relative lack of nerve endings, changes in the tendons are painless unless they involve the surrounding synovial membrane or bursa. Degen-

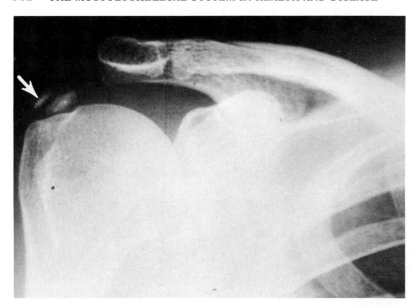

FIG. 25-1. Calcific degeneration in the tendon of the supraspinatus. The radiograph was taken after the calcified material burst through the tendon, and it can be seen extending into the overlying subacromial-subdeltoid bursa **(arrow).**

erative conditions of the tendons are characterized by a deep ache in the affected area, with pain referred into the muscle of the tendon involved. Symptoms are aggravated by use of the involved muscle-tendon unit. Episodes of severe pain may occur from acute inflammation of the synovial sheaths or bursae. On physical examination, the area may show diffuse signs of inflammation, but there is always distinct **point tenderness** over the site of involvement. Squeaking or crepitus may be perceived along the involved tendon sheath. In the case of the long finger flexors at the metacarpophalangeal joint, a phenomenon of catching or triggering may be seen. This occurs when there is a disproportion in the size of the tendon and the fibrous sheath or pulley it traverses. When the flexor muscle contracts, the tendon is drawn through the pulley. When the finger is extended, the flexor tendon may catch proximal to the pulley, requiring additional extensor force to snap the finger into extension (trigger finger, Fig. 15–14).

A tendon undergoing degeneration may rupture under even slight stress. A normal tendon may also rupture if sufficient force is applied. Following an initial stinging, searing pain, there may be little or no discomfort to suggest a significant injury. Diagnosis is made by palpation of the defect or by failure of the tendon to move the appropriate part. Immediate surgical repair is usually the treatment of choice. Tendons may also rupture in advanced rheumatoid arthritis. This most frequently occurs in the extensor tendons of the hand, primarily the ring and little fingers.

CALCIFIC TENDINITIS AND TENOSYNOVITIS

While minor calcific deposits are not unusual in a number of tendons, calcification most commonly occurs at the insertion of the supraspinatus tendon. Any increase in the size of the tendon produces symptoms because of the minimal space between the tuberosity of the humerus and the acromion process. Calcium deposits in this area are repeatedly traumatized by shoulder motion, and the inflammatory process is exacerbated.

Characteristically, the patient complains of aching pain in the shoulder region and has point tenderness over the greater tuberosity of the humerus. Pain is worse at night, and lying on the affected side is virtually impossible. Abduction and medial rotation are restricted and painful. Radiographic evidence of calcification in the supraspinatus tendon is helpful, but calcification may be present without symptoms. Conversely, many patients with symptoms show no evidence of calcification. Relief of symptoms by the injection of a local anesthetic into the involved area corroborates the diagnosis. When any inflammatory or degenerative process in or about the shoulder becomes chronic, a limitation of movement often occurs due to capsular adhesions. This condition, called **frozen shoulder,** can usually be prevented by appropriate range-of-motion exercises.

BURSITIS

An inflammatory reaction may occur in any bursa. Those most commonly involved are located at points of greatest friction, such as the subdeltoid and subacromial bursae at the shoulder, the olecranon bursa at the elbow, the trochanteric bursa at the hip, and the pre- and infrapatellar bursae at the knee. After repeated trauma, these bursae may become distended by effusion, with resulting pain and point tenderness. The term bursitis should be reserved for the acute inflammatory process rather than for chronic tendinitis with secondary bursal irritation.

Occasionally bacteria may enter a bursa from a hematogenous route or, more commonly, from direct extension through the skin, thus producing **septic bursitis.** This condition is most commonly seen in the prepatellar bursa in children. Likewise, infection can enter a tendon sheath and produce **septic tenosynovitis** (see Fig. 15–24).

Aspiration and culture of any fluid are essential to differentiate an aseptic from a septic process. In septic tenosynovitis or bursitis, evacuation of the pus and proper antibiotic treatment are essential. In aseptic inflammatory processes efforts to decrease inflammation through rest and the use of antiinflammatory drugs given locally or systemically are the treatments of choice. Maintenance of the range of motion of the joint is essential.

MYOFASCIAL SYNDROMES

Numerous patients are encountered with aching, tender muscles and with point tenderness at specific sites of tendon insertion, and where nerves penetrate dense fascia. These spots of point tenderness are referred to as **trigger points** and are most characteristic in the back along the spine and in the forearm. Pressure at these sites may produce referred pain segmentally in myotomes. These syndromes are poorly understood, but probably result from chronic overuse, either from repeated activities or from nervous tension. Common trigger areas are the sites of muscle insertion in the occiput, the sacrum, the C7 to T1 spinous processes, and the superior angle of the scapula. Treatment is based on local anesthetic injections, active exercise programs, and efforts to decrease chronic tension and anxiety states.

SUGGESTED READING

Anderson LD: Afflictions of muscles, tendons and tendon sheaths. In Crenshaw AH (ed): Campbell's Operative Orthopedics, 5th ed. St. Louis, CV Mosby, 1971, p 1459
This is a comprehensive account of the operative treatment of afflictions of tendons and tendon sheaths and includes a complete bibliography on the subject, including degenerative conditions.

26
Diseases of the Motor Unit

GEORGE H. KRAFT

A motor neuron cell body, its axon within a peripheral nerve, the neuromuscular junction, and the muscle fibers supplied by the neuron constitute a motor unit, as discussed in Chapters 3 and 4. Any of these structures making up the motor unit may be the target of a variety of pathologic processes. Yet diseases of either muscle fibers or peripheral nerve axons lead to functional impairments which have many similarities.

The hallmark of skeletal muscle and peripheral nerve diseases is **muscle weakness** and **atrophy**. The clinical manifestations, however, differ in two major ways depending on whether the primary pathology affects the muscle or nerve: 1) **In muscle disease there is no loss of sensation while in peripheral nerve disease there may be sensory loss**. Disease processes affecting peripheral motor axons almost always also affect peripheral sensory axons. 2) **Weakness in muscle diseases is usually greatest in proximal muscles while in peripheral nerve diseases the weakness is usually greatest in distal muscles**. In peripheral nerve disease, the dysfunction is greatest in more distal parts of the neuron.

All diseases which primarily affect skeletal muscle are known as **myopathies**. If histologic changes characteristic of a disease can be demonstrated in muscle fibers, or if the cause of the muscle disease can be identified, the myopathy is given a specific name indicative of the histologic changes or associated conditions. If the disorder is inflammatory, it is known as **myositis**; if it is a degeneration of unknown cause with nonspecific pathologic changes the disease is classified as a **dystrophy**.

Disease processes primarily affecting peripheral nerves are known as **neuropathies**. In neuropathies degeneration or dysfunction of lower motor neurons leads to degeneration of the muscle fibers innervated by them. If the disease primarily affects peripheral nerve axons diffusely, the disease is known as a **peripheral neuropathy**. If it affects the motor nerve cell body it is known as a **muscular atrophy**. In neuropathies normal nerve impulses do not pass down the nerve; consequently, the muscle does not function normally and undergoes atrophic changes. Peripheral neuropathies can affect peripheral motor or sensory nerves; in some diseases autonomic nerves are affected as well. Primary pathologic changes may consist of axonal degeneration, demyelination or, in some conditions, both. If axonal degeneration is the primary pathology, secondary demyelination may follow. If extensive enough, primary demyelination may also lead to secondary axonal degeneration.

In addition to the large number of diseases which affect the nerve and muscle, several specific diseases are due to dysfunction of the **myoneural junction**. The major clinical manifestation of these diseases is **fatigability**. These diseases include **myasthenia gravis, myasthenic syndrome,** and **botulism**. The pathophysiology of these disorders has been discussed in Chapter 3.

Myopathies, neuropathies, and diseases of the neuromuscular junction may be primary or may be secondary to a large number of systemic diseases or toxic conditions. The basic **symptom** of nerve and muscle disease is **muscle weakness**. Symptoms may also include **cramps, fatigability, stiffness,** and intermittent (periodic) **paralysis.** Weakness may also be expressed by the patient in terms of such complaints as clumsiness, frequent falling, or difficulty in performing various functions.

Basic **signs** of disorders of nerve or muscle are **flaccidity** (decreased muscle tone), **decreased muscle strength, muscle atrophy** (decreased bulk of muscle), and **hyporeflexia** or **areflexia**. Muscle atrophy follows within weeks after the development of weakness; in chronic disease it generally parallels demonstrable weakness. Hyporeflexia or areflexia may be due either to muscle loss or to peripheral nerve dysfunction. In neuropathies **loss of sensation** and **paresthesia** in distal portions of the legs and arms are generally noted in addition to motor loss.

Diseases of the suprasegmental motor centers and of the descending tracts in the spinal cord or brain stem also result in weakness and some muscle atrophy. Since the motor unit is not directly affected by these diseases, they are not classified as neuropathies. Motor weakness in these conditions is secondary to a reduction in stimuli to the segmental motor neurons. Any muscle atrophy which occurs in these conditions is a **disuse atrophy**. The present chapter is concerned only with diseases which primarily affect the components of the motor unit, and the following chapter will deal with suprasegmental causes of impaired movement.

HISTOPATHOLOGY OF MYOPATHIES AND NEUROPATHIES

Histologic examination of muscle is important in understanding muscle diseases and may be required to confirm a diagnosis. Biopsy of nerves, however, is much less frequently done because of the inevitable anesthesia and/or paralysis which result from removing a portion of nerve for histologic study.

Muscle

The histologic changes found in diseased muscle are muscle fiber degeneration, muscle fiber death, attempts at regeneration, selective loss of type I or type II muscle fibers, complete replacement of muscle by fat and connective tissue, infiltration by inflammatory cells, abnormalities of muscle cell nuclei and mitochondria, excess amounts of lipid droplets, and a number of specific changes in muscle cell architecture seen in light and electron microscope studies (e.g., abnormal central myofibrils, myotubes, specific loss of cross-striations, "fingerprints", zebra bodies, target fibers, and rod bodies). These processes generate various patterns which indicate whether the primary disease process is more compatible with a myopathy or a neuropathy. In some instances of primary muscle disease, the changes are sufficiently unique to permit diagnosis of a specific type of myopathy. **In general, in myopathies pathologic changes are seen diffusely throughout the muscle, whereas in neuropathies clumps of normal appearing or even hypertrophic muscle fibers will be juxtaposed with areas of advanced degeneration.**

In the cross section of a normal muscle four to five nuclei are usually seen at the periphery of each fiber (Fig. 26–1). Muscle cell nuclei multiply and many migrate to the center of the fiber when the muscle becomes diseased. This multiplication is the most frequently observed pathologic change in muscle and is more marked in myopathies than in neuropathies.

In normal muscle, fiber diameter is generally uniform, whereas in myopathies it is highly variable with large and small fibers intermixed (Fig.

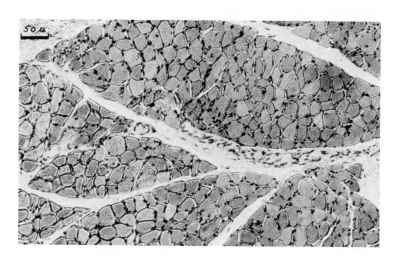

FIG. 26–1. Normal muscle in transverse section. (Hematoxylin and eosin) (Adams RD et al: Diseases of Muscle, 2nd ed. New York, Hoeber, 1962)

26–2). Focal atrophy, termed **perifascicular atrophy**, occurs at the periphery of muscle fiber bundles and is particularly associated with inflammatory myopathies. Also in inflammatory myopathies, as the name implies, infiltration with lymphocytes and phagocytic cells is the characteristic and dominant histologic finding. A less marked inflammatory response is also seen in other diseases of muscle and nerve whenever muscle fibers degenerate. Disruption of the normal pattern of muscle striations occurs in several types of muscle diseases, but is not helpful in differentiating neuropathies from myopathies.

There are two basic muscle fiber types, called type I fibers and type II fibers, as distinguished by the myofibrillar adenosine triphosphatase (ATPase) staining reaction (see Fig. 3–12). Normally muscle fibers of these two types are interdigitated in human muscles. Muscle cell atrophy or hypertrophy can involve either type I or type II fibers or both. A disease producing changes limited to one fiber type is described as a **type specific disease.** Selective atrophy of type I fibers is uncommon and occurs primarily in myotonic dystrophy. Atrophy of type II fibers, however, occurs almost in any disease in which strength is impaired secondary to lesions remote from muscle (i.e., neuropathy or upper motor neuron disease).

Recently a number of new myopathies have been identified by their histologic characteristics. For

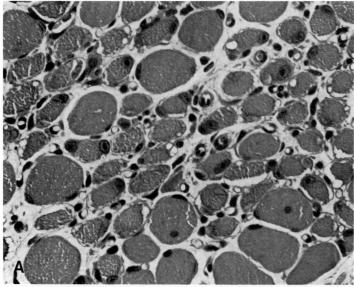

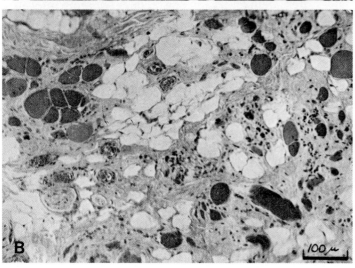

FIG. 26–2. Transverse section of muscle in one of the myopathies (muscular dystrophy). **(A)** Note the variation in the diameter of muscle fibers and the increase in the number of nuclei. Some of the nuclei have been displaced toward the center of the muscle fiber. **(B)** Advanced stage of the same disease shows few and small muscle fibers, areas containing nuclear residue of muscle, and an increased amount of connective tissue and fat cells. **(A,** hematoxylin and eosin × 500; **B,** hematoxylin and van Gieson) **(A,** Aegerter E, Kirkpatrick JA: Orthopedic Diseases, 3rd ed. Philadelphia, Saunders, 1968; **B,** Adams RD et al: Diseases of Muscle, 2nd ed. New York, Hoeber, 1962)

FIG. 26-3. Transverse section of muscle in a neuropathy (chronic polyneuropathy). Note clusters of muscle fibers of varying diameter. Fibers of normal appearance with others showing recent nuclear proliferation are seen next to an area of old atrophy where nuclear residue alone represents muscle substance. Note the presence of fat cells. (Hematoxylin and van Gieson.) (Adams RE et al: Diseases of Muscle, 2nd ed. New York, Hoeber, 1962)

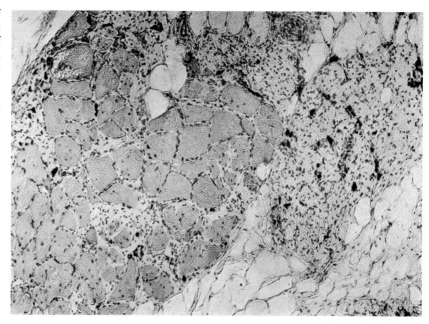

example, central cores of altered myofibrils are pathognomonic of **central core myopathy**. Rod bodies have been found within the cytoplasm of muscle cells in **nemaline myopathy**. Granular or ragged-red muscle fibers, when occurring as a relatively isolated phenomenon, are usually associated with **ophthalmoplegic myopathy** which primarily affects the extraocular muscles.

Muscle biopsy may also be useful in studying diseases of nerve (Fig. 26–3). As pointed out above, nerve disease produces muscle weakness. Similarly, nerve disease will also produce changes in the architecture of skeletal muscle. Often the changes are nonspecific, but in recent onset neuropathy small, atrophic fibers are distributed among fibers of normal size. Atrophy of large segments of muscle (fascicles), called **large group atrophy**, occurs only in chronic denervating diseases. A relative increase in the amount of connective tissue and fat cells occurs in advanced stages of nerve and muscle disease.

Nerve

Nerve biopsies are less frequently used to establish a diagnosis than are muscle biopsies. Whereas a muscle biopsy is relatively innocuous—a small amount of muscle tissue can easily be removed

without any functional loss—and may give direct information about the muscle and the nerve that supplies it, taking a section of nerve for biopsy will denervate the muscle supplied by the nerve or produce an area of anesthesia in the cutaneous distribution of the nerve. In practice, therefore, clinical nerve biopsy, when done, is limited to the sural nerve, which is a sensory nerve.

Neuropathies produce either primary **axonal degeneration** or primary **segmental demyelination.** Demyelination of a secondary nature may also occur along a segment of nerve having undergone axonal degeneration, and in extensive demyelination, secondary axonal changes may occur. Histologically, axonal degeneration is recognized by either a decrease in the cross section diameter of axons or by the complete loss of neuronal tissue and a consequent reduction in the number of axons seen on a cross section of nerve. Demyelination is noted by either a reduction in myelin on a cross section of nerve or by observation of demyelinated regions of a teased nerve fiber preparation (myelin stain).

In diseased nerve, demyelination and remyelination may occur repeatedly. Remyelination may be uncontrolled and thickened myelin sheaths known as **onion bulbs** are produced which are thought to be pathognomonic of this process. In-

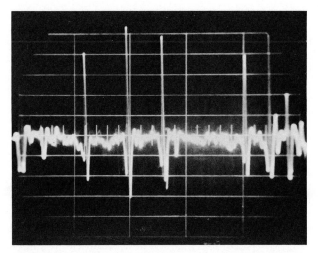

FIG. 26–4. Normal motor unit action potentials. Calibration: each horizontal division 200 μv; each major vertical division 30 msec. Positive deflection is downward. Note that the typical motor unit action potential has three phases with the initial phase positive. Most normal motor unit action potentials are between 1000 and 2000 μv in amplitude. In myopathies the potentials are reduced in amplitude and in neuropathies they are increased in amplitude.

26–4). Electromyography can assess the number of motor units functioning (i.e., the degree of innervation), the type of motor unit action potentials seen (whether they are of the large amplitude, long duration type, typically found in nerve diseases, or the low amplitude, short duration type, typically seen in muscle disease), the ability of patients to control motor units voluntarily, the electrical stability of the muscle cell membrane (positive sharp waves), and can detect involuntary spontaneous events such as fasciculations and fibrillations (Fig. 26–5). **Fasciculations** are spontaneous discharges of entire motor units and are commonly seen in the muscular atrophies, whereas **fibrillations** represent the spontaneous firing of individual muscle fibers and are found in muscle which is either denervated or otherwise pathologically affected. Fasciculation can be noted clinically through the skin, but fibrillations—representing the electrical activity associated with the contraction of a single muscle fiber—cannot. It takes up to 21 days after loss of continuity of axis cylinders for fibrillation potentials to occur.

In myopathies, as individual muscle fibers de-

terruption of an axon leads to its degeneration **(wallerian degeneration)** distal to the site of injury. This takes place over a three-to-five-day period. The axon's metabolic activity requires the integrity of continuity with the nerve cell body situated in the spinal cord or dorsal root ganglion, and when the continuity is interrupted characteristic histologic changes of degeneration follow.

ELECTROMYOGRAPHY AND MUSCLE ENZYMES

The most useful laboratory tests for the investigation of neuromuscular diseases are clinical electromyography and muscle enzyme determinations.

Clinical Electromyography

Clinical electromyography consists of three parts: 1) electromyography (EMG), 2) nerve conduction studies, and 3) repetitive stimulation studies. In **electromyography,** a small needle electrode is inserted into a muscle belly to record the action potentials of individual motor units (MUP) (Fig.

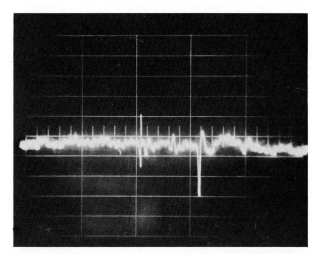

FIG. 26–5. Fibrillation potentials and positive sharp wave. Calibration: each horizontal division 100 μv; each major vertical division 30 msec. Positive deflection is downward. In the middle of the photograph is a fibrillation potential. Fibrillation potentials are biphasic with the initial phase positive. In the right of the picture is a positive sharp wave. Positive sharp waves have an initial positive deflection followed by a low amplitude relatively long duration negative phase.

generate, the number of viable muscle fibers in each motor unit decreases and MUPs are reduced in amplitude and duration. MUPs will also become polyphasic (five or more phases). On the other hand, in neuropathies, the number of muscle fibers innervated by a viable motor neuron increases. This is due to the capture of a few surviving muscle fibers from denervated motor units by the terminal sprouting of an unaffected motor axon. Atrophy of non-reinnervated muscle fibers which are interspersed with the fibers of a viable motor unit leads to a reduction in the over-all diameter of the unit, despite the fact that its population of muscle fibers has been augmented. In effect, the spatial rearrangement of muscle fibers is believed to produce a more compact motor unit. This is thought to produce an increase in the size of the MUPs because the amplitude of the MUP is inversely related to the distance of the contracting muscle fibers from the EMG needle electrode. The rearrangement of muscle fibers also explains, in part, the

characteristic large type grouping seen on histologic sections. Thus, in contrast to myopathies, motor unit action potentials are increased in amplitude and duration in diseases of nerve. As in myopathies, MUPs may be polyphasic also in neuropathies, especially if reinnervation has also occurred. Because there are fewer motor units functioning, when compared with the normal, a reduced number of MUPs will be seen on maximal contraction in neuropathies.

Nerve conduction studies consist of motor and sensory **nerve conduction velocity** determinations, **(NCV),** distal latency measurements and evaluation of the muscle response. NCVs are determined by calculating the conduction velocity (in meters/second) of an electrical impulse along a peripheral nerve (Fig. 26–6). A nerve is stimulated at proximal point and the proximal latency or L_p (time between the stimulus and muscle response) is measured. The nerve is then stimulated at a distal point and the distal latency (L_d) is measured. The

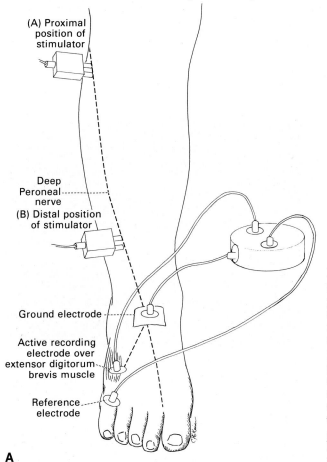

(A) Proximal position of stimulator

Deep Peroneal nerve

(B) Distal position of stimulator

Ground electrode

Active recording electrode over extensor digitorum brevis muscle

Reference electrode

A

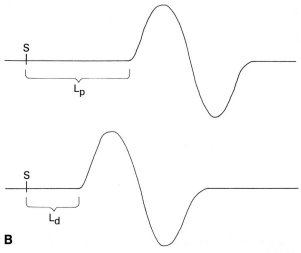

B

FIG. 26–6. (A) Example of routine method for determining motor nerve conduction velocity of the deep peroneal nerve. The active recording electrode is placed over the midportion of the belly of the extensor digitorum brevis muscle, with the reference electrode over the fifth toe. The peroneal nerve is then stimulated at two points. One proximal (A) and the other distal (B). The peroneal nerve underlies the skin in the position of the dotted line in the foot and innervates the extensor digitorum brevis muscle. **(B)** Representation of the trace of the evoked muscle response on an oscilloscope screen with a peripheral nerve stimulated proximally (A) and distally (B). The time of the nerve stimulus is indicated by S, and the times elapsing between the stimuli and the muscle responses are indicated by L_p and L_d.

NCV is calculated by measuring the distance between the two points of stimulation and dividing it by the time taken by the impulse to travel from proximal to distal stimulation points (L_p–L_d). Direct conduction techniques can be used also for sensory NCV determinations.

Nerve conduction velocities are reduced in peripheral neuropathies, whereas they are characteristically normal in myopathies and muscular atrophies of all types. Reduction in axonal diameter results in slowing of nerve conduction, since conduction velocity is directly proportional to myelinated nerve fiber diameter. Segmental demyelination produces an even more striking decrease in NCV because the highly efficient saltatory conduction normally present in myelinated nerves is impaired.

Clinical electromyographic techniques can also be used to study diseases of the myoneural junction. Repetitive nerve stimulation at varying rates will exhaust the acetylcholine mechanism at the neuromuscular junction in these diseases. The amplitude of the muscle response will diminish with the exhaustion of the myoneural junctions and can be quantitated. In different diseases of the myoneural junction, varying rates of stimulation produce characteristic patterns of diminishing muscle response, and these patterns can be useful in identifying the particular type of disorder.

Muscle Enzyme Studies

As muscle fibers undergo degeneration, muscle enzymes are released and become elevated in the systemic circulation. **Creatine phosphokinase (CPK)**, **aldolase**, and **glutamic-oxalacetic transaminase (GOT)** are enzymes most commonly measured for clinical purposes. These enzymes are greatly increased in rapidly progressive muscle diseases such as Duchenne muscular dystrophy and acute polymyositis. They are normal or only moderately elevated in diseases of nerve. However, in far advanced muscle diseases where very little muscle tissue is left to degenerate and release enzymes, muscle enzymes may be either normal or only slightly elevated. CPK is the most sensitive indicator of muscle diseases and may be elevated in mild disease states when other muscle enzymes are normal. Other enzymes which may be elevated in rapidly progressive muscle diseases are lactic dehydrogenase (LDH) and glutamic pyruvic transaminase (GPT).

The function of **creatine** in muscle metabolism

has been discussed in Chapter 3. **Creatinine**, a degradation product of creatine, is excreted in the urine. Muscle, in fact, contributes 95 percent to the total urinary excretion of creatinine. Any condition that results in a significant destruction of muscle fibers (myositis, massive trauma, rapidly progressing muscular dystrophy) or causes a significant reduction in total muscle mass (spinal neurogenic atrophy, late stage muscular dystrophy) may result in: 1) *increase in blood and urine creatine levels* (hypercreatinemia and hypercreatinuria) because creatine is not utilized by muscles to form creatine phosphate and 2) *decrease in urine creatinine level* (hypocreatinuria) because less creatine phosphate is formed and hence less is degraded. Although formerly used in the diagnosis of muscle disease, these tests have been largely superseded by serum muscle enzyme level determinations as enzyme testing has become more widely available.

CLASSIFICATION OF DISORDERS OF SKELETAL MUSCLE AND PERIPHERAL NERVE

Many of the disorders of skeletal muscle and peripheral nerve are incompletely understood and consequently their classifications may change as more information about the diseases is obtained. For example, the disease known as myotonic dystrophy has traditionally been considered to be a primary disease of muscle. Although in this text it will still be considered a muscle disease, there is evidence that it may be a primary disease of nerve with secondary muscle changes. Basic information concerning the etiology and pathogenesis is still lacking for many of the large number of diseases of the motor unit. Classification is according to the genetic basis (when this is known), the clinical course (which may be variable from patient to patient), the pattern of histopathologic changes, the presence of nerve or muscle toxins, characteristic laboratory findings, and association with certain medical diseases or traumatic events.

The major disease categories are the myopathies, neuropathies, spinal muscular atrophies, and myoneural junction diseases. The following list presents some of the more frequently encountered myopathies under a variety of these categories; there are many more muscle diseases and one of the references must be consulted for a comprehensive list.

MYOPATHIES
I. Muscular dystrophies
  A. Rapidly progressive
     Duchenne (pseudohypertrophic) muscular dystrophy
  B. Slowly progressive
     Limb-girdle muscular dystrophy
     Facio-scapulo-humeral (Landouzy-Déjerine) muscular dystrophy
     Myotonic (Steinert's) dystrophy
     Becker muscular dystrophy
II. Congenital myopathies
  A. Slowly progressive
     Nemaline myopathy
  B. Nonprogressive
     Central core diseases
III. Inflammatory diseases of skeletal muscle
  A. Infectious diseases of known etiology
     Parasitic myositis (trichinosis—*Trichinella spiralis)*
  B. Inflammatory myopathies of unknown etiology
     Polymyositis
     Dermatomyositis
  C. Inflammatory myopathies associated with other diseases
     Interstitial (nodular) myositis of rheumatoid arthritis
IV. Myopathies secondary to endocrine and metabolic diseases and muscle membrane dysfunction
  A. Endocrine diseases
     Thyroid myopathy
     Hypothyroidism
     Chronic thyrotoxicosis
     Exogenous steroid (Cushing's myopathy)
  B. Metabolic myopathies
     Primary amyloidosis
     Glycogen storage disease (von Gierke's disease)
  C. Periodic paralyses
     Hypokalemic
     Hyperkalemic
  D. Disorders of muscle cell excitability
     Benign muscle cramps
     Myotonia congenita (Thomsen's disease)

The next list contains a classification of peripheral neuropathies.

PERIPHERAL NEUROPATHIES
I. Hereditary neuropathies
  A. Charcot-Marie Tooth disease
  B. Dejerine-Sottas disease
  C. Roussy-Lévy syndrome

II. Toxic neuropathies
  A. Heavy metals
     Lead
     Arsenic
     Alcohol
  B. Drugs
     Nitrofurantoin (Furadantin)
     Diphenylhydantoin (Dilantin)
     Vincristine
     Isoniazid
  C. Organic compounds
     N-hexane
     Triorthocresyl phosphate
III. Peripheral neuropathies secondary to endocrine metabolic and infectious diseases
  A. Endocrine diseases
     Diabetes mellitus
     Polyneuropathy
     Mononeuropathy
     Hypothyroidism
  B. Metabolic diseases
     Chronic renal insufficiency
     Carcinoma
     Thiamine (vitamin B_1) deficiency
     Riboflavin (vitamin B_2) deficiency
     Pyridoxine (vitamin B_6) deficiency
  C. Infectious diseases
     Diphtheria
     Leprosy
     Herpes zoster
IV. Idiopathic neuropathies
  A. Guillain-Barré syndrome
  B. Shoulder girdle neuropathy

The spinal muscular atrophies can be classified into three major groups.

SPINAL MUSCULAR ATROPHIES
I. Hereditary
  A. Infantile spinal muscular atrophy (Werdnig-Hoffmann disease)
  B. Juvenile spinal muscular atrophy
  C. Spinal muscular atrophy of adults (Aran-Duchenne)
II. Unknown etiology
  A. Motor neuron disease
     Amyotrophic lateral sclerosis
     Primary lateral sclerosis
     Progressive muscular atrophy
III. Poliomyelitis

Finally, **diseases of the myoneural junction** may be classified according to the response to repetitive stimuli.

I. Decrementing response on repetitive stimulation: myasthenia gravis

II. Incrementing response on repetitive stimulation: myasthenic (Eaton-Lambert) syndrome

Although there are some congenital myopathies, the most important groups are 1) the muscular dystrophies, all of unknown etiology and classified by eponyms or by clinical manifestations, 2) inflammatory myopathies (myositis) of unknown etiology, and 3) myopathies secondary to endocrine or metabolic disorders.

Neuropathies fall into four broad groups: 1) hereditary, 2) toxic (due to heavy metals, drugs, or other organic compounds), 3) secondary to a large number of known diseases the most important of which is diabetes mellitus, and 4) idiopathic neuropathies.

Spinal muscular atrophies are diseases of the anterior horn cell. The best understood of these is poliomyelitis caused by a viral infection; others are hereditary or of unknown etiology.

Myoneural junction diseases are not diseases of nerve or muscle *per se*, but represent a dysfunction of the acetylcholine transmitter mechanism.

DIAGNOSIS OF SKELETAL MUSCLE AND PERIPHERAL NERVE DISORDERS

In order to establish a specific diagnosis, given such a large number of possibilities (see preceding lists) with essentially similar clinical manifestations, it is important to pay particular attention to a detailed history, hereditary pattern, and distribution and nature of symptoms and physical signs, as well as determining muscle enzyme levels, obtaining EMG and NCV tests, and often obtaining muscle or even nerve biopsy. There are many reasons for making a correct diagnosis. Although they are self-evident, several examples can be given. It is important to determine whether an asymptomatic person of child-bearing age from a family with an autosomal dominant hereditary neuropathy (e.g., Charcot-Marie-Tooth) has the disease. If found to have the disease, even though subclinical at the time of diagnosis, 50 percent of his or her offspring will have the disease. Such information is obviously important for genetic counseling. As another example, the neuropathy of chronic renal disease is, in part, reversible with improved hemodialysis. The treatment of renal neuropathy, then, first depends on its accurate diagnosis. With regard to muscle diseases, although only a few are treatable, acute polymyositis

may respond to high dose corticosteroid treatment; but first an accurate diagnosis must be made.

Clinical Manifestations

Important historical data include 1) age and sex, 2) onset of weakness, 3) time and course of the progression of weakness, 4) distribution of weakness and loss of function, 5) sensory loss and character of pain, if any, 6) presence or absence of symptoms and signs in other organ systems, 7) family medical history, and 8) evidence of exposure to noxious substances.

In the complete physical examination the following are of special diagnostic value:

1. **Inspection** for the distribution of muscle atrophy and the presence or absence of fasciculations. Fasciculations are very suggestive of spinal muscular atrophy (see Chap. 4.)
2. **Palpation** for muscle tenderness and peripheral nerve hypertrophy. Muscle tenderness is marked in polymyositis. Peripheral nerve hypertrophy is seen in some familial neuropathies and leprosy.
3. **Percussion** of muscle for myotonia. Myotonia is persistent muscle fiber contraction after cessation of a stimulus and is seen in myotonic dystrophy, myotonia congenita, and other myotonic disorders. It is also manifest by delayed relaxation after voluntary contraction.
4. Assessment of **muscle strength** and distribution of weakness. Distal muscle weakness indicates a likely neuropathy whereas proximal weakness most likely signifies myopathy.
5. Testing of **deep tendon reflexes.** These will be reduced or absent in peripheral nerve or muscle diseases, but exaggerated in upper motor neuron diseases.
6. Assessment of **sensation.** As discussed earlier, the presence of sensory loss indicates peripheral nerve disease.
7. Testing of passive joint range of motion to assess **muscle tone** (see Chaps. 4 and 27). Upper motor neuron diseases increase muscle tone, whereas diseases of the motor unit produce decreased tone.

Laboratory Tests

Diagnostic tests consist of muscle enzyme studies, electromyography and nerve conduction measurements, and muscle or nerve biopsy. Testing of the cerebrospinal fluid (CSF) is of no value in the diagnosis of muscle diseases and only of limited value in neuropathies. For example in the Guillain-Barré syndrome, protein in the cerebrospinal fluid may be slightly increased without an increase in the number of cells.

Enzyme Studies. Determination of serum muscle enzyme levels is the simplest of the laboratory tests and generally the most readily available test to differentiate myopathies from neuropathies. The relative value of the various available enzyme tests was discussed earlier in this chapter. The most sensitive enzyme indicator of muscle disease, CPK, may show a slight elevation in some nonaffected carriers of a recessive gene as in the nondystrophic mother of a boy with Duchenne muscular dystrophy.

EMG and NCV. Electromyography and nerve conduction velocity studies are the most important diagnostic tests in distinguishing nerve from muscle disease and in determining the neurophysiologic patterns of these diseases. These tests are noninvasive and can be repeated to assess the progression of disease or response to treatment. They allow for an assessment of the neurophysiologic function of any accessible muscle or nerve, and they reliably demonstrate whether the distribution of the disease is proximal or distal. In peripheral neuropathies NCV studies can identify the segment of the peripheral nerve which is most affected and they can distinguish between motor and sensory nerve involvement. EMG and NCV studies are sensitive diagnostic tools which can detect the earliest changes in both muscle and nerve disease prior to the appearance of unequivocal symptoms and clear-cut physical signs.

Muscle and Nerve Biopsy. The site and method of obtaining a muscle biopsy are of critical importance; tissue should be taken from a muscle which is clinically affected but not paralyzed. Routine and histochemical stains and electron microscopic sections can be employed. Sural nerve biopsy may occasionally be useful in the diagnosis of peripheral neuropathies.

EXAMPLES OF MOTOR UNIT DISEASES

A complete description of all the diseases of skeletal muscle, peripheral nerve, anterior horn cell, and myoneural junction is beyond the scope of this book but representative examples of each major disease category will be discussed briefly. As examples of myopathies, Duchenne muscular dystrophy is chosen along with polymyositis, an inflammatory myopathy. As examples of peripheral neuropathies, Charcot-Marie-Tooth disease, a hereditary neuropathy, is presented together with the Guillain-Barré syndrome, an idiopathic neuropathy. Amyotrophic lateral sclerosis is included as an example of the spinal muscular atrophies, and myasthenia gravis is given as an example of a myoneural junction disease.

Duchenne Muscular Dystrophy

Duchenne muscular dystrophy is the most common and most rapidly progressive of the muscular dystrophies. Duchenne dystrophy is transmitted as a sex-linked recessive trait; the disease is carried by asymptomatic females but the dystrophy is manifested exclusively in males. Onset occurs during the first five years of life, and the disease progresses relentlessly until death in the second decade. The muscles first involved include those of the abdominal wall, the hip extensors, the hip abductors, and the quadriceps. This results in inability to keep up with peers and the first noticeable symptom is usually frequent falling. Calf muscles may be replaced by fatty and fibrous tissue leading to the development of the characteristic pseudohypertrophy seen in the disease. Muscle contractures occur especially in flexors and abductors of the hip and plantar flexors of the foot. Ambulation is characterized by marked lumbar lordosis, side-to-side trunk lurching, and toe-walking.

The diagnosis is made on the basis of clinical findings, genetic history, high muscle enzyme levels during the early stage, and the typical EMG findings (normal numbers of motor unit action potentials having decreased amplitude and duration and increased phasicity). Nerve conduction velocities will be normal.

Although no specific treatment for the muscle loss exists, management of a child with Duchenne dystrophy consists of appropriate exercises to retard contractures and the use of adaptive equipment to maintain functional skills. Female carriers sometimes may be identified by elevated serum levels of the muscle enzyme CPK, and genetic counseling of female siblings and relatives of the patient is therefore important.

Polymyositis

Polymyositis is a myopathy of unknown origin characterized by inflammation of multiple muscles with muscle fiber destruction. The onset is variable; in some patients it is slow and insidious, and in others, acute. The incidence among males and females is approximately equal, and there is an increased frequency of occurrence with carcinoma.

Symmetrical weakness in the proximal muscles of the limb, as well as pain, tenderness, and swelling of these muscles, are characteristic findings in this disease. Neck muscles are also involved, particularly in the acute form. Later, fibrous replacement of muscle causes contractures which may persist even though remission of the active phase occurs. Involvement of the muscles of the jaw, pharynx, and respiration poses a serious threat to life. Fever, malaise, and other systemic symptoms may exist. A characteristic rash may appear on the skin, in which case the disease may be designated as **dermatomyositis.**

Serum muscle enzyme levels are more elevated in acute polymyositis than in muscular dystrophy and can reach the highest levels seen in any disease. The EMG shows much more evidence of membrane instability—fibrillations and positive sharp waves—than with muscular dystrophy. Motor unit action potentials are similar to muscular dystrophy in that they are decreased in amplitude and duration and are polyphasic. Nerve conduction velocities are normal. The histologic demonstration of extensive inflammatory cell infiltration and muscle regeneration helps to differentiate this disorder from the muscular dystrophies.

High doses of corticosteriod therapy may reduce the duration of the acute inflammation in polymyositis. Exercises to maintain the range of motion at joints and to prevent contractures are essential. A search for malignant disease is mandatory in the middle-aged patient.

Charcot-Marie-Tooth Disease

Charcot-Marie-Tooth disease (also known as **peroneal muscular atrophy** and **hereditary motor-sensory neuropathy type I**) is an autosomal dominant disorder. It is the most common hereditary neuropathy. Clinically it is usually apparent by the end of the second decade, with motor loss greater than sensory loss. The weakness is first noted in the feet and patients often have high arched feet. Peripheral nerves may be enlarged and palpable, most notably the greater auricular nerve in the neck.

Histologic section of peripheral nerves demonstrates a reduction in the number of axons in distal nerve segments, a decrease in cross-sectional diameter of remaining axons, and demyelination, most likely secondary to axonal disease. So-called onion-bulb formation of the Schwann sheath around axons is often observed and attributed to the cycle of repeated demyelination and remyelination. Muscle biopsy shows the large group atrophy typical of chronic neuropathic disease. Enzyme levels are generally normal and of little value in the diagnosis, except to exclude muscle disease.

Nerve conduction velocities are strikingly low, especially in the distal portions of peripheral nerves. EMG of an affected muscle shows fibrillations and positive sharp waves as well as a reduced number of increased amplitude, long duration polyphasic voluntary action potentials.

As the disease progresses, muscles of the feet eventually become paralyzed and more proximal muscles become paretic. The disease progresses slowly, affecting the upper limbs in the same manner, but is compatible with a normal life span if adequately managed. Management typically consists of providing bracing for the ankles; canes and other ambulation aids should be used as required.

Because the disease is inherited in an autosomal dominant manner, it is important for members of an affected family to be carefully tested both clinically and by nerve conduction studies. Because it is a dominant trait, the disease is passed on to subsequent generations by an affected parent. Genetic counseling of family members is therefore an important part of management of the disease. If a patient has a disease, even though it is subclinical and can be detected only by careful clinical or nerve conduction velocity studies, 50 percent of his children will inherit the disease.

Guillain-Barré Syndrome

The Guillain-Barré syndrome, also known as **idiopathic polyneuritis**, is a nonhereditary, idiopathic polyneuropathy of acute onset and of unknown etiology. In many cases the disease follows an upper respiratory infection by approximately two weeks. Within a few days of onset a patient may have profound paralysis, including the muscles of respiration. Sensation, however, is usually normal or only slightly affected. With good medical maintenance during this acute phase, neurologic function will improve. In almost all cases there is some degree of residual weakness, the exact degree of which depends upon the extent of axonal loss during the acute stage. For this reason electromyographic studies are of value both as prognostic as well as diagnostic indicators; the presence of large numbers of fibrillation potentials in weakened muscles indicates axonal degeneration and signals a poor prognosis. During the course of the disease, nerve conduction velocities will drop, with the nadir usually occurring several weeks after strength has started to return. Other laboratory tests are usually normal, with the exception of an increase in protein in the spinal fluid without an associated increase in cells (albuminocytologic dissociation).

There is no specific treatment, although corticosteroids have been suggested. During the acute stage, joint range of motion should be maintained, and following the acute stage strengthening exercises should be employed to reverse the disuse atrophy in continually innervated as well as newly reinnervated muscles. Residual weakness can be managed by bracing as well as by ambulation aids and auxiliary devices.

Amyotrophic Lateral Sclerosis

Amyotrophic lateral sclerosis is a relentlessly progressive disease of unknown etiology manifested by degeneration of the anterior horn cells of the spinal cord and the motor cells of the brain stem and cortex. Profound symmetrical weakness and atrophy with diffuse fasciculations are characteristic physical findings. Spasticity and increased tendon reflexes may be noted in the early stages until anterior horn cell destruction is more complete.

Diagnosis is made on the basis of history, clinical examination, and electromyography. Characteristic EMG findings are profuse fibrillations, fasciculations, increased amplitude motor unit action potentials and decreased numbers of motor unit action potentials firing. Nerve conduction velocities are normal.

The disease often begins in the fifth decade, and death usually occurs two to six years from onset and is due to complications of paralysis in the muscles of respiration. No specific treatment exists. Management is directed at maintaining functional skills with adaptive devices and maintaining pulmonary function. The patient and the family should be acquainted with the poor prognosis.

Myasthenia Gravis

As described in Chapter 3, myasthenia gravis is a disease of neuromuscular transmission associated with acetylcholine utilization by muscle receptor sites. The major symptom is fatigability rather than weakness, although in advanced disease true weakness may be significant. A major portion of the fatigability may be reversed through the use of anticholinesterase drugs. The muscles characteristically involved include the muscles of ocular movement, facial expression, mastication, deglutition, and respiration as well as those of the trunk and limbs. A muscle may rapidly weaken after a few repetitions of movement, only to be restored again following a period of rest. The disease may occur at any age after 10 years and has a clinical course that is variable in regard to progression, length of remission, response to anticholinesterase drugs, and number of muscles involved.

The diagnosis is made by the clinical history of muscle weakness following use of a muscle, and reversal of this weakness with the intravenous administration of a short-acting anticholinesterase drug. A progressive decrease in the evoked muscle action potential amplitude during repetitive stimulation of its peripheral nerve (a decrementing response) confirms the diagnosis.

Treatment consists of continued use of anticholinesteraselike drugs. Thymectomy has been shown to be beneficial in some cases and should be considered in each patient but is not always appropriate.

SUGGESTED READING

Adams RD (ed): Diseases of Muscle, 3rd ed. Harper & Row, Hagerstown, 1975
This text covers normal histology, experimental pathology, and diseases of muscle. The emphasis is on pathology.

Dyck PJ, Thomas PK, Lambert EH (eds): Peripheral Neuropathy, Vols 1, 2. Philadelphia, WB Saunders, 1975.
This two-volume set is a definitive and up-to-date review of peripheral neuropathies. The set consists of almost 1400 pages devoted to in-depth study of clinical, histologic, electrodiagnostic and other laboratory information on peripheral neuropathies. It can be highly recommended as a thorough and comprehensive text, and through its excellent index, specific questions can be very easily reviewed.

Goodgold J, Eberstein A (eds): Electrodiagnosis of Neuromuscular Diseases. 2 ed. Baltimore, Williams & Wilkins, 1977
This is a short book, an introduction to clinical electromyography for the student. It is easily read, comprehensive but brief, and can be recommended.

Johnson EW (ed): Practical Electromyography. Baltimore, Williams & Wilkins, 1980
This book presents detailed but practical information on diseases of the motor unit and their diagnosis by clinical electromyographic techniques. The book is recommended for those students who are interested in up-to-date details of the clinical electromyographic abnormalities in motor unit diseases.

Walton JN (ed): Disorders of Voluntary Muscle, 3rd ed. Edinburgh, Churchill-Livingstone, 1974
This text is a very well organized and definitive source for information on diseases of muscle. Its contributors include a number of well-known authorities on muscle diseases. The organization of the book allows the student ready reference to the important aspects of muscle diseases.

27
Impairment of Movement by Suprasegmental Disorders

BARBARA J. deLATEUR

Chapter 4 dealt with the influences suprasegmental motor centers exert on spinal motor neurons (Fig. 4–9), and reference was made to abnormalities of movement and muscle tone which result from interference with these descending impulses. It is important to distinguish the clinical syndromes which are caused by diseases of the spinal motor neuron itself from those that are due to disorders of the suprasegmental centers or their nerve fiber tracts. The former are customarily referred to as *lower motor neuron lesions* while the latter are collectively spoken of as *upper motor neuron lesions*.

Lower motor neuron disorders, discussed in the previous chapter, are characterized by *weakness and muscle atrophy*. In **upper motor neuron lesions,** weakness or even frank paralysis may be present, but muscle atrophy is minimal. The most typical features of suprasegmental disorders as a group are *impairment of control and alteration of muscle tone*. Accordingly, suprasegmental disorders of movement may be classified as hypertonic or hypotonic, on the one hand, and hypokinetic or hyperkinetic on the other. The combinations of these clinical manifestations are largely determined by the anatomic site of the lesions. Before discussing examples of these disorders, normal muscle tone and its pathologic alterations need to be considered.

MUSCLE TONE

Normal Tone

Muscle tone is the resistance offered to passive stretch of that muscle (see Chaps. 4, 7). Tension developed in response to stretch may be static or dynamic, and therefore one may speak of static or dynamic tone in a muscle. Both static and dynamic tone may be the result of active or passive tension in the muscle. Active tension is due to motor unit activity, while passive tension is due to the viscoelastic properties of the muscle–tendon unit.

Static tone is that tension which exists *at the end of a given stretch* and is proportional to the amount of elongation. Passive static tension will diminish with time if the muscle is retained at the same length because the tension in the muscle's stretched elastic element diminishes.

By elongating a tissue to various lengths and measuring the tension at each length, a length-tension diagram may be plotted. In tendon, this static length-tension relationship is entirely passive. The same type of static length–tension relationship may also be determined in muscle (Fig. 3–15). For instance, the Achilles' tendon of a rat may be attached to a device which can measure tension in the muscle–tendon unit at various lengths. If, in addition, the nerve to the gastrocnemius and soleus in blocked, the static length–tension curve obtained will be entirely passive because it is determined only by the viscoelastic properties of the muscle–tendon unit, there being no motor unit discharge (passive tension, Fig. 3–15). The length at which the tension becomes just detectable (i.e., exceeds zero) is defined as the *resting length*. Resting length is not necessarily the same as the length at which the muscle is relaxed or resting in the intact animal, because muscles may relax and be free of motor unit discharge at many lengths.

If, in the same experimental setup, a tetanizing electrical stimulus is applied to the tibial nerve distal to the site of the block, a certain tension will be developed in the muscle. The total static tension (or static tone) will be the sum of the active tension which resulted from the motor unit activity provoked by the stimulus and the passive tension due to stretching the viscoelastic elements (Fig. 3–15). At all lengths shorter than resting length, the passive tension is zero and total tension is therefore equal to active tension alone. Maximum active tension can be developed at the resting length of the muscle, and maximum total tension at or slightly beyond the resting length. Thus the static length–tension relationship may be active or passive or both.

Dynamic tone is the tension developed *during stretch*. Different rates of elongation may yield different dynamic tension curves. At slow rates of stretch, in normal muscle, the tone (tension) is due entirely to passive elements. At faster rates of stretch the active component of the stretch reflex is added. If a sudden, phasic stretch is applied by striking the tendon sharply with a rubber hammer, the tendon jerk will be elicited.

Early work in decerebrate animals led to the notion that muscle tone is normally maintained by a constant, low-frequency discharge of a small proportion of motor units. But it is a basic fact of electromyography that the muscle at rest is electrically silent. In studies on the biceps of humans at rest, no electromyographic (EMG) activity was found for static muscle tension determinations at lengths up to 150 percent of rest length. In studies of dynamic tone, a device was used which measured the torque required to drive the metacarpophalangeal joint of the index finger of normal subjects through its range of motion. In order to assess the active (motor unit) response of the muscle, the required torque was measured before and after nerve block. If the rate of elongation was slower than five cycles per second, no difference was found, indicating an absence of alpha motor neuron discharge as a contributor to dynamic tone. At faster rates of elongation, additional torque was required to overcome the resistance offered by the activated motor units. Furthermore, as explained in Chapter 19, only the soleus maintains an EMG discharge during relaxed standing. This activity disappears, however, when the subject assumes the supine position, even if the soleus is stretched to the same length as when the subject was standing.

In summary, no alpha motor neuron discharge is present in the normal muscle at rest, but is present during a stretch that is rapid enough to initiate a reflex response, or when the muscle is required to neutralize the effect of gravity in order to sustain a posture.

Hypotonia

Static hypotonia exists when the static tension reached at any given position of elongation is less in a given muscle than the static tension at corresponding lengths in a normal muscle. Static hypotonia may occur, for example, in a denervated muscle which has been held chronically in a lengthened position. Static length–tension relationships do not change with acute denervation. If the length–tension curve of the gastrocnemius of the relaxed (anesthetized) rat is plotted and then repeated immediately after section of the tibial nerve, those curves will superimpose. What causes static hypotonia is not a loss of alpha motor neuron discharge, but a secondary change in the elastic properties of the muscle. These elastic changes require several weeks to develop and are position dependent. If the denervated muscle is chronically held in a normal or shortened position, static hypotonia does not develop.

Dynamic hypotonia is present in a muscle if no stretch reflex is elicited when the muscle is elongated at a rate that is ordinarily capable of eliciting a stretch reflex. Dynamic hypotonia is seen in some cerebellar disorders, pure pyramidal lesions (as in experimental section of the pyramids in animals), and in the very acute phase of some mixed suprasegmental disorders such as the stroke syndrome.

Hypertonia

In **static hypertonia** the muscle develops greater than normal resistance or tension to passive stretch. Static hypertonia may be passive or active or both. If a denervated muscle, incapable of contracting voluntarily or reflexly is held in a shortened position for a long time (e.g., the gastrocnemius of a patient confined to bed in the supine position) a contracture will result due to the adaptation of the muscle and its connective tissue to the shortened position.

The tension developed in such a muscle after a stretch is entirely *passive*. The same shortening may occur in the gastrocnemius of a patient with decerebrate rigidity. But in this case there will be an additional *active* component of the static hypertonia which is due to the continuous firing of the uninhibited motor neurons. Such a patient will have dynamic hypertonia as well as static hypertonia.

Dynamic hypertonia is due to the facilitation of alpha motor neurons. Clinically, two types of dynamic hypertonia can be distinguished: *spasticity and rigidity*.

The dynamic hypertonia of **spasticity** is rate dependent, in that measuring length–tension relationships at different rates of stretch will yield different curves. Clinically, this means that the faster one attempts to put the joint through the range of motion, the greater the resistance encountered. Spasticity is associated with increased deep tendon reflexes and the clasp-knife phenomenon (Chap. 4). Where the clasp-knife phenomenon is present, resistance will be highest early in the range of motion and tend to taper off later. This is more likely to be seen in severe spasticity. In milder spasticity, the resistance may increase throughout the range.

In **rigidity,** the hypertonia is more or less constant throughout the range of motion, and usually is independent of the rate of stretch. Thus, the impression is given of *stiffness*, *plastic rigidity*, or *lead-pipe* rigidity. The resistance encountered may be jerky or repetitively variable and is referred to as *cogwheeling*. This phenomenon is frequently associated with tremor, and some authors consider the presence of tremor essential to the definition of cogwheel rigidity. Although rigidity has been discussed under dynamic hypertonia, there is also an element of static, active hypertonia in that there is tonic motor unit activity when the muscle is at any given static length.

NEGATIVE AND POSITIVE SIGNS

The concept of negative and positive signs was introduced by Hughlings Jackson. The disappearance of normal characteristics constitutes a negative sign. A **negative sign** results from destruction of the part of the nervous system which normally mediates that function. Paralysis, weakness, or loss of sensation are negative signs. These are found both in disorders of the lower motor neuron and the upper motor neuron. The appearance of findings not normally present constitutes a positive sign. **Positive signs** occur only in disorders of

the upper motor neuron. The occurrence of a positive sign implies the release from control of some part of the nervous system normally inhibited or influenced by some other part of the nervous system. Destruction of the latter allows the former to function autonomously or with an imbalance of excitatory and inhibitory input. Examples include spasticity and rigidity.

The response to stroking of the skin on the sole of the foot serves to illustrate both negative and positive signs. When a tongue-blade, key, or other such object is drawn firmly along the lateral aspect of the sole of the foot, from posterior to anterior, the toes normally respond, reflexly, by flexion and adduction (flexor plantar response). In a peripheral neuropathy, this response may be absent (absent plantar reflex), a negative sign. On the other hand, in suprasegmental lesions, the response may consist of extension of the great toe, often accompanied by fanning (abduction) of the other toes. Such an extensor plantar response is a positive sign, and it is known as **Babinski's sign.** This sign is perhaps the single most important and useful clinical sign in all of neurology.

Because the pyramidal tracts carry the corticospinal fibers, one would expect lesions of the pyramidal tracts to cause the negative sign of paralysis. This, in fact, occurs. But, in addition, positive signs such as spasticity and Babinski's sign appear. The explanation for the positive signs is that the pyramidal tracts contain, beside the corticospinal fibers, other fibers which are inhibitory to the lower motor neuron. Interruption of the latter removes inhibition, and motor responses to peripheral stimuli become exaggerated and modified. Naturally occurring lesions, particularly those caused by trauma or vascular disorders, involve all types of fibers in an anatomic location, and rarely, if ever, single out only one fiber system.

The clinical examples discussed in the subsequent sections have been selected to illustrate syndromes characterized by hypotonia or hypertonia. Hypotonia is associated with cerebellar disorders, tabes dorsalis, and with certain extrapyramidal syndromes. In the latter, hypotonia is coupled with exaggerated and uncontrolled movements (hyperkinesia). Of the hypertonic syndromes, stroke, the most common example of spasticity, will be discussed, while rigidity will be illustrated with extrapyramidal syndromes other than those falling into the hypotonic–hyperkinetic category. In the hypertonic extrapyramidal lesions, rigidity is associated with the lack of movement or akinesia.

HYPOTONIC SYNDROMES

Cerebellar Disorders

The cerebellum is responsible for the smooth, accurate, coordinated execution of movements. Its connections are schematically summarized in Figures 4–11 and 4–12. The cerebellum receives information from the periphery regarding the actual position and rate of movement of the limbs, plus visual and auditory cues. It also samples information from the motor cortex regarding motor commands, that is, *intended motions*. Comparison of intended versus actual positions and rates of movement prevents gross errors and permits rapid course corrections during a movement. This same system permits the sustaining of the head, trunk, or limbs in any desired posture. Lesions of the cerebellar hemispheres result in decreased tone and the loss of the ability to move in a smooth, coordinated manner. The impairment of performance on the numerous clinical tests is the reflection of these two basic defects.

Of the many disorders affecting the cerebellum, four have been selected for discussion: acute and chronic alcoholic intoxication, Friedreich's ataxia, and paraneoplastic involvement of the cerebellum. It is instructive, however, to deal first with physical signs employed in the diagnosis of all types of cerebellar disorders.

Physical Signs in Cerebellar Disorders. Clinical tests employed in the diagnosis of cerebellar disorders are numerous. Each test evaluates a specific impairment and the label attached to each descriptively conceptualizes the impaired function. There is, of course, extensive overlap of signs in any given patient. The following glossary is, in fact, an impressive illustration of the extensive and profound effect the cerebellum exerts on movement.

DYSSYNERGY. The various muscles which participate in a movement are not coordinated properly, or some groups may not participate at all. For example, the patient could not use reciprocally the arms and legs in an attempt to crawl, or he would fail to flex his knees when he extends his trunk, thus jeopardizing balance and safety.

DYSMETRIA. Inability to execute the appropriate excursion and/or rate of movement required for a specific task. For example, the patient may lift his foot too high when ascending stairs or curbs. When asked to touch the examiner's finger he may go past the finger or (initially) stop short of it, even though he is able to judge the distance and express it in inches.

ATAXIA. Movements are not carried out smoothly. Even though the correct muscles are used in a motion, they do not act harmoniously with the required force and rate of contraction. In the heel–shin test, the patient is asked to slide his heel down the opposite shin. The patient with cerebellar disease jerks the heel medially and laterally, to and fro, as he attempts to follow a straight-line course. The ataxic gait is characterized by jerky, excessive movements of the limbs and trunk. There is, in addition, a very broad base, to keep the center of gravity within the base of support (or, more accurately, to keep the base of support under the widely deviating center of gravity).

INTENTION TREMOR. This is demonstrated particularly well by the finger–nose–finger test. The patient is asked to touch, with the tip of his index finger, his own nose, the examiner's finger, his nose again and repeat the sequence. During this maneuver the examiner moves his own finger from place to place. As the patient's finger approaches that of the examiner, it begins to deviate more and more widely from the desired course. Also, the harder the patient tries to stay on course, the greater the deviation.

ABNORMAL REBOUND. Antagonists fail to prevent or correct overshoot when resistance to the contracting prime movers is removed. For example, if the patient is flexing his elbow against manual resistance supplied by the examiner, who suddenly releases that resistance, the patient may strike himself in the face. In performing this test, the examiner must protect the patient's face with his hand.

DYSDIADOCHOKINESIA. Impairment of performance of rapid, rhythmic, alternating movements. Tapping the foot rapidly against the floor, patting the thigh, pronating and supinating the forearms require the rapid, sequential contraction and relaxation of prime movers and antagonists. Clumsiness of performance of such tests defines dysdiadochokinesia.

HYPOTONIA DURING PASSIVE MOVEMENTS. An easy way to demonstrate this is to shake the patient by the shoulders; there will be excessive arm swing.

PENDULOUS REFLEXES. If, when the patient is seated with the knees flexed and the legs dangling over the edge of the table, a knee jerk is elicited, the leg will swing back and forth in a natural pendulum action until the motion finally decays. This finding is closely related to that of hypotonia and abnormal rebound, and is explained by the failure of the antagonists to dampen the motion.

FALL AWAY IN POSITIONAL TESTING (DRIFT). If the patient is asked to close his eyes and hold his arms outstretched, there will be downward drifting of the arm on the side of the lesion.

ROMBERG'S TEST. The patient is asked to stand with his feet together. His posture becomes uncertain, and he begins to sway. This is worsened if he is asked to close his eyes.

SPEECH DISTURBANCE. There may be staccato, explosive speech, or the speech may be slurred. As with other signs of cerebellar dysfunction, the speech impairment is due to inability to carry out coordinated movements in a fluent manner. Thus, the speech impairment is a *dysarthria*, and not a language disorder.

Acute and Chronic Alcoholism. Perhaps the most common and familiar disorder of the cerebellum is that of acute alcoholic intoxication. The cerebellum is particularly susceptible to the effects of alcohol. All the signs listed above may be present.

Permanent cerebellar damage may develop in chronic alcoholism. However, the cause and effect relationship is not nearly so clear as in acute alcoholic intoxication. It is not known to what extent nutritional and vitamin deficiencies concomitant with chronic alcohol intake contribute to the clinical picture and cerebellar pathology. Pathologically, there exists cortical degeneration in the cerebellum.

Friedreich's Ataxia. Friedreich's ataxia is a member of a group of spinocerebellar degenerations. The syndrome was described by Friedreich in 1861 as a familial disease affecting young patients. Charcot called the disorder "tabetocerebellar," which describes the combination of lesions in the posterior columns of the spi-

nal cord and in the cerebellum. Friedreich's postmortem examinations showed degeneration of the dorsal columns spreading into parts of the lateral columns, plus degeneration of the dorsal roots. Other workers have added to his findings. Some have found loss of the highly characteristic Purkinje cells of the cerebellar cortex. There is also degeneration of the spinocerebellar tracts.

In this disorder, as in other systemic degenerations, it appears that neurons in the involved systems die back gradually from the periphery of the axon to the cell body.

More recently a selective involvement of the group Ia afferents from the muscle spindles has been demonstrated. This is of particular interest because it allows the use of electromyography to assist in confirming the diagnosis. In the previous chapter, it has been pointed out that the EMG is of great use in differentiating myopathies from neuropathies, that is, disorders of peripheral nerves and muscle. But in Friedreich's ataxia, the electromyographer can "get inside" the CNS by utilizing two *late waves*, known as H and F *waves*. Because of their size, Ia afferents are most easily depolarized and can be excited by low threshold stimulation which does not affect smaller fibers in a nerve. Normally, the impulse travels up the Ia afferents, is relayed monosynaptically to the anterior horn cells which transmit an impulse down the motor axon, and this is registered on the EMG as the delayed H wave. This phenomenon, known as the **H-reflex**, is absent or its latency is prolonged in Friedreich's ataxia because of the selective involvement of Ia afferents. The reflex would also be absent, however, in peripheral neuropathies, and in order to rule this out the F-wave phenomenon must be elicited before the EMG diagnosis can be made.

The **F-wave** occurs when the motor nerve is antidromically stimulated so that an action potential is transmitted toward the cell body. The impulse travels up the motor axon and depolarizes the anterior horn cell which then sends an impulse back down the axon, depolarizing some of the muscle fibers, which gives the F-wave. The latency of the F-wave is normal in Friedreich's ataxia. Thus, a prolonged H-reflex in the presence of a normal F-wave provides electrophysiologic confirmation of the diagnosis of Friedreich's ataxia.

Clinical characteristics include ataxia of gait as the most common presenting sign. Clumsiness of the hands appears later, followed by dysarthria. Pes cavus with claw toes may be an early sign, especially if the parents have an older child with

Friedreich's ataxia and are watching the younger children carefully.

Most of the general findings of cerebellar disease described above are found in Friedreich's ataxia. An exception is the pendulous reflex. The tendon jerks are almost always absent, although their presence does not exclude the diagnosis.

Degeneration in the dorsal columns results in loss of position and vibratory sensation and contributes to the ataxia. Although some patients state they can walk equally well in the dark, many find that they do, in fact, rely upon visual cues, and their gait shows deterioration in the dark.

Paraneoplastic Involvement of the Cerebellum. Paraneoplastic disease may involve any part of the central or peripheral nervous system or the neuromuscular apparatus. Paraneoplastic disturbance of the cerebellum is presented as one example. Whereas the exact mechanism of the impairment is not known, something other than direct carcinomatous invasion or metastasis is denoted by paraneoplastic involvement.

The most common pattern is subacute parenchymatous degeneration of the cerebellum. In contrast to the rather specific cerebellar cortical atrophy seen in chronic alcoholism, the lesions in paraneoplastic subacute cerebellar degeneration are diffuse. Loss of Purkinje cells is always a prominent manifestation, with the involvement of other cell types as well. Long tract degeneration of the spinal cord may occur, especially of the spinocerebellar and dorsal column tracts.

The presenting finding is generally that of ataxia, with the patient complaining of unsteadiness of gait. Dysarthria is also a frequent finding. The cerebellar manifestations may precede the tumor manifestations. Careful investigation of the cerebellar disorder may then lead to the discovery of the tumor. In a few cases the clinical and pathological findings are confined to the cerebellum, but in most cases there is evidence of involvement elsewhere in the nervous system, with weakness, wasting, increased or decreased reflexes, sensory changes, and/or dementia.

The tumors most commonly associated with this disorder are lung carcinomas in men and ovarian carcinomas in women. Association with Hodgkin's disease has also been reported.

The disorder cannot be explained by the inanition which often accompanies malignant disease. Paraneoplastic subacute cerebellar degeneration bears a striking resemblance to the disease of scrapie, a viroid disease with hereditary predisposition, which occurs in sheep, but the etiology of the former remains unknown.

Tabes Dorsalis

The disorder is a late manifestation of untreated or inadequately treated syphilis, some 8–12 years after the infection. It receives its name from the wasting of the dorsal columns of the spinal cord which is macroscopically evident. Microscopic examination reveals degeneration of the afferent fibers coming from the dorsal root ganglia to the spinal cord, plus demyelination, axonal degeneration, and glial proliferation in the posterior columns of the cord.

The loss of afferent input from the muscle leads to hypotonia and diminished or absent reflexes. Loss of position sense leads to a steppage gait, characterized by exaggerated flexion of the hip and knee. The steppage gait is adopted to provide ample clearance of the toes to prevent tripping, since the patient cannot tell where his feet are without watching. The gait deteriorates markedly in the dark, and Romberg's sign is positive.

It has been shown that the quadriceps cannot be strengthened with isometric exercise in this disorder, presumably due to lack of sensory feedback regarding the force of contraction.

There is also a diminution in pain sensation, which, together with the hypotonia and loss of position sense, permit uncoordinated, irregular, uncontrolled, and traumatic usage of the joints. This ultimately leads to hypermobility, subluxation, and severe degenerative joint disease with complete destruction of the architecture of the joints (Charcot's joint).

Hyperkinetic–Hypotonic Extrapyramidal Syndromes

Syndromes characterized by involuntary and abnormal movements include chorea, athetosis, ballismus, and dystonia. Muscle tone is usually lower than normal in these conditions, the most consistent exception being dystonia. All these syndromes are associated with lesions of the basal ganglia or of their connections (Chap. 4).

Chorea. Chorea is the term applied to low amplitude, random, jerky movements of the face or limbs. The movements are apparently purposeless and bear no evident relationship to posture or voluntary movement. Pathophysiologically, there is loss of control of the corpus striatum over the globus pallidus and substantia nigra. The corpus striatum is a collective term for the caudate nucleus, putamen, and claustrum. Because of the loss of this control, the substantia nigra transmits the impulses it receives from the premotor cortex in an irregular fashion to the anterior horn cells.

When minimal, the choreiform movements are scarcely noticeable, and may seem only to be the movements of a fidgety or embarrassed person. When severe, they may take the form of marked grimacing and movements which disturb sleep. Hypotonia is frequently present. It may be manifested by a prolonged relaxation of the limb after eliciting a tendon jerk.

Chorea minor, described by Sydenham, is frequently associated with infectious diseases of childhood, particularly rheumatic fever. It tends to be self-limited, disappearing in weeks to months, although some patients are left with residual fidgetiness and tics. There are no definitely documented lesions in chorea minor.

Huntington's chorea, a much more severe and progressive disorder, is inherited as an autosomal dominant and becomes clinically manifest at about 30 to 50 years of age. Pathologically, the lesion involves the caudate nucleus and putamen, although other basal ganglia may also be affected. Pneumoencephalography may reveal the atrophy of the caudate nucleus by showing a loss of convexity normally produced in the lateral wall of the lateral ventricle by the caput of the caudate nucleus.

The movement disorder in Huntington's chorea is accompanied by progressive mental impairment which leads to dementia. The onset and severity of the mental disorder does not parallel the severity of choreiform movements.

Athetosis. In this disorder, movements are characterized as writhing, wormlike. The body may move from one dystonic posture to another, eventually resulting in subluxation of joints because of the extremes of flexion or extension into which joints are forced. The rapidity of movements is less, and their amplitude is greater than in chorea. Intermediate patterns are referred to as choreoathetosis. Voluntary movements and gait are hampered by these underlying involuntary movements.

The disorder is believed to be due to interruption of impulses from the globus pallidus to the thalamus. This results in failure of the latter to relay impulses to the extrapyramidal areas of the premotor cortex, which then transmits unregulated stimuli to the spinal cord and other nuclei.

Athetosis is seen most often in association with cerebral palsy.

Ballismus. Ballismus (derived from the same word as ballistic) refers to wild, centrifugal, throwing movements of the upper or lower limbs. These movements sometimes occur with enough force to injure the patient when he unintentionally strikes an object. When unilateral, it is termed hemiballismus and is caused by a lesion of the opposite subthalamic nucleus.

Dystonia. The dystonic syndromes are characterized by involuntary movements, the duration of which is variable but generally longer than choreiform movements. Moreover, there is faulty timing of contraction and relaxation of prime movers and antagonists.

Spastic Torticollis. This is the most common of the dystonic syndromes and is characterized by prolonged powerful, involuntary contraction of the sternocleidomastoid and trapezius muscles. When asymmetrical, one side gradually overpowers the other, and there is turning of the neck. When symmetrical, there is powerful extension of the head. As with other hyperkinetic disorders, this tends to disappear in sleep. It is caused by an organic lesion of the corpus striatum. Surgical ablation of the dorsal and ventral roots of C1-C4 provides definitive treatment, but with attendant motor and sensory loss. Improvement has been reported with EMG biofeedback, in which the patient regains some voluntary control of the involved muscles.

HYPERTONIC SYNDROMES

Spasticity-Associated Stroke Syndrome

A neurologic deficit of vascular origin and relatively sudden onset is termed a **stroke** or **cerebrovascular accident.** These tend to fall into patterns, according to the vascular territory of the brain in which infarction occurs. The precipitating event may be a subarachnoid or intracerebral hemorrhage or occlusion of a vessel due to an embolus or thrombus. Functional loss resembling the outcome of a cerebrovascular accident may also result from trauma or a tumor, but this is not customarily called a stroke.

Middle Cerebral Artery Syndrome. The most common stroke pattern among patients presenting for rehabilitation is that of infarction in the territory of the middle cerebral artery. This is the largest branch of the internal carotid artery, and its area of supply includes the internal capsule, the corpus striatum, and large areas of the cerebral cortex on the frontal, parietal, and temporal lobes. On the precentral gyrus of the frontal lobe, the middle cerebral artery supplies the motor cortex concerned with most of the body, except the lower limbs, and on the postcentral gyrus a similar territory of the sensory (somesthetic) cortex. Infarction in the motor cortex or in the corticospinal tracts results in *contralateral* **hemiplegia** (loss of voluntary movement) while similar involvement of the sensory cortex or its ascending tracts leads to *contralateral* **hemianesthesia** (loss of sensation).

Not every stroke involves the artery's entire territory of distribution. A small infarct in the branch of the artery which supplies the internal capsule, where corticospinal tract fibers are packed closely, may yield a contralateral hemiplegia with little or no loss of sensation and higher integrative functions. On the other hand, occlusion of a more proximal part of the artery may result, in addition to the contralateral hemiplegia, in sensory loss and extensive impairment of intellectual, perceptual, and memory functions. The exact nature of these deficits is largely dependent on whether the lesion is in the dominant or nondominant hemisphere.

On the side contralateral to the brain lesion, there occur both negative signs, such as paralysis and sensory loss, and positive signs, such as the Babinski sign, increased deep tendon reflexes, and the release of patterns of voluntary and involuntary movements, known as **synergies.** For example, in the lower limb, particularly when the patient is upright, the *extensor synergy* predominates. This consists of extension and adduction at the hip, extension at the knee, and plantar flexion and inversion of the ankle and foot. Although this produces an awkward, circumducted gait, this *positive supporting reflex* makes it possible for some patients to walk who would otherwise have insufficient voluntary motor function to do so.

If the infarction involves extensive cortical areas, then the loss of higher cortical functions, rather than the extent of the paralysis, will be the principal determinant of the patient's ability to learn to communicate, walk, dress, bathe, and feed himself. When the lesion is on the left, which is the dominant side in most individuals, there may be a serious impairment of language (aphasia) and general communicative ability. This is usually readily apparent to the patient, his family, and physician. What may not be so readily apparent is the deficit which occurs when the lesion is on the nondominant (generally the right) side of the brain. There may be serious impairment of perceptual ability and perceptual-motor skills. The patient may not perceive verticality; he may not know how and where to place his center of gravity. He may not be able to plan or carry out a motor sequence in a correct and effective manner. He may neglect and injure the left side of his body. His ability to acquire and retain even simple motor skills may be impaired. Finally, he may be impulsive and unaware of his deficits. In contrast, the right hemiplegic (left brain lesion), with an equally severe paralysis, tends to rapidly acquire the motor skills to become independent in ambulation and self-care, in spite of any language deficit he may have. In teaching these patients, it is best to use verbal instructions for the left hemiplegic, and pantomime for the right hemiplegic.

Anterior Cerebral Artery Syndrome. The anterior cerebral artery supplies the anterior portions of the cerebrum not supplied by the middle cerebral artery, and also supplies all of the medial surface of the hemisphere except for the occipital lobe. This includes the portions of the motor and sensory cortices not supplied by the middle cerebral artery which are concerned chiefly with the lower limbs. The pattern of paralysis is thus the reverse of that in a middle cerebral artery infarct. In a middle cerebral artery infarct, the upper limb is weaker than the lower limb. In an anterior cerebral artery infarct, there is, as a rule, profound weakness of the contralateral lower limb, with relative sparing of the upper limb. In some of these patients the frontal lobe involvement leads to a *paralysis of initiative*. Thus, even though the patients may have the perceptual motor skills to carry out the required self-care tasks, they may not do so unless given repeated external cues by another person. Early after their stroke they may fail to initiate speech. This mutism is sometimes incorrectly diagnosed as aphasia. However, once the patient begins to speak, there is no specific language deficit.

There are statistically significant predictors of outcome in the rehabilitation of stroke patients. However, in any given patient, the power of prediction is low enough so that a therapeutic trial of rehabilitation is warranted in the cooperative patient, in spite of the presence of some unfavorable signs.

Rigidity-Associated Extrapyramidal Syndrome: Parkinson's Syndrome

Parkinson's syndrome is the most common of the extrapyramidal syndromes which exhibit *akinetic rigidity*. In this syndrome, any of the several melanin-bearing basal ganglia may show pathologic changes, but there are always changes in the substantia nigra, which shows atrophy of the ganglion cells and an increase in neuroglia.

The key clinical features of Parkinson's syndrome are rigidity, akinesia, and tremor at rest. Other clinical manifestations can be explained in terms of these basic features.

The aberration of tone in this syndrome can be detected both during a passive movement and afterward. In contrast to spasticity in which the resistance to movement may reach a peak and suddenly decline, there is rigidity in which the examiner perceives a waxy or lead-pipe resistance, more or less throughout the movement of affected joints. There is a ratchety feel known as the cogwheel phenomenon, as if the cogs of two opposing wheels were intermittently catching and releasing throughout the movement range. In addition, there is an increase in resting tone. For example, if the patient is lying in bed supine and the examiner raises the patient's head and shoulders off the bed and then suddenly releases the support, the patient's head and shoulders may stay in the air, as if supported on an invisible pillow. This is the opposite of the rebound phenomenon seen in cerebellar disorders.

The alteration of tone seen in Parkinson's syndrome is thought to be an alpha rigidity. Earlier in this chapter, it was pointed out that the late-wave techniques of electromyography can be used, to some extent, to "get inside" the CNS. Another example is to be found in the study of Parkinson's syndrome. If the submaximal electrical stimulus needed to elicit an H reflex is followed very soon (about 60 msec) by a second such stimulus, the amplitude of the second H wave will be very small, less than 10 percent of the first. As the time between the paired shocks is gradually lengthened,

the ratio of H_2/H_1 gradually increases. In Parkinson's syndrome, this recovery pattern is much faster, reflecting an increase in alpha excitability. Following successful drug or surgical treatment of the syndrome, the recovery pattern reverts toward normal.

Paucity of movement or akinesia in Parkinson's syndrome results from inhibition of primary automatic movements. There is loss of associated arm movements in walking. The face lacks expressiveness (masklike facies); speech is soft, monotonous, and poorly articulated; handwriting is very small (*Parkinsonian micrographia*). Posture of the trunk and the limbs is one of flexion, with inability to adapt suddenly as needed. If the examiner gives the patient a little push, flexing his trunk forward, the center of gravity becomes displaced anterior to the base of support, and the patient will tend to fall forward. To prevent this he will step forward and begin to walk faster and faster, but will not catch up with his center of gravity owing to the trunk retaining its flexion. The patient may actually fall or may catch himself against a wall. This is described as a festinating (Latin, *festina*, make haste) or propulsive gait.

The tremor of Parkinson's syndrome is a resting tremor of about 5 Hz and must be distinguished from postural or intention tremors. In contrast to the latter, resting tremor will diminish during voluntary movement. The characteristic movements of the hands at rest led to the designation of *pill-rolling tremor*, reflecting a time when pills were made by hand, rather than by machine.

Parkinson's syndrome may follow a bout of any type of encephalitis, and has been seen after epidemic encephalitis lethargica. It may also occur as a side effect of drug administration, especially the phenothiazines. It usually remits promptly after drug withdrawal. The term **Parkinson's disease** is reserved for the heredofamilial type of the syndrome. Parkinson's disease is usually inherited as an autosomal dominant.

SUGGESTED READING

Brain RL, Forbes FH Jr: The Remote Effects of Cancer on the Nervous System. New York, Grune & Stratton, 1965 *A collection of essays on the site and type of paraneoplastic disturbances of the central and peripheral nervous system, myoneural junction and muscle. Updated in Norris FH Jr: The remote effects of cancer on the nervous system. Z Neurol 201: 201, 1972.*

DeJong RN: The Neurologic Examination, 3rd ed. New York, Hoeber Division, Harper & Row, 1967
Very detailed, comprehensive (1100 pages) discussion of the manner of carrying out a neurologic examination and of the significance of the findings for lesion localization.

Greenfield JG: The Spino-Cerebellar Degenerations. Oxford, Blackwell Scientific, 1954
The devotion of an entire monograph to this topic allowed the author space to utilize an historical, narrative approach, which lends clarity to an area of neurology in which there is still much uncertainty whether to "lump" or "split" disorders.

Lenman JAR: Clinical Neurophysiology. Oxford, Blackwell Scientific, 1975
Selected normal and disease processes of the central nervous system are discussed in depth, using an experimental approach.

Mumenthaler M: Neurology. Chicago, Year Book Medical, 1977
A concise survey of neuropathologic processes and the neurologic examination.

Stolov WC: The concept of normal muscle tone, hypotonia and hypertonia. Arch Phys Med Rehabil 47: 156, 1966
A systematic exposition of the modern concept of tone, with experimental documentation of all assertions regarding tone and the principal types of deviations from normal.

28
Musculoskeletal Trauma

D. KAY CLAWSON

Musculoskeletal trauma consists of injuries to skin, muscles, tendons, ligaments, nerves, blood vessels, bones, and joints. About 43 percent of the injuries occur in the home, 16 percent in industry, 34 percent in public places including recreational areas, and 7 percent in automobiles. Most tissues have a common response to injury. This response includes inflammation and repair, and these have already been introduced in Chapter 6.

BONE

The common response of bone to trauma is fracture. A bone fractures when its capacity to absorb energy is exceeded. Various types of fractures seen clinically have been duplicated experimentally under controlled conditions of loading. These experimental studies indicate that bone is weaker in resisting tension forces than compression forces (Fig. 28–1A). A large load may be tolerated if applied slowly but may produce a fracture if applied rapidly.

Bone is a dynamic tissue and an *intact blood supply is essential to maintain its normal physical properties*. Physical activity, particularly when it generates compression forces, causes the body to produce more bone. Inactivity results in bone resorption (atrophy). Total loss of blood supply to a bone or segment of a bone produces ischemic necrosis. Ischemic necrosis and bone atrophy (osteoporosis) are both accompanied by a rapid decline in the ability of bone to withstand repetitive loading and set the stage for microscopic or macroscopic fractures. The dynamic, vital aspect of bone must be thoroughly understood to fully comprehend the clinical problems of the musculoskeletal system (Chaps. 2 and 21).

Injury to bone is usually accompanied by significant injury to the surrounding tissues and appreciation of the extent of the soft tissue injury associated with a fracture is essential in the assessment of potential treatment and in prognosis for both healing and functional outcome.

Types of Fracture

The type of fracture depends on the amount and direction of the force. It is possible to analyze the type of force by studying the fracture pattern. A **compression fracture** occurs characteristically in the softer or cancellous bone found in the vertebrae, pelvis, and the epiphyses and metaphyses of long bones. Because cancellous bone has a rich blood supply, and because a compression force produces minimal soft tissue injury, there is little disruption of the fractured bone's blood supply and therefore rapid healing is the usual outcome. **Distraction forces,** on the other hand, rather than fracturing the bone, disrupt and tear the ligaments around the traumatized joint. Exceptions to this rule are the so-called **avulsion fractures**, in which the ligaments remain intact and the bone is literally pulled apart. A direct force acting on a long bone tends to break it transversely or at a short oblique angle, depending upon the direction of force. Unless the force is excessive or recurs repeatedly (as in a fall down a mountain or a ski slope), fractures usually disrupt periosteum and surrounding soft tissues on one side of the bone only (Fig. 28–1A). An intact soft tissue sleeve remains, usually on the opposite side, and is helpful in obtaining and maintaining reduction of the fracture (Fig. 28–1B). If a force is of a rotatory nature, a **spiral fracture** is produced. Because of the nature of the injury, the surrounding tissue trauma is usually incomplete. Unless the soft tissues become interposed between the fragments, they play an important role in maintaining reduction and initiating early fracture healing. If the trauma is se-

407

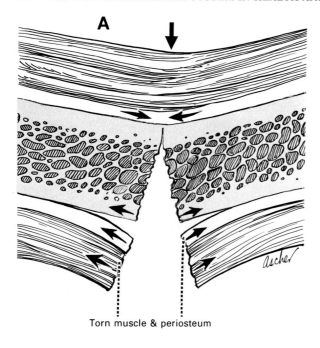

Torn muscle & periosteum

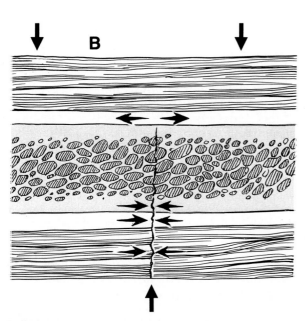

FIG. 28–1. (A) Diagrammatic representation of the relative weakness of bone to withstand tensile force compared to compression force. Bone cortex, periosteum, and the surrounding musculature are disrupted on the side of tension whereas on the side of compression these tissues remain intact. (B) The alignment of the fractured bone can be maintained by three point pressure (large arrows) when there is a periosteal soft tissue sleeve on one aspect of the bone.

vere, the bone may fracture and divide all surrounding soft tissue, or the bone may fragment into numerous pieces. In the latter instance, a **comminuted fracture** is said to have occurred. Fractures are also classified as **closed (simple) fractures,** when the skin remains intact, or **open (compound) fractures,** when the skin is broken and there is communication from the bone to the outside. It should be clear, then, that an understanding of how the injury occurred is helpful in assessing the probable degree of soft tissue damage, which is an important factor in determining treatment and predicting outcome.

Diagnosis of Fractures

Fracture should be suspected whenever there is any history of trauma (in some cases very minimal) and the patient complains of pain when the part is moved or pressed upon. Trauma need not take the form of a single blow, rather, it may be minimal and repetitive, causing only microfractures which eventually may summate and reveal themselves as a macrofracture. These are called **fatigue** or **stress fractures** and are exemplified by tibial and metatarsal fractures of runners. Swelling from hemorrhage and edema usually accompanies fractures and in time this is responsible for the characteristic black and blue discoloration of the overlying skin (ecchymosis). These findings are as true for soft tissue injuries as for bone. A diagnosis of fracture can be firmly established if one feels crepitus (bone grating on bone), but this should never be specifically elicited as it causes increased pain to the patient and may provoke further hemorrhage or soft tissue injury. Fracture can also be diagnosed if there is angulation or motion along a long bone. Many significant fractures would be missed if only the above were used in establishing the diagnosis, and therefore a careful, physical examination must be carried out, looking specifically for point tenderness over bones. Suspicious areas must be x-rayed. Good quality x-rays at least in two planes (anteroposterior and lateral) should be taken for all suspected fractures. *Because of the possibility of multiple injuries of the same bone, it is essential to include in the x-ray the joint above and the joint below the bone involved.*

Fracture Healing

The role of the physician is to assist nature in healing wounds and to prevent deformity. Fracture healing is similar to any other type of wound heal-

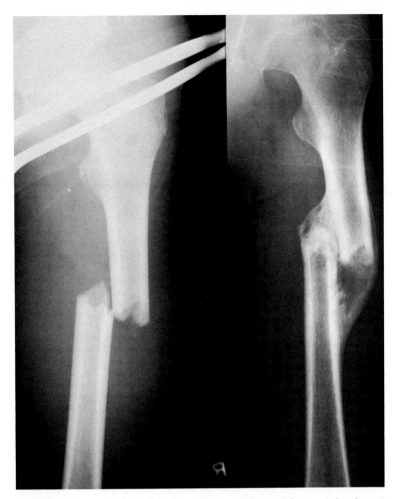

FIG. 28–2. X-rays of a fractured femur (left) and fracture healing 3 months later in the same bone (right). Note bayonet apposition (left) and periosteal and endosteal new bone formation producing a callus (right).

ing, except that osteogenesis occurs to reestablish bone continuity. This was introduced briefly in Chapter 6.

For purposes of discussion, fracture healing can be divided into three stages; however, it must be remembered that these stages overlap. The **first stage** is generally referred to as the **inflammatory stage.** At the time of bone fracture, there will also be disruption of the endosteum and periosteum as well as discontinuity or trauma to the surrounding muscles and blood vessels. The resultant hemorrhage will soon form a blood clot about the fracture site. The fibrin meshwork of the clot is heavily intermixed with red and white blood cells as well as with bone marrow elements and various amounts of debris from devitalized bone or muscle. During the first *12 hours* after injury, polymorphonuclear neutrophilic leukocytes enter the fracture site in increasing numbers. These cells enter the wound from blood vessels which become dilated as a result of the inflammatory response around the fracture. Some *24 hours* later, a second inflammatory cell type appears in the wound, the monocyte. These cells become phagocytic and remove most of the cellular debris and fibrin from the wound. The neutrophil leukocytes initiate the lysis of fibrin and the destruction of the tissue fragments which are then engulfed and removed by the macrophages derived from the monocytes. The role of the blood clot in fracture repair remains unclear. It is likely, however, that blood clot is essential in the healing of most fractures except where the fracture ends are compressed together and are rigidly immobilized. Within *48 to 72 hours* fibroblast-type connective tissue cells appear in the wound, having invaded the fracture site from the adjacent perivascular connective tissue, bone marrow, periosteum, and endosteum. The appearance of these cells is associated with the ingrowth of vascular buds into the area. These cells begin to multiply and some of their progeny have the potential for differentiating into chondroblasts or osteoblasts. Within the first *7 days* the fracture site is similar to any wound, except both fibroblasts and osteoblasts are present.

The **second stage** of fracture healing is described as the **reparative stage.** The fibroblasts and osteoblasts actively engage in the synthesis and secretion of collagen and proteoglycans, which form an integral part of the connective tissue which unites the bone ends and is known as the **callus.** The connective tissue matrix begins to calcify within *14 to 17 days.* Bone mineral (hydroxyapatite) is deposited in the connective tissue matrix, and the process of membranous bone formation is in essence recapitulated (Fig. 28–2).

The exact mechanism of bone induction is unknown. If certain stages of this process are disrupted, for instance loss of hematoma or lack of adequate vascular invasion, the healing process will be delayed. When excessive motion hinders vascular invasion, an excessive amount of cartilaginous callus is produced. If the bone is well immobilized and the blood supply is good, bony union is achieved with relatively little cartilage formation in the callus. The better the blood supply (i.e., oxygenation of the region) the less cartilaginous callus will form. Vascularity of the healing area is therefore of prime importance. *The rate and certainty of fracture healing bear direct relation to the vascularity of the bone and the surrounding soft tissues*:

No blood———→No bone.

As the reparative stage begins to decline, **stage three** or the **remodeling stage** becomes dominant and may continue for many years. The remodeling of bone is largely governed by the mechanical forces acting on the bone (see Fig. 2–16) and is often spoken of as Wolff's law. This law states that bone is laid down along lines of stress and is reabsorbed when stress is absent. Therefore, bone that is not in the direct line of stress becomes reabsorbed by osteoclasts while osteoblasts will continue to lay down new bone along lines of stress. In recent years, the piezoelectric effect has been postulated as an important factor in bone healing and remodeling (see Chap. 2).

While bone may be considered healed when there is mineralized callus bridging the bone ends, its structural strength may be less than normal for months or years, depending on a variety of biomechanical factors.

Local Causes of Delayed and Nonunion

A variety of local and systemic conditions have been implicated in causing delayed union of fracture. The most significant of these factors is **avascularity.** Other local causes include distraction of fracture fragments, inadequate immobilization, loss of blood clot, and infection.

Avascularity. It is now generally recognized that the one common denominator in all causes of delayed or nonunion is the severity of the soft tissue trauma which is directly related to the accessibility of the fracture site to blood vessels. In practically all fractures the broken, bare ends of the bone become avascular and osteocytes die, leaving their lacunae empty. The danger of nonunion increases as larger and larger areas of bone become devested of periosteum, endosteum, and soft tissues. This may be the consequence of the initial trauma or may be caused by surgical intervention (e.g., introduction of metal pins and rods into the medullary cavity). Death of the surrounding muscle or any other factors which interfere with the growth and sprouting of blood vessels in the granulation tissue of the provisional callus will always compromise fracture healing.

Distraction of Fracture Fragments. Different types of separation at the fracture site may occur. When the fragments are aligned but held apart, even slightly, the separation is called **distraction.** This term does not apply when the fragments are separated but overlap. Such a malalignment is called **bayonet apposition** (Fig. 28–2). Bayonet apposition is conducive to rapid fracture healing but results in shortening (Fig. 28–3). Similarly, loss of segments of bone also leads to overall shortening. In each instance, the soft tissues may adapt to the change in bone length (Fig. 28–3B).

Inadequate Immobilization. As a general rule, the more rigid the immobilization the quicker the fracture heals, provided there is no interference

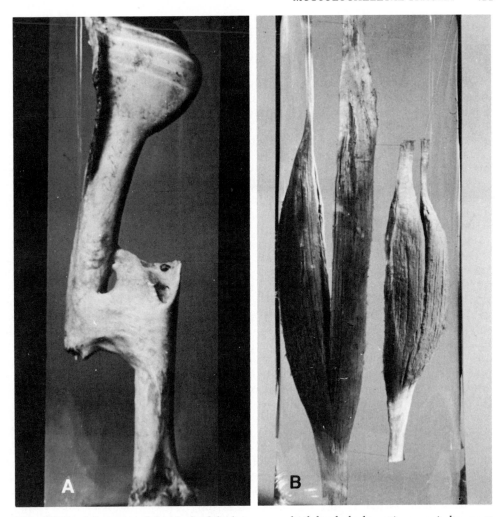

FIG. 28–3. A fracture of the shaft of the humerus which healed a long time ago in bayonet apposition with a considerable degree of shortening **(A).** The different lengths of the two biceps muscles of the same person illustrate the adaptation of soft tissues to long standing shortening of the bone **(B).** (Specimens prepared by John Hunter, Huntarian Museum, Royal College of Surgeons of England, London)

with the vascular supply to the fracture site. The rigidity of immobilization should not prevent stress across the fracture site because stress is essential to the remodeling stage and probably is also important in the reparative stage of fracture healing. The emphasis on immobilization should not be construed to indicate that a fracture will not unite if motion is present. Small amounts of motion are always present with all forms of traction and external fixation and such movement is not detrimental to healing as long as it does not rup-

ture budding capillaries. Early use of the surrounding muscles appears to improve vascularity and accelerate the healing process. Because the forces generated by muscles that span across joints are capable of displacing the segments of the fractured bone, it is necessary to immobilize the joint above and below the fracture. This rule should only be relaxed if specific mechanisms can be devised for neutralizing any muscle action across a joint by positioning or fixation of the injured part. Because of the need for activity to improve fracture healing, a limb should never be immobilized more than is necessary to secure adequate stabilization of the fracture and to prevent deformity.

Loss of Fracture Blood Clot. This is seen most frequently in open fractures, which take longer to heal than their closed counterparts. Loss of fracture blood clot also occurs during open reduction of fractures. When open reduction of the fracture is carried out, it should be done after seven to ten days, when the fracture site is in the stage of vascular invasion and organization. The blood clot is also lost in intraarticular fractures because synovial fluid prevents blood coagulation. Synovial fluid contains fibrinolysins which lyse the clot. Fracture healing will be delayed unless synovial fluid is excluded from the fracture by impaction of the fracture ends.

Infection. If bacterial infection of bone occurs in an open fracture or following operation, delayed or nonunion is almost certain. If an infectious process becomes chronic, the blood supply to the fracture site is reduced, as the scar tissue strangles the small vessels in the immediate vicinity of the fracture. Open fractures are usually associated with serious soft tissue damage which contributes to poor blood supply to the fractured bone. A comminuted fracture renders bone fragments avascular because they are devoid of their soft tissue attachments. These fragments die and become sequestra. The dead bone will be recognized by its increased x-ray density, compared to the surrounding bone which usually becomes somewhat osteoporotic due to hyperemia and disuse. The best treatment for infection is prevention which can be accomplished by minimizing the potential for bacterial contamination, judicious use of prophylactic antibiotics, removal of dead, devitalized tissue from a wound, and adequate immobilization to prevent further soft tissue damage and delayed vascular ingrowth.

No blood———→Impaired defense mechanisms

Systemic Factors Affecting Union

A wide variety of systemic factors have been implicated in delayed bone healing. Most notable of these are high levels of corticosteroids due to endogenous or exogenous origin. On the other hand, absence of male and female hormones may interfere with fracture healing as may abnormally high doses of vitamin A and D as well as a lack of vitamin D. The use of anticoagulants is also suspected to delay bony union but there is no firm evidence as yet for substantiating their effect.

In cases of severe malnutrition or in some endocrine disorders, the union of fractures may be delayed or fail to occur.

Acceleration of Fracture Union

To stimulate bone union, it is necessary to eliminate the causes of delayed and nonunion, and every effort should be made to increase vascularity and nutrition of the area. Weight bearing increases the blood flow in bone and significantly shortens the time required for fracture healing. Muscle activity in the nonweight bearing limb appears to have a similar effect provided it does not cause excessive motion. Recent studies indicate that local electrical currents can stimulate fracture healing. Although these effects may have some application in the treatment of delayed or nonunion, they have not been shown to be clinically applicable in the treatment of fresh fractures. Union can be enhanced by the use of bone grafts. Grafts can 1) act as a supplier of bone cells, 2) serve as an inorganic scaffolding which prevents the invasion of the fracture site by connective tissue and allows the deposition of new bone matrix upon the trabeculae of the graft, and 3) may also function as an inducer of new bone formation owing to the organic component of the graft.

For practical purposes, bone grafts may be divided into four types. An **autograft** is bone taken from the same individual; an **isograft** is bone obtained from an identical twin; an **allograft** is bone transferred from another individual of the same species; and a **xenograft** is bone transferred from one species to another. Only in autogenous and isogenous bone grafts are the cellular elements able to survive and produce new bone directly. The other types of bone grafts may initially promote bone repair but later are usually rejected. *The best bone for grafting is fresh autogenous cancellous bone.* Although in some instances cortical bone may be preferable for providing some degree of internal stability, its osteogenic activity is poor in comparison with cancellous bone.

Intraarticular Fractures

Most bones receive their blood supply from the periosteum and endosteum. When a bone is intraarticular and is covered with cartilage, only the endosteal blood supply is present. In such loca-

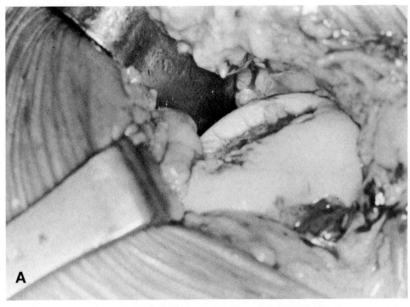

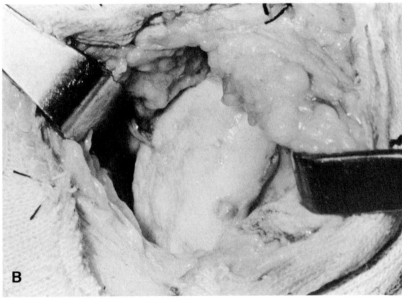

FIG. 28-4. **(A)** Fractured articular cartilage on the femoral condyle involving subchondral bone. Note the height of the articular cartilage and the vascular bony bed at the depth of the fracture. **(B)** The result of healing following the injury shown in **A.** The defect has been filled in by fibrocartilage but the surface is irregular. The irregularities extend over areas of cartilage which show no direct injury in **A** and must be the result of secondary degenerative changes.

tions fracture healing depends entirely on the endosteum. In these instances accurate reduction and rigid fixation of the fracture must be achieved. This is necessary to exclude synovial fluid from the fracture, which has an ability of lysing the blood clot, and to assure access for new blood vessels to cross the fracture site.

Another problem with intraarticular fractures is disruption of congruity in articular surfaces. If these surfaces cannot be reconstructed anatomi-

cally, the friction-free surface is lost and a traumatic arthrosis will result (Fig. 28-4).

Intraarticular fractures must be reduced anatomically if possible. When not possible, early joint motion is the treatment of choice.

When it is not possible to reestablish the congruity of the articular surface, either by manipulation or by direct reconstruction through operative methods, a new though not normal surface can be achieved by instituting early motion. Motion

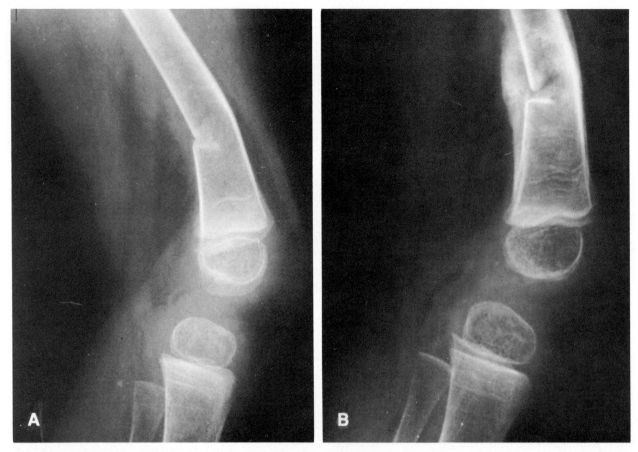

FIG. 28–5. (**A**) Green-stick fracture of the femur in a child suffering from paralysis of the lower limbs. The bones show disuse atrophy (osteoporosis) which predisposed to the fracture which is present only on the concave surface of the bone. (**B**) Six weeks later a large callus is evident which is present in the medullary cavity as well as on the exterior of the cortex, overlying the fracture. Note extensive subperiosteal bone formation. (Courtesy of Dr. Rosalind H. Troupin)

under these circumstances will help the multiple-fragmented pieces of bone to realign in the best possible position and will assist the fibrous tissue to undergo metaplasia into a fibrocartilaginous surface.

Fractures in Children

Healing of fractures in children rarely presents a problem. The periosteum around a growing bone forms a tough sheath in which osteogenic cells may be as many as nine cell layers in thickness, and healing and remodeling are rapid. The long bones in children frequently break like a green willow stick, fracturing the bone and the periosteum on one surface while merely bending the bone on the other surface on which the periosteum remains

intact (Fig. 28–5). The resulting angulation must be reduced but the tendency for this **green stick fracture** to reangulate after reduction requires special attention in its treatment. Trauma plus the inflammatory changes that attend fracture healing result in increased vascularity to the fractured bone and this hyperemia involves also the metaphyseal and epiphyseal regions. The increased vascularity leads to excessive bone growth. In children, a fractured bone tends to grow to a greater length than its unfractured mate. Such an overgrowth must be anticipated and must be taken into account when fractured long bones in children are set. Some overlap between the fracture fragments should be deliberately permitted. This is, of course, not possible in green stick fractures.

Epiphyseal Fractures. Many times epiphyseal injuries are difficult to recognize by x-ray. The normal variations in the time of appearance and fusion of epiphyses in growing children make it essential to *always x-ray the normal limb for comparison.*

The epiphyseal plate is vulnerable to fracture or slip, particularly during a rapid phase of growth. The weakest stratum of the epiphyseal plate is between the zones of cartilage cell hypertrophy and cartilage matrix calcification (see Fig. 2–14). Epiphyseal injuries have been classified by Salter into five classes (Fig. 28–6). This classification is important not only from an academic but also from a clinical point of view.

The **class one fracture** is a slip through the epiphyseal plate without fracture into the epiphysis or metaphysis. The fact that the germinal or growth zone attached to the epiphysis remains undamaged explains why growth disturbances are so rare after the epiphyseal slip is corrected. **Class two injury** is a slip of the epiphyseal plate with an associated fracture through the metaphysis. Such an injury falls into the same prognostic category as class one. **Class three epiphyseal plate slip** is associated with a fracture through the epiphysis. The fact that these fractures also involve the articular surface as well as the growth zone makes the prognosis for this injury much less favorable. Unless anatomically reduced, growth disturbances are common and even with a good reduction the future growth pattern cannot be predicted. In **class four injury** the fracture goes through the epiphysis, the epiphyseal plate, and the metaphysis. These injuries almost invariably result in growth disturbances, although anatomic reduction with firm internal fixation will minimize the growth irregularities. **Class five injury** is a compression or impaction fracture of the epiphyseal plate. This is extremely disruptive and virtually always results in premature arrest of growth.

Management of Fractures

Treatment of fractures requires the care of the soft tissues as well as the repositioning of the fractured bones. Care must always be taken to avoid further injury to surrounding tissues. Generally speaking, most fractures can be reduced by gentle sustained traction *in the direction of the deformity,* which will eventually be in the direction of the long axis of the bone.

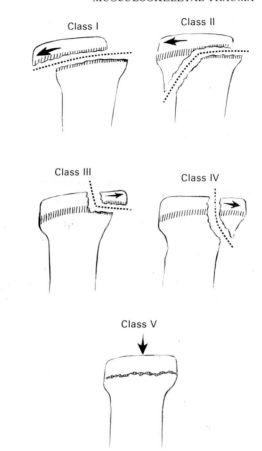

FIG. 28–6. Classification of epiphyseal injuries according to Salter.

Closed Reduction. Closed reduction of fractures is usually the treatment of choice and should be carried out as early as possible. As soon as it is assured that the victim of trauma has an open airway with excellent oxygen exchange and hemorrhage has been controlled, the fracture should either be definitely reduced or at least emergency splints should be applied. Concern with the fractures must be delayed until life-threatening situations have been corrected.

Closed reductions are usually carried out by reversing the mechanism of the original injury. While considerable force may be necessary, it should always be applied gently and slowly, taking care not to stretch or further damage the surrounding vessels and nerves. The reduction should *align the distal fragment to the proximal fragment* as it is usually impossible to manipulate a proximal fragment. Always take advantage of any soft tissue sleeve (Fig. 28–1B) in obtaining the reduction and in maintaining it. This can be best accomplished by applying a three point pressure cast. The rule of "one manipulation for one operator" should always be considered but need not be strictly adhered to. It should, however, be borne in mind that if the first manipulation is unsuccessful in reducing the fracture, repeated attempts are usually not likely to fare better and will increase the amount of damage at the fracture site.

Open fractures can frequently be treated in a manner similar to closed fractures after proper attention to the wound. Proper wound treatment can only be performed in an operating room and includes a careful debridement including all the surrounding soft tissues. The debridement must remove all dead tissue. The area should be cleaned by continuous irrigation delivered from a continuous drip irrigation system or from a mechanical pulsating fluid administrator. As a rule, the skin should not be closed immediately because it is difficult to obtain a completely sterile wound. Therefore, delayed primary closure, three to five days later, is usually considered the safest. Intramuscular or intravenous broad spectrum bactericidal antibiotic coverage commenced prior to debridement and continued for 24 to 72 hours has lowered the incidence of wound infection in open fractures but is not a substitute for careful operative debridement.

Traction. Usually a traction force must be used to align a fracture and to maintain the alignment. The traction is applied as a sustained pull on the skin or by the insertion of a small threaded wire through a distal bone. Various traction techniques are in use and they are most valuable in the management of unstable fractures or fractures that involve joints.

Cast. The fracture may be immobilized by encasing the affected limb or the part in some type of rigid bandaging. The most common type of bandage used is plaster of Paris, but a variety of other forms of immobilizing materials have recently become available. For cast and traction techniques, the *Manual of Acute Orthopaedic Therapeutics* should be consulted which is listed at the end of the chapter.

Internal Fixation. For over 100 years, efforts have been made for providing fracture stability through the use of internal splints, including screws, nails, bolts, and plates. All have some advantages and numerous disadvantages and should be applied only by specialists trained in their use. Metals are not inert in the body and they initiate electrolytic activity which is detrimental to tissue healing. Only the finest of stainless steel, titanium and chrome cobalt vitallium-type alloys are sufficiently inert to permit their use for internal fixation. When these fixation devices can produce immobilization without compromising blood supply, they have advantages in freeing the patient from cumbersome external trappings. Furthermore, they allow earlier movement of the limb and thereby improve blood supply and assure the normal maintenance of joints above and below the fracture. If properly used, the disadvantage of the risk of infection may be outweighed by the advantages of the technique. This is particularly true when the fixation device can be inserted at a distance from the fracture site. Such examples are the pinning of a hip fracture or the closed intramedullary rod inserted into a femur.

The aim of all fracture treatment is the *maintenance of function*. Attention should be given to early exercise. *The treatment to be undertaken in each case should be the one that will restore the functional capacity of the limb as quickly and safely as possible.*

JOINTS

Each component tissue of joints may suffer mechanical injury. The resulting clinical picture as well as the healing process is characteristic of the tissue involved. Joint tissues were discussed in Chapter 5, and Chapters 6 and 22 have dealt with the reaction of these tissues to nonmechanical types of injury. This section considers the consequences of mechanical injury on the tissues of synovial joints.

Articular Cartilage

Articular cartilage may be fractured by a direct blow or by a shearing force. Frequently, this is associated with a fracture of the subchondral bone as well. Since articular cartilage is lacking in nerve supply, the symptoms due to its injury result from the irritation of the surrounding soft tissues.

As noted before, cartilage has a limited capacity for repair, and this may be related to its lack of blood supply. In addition, injured cartilage cells produce lysozymes which hasten the degradation of the cartilage matrix. Hence, most cartilaginous injuries lead eventually to extensive degeneration.

This may, on occasion, be prevented if an osteochondral fragment can be inserted accurately into the defect and contact is made with denuded, subchondral bone. The cartilaginous bone graft will heal and if its cartilage surface is protected during the healing phase, its nutrition will be adequately provided for by the synovial fluid. Minor fissures may remain at the edges of the graft but the joint will usually function effectively for many years.

Injury of articular cartilage is diagnosed by 1) a history of an appropriate injury, 2) irregularity of the cartilaginous surfaces manifested by restricted motion or irregularity perceived in the smooth arc of motion, 3) pain produced by cartilaginous fragments irritating the synovial membrane, and 4) x-ray evidence of a small flake of a bone within a joint which usually indicates an osteocartilaginous injury. The cartilaginous portion of such a fragment is usually much larger than the bony portion visualized on the x-ray.

Cartilaginous injury requires the attention of orthopaedic surgeons. If there is an osteochondral fracture with a loose fragment, this should be replaced and fixed in an anatomic position. When this cannot be accomplished, cartilaginous fragments should be removed from the joint because they will cause synovial irritation and inflammation.

If the injury produced a rutted surface, the adjacent margins of the cartilage should be trimmed, cutting down perpendicularly through the full thickness of the cartilage until vascular bone is reached (Fig. 28–4A). This will allow the filling in of the defect with fibrocartilage which, if partially protected until it becomes mature, can provide a satisfactory surface for movement though it will never be normal (Fig. 28–4B). High dosage of aspirin, as in the treatment of rheumatoid arthritis, may inhibit lysozyme activity, thereby retarding autodegradation of damaged cartilage.

Synovial Membrane

Synovial membrane is damaged in most joint injuries. This delicate structure responds by hemorrhage or effusion into the joint or both. Blood in the joint cavity (hemarthrosis) is irritating to the synovial membrane and may lead to hypervascular synovitis. Blood can only be removed from the joint by phagocytosis in which synovial cells participate. Any large hemarthrosis, therefore, should be treated by aspiration and prevention of repeated hemorrhage. The synovial membrane has excellent reparative properties and apart from arresting bleeding requires no special treatment when torn.

Capsule and Ligaments

When the capsule or ligaments are stressed beyond their normal capacity, they tear. The severity of the tear varies from the rupture of microscopic fibers to the tearing of a gross structure. These tears manifest themselves as **sprains**. It is important to differentiate a complete tear from an incomplete one. The history will not give a clue regarding the completeness of the tear. For the diagnosis of a complete tear it is necessary to demonstrate increased laxity of the joint by subjecting it to stress. A complete tear is confirmed when the joint margins separate under a force applied to the joint which would normally tighten or stress the portion of the capsule or the ligament in question (see Fig. 17–14). The increased laxity may be documented by stress x-rays (see Fig. 8–9).

A sprain is always present if there is pain and swelling about the joint which has been subjected to trauma. The anatomic structures involved may be determined by careful examination for the point of maximum tenderenss. If this is over a known ligament, the diagnosis of a partial tear should be made. If examination can be accomplished prior to soft tissue swelling, it may be possible to note a gap in the ligament or in its place. Such a sign is diagnostic of complete rupture.

Healing of ligaments occurs by fibrous tissue proliferation. This process may be organized or disorganized. **Organized healing** occurs when there are intact collagen fibers or where the ligament has been reconstructed by accurate suturing. Because of the low vascularity of ligaments, healing takes place relatively slowly. **Disorganized healing** occurs when the ends of the ligament are retracted and the fibrous scar formed does not have any specific orientation. In such instances, the healed ligament will be longer than in its normal state. The disorganized fibrous tissue scar may eventually become remodeled in response to the stretches generated by the resumed activity of the joint.

Dislocation. With severe tears, the joint may become dislocated. In a dislocated joint, there is always some injury to the ligaments, capsule, synovial membrane, and frequently articular cartilage, muscle, nerves, and blood vessels. A dislocation should be reduced as soon as possible to take pressure off surrounding tissues. The best results following dislocation are achieved when there is accurate repair of the ligaments. A **subluxation** is an incomplete dislocation.

Management of Joint Injuries

The treatment of a joint injury is based on an accurate diagnosis of the extent of injury. The following considerations should be borne in mind.

1. Dislocated joints must be reduced as quickly and atraumatically as possible in order to prevent disastrous complications from interference with blood supply and nerve function. The ligaments and capsule must be protected by immobilization until healing is complete. If primary function of the joint is motion, early motion must be encouraged in order to avoid contractures. If the primary function of the joint is to provide stability, prolonged immobilization or surgical repair and immobilization are indicated.

2. Complete ligamentous tears require accurate assessment in each anatomic site with respect to joint stability. If the joint is inherently unstable as is the case with the knee, surgical repair of capsule and ligaments is indicated, followed by immobilization for six to eight weeks to ensure healing. If the joint has inherent stability like the hip joint, operative repair of ligaments may not be necessary.

3. Incomplete tears should be treated symptomatically to reduce hemorrhage and edema. Early, protected exercises appear to enhance the rate of healing and also improve early function.

Injury to synovial membrane can best be treated by rest and compression to minimize the hemarthrosis or effusion. Large hemarthroses should be aspirated. The joint should be placed at rest until the synovial membrane can be reconstituted and begins to function normally.

MUSCLE AND TENDON

A muscle may rupture because of overexertion (strain) or direct trauma. It is essential to place the muscle at rest in order to speed healing and minimize excessive scar formation which leads to subsequent contracture. The diagnosis is made through direct observation in an open wound or through palpation of a defect in the muscle over an area of tenderness. Treatment consists of compression dressing, ice, elevation, and rest. The muscle should be immobilized at its resting length.

Complete tendon rupture is more common than complete muscle rupture. Tendons may rupture from direct trauma or following exertion. Spontaneous rupture is unlikely unless degeneration has taken place. Degeneration of musculoskeletal tissues takes place at different rates in different individuals, but starts at approximately the age of 21. Disuse may initiate or accelerate the degenerative process.

Diagnosis is easily established on physical examination. There is a palpable defect in the tendon, and there is loss of the motion produced by the muscle–tendon complex.

Treatment consists of restoring the continuity of the tendon. This is done by surgical repair followed by immobilization until the tendon has healed. The rest period varies from three to eight weeks depending on the size of the tendon and surrounding vascularity.

NERVES

There are three general categories of nerve injury: neuropraxia, axonotmesis, and neurotmesis.

Neuropraxia or Contusion

Contusion of a nerve results in loss of the ability of the cell membrane to repolarize and, hence, inability to conduct across the lesion, despite the fact that all structures are intact. This may last from seconds to 6 weeks, but recovery is complete.

Axonotmesis or Crush

A nerve is crushed when the injury is severe enough to damage the axons to the extent that they undergo distal degeneration. The axon sheaths and neurolemma remain intact. Following the initial degeneration, regrowth occurs down the axon sheath at the rate of approximately 1 mm per day. Recovery may be anticipated after the appropriate time interval.

Neurotmesis or Complete Division

Complete disruption of a nerve requires careful end-to-end suture. Repair can be carried out at the time of injury or secondarily with equally good results, by surgeons skilled in this type of surgery.

A traction injury is a mixed injury with rupture of axon sheaths at various levels along the nerve. This could be considered a neurotmesis, but the perineural connective tissue gives support, and hence, some recovery. Direct repair usually is not practical.

Diagnosis is established by sensory and muscle examination in the area supplied by the nerve. Loss of sweating, skin atrophy, and electrical changes in muscle further substantiate the diagnosis and aid in determining the prognosis.

SUGGESTED READING

Blount WP: Fractures in Children. Baltimore, Williams & Wilkins, 1955
A classic monograph on the special problems of diagnosis and management of injury in the developing individuals. Extensively illustrated.

Conwell HE, Reynolds FC: Key and Conwell's Management of Fractures, Dislocations and Sprains, 7th ed. St. Louis, CV Mosby, 1961
A comprehensive work on diagnosis and management of traumatic injuries of the body. Profusely and well illustrated.

Hartman, JT: Fracture Management. Philadelphia, Lea & Febiger, 1978
Discusses general assessment of the injured patient and the diagnosis and management of injuries in different anatomical regions of the body.

Iversen LD, Clawson DK: Manual of Acute Orthopaedic Therapeutics. Boston, Little, Brown, 1977
A handy manual for students and beginning residents in how to diagnose musculoskeletal injury and how to formulate a treatment plan. A ready reference for techniques of cast and traction application.

Rockwood CA, Green DP: Fractures. Philadelphia, JB Lippincott, 1975
A comprehensive work on the diagnosis and management of fractures presented in two volumes. Well illustrated.

29
Neoplasia

CORNELIUS ROSSE,   D. KAY CLAWSON

Neoplasia is an abnormal proliferative process which exceeds and is not coordinated with the normal rate of proliferation or regeneration in a tissue. This excessive and uncontrolled proliferation persists after the cessation of stimuli that provoked it and proceeds in complete disregard to functional needs, in many instances leading to the death of the individual.

In most tissues the neoplastic process produces a new growth or **neoplasm** which manifests itself as a swelling or tumor. The terms *tumor* and *neoplasm* are not synonymous, however, and should not be used interchangeably, since many tumors are not neoplasms. Also there are neoplasms which do not present as swellings.

Neoplasia may occur in any tissue of the body, and although the basic process is fundamentally the same, the appearance and behavior of neoplasms are characteristic of their tissue of origin. A neoplasm which arises locally from the cells of a given tissue is called a **primary neoplasm. A secondary neoplasm** or **metastasis** is derived from a primary neoplasm but is independent of it, having sequestered in an organ some distance removed from its site of origin. For instance, a primary bone neoplasm in the distal end of the femur (e.g., osteogenic sarcoma) may establish secondaries (metastases) in the lung or in the vertebrae by disseminating its cells via the blood stream. In comparison with neoplasms of other systems, primary neoplasms of the musculoskeletal tissues are uncommon, but the skeleton is a frequent site of metastases.

BENIGN AND MALIGNANT NEOPLASMS

There are as many types of neoplasms as there are cell types in the body. However, it is most important to differentiate between their benign and malignant varieties. A **benign neoplasm** generally retains the recognizable morphologic characteristics of its parent tissue, it may be functional (e.g., produce bone or cartilage matrix, secretions, or hormones), and its growth is usually self-limiting. Benign neoplasms may grow to an enormous size, but they do not invade surrounding tissue nor do they spread to distant sites. They rarely cause death, although they may do so when they compress vital organs. **Malignant neoplasms,** on the other hand, ultimately lead to the death of the individual unless their growth is stopped or they are removed. Unlike their benign counterparts, they invade and metastasize. **Invasion** is a process by which a primary neoplasm infiltrates neighboring structures. **Metastasis** is a process by which neoplastic cells travel in the blood or lymph and establish secondary foci of tumor growth by settling in distant organs. Lymph nodes, lung, liver, and the skeleton are the most common sites of metastases.

Clearly, it is of utmost importance to determine whether a tumor is a benign or malignant neoplasm before it is given time to reveal its true nature by extensive invasion and metastasis. The differentiation between a benign and malignant neoplasm is often difficult and may require considerable experience. The chief distinguishing features are to be sought in the history or clinical course of the lesion, in its radiologic appearance, and in its histopathology.

Clinical Course

Benign neoplasms of musculoskeletal tissues are slow growing tumors which have usually been present for years before the patient seeks advice, complaining of deformity or of symptoms suggesting the compression of structures adjacent to the tumor. They are usually painless and nontender, unless they have been subjected to trauma. Benign

421

neoplasms in bone may produce mechanical weakness predisposing to fracture which may reveal their presence for the first time (see Fig. 8–7B). Most malignant neoplasms of bone and cartilage present as local, painful swellings which gradually increase in size. Pain may not be a feature with malignancy arising in other connective tissues. A malignant tumor, as a rule, is tender and feels warm to touch, which reflects its hypervascularity. Such a tumor may be confused with subacute bacterial infection. With many malignancies there is general ill health.

Radiology

Neoplasms produce focal abnormalities in bone, and x-rays provide important clues whether they are likely to be benign or malignant. Chapter 8 presented the radiologic features of focal bone lesions, and benign, slowly growing tumors (Fig. 8–7A, B) were contrasted with rapidly growing, destructive lesions (Fig. 8–7C, D). As a rule, benign tumors protruding from the surface maintain smooth continuity with the cortex, while most benign tumors situated inside the bone produce a radiolucent lesion with expansion of the cortex. However, there is no erosion or disruption of cortical continuity. A sclerotic shell usually surrounds the lesions. All primary malignant neoplasms in bone produce destruction, and some produce new bone formation and sclerosis as well (Fig. 8–7D). Bone formation is evident subperiosteally as the invading tumor breeches the cortex and elevates the periosteum (Fig. 29–1) and also in the sur-

FIG. 29–1. Osteogenic sarcoma of the distal end of the femur seen in an anteroposterior **(A)** and lateral **(B)** x-ray. Note the typical anatomic site close to the growing end of the bone; the elevation of the periosteum **(white arrows)** where subperiosteal formation of normal bone produced characteristic Codman's triangles. The sunburst appearance, seen particularly in **B,** is due to bone layed down along Sharpey's fibers. Extension of the calcified tumor mass into the surrounding soft tissues beyond the periosteum is well shown in **A (black arrows).**

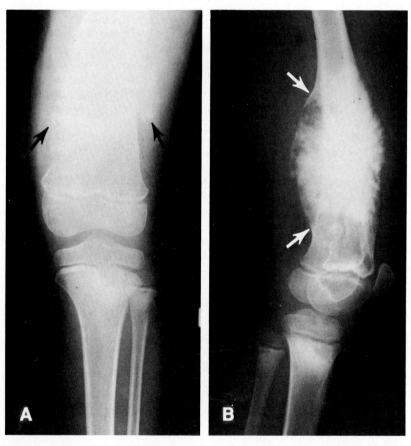

rounding tissues invaded by the tumor (Figs. 8–7D, 8–12A). An invading tumor, whether of bony or of soft tissue origin, tends to blur and obliterate the tissue planes which can normally be defined on plain x-ray films. Most metastases in bone are destructive (Fig. 8–7C) but some may produce sclerosis as well.

Histopathology

A benign tumor, as a rule, is well differentiated and the cell type from which it arose can be determined without difficulty. Malignant neoplasms are poorly differentiated or may lack all signs of differentiation and are, therefore, described as **anaplastic.** Malignant neoplasms of different origin may look alike and often even an experienced pathologist has difficulty in identifying the exact cell type of origin. For the same reason there may be difficulty in distinguishing a primary bone neoplasm from a metastasis.

Histologic evidence of invasiveness is a certain sign of malignancy, but some well encapsulated tumors may be malignant and may metastasize. Cartilage provides an excellent barrier against direct extension of malignant neoplasms. Therefore, when a lesion is seen to cross the articular cartilage or epiphyseal cartilage, it is generally not a neoplasm.

Malignant cells display certain histologic characteristics. They are less adhesive to each other than normal cells and vary greatly in size and shape (pleomorphism). They frequently show diminished cytoplasm with a relative increase in nuclear volume. Malignant cells generally have hyperchromatic nuclei, and there is great variation in nuclear size, shape, and chromatin configuration. They also show an increased number of mitoses, many of which are abnormal.

A **biopsy** is usually performed when malignancy is suspected and the exact type of the neoplasm is in doubt. Radical definitive treatment should not be undertaken until the diagnosis has been independently confirmed by at least two pathologists. A biopsy should be performed by a surgeon who has experience with musculoskeletal neoplasms and can grossly distinguish the tumor from the surrounding reactive tissue. The biopsy has to be sufficiently generous to provide the pathologist with different areas that may show varying degrees of differentiation or matrix formation. Some neoplasms can be identified on frozen section but often the decision has to await routine histologic processing of the tissue.

ETIOLOGY OF NEOPLASMS

The etiology of neoplasia is unknown. Chronic tissue irritation and heredity have been implicated as contributory factors. It has been suggested that some types of neoplasms may have a viral etiology. It is probable that numerous factors are responsible for the origin of most neoplasms. There is evidence that exposure to ionizing radiation (x-rays for instance) increases the risk of cancer. Patients often associate trauma with the appearance of a malignant tumor. This is because a trivial injury may have drawn the patient's attention to the neoplasm. There is no evidence for a causal relationship between trauma and neoplasia.

NEOPLASMS OF MUSCULOSKELETAL TISSUES

The musculoskeletal system is composed largely of connective tissue and, therefore, its primary malignant neoplasms are **sarcomas,** in contrast to **carcinomas** which are malignant neoplasms of epithelial origin. Secondary neoplasms in bone are most frequently carcinomas. The prognosis for malignant neoplasms is variable and is particularly poor for sarcomas.

It is helpful to classify neoplasms according to the tissues from which they arise: neoplasms derived from muscle, bone, cartilage, nerve, and loose connective tissue, as well as neoplasms of vascular, synovial, or bone marrow origin. All neoplasms have a benign and a malignant counterpart. Classification is based, therefore, on the type of cell and its matrix, as well as on the neoplasm's benign or malignant characteristics (Table 29–1).

The various types of neoplasms have a characteristic predilection for different age groups and for different anatomic sites. The sex and racial characteristics are not clear.

Primary Neoplasms of Bone and Cartilage

Practically all cartilage tumors are associated with bones; neoplasia is extremely rare in cartilages that are independent of bones. Therefore, from a clinical point of view, it is practical to consider them together with bone tumors. Primary neoplasms found in bone may be derived from osteoblasts, chondroblasts, fibroblasts, or from their primitive precursors. In addition, osteoclasts can

TABLE 29–1. Primary Neoplasms of Musculoskeletal Tissues*

Benign	Malignant
Bone	
Osteoma	Osteogenic sarcoma (osteo-sarcoma)
Osteochondroma (osteo-cartilaginous exostosis)	
Aneurysmal bone cyst	Giant cell tumor (osteo-clastoma)
Nonosteogenic fibroma	Fibrosarcoma of bone
Osteoid osteoma	
Cartilage	
Chondroma	Chondrosarcoma
Enchondroma	
Ecchondroma	
Osteochondroma (osteo-cartilaginous exostosis)	
Chondroblastoma	
Chondromyxoid fibroma	
Bone Marrow	
	Multiple myeloma
	Ewing's tumor (? endothelial sarcoma)
	Reticulum cell sarcoma
	Hodgkin's disease of bone
Muscle	
Rhabdomyoma	Rhabdomyosarcoma
Loose Connective Tissue	
Fibroma	Fibrosarcoma
Lipoma	Liposarcoma
Hemangioma	Hemangiosarcoma
Neurofibroma	Neurofibrosarcoma
	Synovioma

*For a more comprehensive list consult the references.

also manifest neoplastic change (giant cell tumor). Some neoplasms of the bone marrow present with the clinical picture characteristic of bone tumors and these will be discussed in the subsequent section.

Benign Neoplasms. Osteoma, chondroma, and osteochondroma represent localized, excessive formation of bone, cartilage, or both, respectively. All three present as bony swellings during adolescence and early adult life.

Of the three, **osteochondroma** is the most frequent. The tumor arises from the epiphyseal plate of long bones, and as longitudinal growth proceeds, the swelling gets left behind and appears to migrate along the diaphysis. It protrudes from the bone like a mushroom with its stalk ossified while its cap remains cartilaginous; hence, the tumor is also known as **osteocartilaginous exostosis.** Tumors may be single or multiple. Multiple exostoses are a congenital affection (known also as

diaphyseal aclasis) transmitted by a dominant mutant gene.

An **osteoma** arises by excessive mesenchymal bone formation and is most common on the surface of membrane bones. However, it may occur also subperiosteally on long bones. **Chondromas** occur most frequently in the bones of the hands and feet and may protrude from the surface (**ecchondroma**) or may be enclosed in the bone (**enchondroma**). The latter have a sclerotic shell; they expand the bone and thin out its cortex (see Fig. 8–7A). Chondromas in larger bones may interfere with the epiphyseal plate and predispose to a shortening deformity. **Fibromas** may also develop in bone (see Fig. 8–7B) since bones contain fibroblasts. They are usually discovered on x-rays as incidental findings.

Malignant Neoplasms. Osteogenic sarcoma (osteosarcoma) and chondrosarcoma are the clinically most important malignant neoplasms that produce bone or cartilage. Fibrosarcomas are more rare but areas resembling fibrosarcoma may occasionally be found in osteogenic or chondrosarcomas, which is understandable because all these neoplasms trace their origin from primitive connective tissue cells in bone. Osteogenic sarcoma, twice as common and much more devastating than chondrosarcoma, characteristically affects the 10 to 25-year-old age group, but it may develop in later life as a complication of Paget's disease or as a consequence of exposure to ionizing radiation (e.g., radiation therapy for other lesions). Chondrosarcoma is seen chiefly during middle age. Both tumors are more common in males, as are all malignant neoplasms with the exception of those of the breast and reproductive organs. Osteogenic sarcoma has a much more swift clinical course and a much worse prognosis than chondrosarcoma. Fibrosarcoma has the best prognosis of the three malignant primary bone tumors. Giant cell tumor, though apparently benign for long periods, eventually may turn frankly malignant and is appropriately considered with malignant bone tumors.

Osteogenic sarcoma is found most commonly in the metaphyseal region of long bones, particularly at the more rapidly growing ends (distally in the femur, proximally in the tibia and humerus). The femur is the most frequent site while small bones are rarely involved (Fig. 29–1). As with all malignant bone lesions, the patient complains of bone pain (see Chap. 7) which has been present for a few weeks and is gradually increasing. The pain may be referred to the neighboring joint. A diffuse, firm, tender swelling, which also feels warm, can usually be defined close to the joint. All these signs may suggest an inflammatory lesion which is sometimes not ruled out even by radiologic examination. A biopsy is always mandatory before radical treatment for the suspected sarcoma is undertaken. There may be fever, malaise, weight loss, and general ill health.

The tumor arises from primitive osteoblasts or from primitive connective tissue cells in bone, and in different areas its cells may resemble osteoblasts, chondroblasts, and fibroblasts, although they can be so anaplastic that no distinct cell type can be recognized (Fig. 29–2). Mineralized and unmineralized osteoid, cartilage, and collagenous matrices may be intermixed. In some varieties, neoplastic bone formation dominates the histologic picture, but in others this may be found only by thorough search of an adequate biopsy. Neoplastic bone resembles primitive, woven bone. Normal bone may react by new bone formation to the presence of any neoplasm and this reactive bone may be confused in a biopsy with neoplastic bone.

As a rule, by the time it is examined, the highly vascular tumor has destroyed the cancellous bone of the metaphysis and lysed and burst through the cortex, elevating the periosteum (Fig. 29–1), which is largely responsible for the pain. The neoplasm is highly invasive and metastasizes early and consistently to the lung, more rarely to bone. Regional lymph nodes are usually not involved.

Radiologic findings reflect the pathologic picture (Figs. 8–7D, 29–1). Irregular sclerosis and osteolysis in the metaphysis is associated with cortical erosion and new bone formation under the periosteum as well as in the surrounding soft tissue infiltrated by the tumor, the latter often giving a *"sunburst"* appearance. The earliest radiologic sign may be subperiosteal bone formation revealed by *Codman's triangle* which in itself, of course, is not diagnostic of a neoplasm. The reactive bone produced by the periosteum is histologically normal and not neoplastic.

The differential diagnosis of osteogenic sarcoma is frequently confusing because of the difficulty of differentiating it from reactive bone formation, which may also present as a swelling. Reactive bone formation occurs in fracture repair, following trauma to muscle (myositis ossificans), and around some benign and malignant neoplasms. The differentiation between reactive proliferative bone and neoplasia can be made provided an adequate biopsy is taken to evaluate the entire area.

After the diagnosis is established and treatment instituted (which is amputation of the limb with or without radiation therapy and/or chemotherapy) death occurs in the majority of cases within 18 months due to pulmonary metastases and only a few patients survive for 5 years.

Chondrosarcoma generally affects bones of the trunk, the pectoral and pelvic girdles, and the shafts or upper ends of the humerus, femur, and tibia. In most cases the tumor grows very slowly and often it has been present for years before the patient begins to complain of pain or of a swelling. In half of the cases, chondrosarcoma arises by a malignant change in an enchondroma or in an osteocartilaginous exostosis. Radiologically these tumors are characterized by areas of radiolucency within long bones or, in the case of osteochondrosarcomas, by a radiolucent cap over the ossified stalk of the exostosis. Stippled calcification is commonly seen in these tumors, but cannot be relied on as an indication of the neoplasm's benign

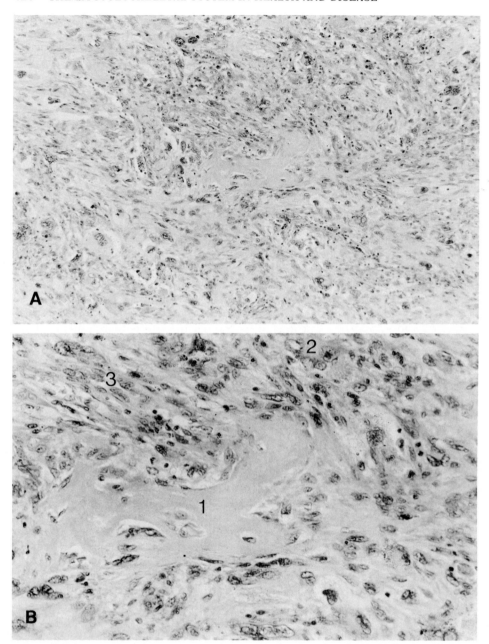

FIG. 29–2. Histologic sections of osteogenic sarcoma. At low magnification **(A)** different tissues may be identified in the same field without any definite pattern of association. At higher resolution **(B)** it is possible to identify areas of osteoid (1), chondroid cells (2), and sheets of fibroblasts (3). In both **A** and **B** note the pleomorphism of the cells, many with hyperchromatic nuclei, characteristic of malignancy.

or malignant nature. The malignant process usually develops after some years. Therefore, whenever there is evidence of clinical or radiologic change, malignant transformation should be suspected and excisional biopsy should be performed by a surgeon who is familiar with these types of neoplasms. Chondrosarcomas metastasize late or not at all, and the prognosis after resection of the tumor is quite favorable.

Fibrosarcoma of bone is thought to be derived from the primitive connective tissue stem cell. It may be a medullary or a periosteal tumor. Though fibrosarcoma of bone can be confused with a very malignant osteosarcoma, its behavior in general is different. The tumor grows slowly and after radical resection it has the best prognosis of all primary bone malignancies. Radiologically it may be confused with a chondrosarcoma, although the stippled calcification is lacking. Pathologically, it is characterized by sheets of malignant fibrous tissue cells and is identical to fibrosarcomas found elsewhere. Left untreated, the tumor will usually metastasize to the lungs. It has a greater incidence of metastases to lymph nodes than other bone sarcomas.

Giant cell tumor or **osteoclastoma** is usually discovered in the metaphysis of long bones within 10–20 years of epiphyseal fusion. The tumor contains a variable density of multinucleate giant cells, most probably derived from osteoclasts, which are intermixed with collagen and anaplastic cells resembling those of a fibrosarcoma (Fig. 29–3). The fact that giant cells are common in bone in a variety of lesions, including osteogenic sarcomas, hyperparathyroidism, aneurysmal bone cysts, as well as in giant cell tumor has led to confusion in the classification and the recognition of this neoplasm. In giant cell tumor there is a characteristic vascular sinusoidal pattern and the giant cells are at times associated with the endothelial cells of the sinuses. While the giant cells are striking, the key to the diagnosis rests in the stromal cells which cannot be distinguished from fibrosarcoma.

Insidious onset of bone pain and swelling or pathologic fracture are the presenting complaints. The most frequently affected sites are the distal ends of the femur and radius, proximal end of the tibia, and the metacarpals, metatarsals, and phalanges. The neoplasm begins in the metaphysis, probably at the time of epiphyseal fusion, and it expands into the epiphysis across the line of fusion, often reaching the articular cartilage. On x-rays, it typically presents as an eccentric osteolytic lesion extending into the epiphysis. Lysis of the cortex is sufficiently slow to permit substantial periosteal bone formation apace with the growth of the tumor so that the bone becomes expanded. There is no marked sclerotic shell delineating the tumor from cancellous bone. While the tumor may appear benign, its growth will speed up eventually in all cases and then the risk of pulmonary metastases becomes high.

Neoplasms of the Bone Marrow

Neoplasia of hematopoietic tissue generally manifests itself in varous forms of leukemia, depending on the cell type primarily involved. Although reactive or malignant hyperplasia of the bone marrow can cause skeletal changes (see Fig. 8–4B) and symptoms due to the skeletal involvement, there are four neoplastic conditions of the bone marrow in which the presence of the neoplasm in bone dominates the clinical picture. These neoplasms are multiple myeloma, Ewing's tumor, reticulum cell sarcoma, and Hodgkin's disease of bone. Only the first two will be discussed because of their relative frequency.

Multiple myeloma or **plasma cell myeloma** afflicts the 50 to 70-year-old age group most frequently, and hence it is important to differentiate it from metastatic carcinoma. It is a neoplastic change in the cell line concerned with the production of plasma cells and occurs at multiple foci in hematopoietic bone marrow or is rapidly disseminated from a single locus.

Multiple myeloma is the most frequent primary neoplasm in bone, and it is fatal in practically all cases within two years of making the diagnosis. The neoplasm manifests itself as multiple, small, osteolytic tumors in the ribs, vertebrae, bones of the pelvic and pectoral girdles, and in the proximal ends of the humerus and femur. These lesions appear on x-rays as punched out radiolucent areas without any sclerosis around their margin. However, approximately one quarter of the cases show no abnormality on x-rays.

The presenting symptoms are insidious development of bone pain, often identified as backache. Bone tenderness may be elicited but there is no swelling. General ill health and anemia are usually evident because the neoplasm replaces normal hematopoietic tissue. Bone marrow biopsy is pathognomonic and reveals an excess of plasma cell-like cells, quite often even when the biopsy is taken from bones lacking any radiologic signs. The

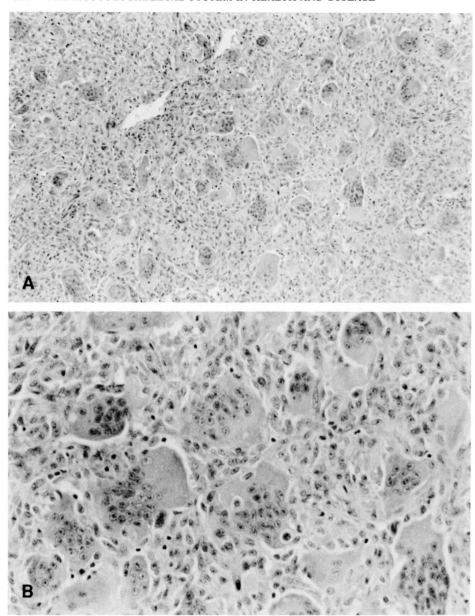

FIG. 29–3. Histologic sections of giant cell tumor shown at different magnifications in **A** and **B**. Large, multinucleated giant cells are randomly scattered throughout the stroma. In **B** some can be seen abutting against sinusoidal spaces. The intervening stroma is homogeneous and resembles fibrosarcoma.

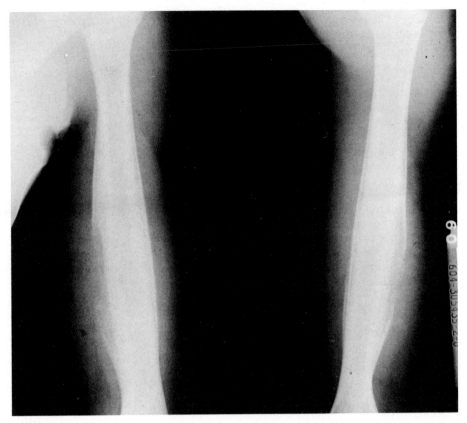

FIG. 29–4. Ewing's sarcoma of the humerus. The x-ray reveals the diffuse nature of the neoplasm which involves the entire medullary cavity. There is characteristic destruction of the cortex and invasion of soft tissues. Subperiosteal new bone formation produced an onion-peel appearance around the circumference of the bone due to repeated elevation of the periosteum.

myeloma produces an excess of abnormal globulins, resulting in an elevated serum globulin level, associated with a characteristically abnormal electrophoretic pattern. In half of the cases, the urine contains a protein known as Bence Jones protein which precipitates at 50°C but dissolves again at 100°C. In many cases the proteinuria leads to renal abnormalities and renal failure.

Ewing's tumor is a highly malignant sarcoma which is nearly always fatal. After multiple myeloma and osteogenic sarcoma, it is the third most common primary bone tumor, and it characteristically afflicts the young. Most patients are between 5–15 years old. The tissue of origin has been presumed to be endothelium in the bone marrow, but this is uncertain.

The white, soft tumor characteristically develops in the medullary cavity of the diaphysis of long bones. It is highly invasive and metastasizes early to the lung and to other bones. The x-ray picture is characterized by bone destruction, lysis of the cortex, and repeated elevation of the periosteum by the invading tumor which results in the deposition of concentric layers of subperiosteal bone in onion-peel fashion (Fig. 29–4). Ossification may also occur around nutrient vessels and Sharpey's fibers stretched between the periosteum and the cortex, giving the sunburst appearance (Figs. 8–12A, 29–1), also seen in osteogenic sarcoma.

The outstanding clinical features are intense bone pain, an exquisitely tender, diffuse, firm swelling, fever, malaise, and leukocytosis. It is readily mistaken for acute osteomyelitis. Biopsy is mandatory before definitive treatment is instituted. Microscopically the tumor has a homogeneous appearance consisting of sheets of uniform, small, anaplastic cells, and many areas of necrosis.

Secondary Neoplasms of Bone

Secondary malignant tumors in bone are much more common than primary neoplasms. They afflict the older age group with the greatest frequency, because in this age group carcinomas have a high incidence. The most common primary neoplasms that metastasize to bone are carcinomas of the lung, breast, prostate, thyroid gland, and kidney. The bones involved are those containing vascular, hematopoietic marrow (see Fig. 8–13), and multiple metastases may be confused with multiple myeloma. As a rule, metastases produce osteolytic lesions with the exception of secondaries from the prostate which may produce sclerosis as well. Bone pain due to metastases may be the first sign of the primary neoplasm (see Fig. 8–13).

Primary Neoplasms of Muscle

Neoplasms of skeletal muscle, called **rhabdomyoma** and **rhabdomyosarcoma,** are rare and often difficult to diagnose even by biopsy.

Primary Neoplasms of Connective Tissue

Benign neoplasms of connective tissue are quite common. They include **fibroma, lipoma, neurofibroma,** and hemangioma. Malignant neoplasms include **fibrosarcoma, liposarcoma,** and **synovial sarcoma.** They may occur at any age. These malignant tumors invade and metastasize despite the fact that they may appear encapsulated. The prognosis for all of them is considerably better than for malignancy in bone.

SUGGESTED READING

Aegerter E, Kirkpatrick JA: Orthopedic Diseases, 3rd ed. Philadelphia, WB Saunders, 1968
Section 4 of this book (Chapters 14–19) deals with tumors and tumor-like processes in the musculoskeletal system. In addition to general consideration of neoplasms in the musculoskeletal system, the various chapters treat the specific neoplasms in considerable detail. The emphasis is on pathology, but clinical and radiologic manifestations are included.
Robbins SL, Angell M: Basic Pathology, 2nd ed. Philadelphia, WB Saunders, 1976
Chapters 3 and 4 present basic concepts of neoplasia. Some neoplasms of the musculoskeletal system are described in Chapter 19.

30
Screening Examination of the Musculoskeletal System

D. KAY CLAWSON, CORNELIUS ROSSE, WALTER C. STOLOV

The foregoing chapters have dealt with assessment of function of different regions of the musculoskeletal system and with the various traumatic and pathologic conditions which may produce a disturbance. The principles outlined have to be applied on a practical level in the physical examination.

The physician should develop a **standard approach** to physical examination of all systems of the body. This is essential for making and recording accurate observations. A standard approach also ensures that essential points of the examination are not overlooked. It is the aim of this chapter to outline such an approach for the musculoskeletal system. While it is recognized that each physician may develop his own routine, a **screening examination** is described which will indicate or exclude functional impairment of the musculoskeletal system. This examination takes only a few minutes to perform and **should form part of the routine examination of all patients.** If an abnormality is revealed, a more detailed examination of the region is indicated, as described in the appropriate chapters.

1. The patient must be disrobed with the exception of shorts and brassiere. A quick inspection allows assessment of body type, abnormal spinal curvatures, deviation from normal limb alignments, and abnormalities of the foot arches and toes. The patient is inspected from the front, from the back, and from the side. Attention is directed to:

    a. Body type and posture
    b. Abnormal spinal curvatures
    c. Deviations from normal alignment of the limbs
    d. Other deformities

2. The patient is asked to walk barefoot to allow detection of any irregularities of gait.

3. The range of motion of the neck is measured in:

    a. Full flexion (normal: chin to chest, Fig. 9–27A)
    b. Extension (normal: the examiner's finger being trapped between the occiput and the C7 spinous process, Fig. 9–27B)
    c. Rotation (normal: greater than 70° from the sagittal plane, Fig. 9–27C)

4. The arms are stretched out horizontally in front of the body with fingers spread to allow checking of symmetry (Fig. 30–1). The power of the intrinsic muscles is assessed by the examiner's attempting to press the fingers together against resistance.

5. The patient abducts the arms fully, placing palms together above the head (Fig. 30–2). Normally the arms touch the ears with the head and cervical spine in the vertical position. The shoulder, acromioclavicular, and sternoclavicular joints are thus tested. A functional range of lateral rotation of the humerus is also demonstrated by the execution of this movement (see Figs. 13–11, 13–12).

6. The arms are brought to the side and the humerus medially rotated to place the hand on the back between the scapulae (see Fig. 13–16). Normally, the hand should reach the level of the inferior angle of the scapula. The range of movement of the elbow is also tested in this manner, and painful afflictions, deformities, and muscle weakness will be revealed. Symmetry of the two sides should be ascertained.

7. The patient grasps the index and the long finger of each of the examiner's hands. The examiner attempts to move the patient's arms in all directions (up, down, laterally, and medially)

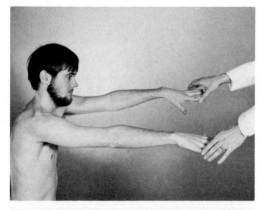

FIG. 30-1. Assessment of intrinsic muscle power in the hands.

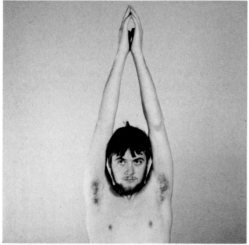

FIG. 30-2. Full abduction of the arms.

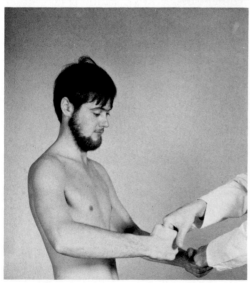

FIG. 30-3. Assessment of muscle power in the major groups of muscles in the upper limb.

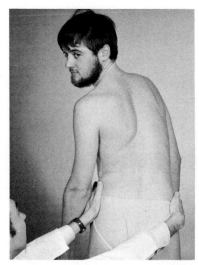

FIG. 30-4. Testing rotation of the spine. The pelvis is stabilized by the examiner. The greatest range of rotation occurs in the thoracic spine.

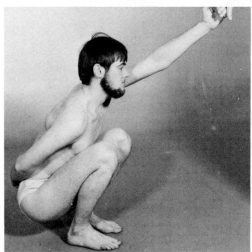

FIG. 30-5. Assessment of joints and muscle power in the lower limbs.

while maximum resistance is offered by the patient (Fig. 30–3). This is an effective though somewhat crude way of assessing strength of the muscles of the hand, wrist, elbow, and even of the shoulder. Pain in any of these joints may result in failure to offer resistance.

8. The patient, standing erect, is inspected again from the back and the following points are checked:

    a. Listing or spinal curvatures

    b. Level of the iliac crests (A difference in level of the two crests may result from leg length inequality, scoliosis, or flexion deformity of the hip)

9. The patient then bends forward, flexing the trunk as far as possible in an attempt to touch the floor while keeping the knees extended. The presence or absence of scoliosis is best demonstrated in this position (see Fig. 9–25).

10. The lumbar spine is further tested by having the patient extend as far back as possible, and the thoracic spine is tested by performing rotation movements (Fig. 30–4).

11. The patient then squats with the feet flat on the floor, knees and hips fully flexed (Fig. 30–5). It may be necessary to hold the patient's hand for more secure balance. This is an excellent test to assess the function of all major joints of the lower

limbs. Watching the manner in which the patient gets down and up gives an accurate impression of the muscle power in the lower limbs.

This completes the screening examination of the musculoskeletal system. This examination will call the physician's attention to the region which has an abnormality, even though the abnormality may be asymptomatic. A neurologic evaluation forms an integral part of the functional assessment of the musculoskeletal system. Although a routine screening examination has been described, a more detailed examination with modifications in the systematic approach may be necessary for the individual patient.

SUGGESTED READING

Hoppenfeld, S: Physical Examination of the Spine and Extremities. New York, Appleton-Century-Crofts, 1976
The most comprehensive description of musculoskeletal examination.

The following two books deal with the systematic approach to the patient and include the evaluation of the musculoskeletal system as well as all other organ systems:

DeGowin, EL, DeGowin RL,: Bedside Diagnostic Examination. 3rd ed. New York, Macmillan Publishing Co. Inc., 1976
Delp, MH, Masnning, RT (eds): Major Physical Diagnosis, 7th Philadelphia, W. B. Saunders Co., 1968

Index